ANP - Polypeptide hormone found
mainly in atrium of many
species of vertebrates.
Released in response to atrial
stretching & ∴ to ↑ B.P.
ANP → ↓ B.P. ① by rapid renal
excretion of Na^+ & ∴ H_2O
(↓ blood vol)
② Relaxes vascular smooth muscle
(VASODILATION)
③ Actions on brain ⎫
④ " " adrenal glands ⎬ ?

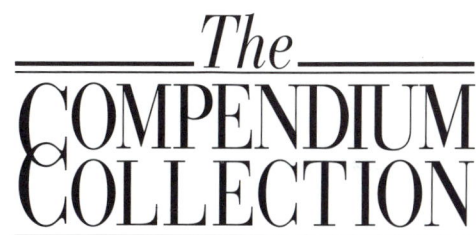

RENAL DISEASE

IN SMALL ANIMAL PRACTICE

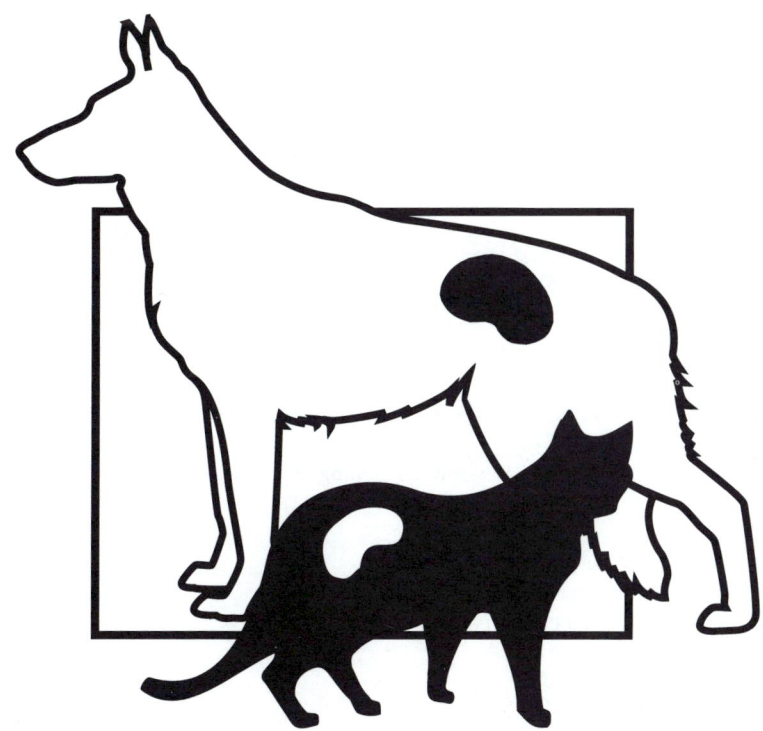

Published by Veterinary Learning Systems
Trenton, New Jersey

ISBN 1-884254-18-7

PREFACE

Dogs and cats are frequently presented to the small animal practitioner for clinical signs resulting from urinary tract disease. This *Compendium Collection* contains a selection of articles, most previously published in the *Compendium on Continuing Education for the Practicing Veterinarian*, which reviews the pathophysiology, diagnosis, and medical treatment of disorders of both the upper and lower urinary tract. This collection fulfills two purposes; first, it can serve as a clinical reference in practice, and second, it can be read and studied for the veterinarian's own continuing education.

Chronic renal failure remains one of the most common causes of morbidity and mortality in geriatric dogs and cats. Its pathophysiology is covered in the articles on *Feline Renal Failure* by Lulich et al, *Azotemia: A Review of What's Old and What's New* by Osborne and Polzin, and *The Pathophysiology of Uremic Bleeding* by Harris and Krawiec. A discussion of some of the specific causes of renal disease can be found in *Feline Idiopathic Polycystic Kidney Disease* by Lulich et al, *Glomerulonephritis in Dogs and Cats* by Jergens, *Bacterial Urinary Tract Infections: Invasion, Host Defenses, and New Approaches to Prevention* by Senior, *Urinary Tract Neoplasms in Dogs and Cats* by Crow, and *Canine Urolithiasis: Diagnosis, Treatment, and Prevention* by Osborne et al. While renal function in affected animals cannot be restored to normal, appropriate medical management, including dietary therapy, can significantly improve the duration and quality of a pet's life. Aspects of therapy of chronic renal failure are discussed in *Drug Metabolism in Renal Failure* by Stern, *Control of Parathyroid Hormone in Chronic Renal Failure* by Mikiciuk and Thornhill, *Clinical Experience with Peritoneal Dialysis in Small Animals* by Carter et al, and *Management of Chronic Renal Failure* by Senior.

Acute renal failure, though less common than chronic, nevertheless remains a diagnostic and therapeutic challenge for the veterinarian. In *Drug-Related Nephropathies*, Brown and Engelhardt discuss one of the more common causes of acute renal failure in small animals. Additional coverage of the causes, diagnosis, and management of this condition are found in the articles on *Acute Renal Failure* by Lane et al, as well as in the previously mentioned article on peritoneal dialysis by Carter et al.

Accurate and timely diagnosis is necessary for appropriate therapy of any medical problem. Medical, laboratory, and diagnostic imaging techniques for the diagnosis of renal disease and renal failure are discussed in *Interpretation of Urine Protein–Creatinine Ratios in Dogs with Glomerular and Nonglomerular Disorders* by Lulich and Osborne, *Polyuria and Polydipsia* by Hughes, *Hematuria: An Algorithm for Differential Diagnosis* by Crow, and *The Excretory Urogram* by Feeney et al.

Lower urinary tract disorders are also common in dogs and cats. Several aspects of these disorders are covered in *Bacterial Urinary Tract Infections* by Senior, *Feline Urologic Signs: A Unifying Hypothesis of Causes* and *Canine Urolithiasis* by Osborne et al, *Urinary Tract Neoplasms* and *Hematuria* by Crow, and *Urinary Incontinence in Geriatric Dogs* by Krawiec and Rubin. Diagnostic imaging techniques for diagnosis of lower urinary tract disease are discussed in *Urethrography and Cystography in Cats* by Johnston et al, *Retrograde Vaginocystography: A Contrast Study for Evaluation of Bitches with Urinary Incontinence* by Leveille and Atilola, and *Cystoscopy in Female Dogs* by Senior.

Renal Tubular Acidosis by Zoran and Jergens and *Developmental Aspects of Fluid and Electrolyte Metabolism and Renal Function* by Fettman and Allen cover some less common but still important clinical information. These articles will be of particular interest to those wishing to broaden their expertise in nephrology.

Linda A. Ross, DVM, MS
Diplomate ACVIM
Associate Dean for Clinical
Programs and
Hospital Director
Tufts University

CONTENTS

RENAL FAILURE

KIDNEY FUNCTION AND DISORDERS

THE URINARY TRACT

CLINICAL SIGNS

DIAGNOSTICS

Acute Renal Failure. Part I. Risk Factors, Prevention, and Strategies for Protection

University of Prince Edward Island, Charlottetown, Prince Edward Island, Canada
India F. Lane, DVM, MS

Colorado State University
Gregory F. Grauer, DVM, MS
Martin J. Fettman, DVM, MS, PhD

KEY FACTS

❑ Acute renal failure may be prevented in patients that are at risk in a hospital setting by identifying such patients and adjusting clinical monitoring and therapy.

❑ Early recognition of impending acute renal failure and therapeutic intervention are facilitated by careful monitoring of urine output and urine characteristics.

❑ Acute renal failure occurs as a result of renal hemodynamic changes or tubular damage caused by nephrotoxic or ischemic insult.

❑ Vasodilators, calcium channel blockers, atrial natriuretic peptide, free radical scavengers, adjustments to diet, and other therapeutic measures show promise for future use in the prevention and treatment of acute renal failure.

Acute renal failure (ARF) is a sudden, severe reduction in renal function. It may be caused by prerenal, postrenal, or intrinsic renal insult. Intrinsic renal insult is generally ischemic or toxic in nature; it can occur as a result of a variety of systemic diseases, injuries, or therapeutic manipulations. Ischemic intrinsic renal insult is the most common cause of acute renal failure in humans; in dogs and cats, intrinsic renal insult resulting from nephrotoxic agents is the most common cause.[1] Acute renal failure carries a guarded prognosis and, despite many years of study and many advances in medical therapy, the overall outcome for patients with the disease has not changed significantly. Before dialysis became available, the mortality rate for humans with acute renal failure exceeded 90%[2–3]; today, with dialytic therapy widely available, the mortality rate is still greater than 50%.[4–6] Because of the potentially devastating results of established acute renal failure, prevention, early recognition, and early intervention are important.

Part I of this two-part series discusses the pathophysiology of acute renal failure, examines the factors that place certain patients at risk, and details methods of early recognition and intervention. Part II discusses diagnosis, management, and prognosis of acute renal failure.

PATHOPHYSIOLOGY

Intricacies of the pathogenesis of ischemic and toxic renal injury are yet to be completely explored. An understanding of these intricacies holds the key to successful intervention in and prevention of cases of acute renal failure.

The general mechanisms of acute renal failure can be categorized as vascular or tubular. Several mechanisms are usually involved in each case of renal dysfunction.[1,7] There are six specific sites of impairment. *Afferent arteriolar vasoconstriction* disrupts glomerular blood flow. Such vasoconstriction is often a physiologic response to decreased effective blood volume caused by

Selected Causes of Acute Renal Failure[1,7]

Vascular or Ischemic
Dehydration
Hemorrhage
Shock
Hypotension
Anesthesia
Surgery
Sepsis
Heart failure
Arrhythmia
Cardiac arrest
Trauma
Renal vascular occlusion
Thromboembolism
Hypertension
Vasculitis
Extensive burns
Hyperthermia
Disseminated intravascular coagulation
Hyperviscosity

Nephrotoxic
Ethylene glycol
Hydrocarbons
Heavy metals
Antimicrobial agents
Angiotensin-converting-enzyme inhibitors
Chemotherapeutic agents
Nonsteroidal antiinflammatory drugs
Thiacetarsamide
Radiocontrast agents
Anesthetic agents
Hemoglobinemia
Myoglobinemia
Hypercalcemia
Snake venom

Other
Glomerulonephritis
Pyelonephritis
Urinary tract obstruction
Leptospirosis
Amyloidosis
Diabetes mellitus

largely modulated by mesangial cell contraction, which can be affected by ischemia, humoral agents, or toxicants. Glomerular permeability may be reduced by toxicant or immunologic injury to podocytes or endothelial architecture.

Decreased glomerular capillary pressure and filtration forces result from *vasodilation of the efferent arteriole*. Damage to tubular epithelial cells disrupts the integrity of the tubular lining and may result in *tubular backleak* of filtrate into the peritubular capillaries and interstitium. Tubular damage also creates cellular casts and debris, which can cause *obstruction of tubular flow*. Tubular flow may be further reduced by interstitial edema and cellular swelling; increased intratubular pressure may exacerbate existing backleak and filtration failure.

Ischemic Injury

Ischemic injury occurs when renal blood flow is attenuated by decreased blood pressure or by renal vasoconstriction. Conditions that result in volume depletion, depressed cardiac output, or sustained systemic hypotension can result in ischemic renal injury (see Selected Causes of Acute Renal Failure).[1,7] Decreased renal blood flow causes a reduction in the amount of oxygen and metabolic substrates available to tubular cells, and this cellular starvation initiates a complicated cycle of events (Figure 1). The adenosine triphosphate (ATP) energy pool is depleted rapidly. Cellular transport mechanisms are affected, particularly the sodium-potassium and sodium-calcium adenosinetriphosphatase (ATPase) pumps.

Increased intracellular concentrations of sodium cause extraction of plasma water and cell swelling, which occludes vascular and tubular lumens.[8] Membrane damage results in excessive calcium influx into renal tubular epithelial cells.[9] The depletion of energy sources depresses calcium efflux from the cell by calcium–adenosinetriphosphatase (Ca–ATPase) dependent transport; calcium processing by mitochondria and the endoplasmic reticulum is subsequently overwhelmed.[9–13] Increased intracellular calcium activates phospholipases, disrupts oxidative phosphorylation in mitochondria, and further constricts renal blood vessels.[11] Thus, intracellular calcium overload acts to perpetuate membrane damage, vasoconstriction, and energy depletion initiated by the ischemic event (Figure 2).

Persistent vasoconstriction and cell swelling create vascular stasis and platelet and red blood cell aggregation.[8] Red blood cells are trapped in the vascular space, occluding as much as 30% of the blood supply to the renal cortex, thereby creating further ischemic injury. Energy substrate delivery remains impaired; adenosine triphosphate restoration cannot occur. De-

dehydration, systemic hypotension, or fluid loss.[1,7] Excessive neurogenic or humoral response to vascular disease, trauma, or systemic injury is also implicated, although involvement of the renin–angiotensin axis is controversial.[7]

Reduced glomerular capillary surface area and *altered intrinsic glomerular filtration properties* also cause dysfunction. Surface area and filtration characteristics are

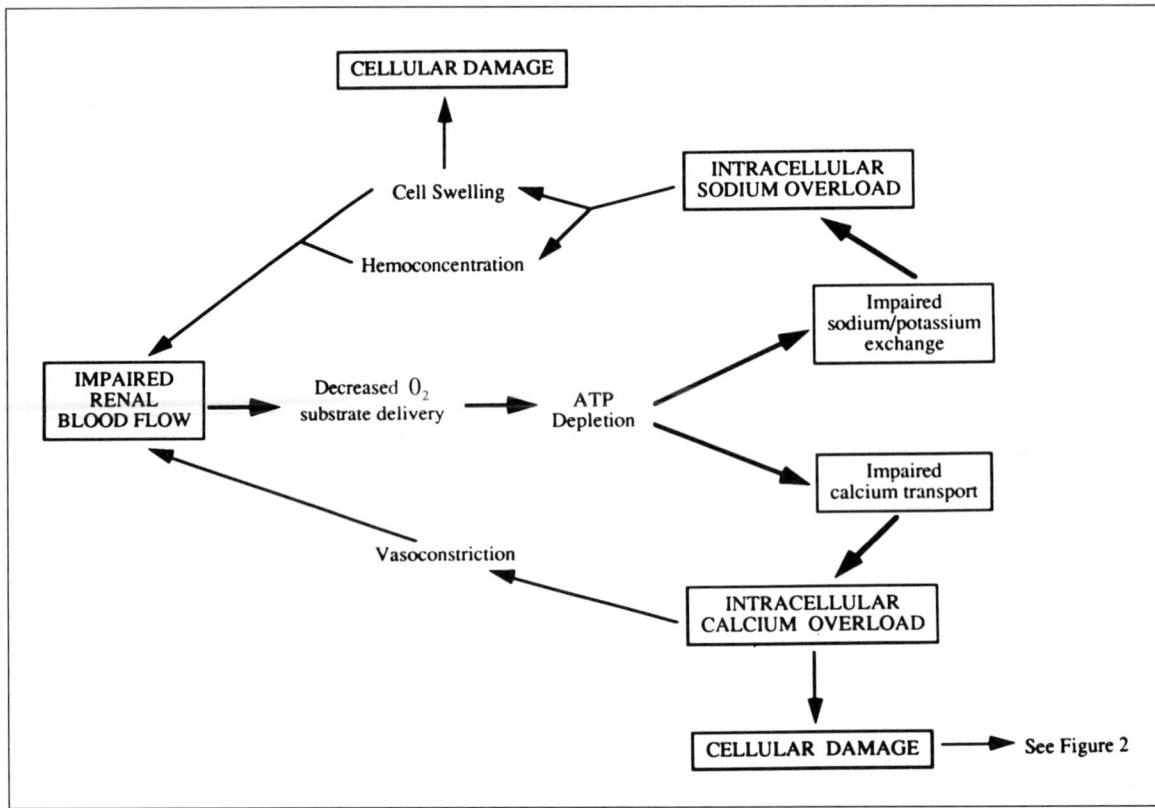

Figure 1—Circulatory and cellular events of ischemic renal injury. *ATP* = adenosine triphosphate.

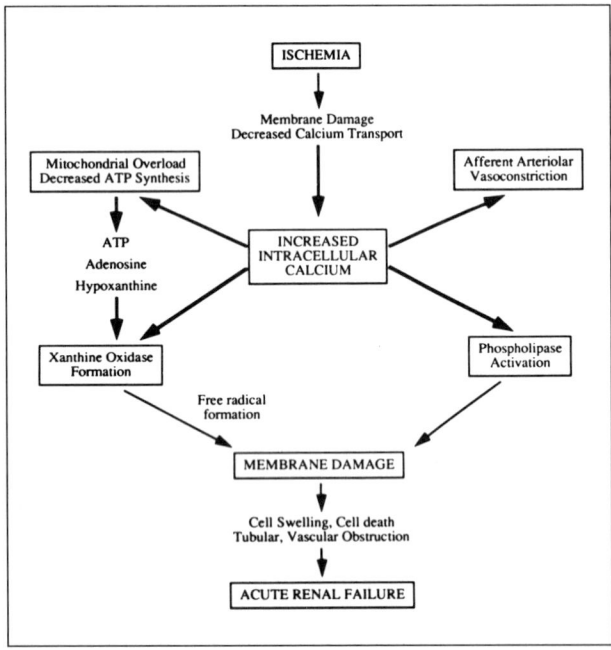

Figure 2—Schematic representation of the role of increased intracellular calcium in ischemic renal injury. *ATP* = adenosine triphosphate.

creased energy production results in membrane damage and oxygen free radical formation. Free radical scavengers are rapidly depleted; damage caused by free radicals contributes to membrane and cellular defects. Leukotrienes, thromboxane A_2, and other chemotactic factors cause infiltration by inflammatory cells and generation of additional inflammatory mediators and vasoactive chemicals.[8]

Nephrotoxic Injury

The kidneys are particularly susceptible to toxic injury for several reasons. They receive 20% of cardiac output, and therefore receive a relatively high proportion of blood-borne toxicants. Each kidney's large glomerular capillary surface area provides a large area for toxicant–endothelial interaction. In the proximal tubule and thick ascending loop of Henle, transport functions and a high metabolic rate make the epithelial cells especially sensitive to toxicants that disrupt energy sources or membrane functions. Tubular epithelial cells may also actively resorb toxicants, allowing such toxicants to accumulate to dangerous levels. The countercurrent mechanism and tubular concentrating functions result in increasing concentrations of toxic substances in the distal portions of the nephron. Finally, biotransformation activity of the kidney may result in local production of metabolites that are more toxic than parent compounds, as is the case with intrarenal oxidation of ethylene glycol.[14,15]

Nephrotoxic injury to the glomerulus can be direct

or immune mediated. Direct nephrotoxic injury includes destruction of capillary surface area by such substances as aminoglycosides; disruption of endothelial integrity and surface barriers by cationic substances, such as doxorubicin hydrochloride, probenecid, and protamine; and mesangial cell proliferation and hypertrophy caused by such substances as azathioprine and penicillamine.

Immunologic injury to the glomerulus occurs secondary to immune complex deposition, systemic lupus-like injury with antinuclear antibody formation, or other hypersensitivity reactions. In humans, such drugs as penicillin, penicillamine, gold salts, and sulfadiazine have been associated with immune complex disease, and procainamide, probenecid, hydralazine, and isoniazid can result in lupus-like syndromes.[14] Immune-complex deposition secondary to other antigens (e.g., *Dirofilaria immitis*) is, however, more common in small animals. Toxicants that disrupt tubular function may also indirectly affect glomerular function. They do so because tubular damage may trigger tubuloglomerular feedback mechanisms and local production of angiotensin II and other mediators that can precipitate hemodynamic and mesangial cell alterations.

Nephrotoxicant-induced tubular injury usually is caused by the effect of a toxicant on epithelial cells. Toxicants attach at luminal or basolateral membrane sites or to intracellular organelles.[1] Cellular function is then disrupted as a result of membrane and transport system damage, interference with energy production and cellular respiration, calcium influx, cell swelling, and cell death.[14]

Nonoliguric Acute Renal Failure

Urine production in cases of acute renal failure is variable. Although oliguria is considered the hallmark of acute renal failure, in many instances urine production is preserved or increased. Nonoliguric acute renal failure may be caused by exposure to such nephrotoxicants as aminoglycosides and cisplatin, or it may occur as a result of milder ischemic events.[16] Impaired tubular responses to antidiuretic hormone (ADH) can contribute to polyuric acute renal failure. Depressed responsiveness to antidiuretic hormone results from reduced medullary hypertonicity or from agents that impair concentrating ability, such as *E. coli* endotoxins, glucocorticoids, and diuretics.[17]

RISK FACTORS

Although prevention of accidental exposure to such nephrotoxic agents as ethylene glycol outside the hospital relies on client education and environmental control, prevention of iatrogenic acute renal failure is aided by the identification of patients at risk (see Risk

---

Risk Factors for Acute Renal Failure

Preexisting Disease
Renal insufficiency
Pancreatitis
Hepatic insufficiency
Diabetes mellitus
Cardiovascular disease
Multiple myeloma
Trauma
Extensive burns
Increasing age

Clinical Conditions
Volume depletion
Electrolyte abnormalities
Hypoalbuminemia
Systemic hypotension
Systemic hypertension
Fever
Sepsis
Anesthesia
Surgery
Radiocontrast media
Nonsteroidal antiinflammatory drugs
Nephrotoxic drugs

Factors for Acute Renal Failure). Trauma, extensive burns, pancreatitis, cardiovascular disease, diabetes mellitus, multiple myeloma, and preexisting renal disease are disorders associated with a high incidence of acute renal failure in humans.[7] Increasing age is considered a risk factor by some researchers[7] but not by others.[18] In humans, a gradual decline in renal blood flow (RBF) and glomerular filtration rate (GFR) occurs with age, probably placing some older patients at increased risk.[19]

Clinical conditions that increase the risk for acute renal failure include dehydration, electrolyte abnormalities, systemic hypotension, hypoalbuminemia, vasculitis, fever, sepsis, prolonged surgery or anesthesia, administration of radiographic contrast media, and use of potentially nephrotoxic agents.[19,20] Surgical procedures in which the renal vasculature is occluded or disrupted result in a high incidence of acute renal failure in humans.[4,7] The most important risk factors in small animals are volume depletion, electrolyte imbalances, anesthesia and surgery, and use of potentially nephrotoxic drugs. Risk factors are additive, and almost any complication occurring in a high-risk patient increases the potential for development of acute renal failure.

Volume depletion is the most significant factor

predisposing patients to acute renal failure, and it is often the only factor that can be prevented or corrected.[7,20] Volume depletion results from renal hypoperfusion, a decreased volume of distribution of nephrotoxic drugs, and decreased tubular flow. Decreased tubular flow potentiates tubular reabsorption, which can increase the intratubular and intracellular concentration of nephrotoxicants.[14] Rapid repletion of circulating blood volume and maintenance of adequate blood pressure in acutely ill or critically ill patients are important. Volume can be replaced by isotonic fluids or colloids. Pressor agents may be used in cases in which severe hypotension does not respond to volume replacement; improved systemic pressure may, however, affect renal vasoconstriction and result in reduced renal blood flow.

With high-risk patients, anesthetic protocols should be adjusted to prevent hypotension or possible nephrotoxicosis. Volume replacement and blood-pressure monitoring are critical. Renal autoregulation can maintain glomerular capillary pressure for short periods, but renal blood flow is compromised when systolic pressure drops below 80 mm Hg for sustained periods.[1] Anesthesia with methoxyflurane occasionally results in acute renal failure in humans if the duration of exposure is prolonged. Nephrotoxicity of methoxyflurane is enhanced by dehydration or concurrent use of nephrotoxic drugs.[21] Dogs seem to be resistant to the effects of methoxyflurane if exposed for only a short time[22]; however, the administration of flunixin meglumine with methoxyflurane anesthesia has been shown to result in acute tubular necrosis.[23]

Electrolyte imbalances, particularly sodium or potassium disturbances, also increase the risk of acute renal failure. Hyponatremia potentiates contrast-media induced acute renal failure in dogs and humans.[24] Hypokalemia, hypocalcemia, hypomagnesemia, and metabolic acidosis enhance gentamicin nephrotoxicity in dog and rat experimental models.[25,26] Electrolyte status should be routinely monitored in high-risk patients and corrected before anesthesia, surgery, contrast imaging procedures, or use of potentially nephrotoxic drugs.

Other specific risk factors for gentamicin nephrotoxicity include old age; dehydration; preexisting renal disease; prolonged duration of therapy; and the concurrent use of cytotoxic drugs, other nephrotoxic agents, or prostaglandin inhibitors.[27] In high-risk patients, the potential dangers of aminoglycoside therapy must be weighed against the benefits. When aminoglycosides are used, therapeutic-drug monitoring allows the clinician to tailor individual dose regimens. Nephrotoxicity increases with elevated trough serum levels (greater than 2 µg/ml for gentamicin; greater than 5 µg/ml for amikacin).[14]

Trough levels can be reduced by decreasing the dose or increasing the dose interval.[27] Recent investigations suggest that increasing the dose interval by a factor arithmetically related to serum creatinine or creatinine clearance values is the most effective way to reduce nephrotoxicity.[28,29] Frequent dosing of gentamicin (every eight hours) may be less efficacious and potentially more nephrotoxic, however, than an equivalent total daily dose given in 12-hour intervals.[29] Other mechanisms of protection in gentamicin therapy are discussed below.

Nonsteroidal antiinflammatory drugs (NSAIDs) may act as nephrotoxicants; administration of such drugs may increase the risk of acute renal failure. Used long term and given in single doses, nonsteroidal antiinflammatory drugs inhibit renal prostaglandin synthesis and decrease urinary prostaglandin excretion by inhibiting cyclooxygenase activity. Prostaglandins, particularly of the E and I series, serve important vasodilatory functions in the kidney; and they influence glomerular filtration rates and solute excretion.[30,31] Prostaglandins also modulate renin release, tubular ion transport, and water balance.[31]

Inhibition of prostaglandin synthesis in the normal kidney does not significantly impair renal function because other regulatory mechanisms compensate for the loss of prostaglandin influence. In diseased kidneys or with the addition of volume depletion or other stressors, however, the vasoconstrictor influences predominate and normal prostaglandin counter-response is required[30] (Figure 3). Anesthesia, surgery, sodium or volume depletion, sepsis, congestive heart failure, nephrotic syndrome, and hepatic disease cause renal function to become more dependent on prostaglandin synthesis; therefore, in such cases, susceptibility to nonsteroidal antiinflammatory drugs is increased.[30] Dogs seem to be particularly sensitive to newer nonsteroidal antiinflammatory drugs, such as ibuprofen or naproxen; reaction may include gastrointestinal ulceration and renal failure.[32] Acute interstitial nephritis and papillary necrosis have also been reported secondary to administration of nonsteroidal antiinflammatory drugs.[30–33]

EARLY RECOGNITION OF RENAL DYSFUNCTION

Acute renal failure occurs in three distinct phases: (1) the induction phase, in which the insult occurs and azotemia, oliguria, or polyuria develop; (2) the maintenance phase, in which established loss of function occurs; and (3) the recovery phase, during which resolution of azotemia, nephron repair, and functional compensation occur.[1] Because therapeutic intervention is most successful when initiated in the induction phase of acute renal failure (which can be very short in duration), early recognition of renal dysfunction can save the patient's life.

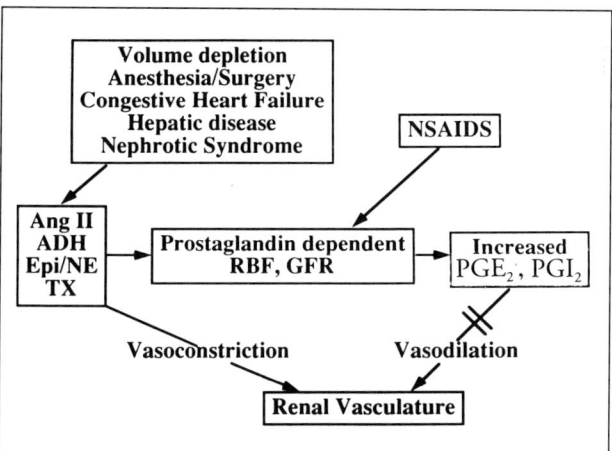

Figure 3—Influence of nonsteroidal antiinflammatory drugs (*NSAIDs*) in conditions in which renal vascular resistance is highly prostaglandin dependent. *Ang II* = angiotensin II, *ADH* = antidiuretic hormone, *Epi/NE* = epinephrine/norepinephrine, *TX* = thromboxane, *RBF* = renal blood flow, *GFR* = glomerular filtration rate, *PGE$_2$* = prostaglandin E$_2$, *PGI$_2$* = prostaglandin I$_2$ (prostacyclin).

In humans, acute renal failure has been defined as an increase in serum creatinine of 0.5 mg/dl/day for two consecutive days.[7] Such relatively small changes are probably often missed or overlooked in veterinary patients. Frequent monitoring of serum creatinine in high-risk patients may allow earlier detection of prerenal or renal azotemia. Monitoring other patient criteria, however, may help to detect renal damage and dysfunction before the development of azotemia.

Physical examination of the patient at risk for acute renal failure should include observation of cardiac rate, rhythm, and pulse quality and assessment of hydration status. Pulse quality and hydration characteristics are outward indexes of hemodynamic status. Frequent recording of body weight, packed cell volume, and plasma total solids helps to detect subtle changes in hydration status. In critically ill patients, direct or indirect monitoring of blood pressure can help to identify hypotension and hypertension, conditions which increase the risk of renal damage. Palpation of the abdomen and kidneys is also important. Kidneys may become enlarged or painful if acute dysfunction and intracapsular swelling occur.

Urine output of critically ill patients should be monitored; it should also be objectively quantified in high-risk patients, using a metabolic cage, intermittent catheterization, or a closed indwelling collection system. Normal urine output should be 1 to 2 ml/hr/kg body weight; significant increases or decreases from normal output may signal acute renal failure. Oliguria (<0.27 ml/hr/kg) or anuria (<.08 ml/hr/kg)[34] requires prompt attention and treatment.

Urine should be assessed at each collection for turbidity or the presence of blood; the urine sediment should be examined daily for red blood cells, white blood cells, casts, renal epithelial cells, and cellular debris. The presence of low–molecular-weight proteins in the urine that normally are freely filtered and then reabsorbed in the proximal tubules is an early marker of acute renal failure. Beta$_2$-microglobulin and retinol binding protein assays have been used in humans as early indicators of proximal tubular damage.[35] In practice, the onset of proteinuria detected by semiquantitative (dipstick or turbidimetric) or quantitative (urine protein/creatinine ratio) methods may indicate early glomerular or tubular damage.

Urinary enzyme activity is a sensitive method of detecting early tubular damage. In cases of tubular damage or necrosis, enzymes such as γ-glutamyl transpeptidase and N-acetyl-β-D-glucoaminidase (NAG) are not filtered normally by the glomerulus but, instead, increase in the urine.[36] Urinary γ-glutamyl transpeptidase originates from the proximal tubular brush border; N-acetyl-β-D-glucoaminidase is present in the proximal tubule lysosomes.[36,37] Urinary γ-glutamyl transpeptidase activity was the earliest known marker of toxicosis reported in studies of gentamicin nephrotoxicity in a dog model.[36] In cases of early gentamicin nephrotoxicity, urinary N-acetyl-β-D-glucoaminidase activity is increased in proportion to tubular damage. Urinary N-acetyl-β-D-glucoaminidase has also been investigated as an early marker for diabetic nephropathy in humans.[37] In a study of experimental organonitrile nephrotoxicity in rats, increases in urinary N-acetyl-β-D-glucoaminidase correlated well with renal morphologic lesions that developed before the onset of azotemia.[38]

Urinary amylase, lysozyme, β-glucuronidase, lactic dehydrogenase, and aspartate transaminase activities also have been investigated in nephrotoxic models.[39–41] False-positive results can occur with severe glomerular damage that results in abnormal filtration into the urine; false-negative results can occur after chronic damage and depletion of enzyme stores.[36] The development of glucosuria or alterations in the fractional excretion of other electrolytes are other early signals of tubular dysfunction.[42]

MECHANISMS OF PROTECTION AND EARLY INTERVENTION

Methods designed to protect the kidneys from acute insults (Table I) attempt to prevent or interrupt the pathophysiologic events that result in acute renal failure. Goals of protective maneuvers are to (1) preserve or restore renal hemodynamics, (2) increase solute excretion, (3) minimize intratubular obstruction, (4) enhance cellular recovery, and (5) reduce toxicity of nephrotoxic agents.[20] Dietary manipulations, va-

TABLE I
Protective Agents in Cases of Acute Renal Failure

Agent	Type of Injury[a]	Timing[a]	Possible Mechanisms
Sodium[42–46]	Toxicant	Prior	Causes volume expansion Increases natriuresis Suppresses RAAS Reduces TGF
Mannitol[55–59]	Toxicant Ischemic	Prior/Post	Causes volume expansion Increases tubular flow, GFR Causes vasodilation Acts as a free radical scavenger
Furosemide[60,62,63]	Toxicant	Prior/Post	Increases renal blood flow Increases tubular flow More effective when used with dopamine
Low-protein diets[46–51]	Toxicant Ischemic	Prior	Reduces renal work Reduces tubular uptake
Atrial natriuretic peptide[24, 65–67]	Ischemic	Initiation	Causes Aa vasodilation May cause Ea vasoconstriction Causes diuresis, natriuresis
Calcium channel blockers[10,12,68–71]	Ischemic Transplant	Prior/Init	Causes Aa vasodilation Prevents calcium overload Prevents membrane damage Prevents reperfusion injury
Free radical scavengers[72,73]	Toxicant Ischemic	Init/Post	Reduces reperfusion injury
ATP-magnesium chloride[76,78]	Ischemic	Initiation	Supplies energy substrate Reduces adenosine accumulation May supply magnesium
Theophylline, Aminophylline[75,77]	Toxicant	Prior	Acts as adenosine receptor blockade
Thyroxin[80]	Toxicant	Initiation	Stimulates renal tubular gluconeogenesis Restores sodium-potassium transport pumps
Thromboxane inhibitors[83]	Ischemic	Init/Post	Reduce vasoconstrictive influence

[a] Type of injury and timing of administration represent best results in experimental models. Selected references are listed for each agent. *ATP* = adenosine triphosphate, *RAAS* = renin-angiotensin-aldosterone system, *TGF* = tubuloglomerular feedback, *GFR* = glomerular filtration rate, *Aa* = afferent arteriole, *Ea* = efferent arteriole.

sodilatory compounds, diuretics, and cytoprotective agents are some treatments that may protect the kidneys from acute renal failure.

Dietary Factors
Sodium

Low-sodium diets have been shown to enhance gentamicin nephrotoxicity.[43] Oral sodium–loading strategies have been beneficial in reducing mortality and cortical gentamicin concentrations in rats.[43] The benefits of sodium loading may involve suppression of intrarenal and plasma renin activity and attenuation of early renin–angiotensin responses. Other manipulations to block renin or angiotensin effects, however, are not uniformly protective after acute renal failure is established.[20] Volume expansion secondary to sodium retention may protect the renal vasculature and may increase the volume of distribution of nephrotoxic drugs, thus reducing their effective serum and tissue concentrations.[43]

Increasing natriuresis, urine volume, and solute excretion before a potential renal insult may also be important to prevent acute renal failure.[44] Saline diuresis has been helpful before the administration of some nephrotoxic agents (cisplatin,[45] amphotericin B[46]) because it results in volume expansion and increased natriuresis. Although sodium loading does not consistently protect against acute renal failure, it is clear that sodium depletion and hyponatremia should be avoided in patients at high risk for acute renal failure.

Protein

The effects of dietary protein on chronic renal disease have been investigated for many years. Recently, however, conditioning with reduced dietary protein has been shown to improve renal function and survival rates in rats subjected to acute ischemic insults[47,48] and uranyl nitrate-,[49] puromycin-[50] and gentamicin-induced[51] acute renal failure. In a model of ischemia, 88% of rats receiving a 5% protein diet and all rats receiving a 0% protein diet survived, whereas only 31% and 7% of rats receiving diets with an average or high level of protein, respectively, survived.[47] Preconditioning with reduced-protein diets had to occur for at least one week before insult to be effective; dietary manipulation immediately after the insult was not protective.[47,48]

In one study in which rats were given nephrotoxic doses of gentamicin, animals that were preconditioned with a low-protein diet showed improved creatinine clearance, decreased enzymuria, and decreased renal cortical concentrations of gentamicin compared with animals that received diets with an average or high protein content.[51] In another study, low-protein conditioning again improved survival in rats treated with gentamicin; however, significant protection was also provided by preconditioning the rats with a high-protein diet, and then switching them to a low-protein diet at the time of gentamicin administration.[52]

Low protein intake may downshift renal work by reducing renal blood flow and glomerular filtration rate. A low-protein diet reduces tubular metabolic work, thus perhaps decreasing tubular uptake of gentamicin. In one study in dogs, however, conditioning with a high-protein (26%) diet before and during gentamicin administration reduced nephrotoxicity[53] and enhanced gentamicin clearence[54] compared with such functions in dogs fed diets that were 13% or 9% protein.

The effects of dietary protein conditioning on susceptibility to renal failure may depend on the nephrotoxicant involved, because high protein intake is protective in models of mercuric chloride toxicity, even with short-term conditioning.[55] Evaluation of dietary protein conditioning in dogs before and after renal ischemia or nephrotoxicant-induced renal injury may have important clinical implications.

Diuretics and Vasodilators

Diuretics have long been used in cases of acute renal failure to combat oliguria. Mannitol, an osmotic diuretic, serves to increase intravascular volume, increase tubular fluid flow, and prevent tubular obstruction and collapse. Mannitol also acts as a renal vasodilator, improving renal blood flow and glomerular filtration rate, if given early in acute renal failure.[56-58] The vasodilatory effects of mannitol may be mediated by renal prostaglandins[57] or by the release of atrial natriuretic hormone.[58] Hypertonic mannitol solutions help reduce cellular swelling in cases of acute renal failure and thus prevent tubular obstruction and cell death. Cellular protection may also be afforded by the free radical scavenging properties of mannitol and its influence on prevention of mitochondrial calcium accumulation.[57]

Experimentally, mannitol has proven protective against acute renal failure in ischemic models[59,60] and toxicant-induced models including glycerol, methemoglobin, cisplatin, and amphotericin B.[57] Mannitol is used in humans to protect against acute renal failure during high-risk surgeries, radiocontrast procedures, and use of amphotericin B and cisplatin.[57]

Furosemide also acts to increase renal blood flow and tubular flow, but it does not significantly influence glomerular filtration rate. Enhanced diuresis created by furosemide may resolve oliguria, but it does not seem to affect recovery or survival.[57] Furosemide seems to be more effective in inducing diuresis when it is used in combination with dopamine infusion.[61] The intravenous infusion of dopamine at low dosages (1 to 3 µg/kg/min) acts via renal dopaminergic receptors to increase renal blood flow, glomerular filtration rate, and sodium excretion in normal kidneys. Low-dose dopamine alone may also improve renal function in cases of acute renal failure.[62] Furosemide has been protective in some models of ischemia,[63-65] but mixed results have been obtained from its use with nephrotoxicants. Both furosemide and dopamine are most effective when administered soon after onset of renal failure. Furosemide in combination with gentamicin actually enhances nephrotoxicity, probably by creating volume depletion.[65]

Atrial Natriuretic Peptide

Atrial natriuretic peptide (ANP) counterbalances the vasoconstrictive activity of catecholamines and angiotensin II. Atrial natriuretic peptide release results in vasorelaxation, diuresis, and natriuresis.[66] It seems to preserve renal blood flow and glomerular filtration rate during ischemia and volume depletion by causing afferent arteriolar vasodilation and, possibly, efferent arteriolar vasoconstriction.[67]

In a canine model of norepinephrine-induced acute

renal failure, atrial natriuretic peptide infusion resulted in better protection of renal blood flow and creatinine clearance than did dopamine infusion; elevations in systemic blood pressure and total vascular resistance were attenuated.[66] Natriuretic peptide, used in a model of ischemia in rats, improved glomerular capillary pressure and afferent arteriolar blood flow resulting from a decrease in afferent arteriolar resistance were documented.[68] In another study, atrial natriuretic peptide preserved renal function in dogs with congestive heart failure receiving iodinated radiocontrast media.[24] Atrial natriuretic peptide infusion was not found, however, to be significantly more protective than mannitol in a clinical trial of humans at high risk of acute renal failure during angiography procedures.[58]

Calcium Channel Blockers

Increased intracellular calcium concentrations secondary to ischemic or nephrotoxicant-induced injury cause membrane and cytoskeletal damage, deranged cellular metabolism, and sustained vasoconstriction in the injured kidney.[10,12] Calcium channel blockers (CCBs, calcium-entry blockers) exert a cytoprotective and vasodilatory effect if given before or early in the course of ischemia.[10–12]

In a normal animal, calcium channel blockers increase renal blood flow, glomerular filtration rate, urine flow, and electrolyte excretion.[10] Hemodynamic alterations result from a decrease in afferent arteriolar resistance and are accentuated if preexisting vascular tone is high.[10]

The protective mechanisms of calcium channel blockers in acute renal failure may involve preservation of renal blood flow or cytoprotective effects, including the prevention of mitochondrial calcium overload and reperfusion injury.[10,13,69,70] An interaction between calcium channel blockers and tissue magnesium also seems to be important. In a model of ischemic injury in guinea pigs in which verapamil infusion was protective, the significant difference between treated and untreated animals was the preservation of tissue magnesium levels.[71] Interfering with the effects of calcium may preserve membrane integrity and therefore prevent loss of tissue magnesium.[71]

Calcium channel blockers have been protective in models of ischemic acute renal failure in dogs.[72] Calcium channel blockers have also improved glomerular filtration rate in transplanted kidneys in dogs, and they are used clinically to help prevent acute renal failure in transplanted kidneys in humans.[69] It seems that calcium channel blockers improve graft function slightly and may protect transplanted kidneys from cyclosporine toxicity,[10] but improved graft survival has not been demonstrated.[69] Protection in ischemic acute renal failure models was best when calcium

channel blockers were administered via intraarterial or intrarenal infusion before and after the insult,[10,69] a frequency that may limit their practicality and effectiveness in clinical cases of acute renal failure. Finally, although promising results have been observed in many experimental models, infusion of calcium channel blockers may have systemic hypotensive and cardiodepressant effects that could decrease renal blood flow.

Free Radical Scavengers

Hypoxia, membrane damage, adenosine triphosphate degradation, and reperfusion can result in free radical formation, which creates further membrane damage.[8,9,73] During ischemia, tissue adenosine triphosphate is used rapidly and adenosine degradation to hypoxanthine occurs. Xanthine dehydrogenase is converted to xanthine oxidase, which preferentially metabolizes hypoxanthine to free radicals. Xanthine oxidase formation is also enhanced by elevated intracellular calcium concentration. When oxygen reappears, a burst of free radical production occurs. Intermediates of oxygen, including superoxides, hydroxyl radicals, and singlet oxygen, are toxic to mitochondria and cell membranes.[73]

Free radical scavengers have been protective in ischemic, aminoglycoside-induced, and glycerol-induced acute renal failure models.[75] In one study, increased lipid peroxidation and depressed glutathione peroxidase activity occurred after renal ischemia in rats fed a diet deficient in vitamin E and selenium—both natural free radical scavengers.[75] Superoxide dismutase, which metabolizes hydroxyl radicals to hydrogen peroxide, and allopurinol, which inhibits xanthine oxidase and reduces peroxide formation, have been shown to be protective by reducing reactive oxygen metabolites in some models.[75] Superoxide and hydroxyl radical scavengers, however, did not attenuate renal dysfunction in a recent model of endotoxin-induced acute renal failure in rats.[74]

Adenosine Nucleotides

Elevations in tissue adenosine concentrations occur after adenosine triphosphate degradation in renal ischemia, and infusion of adenosine into the interstitium of rat kidneys has resulted in decreased glomerular filtration rate.[76] Adenosine may be responsible for tubuloglomerular feedback and renal vasoconstriction after ischemia.[77] Adenosine receptor blockade with theophylline[76] or aminophylline[78] has been shown to reverse the effects of adenosine.

Postischemic infusion of adenine nucleotides (adenosine triphosphate, adenosine diphosphate, and adenosine monophosphate) combined with magnesium chloride in rats enhanced renal recovery, possibly by reducing adenine catabolism and adenosine production.[77] Adenosine triphosphate with magnesium chloride may also protect the kidney from ischemia by promoting prostaglandin synthesis or by acting as an intracellular energy source; the influence of magnesium may, again, be important. In one study involving dogs, however, adenosine triphosphate with magnesium chloride actually enhanced toxicity of cisplatin.[79]

Other Mechanisms

The effect of many other vasodilatory and cytoprotective agents in cases of acute renal failure are being investigated. Magnesium apparently plays a role in the protection afforded by calcium channel blockers, and it may have an influence on the effects of adenosine triphosphate-magnesium chloride infusion.[71,77] High magnesium intake is also protective against gentamicin toxicity.[80] Magnesium and calcium compete with gentamicin for binding sites at the renal tubular brush border.[80,81] Magnesium and calcium will probably be important components in dietary protection against acute renal failure. Attention to plasma magnesium levels is warranted with the use of aminoglycosides. Thyroxin administration has been protective in several toxicant-induced acute renal failure models in rats, possibly because of its role in the stimulation of gluconeogenesis and restoration of sodium-potassium pumps in renal tubular epithelial cells.[82] Vasodilatory substances, such as β-adrenergic antagonists,[83] synthetic vasodilatory prostaglandins,[84] and thromboxane synthetase inhibitors,[84] may also prove to be useful in the intervention of acute renal failure.

About the Authors

Dr. Lane is affiliated with the Department of Companion Animals, Atlantic Veterinary College, University of Prince Edward Island, Charlottetown, Prince Edward Island, Canada. Dr. Grauer is affiliated with the Department of Clinical Science and Dr. Fettman is affiliated with the Department of Pathology at the College of Veterinary Medicine and Biomedical Sciences, Colorado State University, Fort Collins, Colorado.

REFERENCES

1. Chew DJ, Dibartola SP: Diagnosis and pathophysiology of renal disease, in Ettinger SJ (ed): *Textbook of Veterinary Internal Medicine*, ed. 3. Philadelphia, WB Saunders Co, 1989, pp 1893–1961.
2. Byrick RJ, Rose DK: Pathophysiology and prevention of acute renal failure; the role of the anaesthetist. *Can J Anaesth* 37:457–467, 1990.
3. Guly UM, Turney JH: Post-traumatic acute renal failure, 1956–1988. *Clin Nephrol* 34:79–83, 1990.
4. Cioffi WG, Ashikaga T, Gamelli RL: Probability of surviv-
ing postoperative acute renal failure; development of a prognostic index. *Ann Surg* 200:205–211, 1984.
5. Maher ER, Robinson KN, Scoble JE, et al. Prognosis of critically ill patients with acute renal failure; APACHE II score and other predictive factors. *Q J Med* 72:857–866, 1989.
6. Liano F, Garci-Martin F, Gallego A, et al. Easy and early prognosis in acute tubular necrosis: A forward analysis of 228 cases. *Nephron* 51:307–313, 1989.
7. Wilkes BM, Mailloux LU: Acute renal failure; pathogenesis and prevention. *Am J Med* 80:1129–1136, 1986.
8. Mason J: The pathophysiology of ischemic acute renal failure; a new hypothesis about the initiation phase. *Renal Physiol* 9:129–147, 1986.
9. Weinberg J: The cell biology of ischemic renal injury. *Kidney Int* 39:476–500, 1991.
10. Chan L, Schrier RW: Effects of calcium channel blockers on renal function. *Annu Rev Med* 41:289–302, 1990.
11. Hume HD: Role of calcium in pathogenesis of acute renal failure. *Am J Physiol* 250:F579–F589, 1986.
12. Schrier RW, Arnold PE, Van Putten VJ, Burke TJ: Cellular calcium in ischemic acute renal failure: Role of calcium entry blockers. *Kidney Int* 32:313–321, 1987.
13. Schrier RW: Role of calcium channel blockers in protection against experimental renal injury. *Am J Med* 90 (Suppl 5A):21S–25S, 1991.
14. Brown SA, Engelhardt JA: Drug-related nephropathies. Part I. Mechanisms, diagnosis, and management. *Compend Contin Educ Pract Vet* 9(2):148–160, 1987.
15. Weening JJ: Mechanisms leading to toxin-induced impairment of renal function, with a focus on immunopathology. *Toxicol Lett* 46:205–211, 1989.
16. Anderson RJ, Linsa SL, Berns AS, et al: Nonoliguric acute renal failure. *N Engl J Med* 296:1134–1138, 1977.
17. Anderson RJ, Schrier RW: Clinical spectrum of oliguric and nonoliguric acute renal failure, in Brenner BM, Stein H (eds): *Acute Renal Failure*. New York, Churchill Livingstone, 1980, pp 3, 4.
18. Rasmussen HH, Pitt EA, Ibels LS, McNeil DR: Prediction of outcome in acute renal failure by discriminant analysis of clinical variables. *Arch Intern Med* 145:2015–2018, 1985.
19. Cowgill LD: Acute renal failure, in Bovee KC (ed): *Canine Nephrology*. Media, PA, Harwal Publishing Co, 1984, pp 405–438.
20. Mandal AK, Lightfoot BO, Treat RC: Mechanisms of protection in acute renal failure. *Circ Shock* 11:245–253, 1983.
21. Mazze RI: Methoxyflurane nephropathy. *Environ Health Perspect* 15:111–119, 1976.
22. Pedersoli WM: Serum flouride concentration, renal and hepatic function test results in dogs with methoxyflurane anesthesia. *Am J Vet Res* 38:949–953, 1977.
23. Mathews K, Doherty T, Dyson D, Wilcock B: Renal failure in dogs associated with flunixin meglumine and methoxyflurane anesthesia. *Vet Surg* 16:323, (abstract) 1987.
24. Margulies KB, McKinley LJ, Cavero PG, Burnett JC: Induction and prevention of radiocontrast-induced nephropathy in dogs with heart failure. *Kidney Int* 38:1101–1108, 1990.
25. Brinker KR, Bulger RE, Dolgan DC, et al: Effect of potassium depletion on gentamicin nephrotoxicity. *J Lab Clin Med* 98:292–301, 1981.
26. Hsu CH, Kurtz TW, Easterling RE, Weller JM: Potentiation of gentamicin nephrotoxicity by metabolic acidosis. *Proc Soc Exp Biol Med* 46:894–897, 1974.
27. Cooper K, Bennett WM: Nephrotoxicity of common drugs used in clinical practice. *Arch Intern Med* 147:1213–1218, 1987.
28. Rogers RA, Hanna AY, Riviere JE: Dose response studies of

gentamicin nephrotoxicity in rats with experimental renal dysfunction. III. Effects of dosage adjustment method. *Res Commun Chem Path Pharm* 57:301–311, 1987.

29. Frazier DL, Riviere JC: Gentamicin dosing strategies for dogs with subclinical renal dysfunction. *Antimicrob Agent Chemother* 31:1929–1934, 1987.

30. Patrono C, Dunn MJ: The clinical significance of inhibition of renal prostaglandin synthesis. *Kidney Int* 32:1–12, 1987.

31. Clive DM, Stoff JS: Renal syndromes associated with non-steroidal antiinflammatory drugs. *N Engl J Med* 310:563–571, 1984.

32. Spyridakis LK, Bacia JJ, Barsanti JA, Brown SA: Ibuprofen toxicosis in the dog. *JAVMA* 189:918–919, 1986.

33. Rubin SI: Nonsteroidal antiinflammatory drugs, prostaglandins, and the kidney. *JAVMA* 188:1065–1068, 1986.

34. English PB: Acute renal failure in the dog and cat. *Aust Vet J* 50:384–392, 1974.

35. Roberts DS, Haycock GB, Dalton RN, et al: Prediction of acute renal failure after birth asphyxia. *Arch Dis Child* 65:1021–1028, 1990.

36. Greco DS, Turnwald GH, Adams R, et al: Urinary gamma-glutamyl transpeptidase activity in dogs with gentamicin-induced nephrotoxicity. *Am J Vet Res* 46:2332–2335, 1985.

37. Stolarek I, Howey JE, Fraser CG. Biological variation of urinary N-acetyl-β-D-glucosaminidase: Practical and clinical implications. *Clin Chem* 35:560–563, 1989.

38. Gould DH, Fettman MJ, Daxenbichler ME, Bartuska BM: Functional and structural alterations of the rat kidney induced by the naturally occurring organonitrile 25-1-cyano-2-hydroxy-3,4 epithiobutane. *Toxicol Appl Pharmacol* 78:190–201, 1985.

39. Aderka D, Tene M, Graff E, Levo Y: Amylase-creatinine clearance ratio: A simple test to predict gentamicin nephrotoxicity. *Arch Intern Med* 148:1093–1096, 1988.

40. Szczech GM, Carlton WW, Lund JE: Determination of enzyme concentrations in urine for diagnosis of renal damage. *JAAHA* 10:1093–1096, 1974.

41. Hardy ML, Hsu RC, Short CR: The nephrotoxic potential of gentamicin in the cat; enzymuria and alterations in urine concentrating ability. *J Vet Pharmacol Ther* 8:382–392, 1985.

42. Garry F, Chew DJ, Hoffsis GF: Urinary indices of renal function in sheep with induced aminoglycoside nephrotoxicosis. *Am J Vet Res* 51:420–427, 1990.

43. Bennett WM, Hartnett MN, Gilbert D, et al: Effect of sodium intake on gentamicin nephrotoxicity in the rat. *Proc Soc Exp Biol Med* 151:736–738, 1976.

44. Vari RC, Natarajan LA, Whitescaver SA, et al: Induction, prevention and mechanisms of contrast media induced acute renal failure. *Kidney Int* 33:699–707, 1988.

45. Ogilvie GK, Krawiec DR, Gelberg HB, et al: Evaluation of a short-term saline diuresis protocol for the administration of *cis*-platinum. *Am J Vet Res* 49:1076–1078, 1988.

46. Gerkens JF, Branch RA: The influence of sodium status and furosemide on canine acute amphotericin B nephrotoxicity. *J Pharmacol Exp Ther* 214:306–311, 1980.

47. Andrews PM, Bates SB: Dietary protein prior to renal ischemia dramatically affects postischemic kidney function. *Kidney Int* 30:299–303, 1986.

48. Andrews PM, Bates SB: Dietary protein prior to renal ischemia and postischemic kidney function. *Kidney Int* 32(Suppl 22):576–580, 1987.

49. Andrews PM, Bates SB: Effects of dietary protein on uranyl-nitrate-induced acute renal failure. *Nephron* 45:296–301, 1987.

50. Marinides GN, Groggel GC, Cohen AH, Border WA: Enalapril and low protein diet reverse chronic puromycin aminonucleoside nephropathy. *Kidney Int* 37:749–757, 1990.

51. Whiting PH, Power DA, Petersen J, et al: The effect of dietary protein restriction on high dose gentamicin nephrotoxicity in rats. *Br J Exp Path* 69:35–41, 1988.

52. Andrews PM, Bates SB: Dietary protein as a risk factor in gentamicin nephrotoxicity. *Renal Failure* 10:153–159, 1987–1988.

53. Grauer GF, Behrend EN, Greco DS, et al: Effects of dietary protein conditioning on gentamicin-induced nephrotoxicity in dogs. *J Am Soc Nephrol* 3:724, (abstract) 1992.

54. Behrend EN, Grauer GF, Greco DS, et al: Effects of dietary protein conditioning on gentamicin pharmokinetics in dogs. *J Am Soc Nephrol* 3:720, (abstract) 1992.

55. Andrews PM, Chung EM: High dietary protein regimens provide significant protection from mercury nephrotoxicity in rats. *Toxicol Field Pharmacol* 105:288–304, 1990.

56. Finn WF: Diagnosis and management of acute tubular necrosis. *Med Clin North Am* 74(4):873–892, 1990.

57. Burnier M, Schrier RW: Protection from acute renal failure. *Adv Exp Med Biol* 212:275–283, 1986.

58. Kurnik BR, Weisberg LS, Cuttler IM, Kurnik PB: Effects of atrial natriuretic peptide versus mannitol on renal blood flow during radiocontrast infusion in chronic renal failure. *J Lab Clin Med* 116:27–35, 1990.

59. Johnston PA, Bernard DB, Perrin NS, et al: Prostaglandins mediate the vasodilatory effect of mannitol in the hypoperfused rat kidney. *J Clin Invest* 68:127–133, 1981.

60. Burke TJ, Cronin RE, Duchin KL, et al: Ischemia and tubule obstruction during acute renal failure in dogs: Mannitol in protection. *Am J Physiol* 238:F305–F314, 1980.

61. Lindner A: Synergism of dopamine and furosemide in diuretic-resistant, oliguric acute renal failure. *Nephron* 33:121–126, 1983.

62. Parker S, Carlon GC, Isaacs M, et al: Dopamine administration in oliguria and oliguric renal failure. *Crit Care Med* 9:630–632, 1981.

63. DeTorrente A, Miller PD, Cronin RE, et al: Effects of furosemide and acetylcholine in norepinephrine-induced acute renal failure. *Am J Physiol* 235:F131–F136, 1978.

64. Kramer HJ, Schuurmann J, Wasserman C, Dusing R: Prostaglandin-independent protection by furosemide from oliguric ischemic renal failure in conscious rats. *Kidney Int* 17:455–464, 1980.

65. Adelman RD, Spangler WL, Beasom F, et al: Furosemide enhancement of experimental gentamicin nephrotoxicity: Comparison of functional and morphological changes with activities of urinary enzymes. *J Infect Dis* 140:342–352, 1979.

66. Aikawa N, Wakabayashi GO, Masakazu U, Shinozawa Y: Regulation of renal function in thermal injury. *J Trauma* 30:S174–S178, 1990.

67. Flier JS, Underhill LH: Atrial natriuretic hormone, the renin-aldosterone axis, and blood pressure electrolyte homeostasis. *N Engl J Med* 315:1330–1340, 1985.

68. Conger JD, Falk SA, Yuan BH, Schrier RW: Atrial natriuretic peptide and dopamine in a rat model of ischemic acute renal failure. *Kidney Int* 35:1126–1132, 1989.

69. Russell JD, Churchill DN: Calcium antagonists and acute renal failure. *Am J Med* 87:306–315, 1989.

70. Blau A, Shulman L, Eliahou HE: Calcium channel blockers and experimental acute renal failure. *Isr J Med Sci* 26:334–336, 1990.

71. Widener LL, Mela-riker LM: Verapamil pretreatment preserves mitochondrial function and tissue magnesium in the

ischemic kidney. *Circ Shock* 13:27–37, 1984.

72. Burke TJ, Arnold PE, Gordon JA, et al: Protective effect of intrarenal calcium membrane blockers before or after renal ischemia; functional, morphological and mitochondrial studies. *J Clin Invest* 74:1830–1841, 1984.

73. Canavese C, Stratta P, Vercellone A: The case for oxygen free radicals in the pathogenesis of ischemic acute renal failure. *Nephron* 49:9–15, 1988.

74. Nath KA, Paller MS: Dietary deficiency of antioxidants exacerbates ischemic injury in the rat kidney. *Kidney Int* 38:1109–1117, 1990.

75. Walker PD, Shah SV: Reactive oxygen metabolites in endotoxin-induced acute renal failure in rats. *Kidney Int* 38:1125–1132, 1990.

76. Pawlowska D, Granger JP, Knox FG: Effects of adenosine infusion into renal interstitium on renal hemodynamics. *Am J Physiol* 252:F678–F682, 1987.

77. Siegel NJ, Glazier WB, Chaudry IH, et al: Enhanced recovery from acute renal failure by the postischemic infusion of adenine nucleotides and magnesium chloride in rats. *Kidney Int* 17:338–349, 1980.

78. Gerkens JF, Heidemann HT, Jackson EK, Branch RA: Effect of aminophylline on amphotericin B nephrotoxicity in the dog. *J Pharmacol Exp Ther* 224:609–613, 1983.

79. Hardie EM, Pose RL, Hoopes PJ: ATP–MgCl$_2$ increases cisplatin toxicity in the dog and rat. *J Appl Toxicol* 12:369–375, 1992.

80. Wong NL, Magil AB, Dirks JH: Effect of magnesium diet in gentamicin-induced acute renal failure in rats. *Nephron* 51:84–88, 1989.

81. Humes HD, Sastrasinh M, Weinberg JM: Calcium is a competitive inhibitor of gentamicin-renal membrane binding interactions and dietary calcium supplementation protects against gentamicin nephrotoxicity. *J Clin Invest* 73:134–147, 1984.

82. Siegel NJ, Gaudio KM, Katz LA, et al: Beneficial effect of thyroxin on recovery from toxic acute renal failure. *Kidney Int* 25:906–911, 1984.

83. Chevalier RL, Finn WF: Effects of propranolol on postischemic acute renal failure. *Nephron* 25:77–81, 1980.

84. Grekas D, Kalekou H, Tourkantonis A: Effect of prostaglandin E$_2$ (PGE$_2$) in the prevention of acute renal failure in anesthetized dogs; in situ renal preservation. *Renal Failure* 11:27–31, 1989.

85. Benabe JE, Klahr S, Hoffman MK, et al: Production of thromboxane A$_2$ by the kidney in glycerol induced acute renal failure in the rabbit. *Prostaglandins* 19:333–347, 1980.

UPDATE

Angiotensin converting enzyme (ACE) inhibitors such as captopril, enalapril, and lisinopril are now widely used in the management of congestive heart failure in dogs. As an inhibitor of the production of the potent vasopressor angiotensin II (which stimulates the secretion of aldosterone, a hormone that prompts water and sodium retention), the ACE agent fosters balanced vasodilation and enhances sodium and water excretion. In the glomerulus, angiotensin II blockade can cause preferential dilation of the efferent arteriole, a loss of glomerular capillary pressure, and a reduction in the glomerular fil-

tration rate.[1] This vasodilatory effect is most prominent in diseased or poorly perfused kidneys. Poor renal perfusion is a common complication among heart failure patients, particularly those receiving diuretics. Progression of azotemia or acute renal failure may be observed. Renal function should be monitored following the initiation of ACE inhibitor therapy in dogs. Adjusting the dosage of the ACE inhibitor and/or diuretic agent(s) administered usually is sufficient to attenuate azotemia; more intensive support is required in some cases. Azotemia that develops early in the course of enalapril therapy may resolve over time in some cases, presumably because of improvements in peripheral perfusion.[2]

In dogs, acute renal failure has also been described as a significant component of some infectious diseases, including bacterial endocarditis and rickettsial diseases.[3,4] Bacterial endocarditis may cause renal thrombosis or infarction, or inflammatory lesions such as glomerulonephritis or pyelonephritis.[4] Rickettsial organisms (e.g., the etiologic agents in Rocky Mountain spotted fever or canine ehrlichiosis) create a variety of clinical signs, including those associated with the consequences of diffuse vasculitis. Direct or immune-mediated damage to endothelial cells may extend to the renal circulation and result in acute failure.[3] In these cases, clinical signs of the infectious disorder may predominate and biochemical changes reflect renal involvement. Dogs with multisystemic disease should be monitored, as they are at high risk of acute renal failure. Support of the circulating blood volume and of renal perfusion—in addition to specific treatment of the primary disease—are important.

Ongoing investigations into the prevention and treatment of acute renal failure are focused on agents that influence renal hemodynamics and agents that influence cellular repair. Vasodilatory agents under investigation include low-dose norepinephrine, clonidine, propranolol, and endothelin antagonists. The infusion of norepinephrine (a catecholamine) at low dosages appears to selectively vasoconstrict the efferent arteriole and improve glomerular capillary pressure, filtration fraction, and urine output; higher dosages also constrict the afferent arteriole.[5] The effect of low-dose norepinephrine in ischemic acute renal failure may be enhanced by the concurrent infusion of dopamine.[6] Administration of clonidine or propranolol (a beta blocker) may improve renal recovery by improving renal microcirculation.[7] Endothelin is a regulatory peptide secreted from endothelial cells in response to hypoxia. In addition to its multiple effects on renal function, endothelin is a potent vasoconstrictor, and endothelin-neutralizing antibodies have been effective in reversing renal dysfunction in an ischemic model of acute renal failure.[8,9]

Dietary manipulation of eicosanoid production may enhance renal vasodilatory mechanisms by reducing the

(continues on page 83)

Acute Renal Failure. Part II. Diagnosis, Management, and Prognosis*

University of Prince Edward Island
India F. Lane, DVM, MS

Colorado State University
Gregory F. Grauer, DVM, MS
Martin J. Fettman, DVM, MS, PhD

A cute renal failure (ARF) is a sudden, severe reduction in renal function. The condition is often life threatening. In some cases, however, renal lesions associated with acute renal failure are reversible; adequate renal function can be regained with appropriate supportive care.

Part I of this presentation reviewed the pathophysiology of acute renal failure, identification of patients at risk for the development of acute renal failure, and potential strategies for prevention and treatment of the condition.

In Part II, diagnosis and management of acute renal failure are reviewed. Acute versus chronic renal failure, prerenal azotemia, and postrenal azotemia are emphasized; fluid therapy as a general consideration of management is also discussed.

DIAGNOSIS
Acute Versus Chronic Renal Failure

Prerenal azotemia, postrenal azotemia, and both acute and chronic renal failure can lead to such clinical signs as lethargy, depression, anorexia, vomiting, diarrhea, and dehydration. The more severe signs of uremia (including stupor; coma; hemorrhage; oral ulcerations; and, occasionally, seizures) are usually not observed in cases of prerenal azotemia. Such signs may, however, be associated with postrenal azotemia and acute and chronic renal failure.[1]

Diagnosis of renal failure (Figure 1) is made when azotemia is accompanied by isosthenuria (urine specific gravity 1.008 to 1.012) or minimally concentrated urine (urine specific gravity 1.013 to 1.029 in dogs, 1.013 to 1.034 in cats). Other clinicopathologic abnormalities found in cases of renal failure include anemia, electrolyte imbalances, and metabolic acidosis.

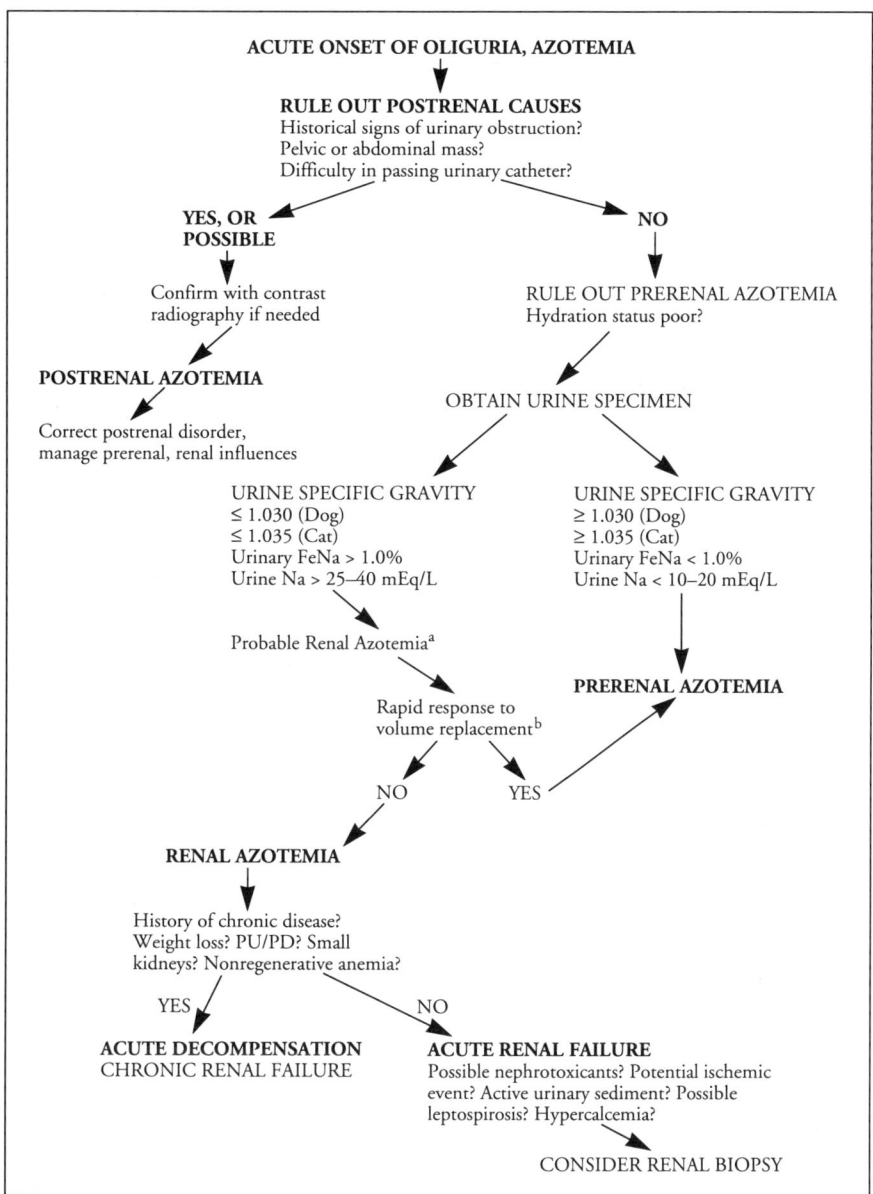

Figure 1—Diagnostic algorithm for the assessment of animals with suspected acute renal failure. (*a*) Impaired concentrating ability exists and is most likely caused by renal parenchymal lesions; however, other causes of impaired tubular concentrating ability (e.g., diuretic administration, hypoadrenocorticism, hypercalcemia, pyometra, and renal medullary washout) must be considered. (*b*) Entails a marked increase in urine production and rapid resolution of azotemia. FE_{Na} = Excreted fraction of filtered sodium, Na = sodium, *PU/PD* = polyuria/polydipsia.

Such findings as previous weight loss or episodes of illness; polyuria; polydipsia; pale mucous membranes; and small, irregular kidneys may be indicative of chronic renal failure.[2,3] A young animal in good body condition without a history of illness that exhibits clinical signs is more likely to have acute rather than chronic renal failure, unless the breed is known to have a high incidence of juvenile renal disease. A history of nephrotoxic drug use, toxicant exposure, trauma, or potential ischemic insult (as discussed in Part I) may indicate that acute renal failure is involved.

In cases of acute renal failure, the kidneys may be painful or enlarged. Clinical signs are often more severe than they are in a patient with chronic renal failure at the same level of dysfunction.

Hyperkalemia and severe metabolic acidosis are most likely to occur in cases of acute renal failure, whereas nonregenerative anemia, normokalemia, hypokalemia, and mild metabolic acidosis are suggestive of chronic renal failure.[2,4] Hyperkalemia and severe azotemia are less likely to occur in animals with nonoliguric acute renal failure.[5] Proteinuria and the presence of granular casts and renal epithelial cells and debris are indicative of acute renal damage.[2,4]

Dogs and cats with chronic renal failure may exhibit an apparently acute onset of clinical signs or an acute exacerbation of the disease (sometimes called *acute-on-chronic* renal failure). In such cases, the distinction between acute and chronic disease may require renal biopsy. Initial management for prerenal azotemia, acute renal failure, and acute-on-chronic disease is similar; the long-term prognoses, however, may differ significantly.

Prerenal Azotemia

Many extrarenal disorders can cause hypovolemia or hypotension and thereby result in reduced renal perfusion, reduced glomerular filtration, and prerenal azotemia. In such cases, urine concentrating ability is usually maintained (urine specific gravity >1.030 in dogs, >1.035 in cats). If urine concentrating ability is impaired by other influences, such as hyperadrenocorticism or hypoadrenocorticism, pyometra, liver disease, hypotonic dehydration, and diuretics, distinguishing between prerenal and renal azotemia can be difficult.[6,7] Under such circumstances, other assessments of urine composition may facilitate diagnosis.

Urinary sodium concentration can be measured; it is generally less than 10 to 20 mEq/L in cases of prerenal azotemia, because sodium retaining ability remains. Urinary sodium concentrations can be variable in dogs; the fractional excretion of sodium (FE_{Na} = [$Urine_{Na}$/$Plasma_{Na} \times Plasma_{Cr}$/$Urine_{Cr} \times 100$]) is therefore a more accurate reflection of sodium conservation. In cases of prerenal disorders with adequate tubular function, fractional excretion of sodium is generally less than 1%. Urinary sodium concentrations greater than 25 mEq/L and fractional excretion of sodium values greater than 1% are indicative of renal failure.[3,8,9]

Interpretation of the fractional excretion of sodium may be invalid in cases with such conditions as congestive heart failure, hepatic failure, or nephrotic syndrome. In such cases, excretion of sodium is impaired, and retention of sodium may persist despite renal dysfunction.[9] Other urinary indexes supporting a diagnosis of prerenal azotemia include urine osmolality significantly greater than plasma osmolality (ratio >5 to 6:1) and high urine-to-plasma creatinine ratio (>20:1).[8]

In humans, urinary sodium excretion and urine-to-plasma creatinine values are combined to give a renal failure index (RFI). The renal failure index is determined by the formula $urine_{Na}$/$urine_{Cr}$/$plasma_{Cr}$.[8] Renal failure index values greater than 1.0 are consistent with oliguric acute renal failure; renal failure index values less that 1.0 are indicative of prerenal azotemia.[3,8] In one group of human patients, however, renal failure index values were not found to be reliable indicators of acute renal failure.[10]

Azotemia and clinical signs of prerenal dysfunction should resolve rapidly with correction of volume deficits and restoration of renal perfusion. Initial fluid therapy for azotemic patients is thus designed to rapidly replace fluid deficits and reduce prerenal influences.

Postrenal Azotemia

Trigonal or urethral obstruction and upper or lower urinary tract rupture lead to postrenal azotemia. Lower urinary tract obstruction should be suspected if a history of strangury, dysuria, or complete anuria is reported.[3] Obstruction of the urethra or bladder neck can usually be ruled out by the passage of a urinary catheter. Passage of a catheter also provides an opportunity to obtain urine specimens for specific-gravity determination and other analyses.

Although unilateral obstruction of the renal pelvis or ureter generally does not result in azotemia, upper urinary tract obstruction should be suspected when demonstrable abdominal pain, abdominal masses, or a history of nephroliths is present. Urine sediment may contain evidence of crystals or inflammatory cells. Survey radiographs can be used to assess renal size, shape, and symmetry, as well as to rule out radiodense calculi and mass lesions. Renal ultrasonography may reveal hydronephrosis, hydroureter, nephroliths, or renal masses. Excretory urography or computed tomography might be necessary to completely rule out upper urinary tract disease.[2,4]

The possibility of urinary tract rupture should be considered in cases involving abdominal or pelvic trauma. Hematuria, swelling of the inguinal or perineal area, and abdominal distension are signs suggestive of urine leakage. Peritoneal fluid with a creatinine concentration greater than serum creatinine concentration is supportive of urine leakage, but a contrast radiograph is the best tool for confirming and localizing the rupture site.

MANAGEMENT
General Considerations

When acute renal failure is suspected (Figure 2), use of potentially nephrotoxic drugs should be discontinued. If a toxicant is the suspected cause of acute renal failure, nonspecific therapy to reduce further absorption of the agent should be instituted, including gastric lavage and/or administration of acti-

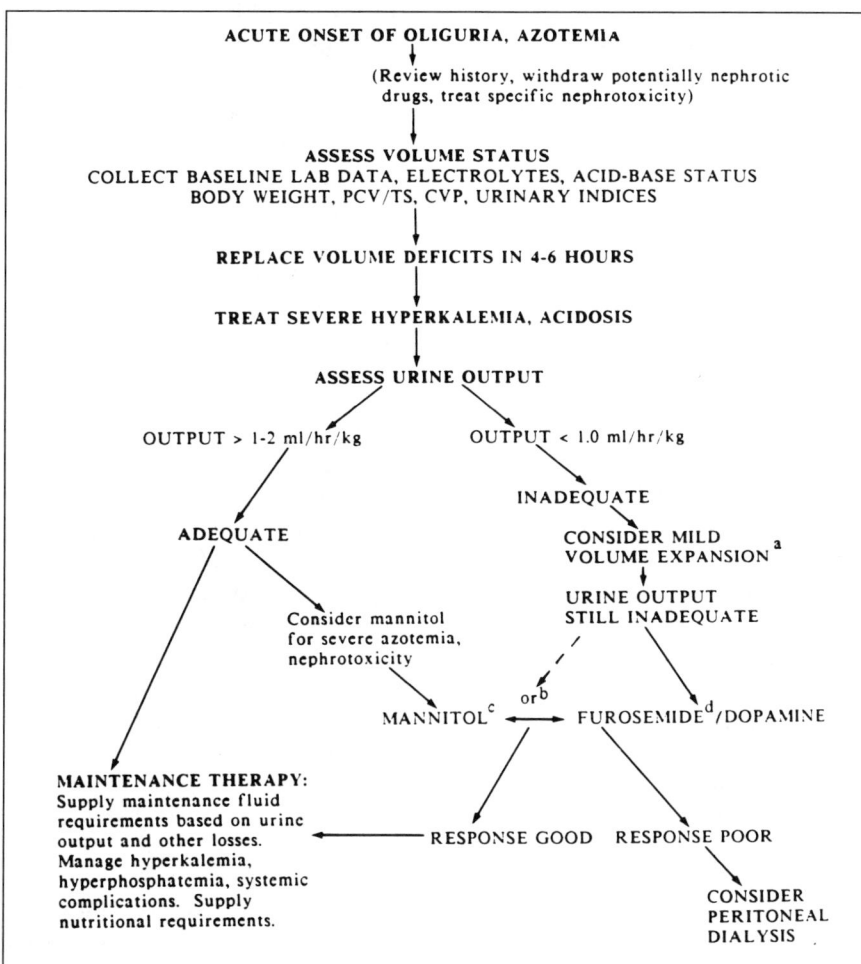

Figure 2—Therapeutic algorithm for management of animals with suspected acute renal failure. (*a*) If no evidence of overhydration exists, there is no increase in central venous pressure. (*b*) If one regimen is unsuccessful, the other may be attempted. (*c*) Avoid in cases with evidence of overhydration. (*d*) Avoid in cases of gentamicin nephrotoxicity. *PCV* = packed cell volume, *TS* = total solids, *CVP* = central venous pressure.

vated charcoal and cathartics. Specific antidotes should be administered if the toxicant is known (e.g., ethylene glycol).

If possible, underlying diseases, such as hypoadrenocorticism, pyometra, and hepatic disease, should be managed specifically. Treatable intrinsic renal disorders, such as leptospirosis and pyelonephritis, should be identified and appropriate management initiated. Obstructions to urine flow should be removed. Supportive therapy is designed to provide time for nephron repair, regeneration, and compensation.[2-4]

Fluid Therapy

Fluid therapy remains the mainstay of treatment for acute renal failure. The goals of fluid therapy are to correct fluid and electrolyte imbalances, improve renal hemodynamics, increase tubular flow, and initiate diuresis. Fluid needs in cases of acute renal failure are such that intravenous infusion is required. Jugular catheters allow administration of fluid loads, facilitate frequent blood sampling, and supply access for central venous pressure (CVP) measurement.

Fluid deficits should be replaced intravenously during the first four to six hours of treatment.[2,4] A 0.45% saline and 2.5% dextrose solution or 0.9% saline solution can be used initially. The amount of fluid required to restore extracellular fluid deficits can be calculated by multiplying the estimated percentage of dehydration by the patient's body weight in kilograms (e.g., for a dog that weighs 10 kilograms and is 5% dehydrated: 0.05 × 10 kg = 0.5 kg = 0.5 liters, or 500 ml).[11] The fluid rate should be reduced in animals with known or suspected cardiovascular dysfunction.

TABLE I
Potassium Supplementation in the Management of Renal Failure

Measured Serum Potassium Concentration	Amount of Potassium Chloride to be Added to Each Liter of Fluid Administered[a] (mEq)
3.5–4.0	20
3.0–3.5	30
2.5–3.0	40
2.0–2.5	60
<2.0	80

[a]Do not exceed an administration rate of 0.5 mEq/kg/hr.

During the rehydration phase, the animal should be carefully monitored for urine output and overhydration. Frequent monitoring of body weight, central venous pressure, packed cell volume, and plasma total solids helps to detect early overhydration.[12] Physical manifestations of overhydration include increased bronchovesicular sounds, tachycardia, restlessness, chemosis, and serous nasal discharge. Auscultation of overt crackles and wheezes is usually a late sign of overhydration with established pulmonary edema.

If overhydration is not apparent after rehydration, a moderate fluid challenge may help to improve urine flow. Because remaining deficits may be difficult to detect clinically, volume expansion with fluids equivalent to an additional 3% to 5% body weight can be administered to facilitate rehydration and improve renal perfusion.[4] If volume expansion is attempted, however, close observation for signs of overhydration is necessary.

Once diuresis has been established (urine output of 1 to 2 ml/kg/hr), and in cases of nonoliguric acute renal failure, fluid therapy should be tailored to match urine volume and other losses. Such losses include insensible losses (e.g., water loss resulting from respiration) and continuing losses (e.g., fluid loss resulting from vomiting, diarrhea, or hemorrhage). Insensible losses are estimated at 20 ml/kg/day. Urine output is quantitated for six- to eight-hour intervals; the amount is replaced during an equivalent time period. Ongoing gastrointestinal losses are also replaced. If hyperkalemia is not present and diuresis has ensued, polyionic maintenance fluids (e.g., lactated Ringer's solution) can be used.

In the recovery phase of acute renal failure, urine volume and electrolyte losses can be great. Maintenance potassium requirements should be administered in fluids based on serum potassium measurements as given in Table I.

Treatment of Hyperkalemia and Metabolic Acidosis

In cases of oliguric acute renal failure, hyperkalemia and metabolic acidosis often develop. Mild to moderate imbalances are often resolved with appropriate fluid therapy; however, hyperkalemia and severe metabolic acidosis can be life threatening and should be treated specifically.

Serum potassium concentrations greater than 6.5 to 7 mEq/L can cause cardiac conduction disturbances and electrocardiographic changes, including peaked T waves, bradycardia, prolonged P–R intervals, widened QRS complexes, and loss of P waves. Severe hyperkalemia can also precipitate atrial standstill, idioventricular rhythms, ventricular tachycardia, fibrillation, and asystole.[13,14]

Moderate hyperkalemia is largely resolved by administration of potassium-free fluids (dilution) and improvement of urine flow (increased excretion). Severe hyperkalemia (K^+ >7 to 8 mEq/L) or hyperkalemia resulting in cardiotoxicity should be treated by administering 10% calcium gluconate (0.5 to 1.0 ml/kg given intravenously during a period of 10 to 15 minutes)[2,14,15] or sodium bicarbonate (0.5 to 2 mEq/kg given intravenously during a period of 20 to 30 minutes, or as calculated to correct metabolic acidosis).[14,15]

Calcium ions counteract the cardiotoxic effects of excess potassium without lowering serum potassium; therefore, calcium treatment is reserved for cases in which immediate treatment of cardiac disturbances is required. Treatment of acidosis with bicarbonate facilitates the entry of potassium into cells. Glucose and insulin can also be used in emergency situations to increase intracellular shifting of potassium. Insulin is administered at a dose of 0.1 to 0.25 U/kg followed by a glucose bolus of 1 to 2 grams per unit of insulin given.[12] Blood glucose monitoring should be maintained for several hours after administration of insulin because hypoglycemia can occur. The effects of a calcium, bicarbonate, or glucose and insulin regimen are, however, short-lived; maintenance therapy, such as fluid diuresis or dialysis, must be initiated to ultimately maintain potassium excretion.[11]

Mild to moderate metabolic acidosis also commonly resolves with fluid therapy; specific treatment is rarely necessary unless blood pH is less than 7.10 to 7.15 or total carbon dioxide measures less than 10 to 12 mEq/L.[2,4] Bicarbonate requirements can be calculated using the base deficit determined from arterial blood or an estimated base deficit (body weight [kg] × 0.5 × base deficit or [20 – T CO_2] = mEq bicarbonate required).[12] Optimally, one half of the calculated bicarbonate dose should be administered slowly during a period of 15 to 30 minutes, after which

TABLE II
Pharmacologic Agents and Dose Regimens Used in Treatment of Acute Renal Failure[2,12,21,28]

Drug	Action	Dose Regimen	Comments	Contraindications, Possible Complications
Furosemide	Loop diuretic	D, C: 2–6 mg/kg every 6–8 hours IV	Incrementally increase dose every 1 hour up to 6 mg/kg if urine output remains poor; efficacy improved with concurrent administration of dopamine	Dehydration, hypokalemia, aminoglycoside nephrotoxicity
Mannitol	Osmotic diuretic	D, C: 0.25–1.0 g/kg (10%–25% solution)	Administer as slow bolus over 15–20 minutes; can be repeated every 4–6 hours or administered as infusion (8%–10% solution) if effective	Dehydration, cardiopulmonary insufficiency, overhydration, elevated central venous pressure, intracranial hemorrhage
Dextrose	Osmotic diuretic	D, C: 25–50 ml/kg over 1–2 hours IV (10%–20% solution); repeat every 8–12 hours	Test initial urine for glucose and continue to monitor urine output; adjust maintenance fluid therapy administered between boluses to supply total daily calculated requirements	Discontinue infusion if glucosuria is not present or if adequate urine output does not occur after approximately half the recommended dose is administered
Dopamine	Renal vasodilator	D, C: 1–3 µg/kg/min CRI	Dilute in normal saline, 5% dextrose or lactated Ringer's solution; avoid dilution in alkaline solution; avoid additional additives in solution; efficacy improved if combined with furosemide	Hyperkalemia; may be arrhythmogenic
Sucralfate	Gastrointestinal protectant	D: 0.5–1.0 g every 6–8 hours PO C: 0.25–0.5 g every 8–12 hours PO	Separate administration from concurrent dosing of antacids by 30 minutes to 1 hour	Constipation is a possible side effect
Cimetidine	H_2-receptor antagonist	D: 5–10 mg/kg every 6–8 hours IV or PO C: 2.5–5 mg/kg every 12 hours IV or PO	Administer slowly when given IV	Reduce dose in cases involving hepatic disease
Ranitidine	H_2-receptor antagonist	D: 2 mg/kg every 8–12 hours IV or PO C: Not established	Same as for cimetidine	Reduce dose in cases involving renal disease
Metoclopromide	Antiemetic (antidopaminergic)	D, C: 0.2–0.5 mg/kg every 8 hours PO, SQ, or IV, or 1–2 mg/kg 24 hours CRI	Acts at CRTZ. Enhances gastric emptying	Avoid in epileptics; high doses may cause mental disturbances
Trimethobenzamide	Antiemetic (antihistamine-like)	D: 3 mg/kg every 8 hours IM C: Not established	Acts at CRTZ	

D = dog, *C* = cat, *CRI* = constant rate infusion, *IV* = intravenously, *IM* = intramuscularly, *PO* = orally, *SQ* = subcutaneously, *CRTZ* = chemoreceptor trigger zone.

acid–base parameters should be reassessed.[12] Over-zealous bicarbonate administration can result in ionized calcium deficits, paradoxic cerebrospinal fluid acidosis, and cerebral edema.[4,12]

Treatment of Oliguria

Oliguria is defined as urine output less than 0.27 ml/kg body weight/hr[16]; however, after rehydration, urine output less than 1 to 2 ml/kg/hr is inadequate. If oliguria persists, additional pharmacologic manipulation with diuretics or vasodilators is necessary. Furosemide given in increasing doses (2 to 6 mg/kg; see Table II) has been advocated as an initial treatment for oliguria. Single, high-dose regimens (200 to 500 mg)[8,17] are used in humans to initiate urine flow. Apparently, however, mannitol[18] or dopamine in combination with furosemide[19] is a better choice than furosemide alone to initiate diuresis and possibly increase glomerular filtration rate.

Mannitol (10% or 20% solution) is administered at 0.5 to 1.0 g/kg as a slow bolus during a period of 15 to 20 minutes[2,4,12] (Table II). Urine output should improve within one hour of administration if the agent is effective. A second bolus may be administered, but doing so considerably increases the potential for volume overexpansion and complications, such as pulmonary and tissue edema.

As an osmotic agent, mannitol acts to increase tubular flow and help prevent tubular obstruction or collapse.[8,18] It is also a weak renal vasodilator, in which capacity its effect may be mediated by prostaglandins or atrial natriuretic peptide.[20] Mannitol acts as a scavenger of oxygen-derived free radicals that sometimes form after ischemia and reperfusion (see Part I).[8] Thus, mannitol should increase urine output and perhaps have a mild positive effect on glomerular filtration rate.

Hypertonic (10% to 20%) glucose, another osmotic agent, has been suggested as an alternative therapy to mannitol.[21] Its effects in initiating tubular flow and urine output are similar to those of mannitol. Solutions of 10% or 20% dextrose are easily formulated and supply metabolizable energy. Hypertonic dextrose is administered as an intermittent slow bolus of 25 to 50 ml/kg (see Table II), given during the course of one to two hours, two to three times daily.[21] A potential advantage of administration of hypertonic glucose is that urine can be monitored early after the start of therapy and the infusion can be stopped before the risk of overhydration is incurred. The detection of glucose in the urine should not preclude monitoring urine output; glucosuria can occur without a significant increase in urine production.

Hypertonic glucose lacks certain beneficial effects of mannitol, including vasodilation and oxygen-derived–free radical scavenging.[8] Mannitol may also be a better osmotic agent, because it is not metabolized or resorbed by renal tubules.

Dopamine (Table II) combined with furosemide should be used in overhydrated patients instead of osmotic agents; it may be effective when osmotic diuresis fails. Low-dose dopamine infusion (1 to 3 µg/kg/min) causes renal vasodilation and preserves renal and splanchnic blood flow.[22] Increases in glomerular filtration and sodium excretion may also occur.[8] Although when given in low doses dopamine has minimal systemic effects, it can be arrhythmogenic; electrocardiographic monitoring is therefore advised when dopamine is administered. The half-life of dopamine is extremely short; if arrhythmia is observed, discontinuing dopamine infusion should result in rapid resolution of the arrhythmia.

When furosemide therapy is combined with dopamine infusion, the likelihood of inducing diuresis is increased.[19] Furosemide has been shown to exacerbate gentamicin toxicity[23]; its use should probably be avoided in cases of acute renal failure caused by aminoglycoside use.

Initiation of diuresis facilitates the management of acute renal failure by lowering serum urea nitrogen and potassium concentrations and reducing the risk of overhydration. The increase in urine production, however, is usually the result of decreased tubular reabsorption of water with no real increase in glomerular filtration rate.[2]

Systemic Complications

In cases of acute uremia, gastrointestinal signs occur most frequently. Nausea, anorexia, vomiting, hematemesis, diarrhea, and oral ulcerations are common.[24–26] Intussusceptions occasionally develop in uremic patients.[24] Uremic stomatitis, characterized by oral ulcerations, discoloration or sloughing of the tip of the tongue, and fetid breath, is seen most frequently with chronic disease but may also develop with severe acute uremia. The oral lesions may be a result of the caustic effects of ammonia produced locally by the action of bacterial ureases. It is also possible that mucosal damage is simply a manifestation of a more generalized disruption of gastrointestinal mucosa.[24,26]

In humans, oral lesions are aggravated by periodontal disease; good oral hygiene may reduce the severity of oral ulceration.[24] Severe pain from oral ulceration can be relieved by topical administration of compounds containing lidocaine.

Hemorrhagic or ulcerative gastritis that leads to anorexia and vomiting is commonly induced by uremia. Lesions may be caused by local irritation from high levels of ammonia or an altered gastric mucosal barrier. Increased urea concentrations may also alter the gastric mucosal barrier.[24,25] Renal failure results in decreased clearance of gastrin, which may precipitate hypergastrinemia and increased gastric acid production, two conditions that can exacerbate gastric lesions.[25] Pathologic findings include edema, mastocytosis, fibroplasia and mineralization in the lamina propria, and arteriolar lesions in the submucosa.[27]

Vomiting caused by gastritis can be controlled to a certain extent by administration of histamine (H$_2$ receptor) blockers, cimetidine (5 to 10 mg/kg given orally every 6 to 8 hours), or ranitidine (2 mg/kg given orally every 8 to 12 hours; see Table II), agents which reduce gastric hydrochloric acid production. Sucralfate (0.5 to 1.0 gram given orally every 6 to 8 hours; see Table II), a gastrointestinal protectant, is administered to coat existing gastric and intestinal mucosal ulcerations. Sucralfate dissociates in the stomach to aluminum hydroxide and sucrose octasulfate, a viscous substance that forms a complex with gastrointestinal mucosa and preferentially adheres to ulcerated areas. Sucralfate also protects the mucosa from gastric acid penetration, inactivates pepsin, and adsorbs damaging bile acids.[28]

In cases of uremia, the large and small bowel are affected by increased serum urea concentrations. Diarrhea results from enterocolitis, partial malabsorption of proteins and carbohydrates, altered bile salt metabolism, and bacterial overgrowth.[1,24–26] Finally, vasculitis and coagulation abnormalities induced by uremia can create severe generalized gastrointestinal hemorrhage.[24,25]

Vomiting can also result from direct stimulation of the chemoreceptor trigger zone (CRTZ) by uremic toxins, such as guanidines.[24] Effects of these toxins can be reduced by administration of centrally acting antiemetics, such as metoclopramide or trimethobenzamide (Table II), which act at the chemoreceptor trigger zone. Because α-adrenergic blockade can result in significant vasodilation and hypotension, phenothiazine compounds (e.g., chlorpromazine) that act at both the emetic center and the chemoreceptor trigger zone should be avoided unless adequate hydration and blood pressure have been restored.

Critically ill uremic patients are highly susceptible to infection; septicemia or other infections are major causes of death in humans with renal failure.[3] Depressed leukocyte function and depressed cellular immunity have been documented.[1,29,30] In cases of uremia, production of chemotactic factors as well as polymorphonuclear chemotactic responses are depressed. Lymphocyte numbers and activity are also depressed.[29,30] Recently, defects in macrophage receptor functions[31] and monocyte responsiveness[32] have been documented in humans with end-stage renal

failure. Metabolic acidosis, altered mucosal barriers, and malnutrition can contribute to weakened host defenses.[1] Humoral immunity appears to be less significantly affected by uremia.[29,30]

Prevention of infection is essential in uremic patients; strict aseptic techniques should be used when placing vascular and urinary catheters, administering parenteral medications, and caring for wounds. If urine output is in question, the use of metabolic cages or intermittent catheterization is preferred over placement of indwelling urinary catheters. If peritoneal dialysis is used, infection becomes an even greater concern; peritonitis can be a serious complication.[33,34] Careful attention should therefore be paid to protocol and asepsis when peritoneal dialysis is used.

Other complications in cases of acute renal failure include hemorrhage and neurologic dysfunction. The bleeding tendency in uremic humans is still not completely understood, but it is characterized by an increased bleeding time and altered platelet function. Undetermined uremic compounds produce defects in platelet aggregation, platelet adhesiveness, and platelet factor 3 release in humans; such conditions are reversed by dialytic therapy.[29,30] Limited studies have found whole-blood platelet aggregation in uremic dogs to be normal, however.[35]

Hemorrhage is best managed by decreasing the severity of uremia, although some animals may require transfusions if significant blood loss occurs. Administration of cryoprecipitate,[36] desmopressin (DDAVP),[37] and other vascular factors[38] has recently been shown to alleviate the bleeding tendency in some humans with uremia.

Neurologic abnormalities associated with uremia include encephalopathic signs and peripheral neuropathy.[1,39,40] Uremic encephalopathy occurs in humans when the glomerular filtration rate (GFR) falls below 10% of the normal rate.[40] Clinical signs in such cases include sluggishness; confusion; disorientation; hallucinations; vertigo; ataxia; clonus; and centrally mediated anorexia, nausea, and vomiting.[40] In dogs, tremors, head bobbing, and seizures are reported.[41]

Alterations in calcium levels in the brain have been documented in humans and dogs, and it is speculated that increased calcium entry is facilitated by parathyroid hormone (PTH).[40] In rats, alterations in brain metabolism and energy use have also been observed; other uremic toxins may play a role in the cause.[40] A peripheral neuropathy associated with uremia is also seen in humans and is more likely to be clinically evident in chronic end-stage renal disease. This distal polyneuropathy is characterized clinically by sensory changes in distal limbs and depressed distal reflexes. Motor-nerve conduction velocities are variably reduced. Although similar electrophysiologic changes can be documented in humans with acute renal failure, clinical signs are usually not apparent.[40] Control of uremia is the best method of management of neurologic dysfunction. Seizures may be managed with low-dose diazepam.

Nutritional support must be maintained in animals with acute renal failure. Many such animals cannot tolerate oral intake or cannot consume enough calories to compensate for severe illness. Ongoing catabolic processes then increase the burden of nitrogenous wastes presented to the kidneys.[42] Enteral or parenteral feeding can be considered for these patients. The goal of nutritional therapy in uremic patients is to supply caloric requirements using adequate carbohydrate sources and to supply amino acids or protein sources in an amount that can maintain nitrogen balance but avoid excessive protein load on the damaged kidneys.[42] Ideally, protein should be supplied as amino acids; essential amino acid supplementation has been shown to improve survival in anephric dogs.[43]

Suggested protein requirements for uremic dogs are 0.3 g/kg/day of a basic amino acid solution[42] or 2.2 g/kg/day total protein. Diets should be moderately restricted in phosphorus; intestinal phosphate binders may be needed to control hyperphosphatemia.[4] Methods of enteral and parenteral feeding in dogs and cats have been described.[44,45]

Renal Biopsy

Histologic evaluation of renal tissue is often important in cases of acute renal failure to establish an accurate diagnosis and prognosis for return of renal function. Renal biopsy should be considered in cases in which a definitive diagnosis is required, heavy proteinuria is present, diffuse systemic disease is suspected, or when the type of renal failure (acute or chronic) cannot be established.[4] Biopsy is also indicated when conservative methods of treatment have failed, when oliguria cannot be corrected after one to two days of therapy, or when severe uremia or hyperkalemia persist for long periods.[2,13]

Histologic evidence of tubular regeneration and intact tubular basement membranes are considered good prognostic indicators of reversibility; extensive tubular necrosis and interstitial mineralization with disrupted basement membranes are poor prognostic signs.[2,46] In one group of humans with acute renal failure, renal biopsy results altered the diagnosis in 44% of cases for which a biopsy was obtained.[47] Specific therapy was altered in 37% of such cases, particularly when glomerular disease or interstitial nephritis was identified.[47]

Biopsies are most helpful when performed early in the course of treatment and should always be performed if intensive therapeutics, such as dialysis, are considered. Surgical; laparoscopic; and blind, keyhole, or percutaneous approaches guided by ultrasonography have been described.[48–51] Various percutaneous and laparascopic techniques apparently produce similarly adequate tissue samples.[51]

Serious complications of biopsies are rare. Transient hematuria and occasional incidences of hydronephrosis are reported with needle biopsies.[52] More severe complications, including perirenal hemorrhage or urine leakage, are possible. An open wedge biopsy can be obtained if a dialysis catheter is placed surgically for initiation of peritoneal dialysis. Coagulation parameters, including the platelet count, mucosal bleeding time, and such tests of coagulation as activated clotting time, activated partial thromboplastin time (APTT), and/or one-stage prothrombin time (OSPT) should be performed before renal biopsy.

Peritoneal Dialysis

Dialytic therapy should be considered when initial fluid and diuretic therapy have not been successful in relieving oliguria or uremia. Dialysis can also be used to manage overhydrated patients and to hasten elimination of certain toxicants.[53]

Dialysis must be undertaken early in the course of acute renal failure if it is to be helpful. Hemodialysis is costly and technically demanding, requiring specialized equipment and trained personnel. Peritoneal dialysis can be equally effective and does not require a great deal of specialized equipment or training. The procedure is still expensive and labor intensive,[33] however, and it should not be undertaken without serious consideration of the financial and time commitments involved. The procedure for peritoneal dialysis has been described in the literature[53] and can be accomplished at an experienced 24-hour treatment center or at referral teaching hospitals.

PROGNOSIS

Once acute renal failure is established, treatment is intensive and costly, particularly if dialytic therapy is considered. Because high mortality is associated with acute renal failure, it is helpful to have an accurate prognosis before aggressive therapy is considered.

In general, nonoliguric acute renal failure has a better prognosis than oliguric acute renal failure because hyperkalemia is less likely to be present and the tendency for overhydration to occur is minimized. Nephrotoxicant-induced acute renal failure may have a better prognosis than acute renal failure resulting from ischemia and other causes because tubular basement membranes frequently remain intact following nephrotoxicant-induced damage. Certainly, exceptions to these generalities occur, depending on the degree of damage and dysfunction.

Many prognostic factors have been investigated in humans with acute renal failure. Univariate and multivariate discrimination score systems exist to give a prognosis for survival in individual cases.[54–57] Significant variables contributing to a poor prognosis include preexisting cardiac disease, renal disease, neoplasia, pancreatitis, acute trauma, and such complications as oliguria, respiratory failure, coma, and sepsis.[54–56] The number of complications and number of organ systems failing also correlates with outcome.[54,55,57,58] Mortality is highest in surgical patients (>80%), primarily because of complications and multiple organ-system failure.[54,57,59] The severity of azotemia and the interval before the start of dialysis in surgical patients have been shown to be important,[54] a finding that emphasizes the need for early recognition and treatment.

Age of the patient was a significant factor in several studies, with mortality increasing progressively in human patients over 50 years of age.[54,59] Overall, the conditions most frequently associated with mortality in several studies were hypotension, neurologic coma, and respiratory failure.[57,58] Death, however, is often caused by the initial disease or secondary complications of the condition other than uremia.

Variables affecting humans can be applied to veterinary medical patients. In general, prognosis in cases of acute renal failure is affected by the severity of renal dysfunction, the extent of histologic damage, and the response to treatment. Awareness of the severity of underlying disease, mental status, significant complications, and status of other organ systems should help the clinician to formulate an early prognosis in individual cases. Histologic assessment of renal tissue and the effectiveness of early management may provide a better prognosis for survival as time progresses. In dogs and cats that survive to reach the recovery phase, adequate (although subnormal) renal function is usually recovered.

About the Authors

Dr. Lane is affiliated with the Department of Companion Animals, Atlantic Veterinary College, University of Prince Edward Island, Charlottetown, Prince Edward Island, Canada. Dr. Grauer is affiliated with the Department of Clinical Science and Dr. Fettman is affiliated with the Department of Pathology at the College of Veterinary Medicine and Biomedical Sciences, Colorado State University, Fort Collins, Colorado.

REFERENCES

1. Bovee KC: Metabolic disturbances of uremia, in Bovee KC (ed): *Canine Nephrology*. Media, PA, Harwal Publishing Co, 1984, pp 555–612.

2. Grauer GF: Acute renal failure, in Allen DG (ed): *Small Animal Medicine*. Philadelphia, JB Lippincott Co, 1991, pp 595–604.

3. Brezis M, Rosen S, Epstein FH: Acute renal failure, in Brenner BM, Rector FC (eds): *The Kidney*, ed 3. Philadelphia, WB Saunders Co, 1986, pp 735–799.

4. Polzin D, Osborne C, O'Brien T: Diseases of the kidney and ureters, in Ettinger SJ (ed): *Textbook of Veterinary Internal Medicine*, ed 3. Philadelphia, WB Saunders Co, 1989, pp 1963–2046.

5. Anderson RJ, Linas SC, Berns AS, et al: Nonoliguric acute renal failure. *N Engl J Med* 296:1134–1138, 1977.

6. Feldman EC, Nelson RW: *Canine and Feline Endocrinology and Reproduction*. Philadelphia, WB Saunders Co, 1987, pp 1–28.

7. Tyler RD, Qualls CW, Heald RD: Renal concentrating ability in dehydrated hyponatremia dogs. *JAVMA* 191:1095–1100, 1987.

8. Finn WF: Diagnosis and management of acute tubular necrosis. *Med Clin North Am* 74:873–892, 1990.

9. Zarich SZ, Fang LST, Diamond JR: Fractional excretion of sodium; exceptions to its diagnostic value. *Arch Intern Med* 145:108–112, 1985.

10. Durakovic Z, Durakovic A, Durokovic S: The lack of clinical value of laboratory parameters in predicting outcome in acute renal failure. *Ren Fail* 11:213–219, 1989–1990.

11. Muir WM, DiBartola SP: Fluid therapy, in Kirk RW (ed): *Current Veterinary Therapy. VIII. Small Animal Practice*. Philadelphia, WB Saunders Co, 1983, pp 28–40.

12. Kirby R: Acute renal failure as a complication in the critically ill animal. *Vet Clin North Am Small Anim Pract* 19:1189–1208, 1989.

13. Tilley LP: *Essentials of Canine and Feline Electrocardiography*, ed 2. Philadelphia: Lea & Febiger, 1985, pp 232–233.

14. Willard MD: Treatment of hyperkalemia, in Kirk RW (ed): *Current Veterinary Therapy. IX. Small Animal Practice*. Philadelphia, WB Saunders Co, 1987, pp 94–101.

15. Cowgill LD: Acute renal failure, in Bovee KC (ed): *Canine Nephrology*. Media, PA, Harwal Publishing Co, 1984, pp 405–438.

16. English PB: Acute renal failure in the dog and cat. *Aust Vet J* 50:384–392, 1974.

17. Rose BD: Diuretics. *Kidney Int* 39:336–352, 1991.

18. Burnier M, Schrier RW: Protection from acute renal failure. *Adv Exp Med Biol* 212:275–283, 1986.

19. Lindner A: Synergism of dopamine and furosemide in diuretic-resistant, oliguric acute renal failure. *Nephron* 33:121–126, 1983.

20. Kurnik BR, Weisberg LS, Cuttler IM, Kurnik PB: Effects of atrial natriuretic peptide versus mannitol on renal blood flow during radiocontrast infusion in chronic renal failure. *J Lab Clin Med* 116:27–35, 1990.

21. Finco DR, Low DG: Intensive diuresis in polyuric renal failure, in Kirk RW (ed): *Current Veterinary Therapy. VII. Small Animal Practice*. Philadelphia, WB Saunders Co, 1980, pp 1091–1093.

22. Parker S, Carlon GC, Isaacs M, et al: Dopamine administration in oliguria and oliguric renal failure. *Crit Care Med* 9:630–632, 1981.

23. Adelman RD, Spangler WL, Beasom F, et al: Furosemide enhancement of experimental gentamicin nephrotoxicity: Comparison of functional and morphological changes with activities of urinary enzymes. *J Infect Dis* 140:342–352, 1979.

24. Osborne CA, Stevens JB, Polzin DJ: Gastrointestinal manifestations of urinary diseases, in Anderson NV (ed): *Veteri-*

nary Gastroenterology. Philadelphia, Lea & Febiger, 1980, pp 681–704.

25. Strombeck DR, Guilford WG: *Small Animal Gastroenterology,* ed 2. Davis, CA, Stonegate Publishing Co, 1990.
26. Chew DJ, DiBartola SP: Diagnosis and pathophysiology of renal disease, in Ettinger SJ (ed): *Textbook of Veterinary Internal Medicine,* ed 3. Philadelphia, WB Saunders Co, 1989, pp 1893–1961.
27. Cheville NF: Uremic gastropathy in the dog. *Vet Pathol* 16:292–309, 1979.
28. Papich MG: Medical therapy for gastrointestinal ulcers, in Kirk RW (ed): *Current Veterinary Therapy. X. Small Animal Practice.* Philadelphia, WB Saunders Co, pp 911–918.
29. Anagnostou A, Kurtzman NA: Hematological consequences of renal failure, in Brenner BM, Rector FC (eds): *The Kidney,* ed 3. Philadelphia, WB Saunders Co, 1986, pp 1631–1656.
30. Fried W: Hematologic complications of chronic renal failure. *Med Clin North Am* 62:1363–1379, 1978.
31. Ruiz P, Gomez F, Schrieber AD: Impaired function of macrophage Fc gamma receptors in end-stage renal disease. *N Engl J Med* 322:717–722, 1990.
32. Gibbons RA, Martinez OM, Garovoy MR: Altered monocyte function in uremia. *Clin Immunol Immunopath* 56:66–80, 1990.
33. Carter LJ, Wingfield WE, Allen TA: Clinical experience with peritoneal dialysis in small animals. *Compend Contin Educ Pract Vet* 11(11):1335–1343, 1989.
34. Thornhill JA: Therapeutic strategies involving antimicrobial treatment of small animals with peritonitis. *JAVMA* 185:1181–1184,1984.
35. Forsythe LT, Jackson ML, Meric SM: Whole blood platelet aggregation in uremic dogs. *Am J Vet Res* 50:1754–1757, 1989.
36. Triulzi DJ, Blumberg N: Variability in response to cryoprecipitate treatment for hemostatic defects in uremia. *Yale J Biol Med* 63:1–7, 1990.
37. Vigano GL, Mannucci PM, Lattuada A, et al: Subcutaneous desmopressin (DDAVP) shortens bleeding time in uremia. *Am J Hematol* 31:32–35, 1989.
38. DiPaolo N, Capotondo L, Rossi P, et al: Bleeding tendency of chronic uremia improved by vascular factor. *Nephron* 52:268–272, 1989.
39. Raskin NH, Fishman RA: Neurologic disorders in renal failure (part I). *N Engl J Med* 294:143–148, 1976.
40. Arieff AI: Neurologic manifestations of uremia, in Brenner BM, Rector FC (eds): *The Kidney,* ed 3. Philadelphia, WB Saunders Co, 1986, pp 1731–1758.
41. Wolf AM: Canine uremic encephalopathy. *JAAHA* 16:735–738, 1980.
42. Finco DR, Barsanti JA: Parenteral nutrition during a uremic crisis, in Kirk RW (ed), *Current Veterinary Therapy. VIII. Small Animal Practice.* Philadelphia, WB Saunders Co, 1983, pp 994–996.
43. Van Buren CT, Dudrick SJ, Dworkin L, et al: Effects of intravenous essential L-amino acids and hypertonic dextrose on anephric beagles. *Surg Forum* 23:83–84, 1972.
44. Wheeler SL, McGuire BH: Enteral nutrional support, in Kirk RW (ed): *Current Veterinary Therapy. X. Small Animal Practice.* Philadelphia, WB Saunders Co, 1989, pp 30–37.
45. Lippert AC, Armstrong PJ: Parenteral nutritional support, in Kirk RW (ed): *Current Veterinary Therapy. X. Small Animal Practice.* Philadelphia, WB Saunders Co, 1989, pp 25–30.
46. Maxie MG: The urinary system, in Jubb KV, Kennedy PC, Palmer N (eds): *Pathology of Domestic Animals,* ed 3. Orlando, FL, Academic Press, 1985, pp 343–411.

47. Richet G: When should renal biopsy be done in acute uremia? *Kidney Int* 28(Suppl 17):S152–S153, 1985.
48. Hager DA, Nyland TG, Fisher P: Ultrasound-guided biopsy of the canine liver, kidney and prostate. *Vet Radiol* 26:82–88, 1985.
49. Grauer GF, Twedt DC, Mero KN: Evaluation of laparoscopy for obtaining renal biopsy specimens from dogs and cats. *JAVMA* 183:677–679, 1983.
50. Osborne CA, Finco DR, Low DG, et al: Percutaneous renal biopsy in the dog and cat. *JAVMA* 151:1474–1480, 1967.
51. Wise LA, Allen TA, Cartwright M: Comparison of renal biopsy techniques in dogs. *JAVMA* 195:935–939, 1989.
52. Jeraj K, Osborne CA, Stevens JB: Evaluation of renal biopsy in 197 dogs and cats. *JAVMA* 181:367–369, 1982.
53. Parker HR: Peritoneal dialysis and hemofiltration, in Bovee KC (ed): *Canine Nephrology.* Media, PA, Harwal Publishing Co, 1984, pp 723–754.
54. Cioffi WG, Ashikaga T, Gamelli RL: Probability of surviving postoperative acute renal failure; development of a prognostic index. *Ann Surg* 200:205–211, 1984.
55. Rasmussen HH, Pitt EA, Ibels LS, McNeil DR: Prediction of outcome in acute renal failure by discriminant analysis of clinical variables. *Arch Intern Med* 145:2015–2018, 1985.
56. Lien J, Chan V: Risk factors influencing survival in acute renal failure treated by hemodialysis. *Arch Intern Med* 145:2067–2069, 1985.
57. Liano F, Garci-Martin F, Gallego A, et al: Easy and early prognosis in acute tubular necrosis: A forward analysis of 228 cases. *Nephron* 51:307–313, 1989.
58. Smithies MN, Cameron JS: Can we predict outcome in acute renal failure? *Nephron* 51:297–300, 1989.
59. Wilkes BM, Mailloux LU: Acute renal failure; pathogenesis and prevention. *Am J Med* 80:1129–1136, 1986.

UPDATE

The preceding text outlined the principles of early treatment of acute renal failure, emphasizing restoring volume requirements, achieving diuresis, and correcting early metabolic complications. Patients that survive the early phase of dysfunction require long periods of maintenance therapy. In these cases, attention to fluid therapy remains important, as urine volume and metabolic needs can be variable. Monitoring of urine output, acid–base status, and electrolyte status must be continued.

The patient's fluid requirements are based on estimates of the volume required to:

- Replace persistent volume deficits
- Supply maintenance needs for typical sensible and insensible losses
- Replace ongoing losses due to vomiting, diarrhea, bleeding, or polyuria.

In dogs and cats with acute renal failure, losses due to urine output will be most variable. Therefore, fluid requirements in acute renal failure patients are best determined by calculating volumes required to:

(continues on page 124)

Management of Chronic Renal Failure in the Dog

University of Florida
David F. Senior, BVSc

From a diagnostic standpoint, azotemia must be classified according to cause—prenal, renal, or postrenal; once the presence of renal azotemia is established, acute renal failure (ARF) must be differentiated from chronic renal failure (CRF). Although renal function in patients with ARF may improve over time with appropriate treatment, the reduced glomerular filtration rate (GFR) observed with CRF is irreversible, with no chance of improvement. Furthermore, in patients with CRF, GFR tends to decline as renal lesions become progressively more severe. Patients with CRF tend to develop the characteristic uremic syndrome, the major clinical features of which are listed in Table I. Compensation for loss of renal function in CRF is so effective that few, if any, of these clinical features become evident until more than 60% of functional renal mass is lost. Further losses cause signs to develop, but individual dogs may be either excruciatingly sensitive or highly resistant to the detrimental effects of a certain degree of azotemia and, therefore, the number of signs exhibited will vary from patient to patient. Only dogs with advanced CRF show most or all of the features listed in Table I.

The causes of many of the clinical manifestations of the uremic syndrome remain unknown, but signs generally can be attributed to (1) the effects of metabolites that accumulate in the body because of reduced GFR (uremic toxins), and (2) compensatory physiological adjustments that maintain external balance of body fluids but cause adverse side effects. The clinician's goals in management of patients with CRF are threefold: (1) to identify and eliminate, if possible, insults that directly contribute to renal damage; (2) to provide special diets and treatments to increase vigor and the feeling of well-being; and (3) to prevent the intrinsic progression of chronic renal disease. Effective management of CRF is based on an understanding of the pathogenesis of the uremic syndrome.

PATHOPHYSIOLOGY OF CRF IN DOGS

As GFR in patients with CRF progressively falls, the tubular changes required to maintain external balance in response to altered nutrient intake become progressively greater. Thus, an animal with one-tenth normal GFR must undergo 10 times the normal change in fractional excretion of sodium

TABLE I
Major Clinical Features of the Uremic Syndrome in Dogs with CRF

History	*Clinical Signs*	*Laboratory Results*
Reduced appetite	Hypothermia	High BUN
Weight loss	Hypertension	High serum creatinine
Poor condition of coat	Rubber jaw	Hyperphosphatemia
Reduced exercise tolerance	Oral ulcers	Mild hyperglycemia
Vomiting	Pale mucous membranes	Metabolic acidosis
Increased thirst		Increased anion gap
Increased urine volume		Nonregenerative anemia
Nocturia		Isosthenuria
Dark stools		Proteinuria
Tremors		
Seizures		

when dietary sodium intake is increased or decreased. This phenomenon is known as the *magnification effect* and is responsible for the inability of uremic patients to handle stress (i.e., changes in the external environment that require changes in renal function).[1]

Gastrointestinal Signs

Gastrointestinal signs of CRF include oral ulceration, vomiting, and melena (Figure 1). The oral ulcerations are shallow and tend to occur on mucous membranes adjacent to contact points such as the teeth. Shallow erosions also develop in the stomach and small intestinal mucosa, contributing to gastrointestinal blood loss and melena. Occasionally, severely azotemic animals develop necrosis of the tip of the tongue, soft palate, and lip protrusions.

Shallow oral ulcerations may be due in part to excessive amounts of oral ammonia, caused by the action of urease-producing bacteria on the increased salivary urea of CRF. Ammonia is known to affect the coating of glycosaminoglycans that protect the mucous membranes, but the precise cause of oral ulceration remains obscure.[2] The large tissue sloughs of the tongue and soft palate may be due to a major vascular event such as peripheral vasculitis with vasoconstriction, venous occlusion, and subsequent ischemic necrosis—although this fairly rare phenomenon has not been investigated.

Superficial mucosal erosions of the stomach and small intestine may be caused by high levels of urea that reduce the protection provided by gastrointestinal mucus against the adverse effects of luminal digestive juices. Also, the hypergastrinemia seen in CRF in dogs may contribute to excessive gastric acid production, thereby exacerbating the tendency to develop gastrointestinal ulceration.[3] Although serum gastrin levels are elevated in CRF, excessive gastric

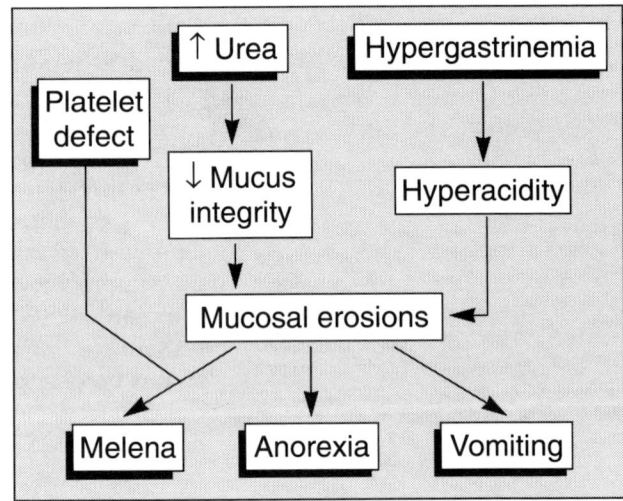

Figure 1—Pathogenesis of gastrointestinal signs in CRF.

acid production has not been documented. Inhibition of gastrin activity may occur at the gastrin receptor level or may be an intracellular postreceptor event. Despite confusion concerning the role of hypergastrinemia in gastrointestinal ulceration, administration of H_2 antihistamine to dogs with CRF tends to suppress vomiting and increase appetite (Figure 2).[3] Gastrointestinal blood loss from superficial mucosal erosions may be exacerbated by impaired hemostasis caused mainly by altered platelet function.

Anemia

Several factors contribute to the normocytic, normochromic anemia observed in CRF in the dog (Figure 3). Elevated erythrocyte 2,3-diphosphoglycerate (2,3-DPG) levels, reduced renal erythropoietin production, direct inhibition of hematopoiesis, decreased erythrocyte life span, and increased gastrointestinal

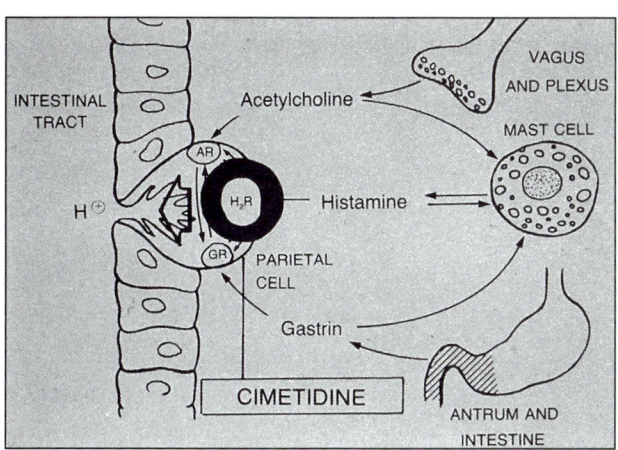

Figure 2A

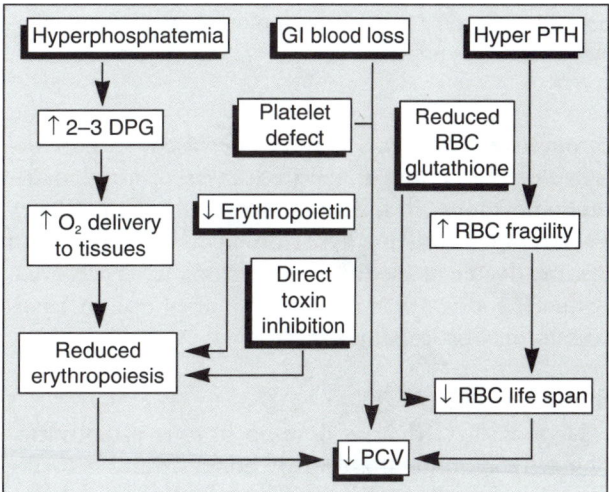

Figure 2B

Figure 2—(**A**) Role of gastric acid production and (**B**) effect of H_2 histamine receptor antagonists.

blood loss due to a platelet function defect all may contribute to anemia in CRF.[4-7] The anemia of CRF may be partly physiological. Hyperphosphatemia observed in late CRF leads to increased erythrocyte 2,3-DPG levels, causing the oxygen-hemoglobin dissociation curve to shift to the right, thereby facilitating oxygen delivery to peripheral tissues.[4] Enhanced peripheral oxygen delivery tends to reduce erythropoiesis, and a lower-than-normal hematocrit with no detrimental effect on tissue oxygenation would be expected.

Renal erythropoietin production is reduced in CRF, and replacement treatment with recombinant erythropoietin in human patients causes a dramatic correction of erythropoiesis and a return to a nearly normal hematocrit.[5] Unknown substances in uremic serum appear to directly inhibit erythropoiesis in bone marrow. Although elevated levels of parathyroid hormone (PTH) may play a role, the precise mechanism remains obscure.[6]

Erythrocyte life span can be reduced to one-half normal in human uremic patients.[8] Red cell osmotic fragility is increased and the red cell membrane appears to develop reduced deformability.[8] In dogs, the stability and integrity of the erythrocyte membrane may be adversely affected, in turn, by elevated plasma PTH levels, leading to increased intracellular Ca^{++} that subsequently affects spectrin-actin in the cytoskeletal network of erythrocytes.[8] Furthermore, uremic serum appears to inhibit the intracellular pentose phosphate shunt in erythrocytes, causing reduced glutathione levels and reduced resistance to oxidative hemoglobin changes.[9]

In uremic humans, primary hemostasis is impaired because of changes in vessel wall contraction, reduced platelet adherence to the injured vessel wall, reduced platelet aggregation, and poor formation and stabilization of fibrin clots.[10] Platelets are intrinsic to pri-

Figure 3—Pathogenesis of anemia in CRF.

mary hemostasis and several factors may contribute to altered platelet function. Reduced platelet serotonin, adenosine diphosphate (ADP) and thromboxane A_2 production, increased vessel wall prostaglandin I_2 (PGI_2) production, and changes in von Willebrand's factor have all been documented and could contribute to platelet dysfunction.[10]

Polyuria and Polydipsia

Dogs with CRF develop increased thirst and urine output owing to a urine concentration defect whereby they are unable to produce urine much above 300 mOsm/kg • H_2O (specific gravity=1.010) even when they are dehydrated. The urine concentration defect appears to result from several factors, including the high tubular fluid flow rate in remaining nephrons that impairs the development of medullary interstitial hypertonicity.[1,11] Furthermore, medullary blood flow

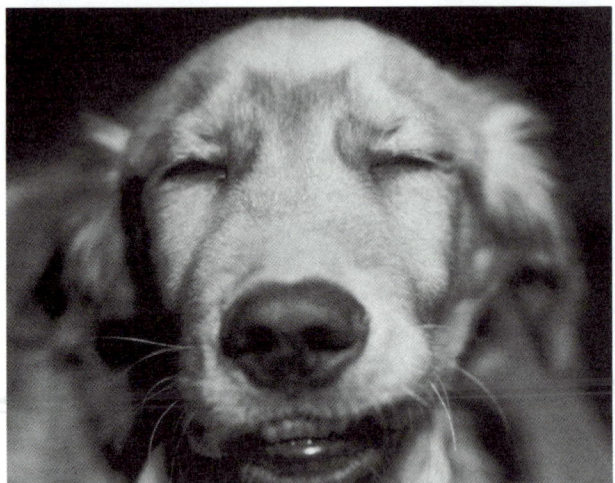

Figure 4A

Figure 4—(**A**) Thickened maxillae and (**B**) maxillary hemorrhagic fibrous osteodystrophy surrounding the carnaissial tooth root in a seven-month-old golden retriever puppy with renal hypoplasia.

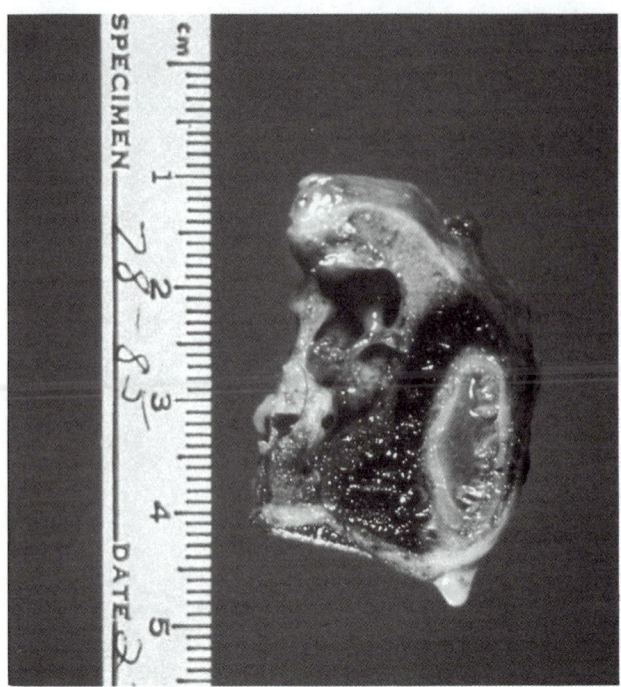

Figure 4B

through the vasa recta may be increased, in part because of the action of elevated levels of atrial natriuretic hormone, thus further dissipating the tendency to develop medullary hypertonicity.[12,13] Finally, even if some degree of medullary hypertonicity is achieved, collecting duct permeability in response to vasopressin may be impaired.[14]

Bone Disease

Dogs with CRF may develop fibrous osteodystrophy with demineralization of bone. Young growing dogs with CRF tend to develop thickened maxillae with zones of hemorrhagic fibrous tissue around the tooth roots (Figure 4). Adult dogs with long-standing CRF may develop rubber jaw, although only a small proportion of dogs with CRF are affected so severely (Figure 5).

The bone disease of CRF is caused by renal secondary hyperparathyroidism, impaired renal production of 1,25-dihydroxycholecalciferol [1,25-$(OH)_2D_3$], impaired gastrointestinal calcium absorption, and chronic metabolic acidosis (Figure 6).

As GFR progressively declines, phosphate tends to be retained. Consequently, high dietary phosphate intake and, eventually, hyperphosphatemia, tend to inhibit the renal enzyme α-hydroxylase, which catalyzes the metabolic step leading to the production of 1,25-$(OH)_2D_3$.[15,16] Reduced levels of 1,25-$(OH)_2D_3$ cause calcium malabsorption. The tendency toward hypocalcemia caused by either calcium malabsorption or phosphate retention stimulates the production of PTH.[17] Reduction of the normal suppressive action of 1,25-$(OH)_2D_3$ on PTH production also

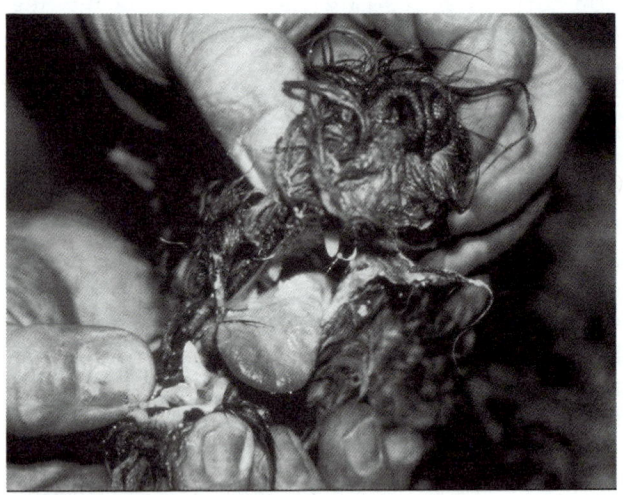

Figure 5—Severe rubber jaw in a seven-year-old miniature schnauzer with chronic renal failure.

contributes to increased plasma PTH levels.[16] Initially, the phosphaturic and hypercalcemic effects of PTH maintain normophosphatemia and normocalcemia, but once GFR falls below about 30% of normal, the tubular adaptations in response to PTH approach their limit and hyperphosphatemia develops.[17] Normal serum ionized calcium usually is preserved even in advanced CRF, although occasionally hypocalcemia or hypercalcemia occurs.

Dogs with CRF develop metabolic acidosis because of reduced renal reabsorption of filtered bicarbonate (HCO_3) and reduced secretion of hydrogen ion

↓ P if on Prestricted diet.

METABOLIC ACIDOSIS ∴ ↓ H⁺ BUFFERS ie. ↓ AMMONIA

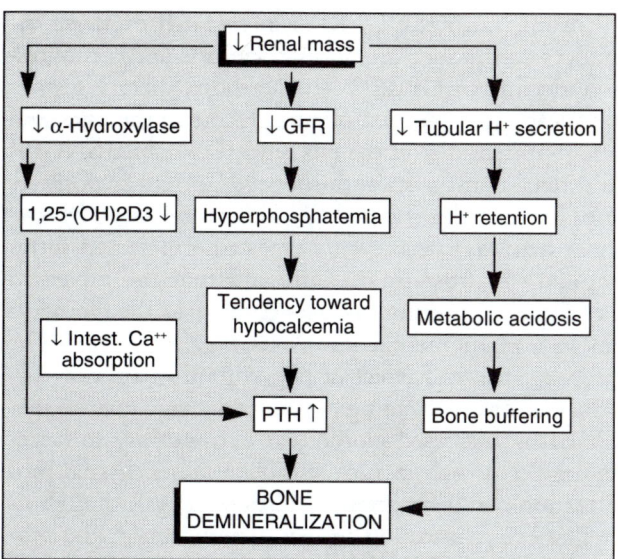

Figure 6—Pathogenesis of metabolic bone disease in CRF.

GFR↓
↓
P
retention
↓
HyperP
↓
-ve
1,25
(OH)₂D₃
(∴ α
hydroxylase
inhibited)
↓
HYPO
CALCAEMIA
↓
↑ PTH

(H⁺).[1] Impaired HCO_3 reabsorption is probably caused by several factors, including solute diuresis, high fractional excretion of sodium, and high levels of PTH.[18] Total renal H⁺ secretion is reduced because of limited tubular production of ammonia. Because tubular ammonia acts as a buffer for secreted H⁺, reduced ammonia production, caused by reduced functional renal mass, limits H⁺ excretion.[1] Acid excretion may be further impaired when dogs with CRF are fed a very low-phosphate diet, because phosphate acts as an intratubular buffer for secreted H⁺.[19] When intratubular phosphate buffer levels are reduced, excretion of titratable acid is impaired. When dietary intake of acidogenic food (e.g., meat protein) remains high, dogs with CRF develop a positive H⁺ balance, and retained H⁺ is buffered by bone. By buffering H⁺, bone tends to lose calcium carbonate, and bone demineralization of CRF may be increased.

Thus, metabolic bone disease in CRF is due to a complex array of dysfunctions involving PTH, 1,25-$(OH)_2D_3$, phosphate retention, calcium malabsorption, and impaired renal control of acid–base balance. Some of the precise details concerning the pathogenesis of metabolic bone disease remain controversial. Interestingly, metabolic acidosis has several positive aspects. The resulting mild acidemia tends to shift the oxygen–hemoglobin dissociation curve to the right, allowing better oxygen delivery to peripheral tissues and a tendency to shift plasma calcium to the ionized active form, thus offsetting the tendency toward hypocalcemia.

Hypertension

The incidence of hypertension in dogs with CRF appears to be about 60% overall and closer to 80% in dogs with glomerulonephropathy.[20,21] In most instances, the degree of hypertension is relatively mild and appears to have little effect on the progression of renal disease. A small proportion of dogs, however, suffers from severe hypertension that induces a progressive decline in kidney function.[22] Extreme hypertension may be the primary cause of CRF, or it may develop secondary to CRF but subsequently become severe enough to contribute significantly to the rate of progression of renal disease.

Hypertension can be caused by several factors, including sodium retention, increased extracellular fluid volume, increased norepinephrine levels, and both ischemia and impaired suppression of the juxtaglomerular apparatus leading to excessively high production of renin.[23] Furthermore, the cardiovascular responses to sodium retention, angiotensin II, and norepinephrine may be altered in CRF patients in such a way as to sustain hypertension.[23]

Immunodeficiency

Impairment of cell-mediated and humoral immunity can be demonstrated in human uremic patients, but the precise cause remains obscure.[24] Affected dogs may be susceptible to infections, but severe immunodeficiency is not usually apparent.

Glucose Intolerance

The mild hyperglycemia often observed in dogs with CRF is probably a result of postinsulin-receptor inhibition of carbohydrate utilization.[25]

Neurologic Signs

Tremors, seizures, weakness, and depression are all observed in dogs with CRF. Uremic encephalopathy and neuropathy are well recognized phenomena in human patients and experimental animals.[26,27] In experimental ARF in dogs, slowing of electroencephalograph patterns, increased calcium levels in the brain, and reduced motor nerve conduction velocity have been observed.[8] These changes are thought to be mediated in part by hyperparathyroidism and may have some relevance to the neurologic signs observed in dogs with CRF.[8]

Uremic Toxins

Many substances that accumulate in the plasma of uremic patients have been investigated as potential uremic toxins (Table II).[28] The actions and interactions of many different toxins appear to be necessary to produce all of the signs of the uremic syndrome.

Progression

Once CRF is established, GFR tends to decline progressively, regardless of the primary cause and

TABLE II
Substances that Accumulate in the Plasma of Uremic Patients and Are Thought to Act as Uremic Toxins

Toxin	Proposed Effect in Uremia
Guanidine compounds (e.g., methylguanidine)	Weight loss Altered platelet factor 3 function
Aliphatic amines	Inhibitiion of NA, K-ATPase Stimulation of histamine release from mast cells Possible inhibition of PTH and insulin action
Polyamines (e.g., spermine spermidine, etc.)	Inhibition of erythropoiesis
Myoinositol	Decreased never conduction velocity
Middle molecules	Confusing, but many effects are possible
Parathyroid hormoe	Neurologic dysfunction Reduced erythropoiesis Reduced red cell life span
Cyanate	Hypothermia Lethargy Anorexia Diarrhea Seizures

even if the primary cause no longer exists. Several factors are known to exacerbate progressive loss of renal function in dogs, including pyelonephritis, outflow obstruction (e.g., renal calculi), hypercalcemia, and extreme hypertension—although most of these would be regarded as primary causes of CRF.

Recently, considerable interest has developed in identifying causes of CRF progression that may be intrinsic to the uremic environment. In rats with experimental CRF, increased single-nephron ammonia production with elevated levels of ammonia in tissues appears to activate complement C3, inducing a cellular infiltrate and tissue damage.[29,30]

Hyperphosphatemia with a calcium phosphate product greater than 60 mg/dl[2] tends to induce soft tissue mineralization in several target tissues, including the stomach, heart, intercostal muscles, and kidneys.[2,31] Renal mineralization causes further loss of renal function in CRF, and a phosphate-restricted diet appears to protect against loss of kidney function as a result of hyperphosphatemia in rats and dogs and against renal mineralization in cats.[32,34]

Studies on mice with congenital diabetes mellitus fed ad libitum and rats with CRF fed a high-protein diet suggest that the high single nephron glomerular filtration ratio (SNGFR) seen in both of these instances can induce glomerular sclerosis and a progressive decline in GFR.[35,36] Furthermore, dietary restriction leading to reduced plasma glucose in the mice and a low-protein diet in the rats tended to reduce SNGFR and renal damage in both models. Current hypotheses propose that the elevated SNGFR is mediated by vascular hemodynamic events that cause increased intracapillary hydrostatic pressure and that the increased net filtration pressure induces damage to the glomerulus in a phenomenon known as *hyperfiltration*.[37] The precise cause and effect of hyperfiltration are not currently understood, but glomerular damage may be mediated by increased glomerular permeability to larger molecules, which in turn stimulate mesenchymal proliferation and infiltration of macrophages. Although simultaneous protection against hyperfiltration and progression of CRF by a low-protein diet has been well demonstrated in experimental rats, a similar phenomenon has yet to be demonstrated in dogs.[38–41]

MANAGEMENT OF CRF IN DOGS

When developing a management plan for dogs with CRF, attention must be given to identifying and controlling causes of renal damage such as pyelonephritis, hypercalcemia, hyperphosphatemia, outflow obstruction, hypertension, and immune-mediated disease. Owners must be advised of their pets' limited adaptability to rapid changes in environment and diet. Because CRF cannot be cured, clinical management should aim at suppressing clinical signs and limiting further renal damage.

The basis of clinical management of CRF involves dietary adjustment and control of anorexia, vomiting, azotemia, hyperphosphatemia, metabolic acidosis, anemia, and hypertension (Table III). Nutrition is the primary basis of CRF management, although several aspects of nutritional adjustment remain controversial. Fresh clean water must be available at all times, and the diet should provide 70 to 110 kcal/kg BW/day of metabolizable energy. Greater energy levels per kilogram of body weight are required to maintain body weight in smaller breeds, and lower levels are required in larger breeds.

Protein Restriction

In experimental studies, dogs with CRF that were fed a low-protein diet appeared stronger and more lively and had healthier coats than dogs with CRF that were fed a normal canine diet.[40] The improvement could be due to reduced accumulation of urea as well as a wide variety of protein metabolites that contribute to the uremic syndrome. Low-protein diets fed to dogs with CRF reduced GFR, proteinuria, and renal histological changes seen on light microscopy, al-

TABLE III
Medical Management of Chronic Renal Failure

Strategy	*Goals of Treatment*
Dietary Adjustment	
Ad lib water	
Energy 70–110 kcal/kg/day	
Low-protein	BUN < 80 mg/dl
Low-phosphate	PO4 < 6.0 mg/dl
Low-sodium	Control hypertension
Antiemetics	Control vomiting
Cimetidine	
Metaclopramide	
Trimethobenzamide	
Phosphate Binders	PO4 < 6.0 mg/dl
Aluminum hydroxide	
Alkalinizers	HCO3 > 17 mEq/L
Bicarbonate	
Citrate	
Antihypertensives	BP < 150 / <100
Furosemide	
Propranolol	
Diltiazem	
Captopril	
Erythropoietics	PCV > 25%
Epoetin alfa (recombinant)	
Anabolic steroids: nandrolone	

though electron microscopic (EM) examination of tissues revealed no significant difference between the morphological features of dogs on low- and normal-protein diets.[39,40,42] Low-protein diets reduce the solute load that must be excreted. Because urine osmolality is fixed, low-protein diets reduce urine volume, and owners note that nocturia tends to diminish or cease. Studies indicated that if protein restriction were too severe, several problems occurred, including failure to thrive, weight loss, anemia, hypoalbuminemia, and metabolic acidosis.[43,44] These problems may not have been solely caused by reduced dietary protein, because the diets also were severely restricted in phosphate and several other nutrients.

Moderate protein restriction is recommended for dogs with mild to moderate CRF (creatinine 4.5 mg/dl). Approximately 2 to 2.2 g/kg/day of high-biologic-value protein, such as egg protein and muscle meat, should be fed to such dogs. Dogs fed egg protein exclusively, concurrent with a low-phosphate diet, tend to develop metabolic acidosis, so the additional phosphate in muscle meat protein may be preferable with very low-protein diets.[19,44] For dogs

with more advanced renal failure, protein intake can be reduced gradually to below 2 g/kg/day, but diets containing less than 1.6 g/kg/day are less successful, and the patient should be observed carefully for appetite and weight loss, hypoproteinemia, and anemia.

Phosphate Restriction

Phosphate absorption can be limited with a low-phosphate diet and phosphate binders, if necessary. Restricted phosphate absorption has several beneficial effects, including reduced accumulation of phosphate in plasma, reduced soft tissue mineralization, and reduced metabolic bone disease caused by renal secondary hyperparathyroidism.[32-34] Severe phosphate restriction impairs excretion of titratable acid in dogs and predisposes them to metabolic acidosis.[19] In most instances, low-protein diets are also low in phosphate, so that restriction of one results in restriction of both. The goal should be to reduce serum phosphate levels to less than 6.0 mg/dl.

Phosphate Binding and Calcium Supplementation

If dietary phosphate restriction alone fails to reduce serum phosphate to the desired level, phosphate binders such as aluminum hydroxide or aluminum carbonate can be given orally. Phosphate binders should be given with meals and are only effective when given concurrently with a low-phosphate diet.[45] Although the liquid suspensions of these salts appear to be more effective (Alterna-GEL®, Liquid—Stuart Pharmaceuticals, 600 mg/5 ml; Basaljel® extra strength liquid—Wyeth Laboratories, 1,000 mg/5 ml), dogs dislike their taste and texture, and owners may be more successful with aluminum hydroxide tablets (Amphojel®—Wyeth Laboratories, 300 mg and 600 mg tablets) or aluminum carbonate capsules (Basaljel®—Wyeth Laboratories, equivalent to 500 mg Al(OH)₃ capsules). The suggested dose is 10 to 30 mg/kg three times daily with serum phosphate monitored at 10 to 14 day intervals. Once serum phosphate levels are normal, calcium carbonate has been used in human uremic patients as the oral binding agent.[46] This approach combines the provision of more calcium for absorption with effective gastrointestinal phosphate binding. Because reduced plasma ionized calcium is one of the stimuli for hyperparathyroidism, the use of calcium carbonate as the phosphate binder may be effective in reducing hyperparathyroidism. Calcium carbonate (Tums®—Norcliff Thayer, 500 mg tablets) can be given to dogs at 100 mg/kg/day initially; serum calcium and phosphate levels must be carefully monitored. The dose should then be adjusted according to individual patient response to achieve normocalcemia and normophosphatemia. Calcium salts should be given as phosphate binders only after the serum phosphate level has been reduced to 6 mg/dl or lower, because hypercalcemia combined with hyperphosphatemia will lead to rapid soft tissue mineralization and further damage of renal tissue.

Vitamin D Supplementation

One cause of renal secondary hyperparathyroidism is impaired renal production of $1,25-(OH)_2D_3$ with reduced intestinal calcium absorption. Replacement of $1,25-(OH)_2D_3$ with calcitriol (Rocaltrol®—Roche Laboratories, 0.25 µg and 0.5 µg capsules) at 0.03 to 0.06 µg/kg/day or dihydrotachysterol (DHT®—Roxane Laboratories, 0.125 mg, 0.2 mg, and 0.4 mg tablets; 0.2 mg/ml liquid) at 0.01 mg/kg/day may return intestinal calcium absorption to normal.[47] This strategy is useful only if serum phosphate levels are less than 6 mg/dl. Serum ionized calcium levels should be monitored every 1 to 2 days for the first 7 to 10 days of treatment so that hypercalcemia is not inadvertently induced.

Sodium Restriction

The quantity of sodium in the diet should be reduced even in animals that are not overtly hypertensive. Very high dietary sodium levels in CRF, a common practice used by veterinarians in the past to induce diuresis, should be avoided because severe hypertension with retinal detachment has been observed frequently with such feeding.[21] Severe sodium restriction may also be dangerous because dogs with CRF may have limited ability for renal sodium retention, so that low-sodium diets could cause reduced extracellular fluid volume leading to reduced GFR with exacerbation of azotemia. In the absence of marked hypertension, about one-half the sodium of a normal diet should be provided (0.5 to 0.6 mg/kcal in food or 30 to 45 mg/kg body weight/day). Most uremic patients can handle a fairly wide range of the quantity of minerals in their diet, including sodium, but dietary adjustments require exaggerated changes in tubular function to maintain external balance; such changes may take a prolonged time. Sudden reduction of sodium intake without rapid reduction of renal sodium excretion will result in negative sodium balance, reduced ECF volume, and reduced GFR, which may cause sudden worsening of azotemia. In dogs with CRF, rapid reduction of renal sodium excretion may not be possible, so dietary adjustment should be gradual, particularly in advanced CRF.

Bicarbonate Supplementation

Metabolic acidosis is frequently observed when diets of dogs with CRF are severely restricted in protein and phosphate.[19,43,44] Metabolic acidosis causes hyperventilation and limits exercise tolerance. Alkaline supplementation should be provided if plasma HCO_3 is less than 15 mEq/L; the goal is to maintain levels in the range of 15 to 20 mEq/L. An initial dosage of sodium bicarbonate at 8.8 to 11 mg/kg two to three times daily can be used, and subsequent supplementation can be adjusted based on regular 2 to 4 week monitoring of plasma bicarbonate levels. Potassium citrate, calcium carbonate, or calcium lactate may be preferable if strict sodium restriction is necessary. The provision of a metabolic buffer may reduce excessive renal ammonia production and limit the toxic effects of subsequent complement activation.[30]

Vitamin Supplementation

Supplementation with B-complex and C vitamins is used in human uremics, and similar recommendations are made for dogs, even though definitive data regarding requirements are not available. Human patients with CRF tend to become deficient in folate, pyridoxine, and ascorbate.[48] Most commercial low-protein dog foods designed for feeding animals with renal failure are replete with B-complex and C vitamins. (It is not known if vitamin C is required in dogs with chronic renal failure.) Supplementation with a standard daily vitamin preparation is recommended only for dogs whose diet consists entirely of home-cooked food.

Appetite Enhancement and Antiemetics

One of the biggest problems associated with feeding canine CRF patients is the control of anorexia and vomiting. Animal CRF patients with finicky appetites are a supreme challenge. Uremic toxins appear to stimulate the medullary emetic chemoreceptor trigger zone, and elevated plasma gastrin levels seem to contribute to the shallow gastric erosions observed in CRF.[3,49] Several strategies have been devised to induce affected dogs to eat, but sometimes none are effective.

Food is usually more palatable if it is warmed or if its texture is familiar. More food may be consumed each day if frequent small meals rather than one or two large meals are provided. Adding chicken fat to meals may increase their palatability. The H_2-histamine antagonist drugs are often effective antiemetics. Cimetidine hydrochloride (Tagamet®—Smith Kline & French, 300 mg tablets) can be given at 5 to 10 mg/kg orally three to four times daily. Ranitidine hydrochloride (Zantac®—Glaxo Pharmaceuticals, 50 mg and 100 mg tablets) can be given at 2 mg/kg orally three times daily. Motility disturbances can be corrected with metoclopramide (Reglan®—A. H. Robins, 5 mg and 10 mg tablets; 1 mg/ml syrup) given at 0.2 to 0.4 mg/kg orally 30 minutes before meals three to four times daily. Metoclopramide is a centrally acting antiemetic that promotes gastric emptying. Other centrally acting antiemetics can be used, but care must be taken with their dosages because they tend to cause drowsiness. Among the most useful are trimethobenzamide (Tigan®—Beecham Laboratories, 100 mg and 250 mg capsules; 200 mg suppositories) given at 3 mg/kg orally three times daily; prochlorperazine (Compazine®—Smith Kline & French, 5 mg and 10 mg tablets; 10 mg, 15 mg, and 30 mg Spansule® capsules; 1 mg/ml syrup) given at 0.13 mg/kg orally three to four times daily; and chlorpromazine (Thorazine®—Smith Kline & French, 10 mg and 25 mg tablets; 30 mg and 75 mg Spansule®, capsules; 2 mg/ml syrup) given at 3.3 mg/kg orally one to four times daily. Long-term use of the centrally acting antiemetics is best avoided, and the dose may have to be reduced to avoid excessive sedation. Direct appetite stimulants have limited usefulness because they also cause sedation. Oxazepam (Serax®—Wyeth Laboratories, 10 mg, 15 mg, and 30 mg capsules) can be given at 0.1 mg/kg orally once daily. Flurazepam (Dalmane®—Roche Products, 15 mg and 30 mg capsules) can be given at 0.22 to 0.44 mg/kg orally every four to seven days. Diazepam (Valium®—Roche Products, 2 mg, 5 mg, and 10 mg tablets) can be given at 2.5 to 10 mg orally one to two times daily. These drugs may cause sedation, and, although they are marginally effective appetite stimulants in cats, they are of questionable value in azotemic dogs.

Erythropoietics

The anemia of CRF is best treated with recombinant erythropoietin (Epogen®—Amgen, 2,000 U/ml and 4,000 U/ml injectable, 1 ml vials).[50] Although the dose rate for dogs is not currently known, the human dose is 50 to 100 U/kg subcutaneously three times weekly. Recombinant erythropoietin, however, is expensive. An alternative is nandrolone decanoate (Deca-Durabolin®—Organon, 50 mg/ml injectable, 2 ml vials) given at 1.0 to 1.5 mg/kg intramuscularly weekly. Nandrolone is sluggishly effective in human CRF patients at correcting anemia but has not been tested for efficacy in dogs.[51] It is purported to stimulate erythropoietin production in the damaged kidneys and commit pluripotential stem cells in the bone marrow into the erythropoietic line. Other anabolic steroids, such as stanozolol (Winstrol® V—Winthrop, 2 mg tablet; 50 mg/ml injectable) given at 1 to 4 mg orally twice daily or 25 to 50 mg intramuscularly weekly have been suggested, although in other species they have not been as effective as nandrolone.

Antihypertensives

Antihypertensive agents have been used in dogs with CRF, although at present their use has been associated with neither a decrease in the rate of progression of CRF nor an increase in chance of survival.[52] The usual strategies for CRF management include stepwise implementation of a sodium-restricted diet, diuretics, beta blockers, and then vasodilators. The most effective approach in dogs with CRF, however, is thought to include gradual implementation over three to four weeks of a sodium-restricted diet (0.5 to 0.6 mg/kcal in food or 10 mg/kg body weight/day) followed by or combined with an angiotensin-converting enzyme inhibitor such as captopril (Capoten®—Squibb, 25 mg, 50 mg, and 100 mg tablets) given at 0.5 to 2 mg/kg 2 to 3 times daily.[32] This dose should be less in dogs with extremely low GFR, and treated animals should be observed carefully for adverse effects such as exacerbated azotemia and shock. Calcium channel blockers may be useful as vasodilators for hypertension; for example, nifedipine (Adalat®—Miles, 10 mg and 20 mg capsules) may be effective if given at 1 to 2 mg/kg three times daily. Blood pressure should be monitored carefully.

Dose Adjustment in CRF

Adverse side effects are seen more frequently when drugs are given to animals with CRF.[53,54] Many drugs are excreted primarily by the kidneys, and these drugs will tend to accumulate if normal doses are given. Furthermore, drug distribution and protein binding are altered in azotemia so that side effects are enhanced. Veterinarians should have a high degree of awareness of the potential for adverse reactions when treating azotemic animals, and medications should be withdrawn if untoward effects are suspected. Drugs that are excreted primarily by a nonrenal system are less likely to cause a problem. Drugs that are excreted primarily by the kidneys may be (1) innocuous even at very high blood levels and therefore not a problem; (2) toxic at high plasma concentration; or, most dangerously (3) nephrotoxic at high plasma concentration. Dose adjustment ideally should be based on measured drug blood levels or on creatinine clearance if the drug is excreted primarily by the kidneys. As these data are not readily available in most clinical situations, clinicians can adjust the dose according to the serum creatinine level. The dose amount can remain normal if the dose interval is multiplied by the serum creatinine level (in mg/ml), or the dose interval can remain the same as usual if the dose amount is divided by the serum creatinine. Drugs that require dose adjustment include aminoglycosides, penicillins, cephalosporins, digoxin, and trimethoprim/sulfamethoxazole.

Monitoring Progression

A plot of the reciprocal of serum creatinine against time has been touted as an effective means of determining the rate of progression of renal disease in dogs with CRF.[55] The method has not held up well under close scrutiny in human patients, and there is considerable doubt about its accuracy in dogs.[56] Accurate assessment of GFR in uremic dogs currently requires more accurate and often more cumbersome clearance methods better suited to the research setting than to individual patients.

In conclusion, veterinarians should set definite physical and physiological goals when managing dogs with CRF. Repeated evaluation of body weight, appetite, general appearance, blood urea nitrogen, serum phosphate and bicarbonate, packed cell volume, urine sediment, and blood pressure at regular intervals should provide sufficient information upon which to base management decisions. Very frequent evaluation may be required in the early phases of treatment.

ABOUT THE AUTHOR

David F. Senior, BVSc
Diplomate, ACVIM
Department of Small Animal Clinical Sciences
College of Veterinary Medicine
University of Florida
Gainesville, Florida

REFERENCES

1. Valtin H: Renal dysfunction: Mechanisms involved in fluid and solute imbalance. Boston, Little, Brown and Co, 1979.
2. Parsons CL, Stauffer C, Mulholland SG: Effect of ammonium on bacterial adherence to bladder transitional epithelium. *J Urol* 132:365–366, 1984.
3. Thornhill JA: Control of vomiting in the uremic patient, in Kirk RW (ed): *Current Veterinary Therapy VIII*, Philadelphia, WB Saunders Co, 1983, pp 1022–1025.
4. Mitchell TR, Pegrum CD: The oxygen affinity for hemoglobin in chronic renal failure. *Br J Haematol* 21:463–472, 1971.
5. Eschbach JW, Egrie JC, Downing MR, et al: Correction of the anemia of endstage renal disease with recombinant human erythropoietin: Results of a phase I and II clinical trial. *N Engl J Med* 316:73–78, 1987.
6. Massry SC: Pathogenesis of the anemia in uremia: Role of secondary hyperparathyroidism. *Kidney Int* 24:5204–5207, 1983.
7. Remuzzi G, Pusiner F: Coagulation defects in uremia. *Kidney Int* 33(Suppl 24):S13–S17, 1988.
8. Massry SC: Parathyroid hormone as a uremic toxin, in Massry SC, Glassock RJ (eds): *Textbook of Nephrology*, ed 2. Baltimore, Williams & Wilkins, 1989, pp 1126–1144.
9. Kock KM: Anemia, in Massry SC, Glassock RJ (eds): *Textbook of Nephrology*, ed 2. Baltimore, Williams and Wilkins, 1989, pp 1199–1204.
10. Remuzzi G: Bleeding and coagulation abnormalities, in Massry SG, Glassock RJ (eds): *Textbook of Nephrology*, ed 2. Baltimore, Williams and Wilkins, 1989, pp 1205–1209.
11. Bricker NS, Fine LG: The renal response to progressive nephron loss, in Brenner BM, Rector FC (eds): *The Kidney*, ed 2. Philadelphia, WB Saunders Co, 1981, pp 1056–1096.
12. Carriere S, Wong NLM, Dirks JH: Redistribution of renal blood flow in acute and chronic reduction of renal mass. *Kidney Int* 3:364–371, 1973.
13. Maack T, Camargo MJF, Kleinerd HD, et al: Atrial natriuretic factor: Structure and functional properties. *Kidney Int* 27:607–615, 1985.
14. Tannen RL, Regal EM, Dunn MJ, et al: Vasopressin-resistant hyposthenuria in advanced chronic renal disease. *N Engl J Med* 180:1135–1141, 1969.
15. Slatopolsky E, Caglar S, Gradowska L, et al: On the prevention of secondary hyperparathyroidism in experimental chronic renal disease using "proportional reduction" of dietary phosphorus intake. *Kidney Int* 2:147–151, 1972.
16. Massry SG: Divalent ion metabolism and renal osteodystrophy, in Massry SG, Glassock RJ (eds): *Textbook of Nephrology*, ed 2. Baltimore, Williams and Wilkins, 1989, pp 1278–1311.
17. Slatopolsky E, Caglar S, Pennell JP, et al: On the pathogenesis of hyperparathyroidism in chronic renal insufficiency in the dog. *J Clin Invest* 50:492–499, 1971.
18. Bourjoignie JJ: Patients with chronic renal failure, in Massry SG, Glassock RJ (eds): *Textbook of Nephrology*, ed 2. Baltimore, Williams and Wilkins, 1989, pp 1263–1270.
19. Hulter HN: Hypophosphaturia impairs the renal defense against metabolic acidosis. *Kidney Int* 26:302–307, 1984.
20. Weiser MG, Spangler WL, Gribble DH: Blood pressure measurement in the dog. *JAVMA* 171:364–368, 1977.
21. Cowgill LD, Kallet AJ: Recognition and management of hypertension in the dog, in Kirk RW (ed): *Current Veterinary Therapy VIII*. Philadelphia, WB Saunders Co, 1983, pp 1025–1028.
22. Bovee KC, Littman MP, Crabtree BJ, et al: Essential hypertension in a dog. *JAVMA* 195:81–86, 1989.
23. Weidmann P: Hypertension, in Massry SG, Glassock RJ (eds): *Textbook of Nephrology*, ed 2. Baltimore, Williams and Wilkins, 1989, pp 1182–1194.
24. Anagnostou A, Kurtzman NA: Hematological consequence of renal failure, in Brenner BM, Rector FC (eds): *The Kidney*, ed 3. Philadelphia, WB Saunders Co, 1986, pp 1361–1656.
25. Pabico RC: Pericarditis, in Massry SG, Glassock RJ (eds): *Textbook of Nephrology*, ed 2. Baltimore, Williams and Wilkins, 1989, pp 1171–1177.
26. Arieff AI: Neurological manifestations of uremia, in Brenner BM, Rector FC (eds): *The Kidney*, ed 3. Philadelphia, WB Saunders Co, 1986, pp 1731–1756.
27. Raskin NH, Fishman RA: Neurological disorders in renal failure. *N Engl J Med* 294:143–148, 1976.
28. Bergstrom J, Furst P: Uremic toxins. *Kidney Int* 13:(Suppl 8):S9–S12, 1978.
29. Nath KA, Hostetter MK, Hostetter TH: Pathophysiology of chronic tubulointerstitial disease in rats: Interactions of dietary acid load, ammonia and complement C3. *J Clin Invest* 76:667–675, 1985.
30. Nath KA, Hostetter MK, Hostetter TH: Ammonia complement interaction in the pathogenesis of progressive renal injury. *Kidney Int* 36:(Suppl 27):552–554, 1989.
31. Bovee KC: Metabolic disturbances of uremia, in Bovee KC (ed): *Canine Nephrology*. Philadelphia, Harwell, 1984, pp 555–612.
32. Ibels LS, Alfrey AC, Haut L, et al: Preservation of function

in experimental renal disease by dietary restriction of phosphate. *N Engl J Med* 298:122–126, 1978.

33. Brown S, Finco D, Crowell W, et al: Beneficial effect of moderate phosphate restriction in partially nephrectomized dogs on a low protein diet. *Kidney Int* 31:380(abst), 1987.

34. Ross LA, Finco DR, Crowell WA: Effect of dietary phosphorus restriction on the kidneys of cats with reduced renal mass. *Am J Vet Res* 43:1023–1026, 1982.

35. Hostetter TH, Olson JL, Rennke HG, et al: Hyperfiltration in remnant nephrons: A potentially adverse response to renal ablation. *Am J Physiol* 241:F85–F93, 1981.

36. Olson JL, Hostetter TH, Rennke HG, et al: Altered glomerular permselectivity and progressive sclerosis following extreme ablation of renal mass. *Kidney Int* 22:112–126, 1982.

37. Brenner BM: Nephron adaptation to renal injury or ablation. *Am J Physiol* 249:F324–F337, 1985.

38. Bovee KC, Kronfeld DS, Ramberg C, Ct al: Long-term measurement of renal function in partially nephrectomized dogs fed 56, 27, or 19 percent protein. *Invest Urol* 16:378–384, 1979.

39. Robertson JL, Goldschmidt M, Kronfeld DS, et al: Long-term renal responses to high dietary protein in dogs with 75 percent nephrectomy. *Kidney Int* 29:511–519, 1986.

40. Polzin DJ, Osborne CA, Hayden DW, et al: Influence of reduced protein diets on morbidity, mortality, and renal function in dogs with induced chronic renal failure. *Am J Vet Res* 45:506–517, 1984.

41. Bourgoignie JJ, Gavellas G, Martinez E, et al: Glomerular function and morphology after renal mass reduction in dogs. *J Lab Clin Med* 109:380–388, 1987.

42. Polzin DJ, Osborne CA, Hayden DW, et al: Effects of modified protein diets in dogs with chronic renal failure. *JAVMA* 183:980–986, 1983.

43. Polzin DJ, Osborne CA, Stevens JB, et al: Influence of modified protein diets on the nutritional status of dogs with induced chronic renal failure. *Am J Vet Res* 44:1694–1702, 1983.

44. Polzin DJ: The importance of egg protein in reduced protein diets designed for dogs with renal failure. *J Vet Intern Med* 2:15–21, 1988.

45. Finco DR, Crowell WA, Barsanti JA: Effects of three diets on dogs with induced chronic renal failure. *Am J Vet Res* 46:646–653, 1985.

46. Slatopolsky E, Weerts C, Lopez-Hilker S, et al: Calcium carbonate as a phosphate binder in patients with chronic renal failure undergoing dialysis. *N Engl J Med* 315:157–161, 1986.

47. Peterson ME: Hypoparathyroidism, in Kirk RW (ed): *Current Veterinary Therapy IX*. Philadelphia, WB Saunders Co, 1986, pp 1039–1045.

48. Kopple JD: Chronic renal failure: Nutritional and nondialytic management, in Glassock RJ (ed): *Current Therapy in Nephrology and Hypertension*. St Louis, CV Mosby, 1984, pp 252–260.

49. Borison HL, Hebertson LM: Role of medullary emetic chemoreceptor trigger zone in post-nephrectomy vomiting dogs. *Am J Physiol* 197:850–852, 1959.

50. Eschbach JW: The anemia of chronic renal failure: Pathophysiology and the effects of recombinant erythropoietin. *Kidney Int* 35:134–148, 1989.

51. Dainiak N: The role of androgens in the treatment of chronic renal failure. *Semin Nephrol* 5:147–154, 1985.

52. Ross LA, Labato MA: Use of drugs to control hypertension in renal failure, in Kirk RW (ed): *Current Veterinary Therapy X*. Philadelphia, WB Saunders Co, 1989, pp 1201–1204.

53. Senior DF: Drug therapy in renal failure. *Vet Clin North Am* 9:805–817, 1979.

54. Riviere JE: Calculation of dosage regimens of antimicrobial drugs in animals with renal and hepatic dysfunction. *JAVMA* 185:1094–1097, 1984.

55. Allen TA, Jaenke RS, Fettman MJ: A technique for estimating progression of chronic renal failure in the dog. *JAVMA* 190:866–868, 1987.

56. Walser M, Drew HH, LaFrance ND: Reciprocal creatinine slopes often give erroneous estimates of progression of chronic renal failure. *Kidney Int* 36(Suppl 27):581–585, 1989.

Feline Renal Failure: Questions, Answers, Questions*

KEY FACTS

- Advancing age is a risk factor for renal failure in cats.
- To detect renal failure before the development of uremia, we recommend evaluation of serial serum creatinine concentrations and results of urinalyses in all cats older than 8 to 10 years of age.
- Short-term and long-term prognoses for cats with renal failure should be determined on the basis of serial serum creatinine values.
- Supportive and symptomatic therapy for cats with renal failure should be initiated in a stepwise fashion. For example, dehydration, hyperphosphatemia, and mild acidemia should be corrected by fluid replacement and dietary modification before determining the need for intestinal phosphorus binders and alkali therapy.

University of Minnesota
Jody P. Lulich, DVM, PhD
Carl A. Osborne, DVM, PhD
Timothy D. O'Brien, DVM, PhD
David J. Polzin, DVM, PhD

"THE STUDY of the causes of things must be preceded by the study of things caused."

Hughlings Jackson

HOW IMPORTANT IS RENAL FAILURE IN CATS?
Prevalence of Feline Renal Failure at Veterinary Colleges in North America

Between 1980 and 1990, 189,371 cats were examined at 23 veterinary colleges in North America.[a] Of 189,371 cats, renal failure was diagnosed in 2228. Based on these numbers, the prevalence of renal failure in cats was 1.18%.[1] In other words, 12 cases of renal failure were recognized for every 1000 cats admitted. The frequency of renal failure in male cats was similar to that in females (Table I). Compared with the average, however, renal failure was recognized more than twice as often in the following breeds: Maine Coon, Abyssinian, Siamese, Russian Blue, and Burmese (Table II).

The prevalence of renal failure in cats is increasing (Figure 1). For every 1000 cats evaluated in 1980, four had renal failure regardless of age. By 1990, the number of reported cases of renal failure quadrupled; 16 cases were identified for every 1000 cats examined.

Of 2228 cases of feline renal failure diagnosed between 1980 and 1990, 63% of the cats were 10 years of age or older (Figure 2). In 1980, 42 cases of renal failure were diagnosed for every 1000 cats 10 years of age or older; by 1990, this number increased to 77 per 1000. For cats older than 15 years of age, 126 cases were diagnosed for every 1000 cats examined in 1980 and 153 cases for every 1000 in 1990. The increase in prevalence of renal failure in aging cats may reflect an increase in veterinary care sought by owners as well as greater efforts by veterinarians to detect renal failure. Whatever the reason, these findings emphasize the importance of renal failure in older cats.

Prevalence of Feline Renal Failure at the University of Minnesota

Between 1980 and 1990, 8928 cats were examined at the University of Minnesota Veterinary Teaching Hospital (UMVTH). Of these 8928 cats, renal failure was diagnosed in 273. The prevalence of renal failure was 3.05%. In 1980, five cases were diagnosed for every 1000 cats examined (Figure 1). By 1990, the number of affected cats

*Supported in part by a grant from Mark Morris Associates, Topeka, Kansas.

[a]Veterinary Medical Data Base, Purdue University, West Lafayette, Indiana.

TABLE I
Prevalence of Renal Failure Identified in Cats of Different Genders[a]

Gender	Female		Male		Unknown	
	%	No.	%	No.	%	No.
Intact	0.42	205 of 49,273	0.52	256 of 48,697	NA	NA
Neutered	1.9	814 of 42,940	2.1	943 of 44,467	NA	NA
Unknown	2.4	2 of 82	NA	NA	NA	NA
Total	1.1	1,021 of 92,295	1.3	1,199 of 93,164	0.20	8 of 3,912

[a]From 1980 through 1990, 189,371 case records from 23 veterinary colleges in North America entered into the Veterinary Medical Data Base, Purdue University.

TABLE II
Prevalence and Risk of Renal Failure Identified in Cats of Different Breeds[a]

Breed	Prevalence		Risk	
	%	No.	Odd's Ratio	95% CI[b]
Main Coon	2.88	9 of 312	2.44:1	1.18 to 4.88[c]
Abyssinian	2.85	22 of 771	2.42:1	1.54 to 3.77[c]
Siamese	2.77	354 of 12,770	2.6:1	2.31 to 2.93[c]
Russian Blue	2.57	8 of 311	2.17:1	1 to 4.51
Burmese	2.45	19 of 776	2.07:1	1.27 to 3.32
Balinese	2.14	4 of 187	NA[d]	NA
Japanese Bobtail	2.0	1 of 50	NA	NA
Angora	1.89	3 of 159	NA	NA
Persian	1.66	82 of 4,932	1.40:1	1.11 to 1.76[c]
Himalayan	1.61	43 of 2,664	1.35:1	0.98 to 1.85
Scottish Fold	1.49	1 of 67	NA	NA
Colorpoint Shorthair	1.32	2 of 152	NA	NA
Rex	1.12	2 of 179	NA	NA
Tonkinese	1.1	1 of 91	NA	NA
Mixed (includes Domestic Longhair)	1.09	738 of 67,703	0.85:1	0.78 to 0.93[c]
American Domestic Shorthair	0.96	932 of 96,646	0.64:1	0.59 to 0.70[c]
Manx	0.56	6 of 1,071	0.46:1	0.19 to 1.06
Birman	0.49	1 of 205	NA	NA

[a]From 1980 through 1990, 189,371 case records from 23 veterinary colleges in North America entered into the Veterinary Medical Data Base, Purdue University. Breeds of cats examined in which renal failure was not recognized were American Wirehair (2), Bombay (22), British Blue (42), British Shorthair (6), Chartreaux (5), Egyptian Mau cat (39), Exotic Shorthair (61), Harlequin (1), Havana Brown (26), Longhair Manx (20), Korat (20), Maltese (23), Manxamese (6), Ocicat (22), Oriental Shorthair (4), Ragdoll (2), Snowshoe (1), and Somali (13).
[b]CI = Confidence interval.
[c]Statistically significant (*p* value < 0.05).
[d]NA = Not applicable because small numbers of affected cats precluded meaningful statistical interpretation of results.

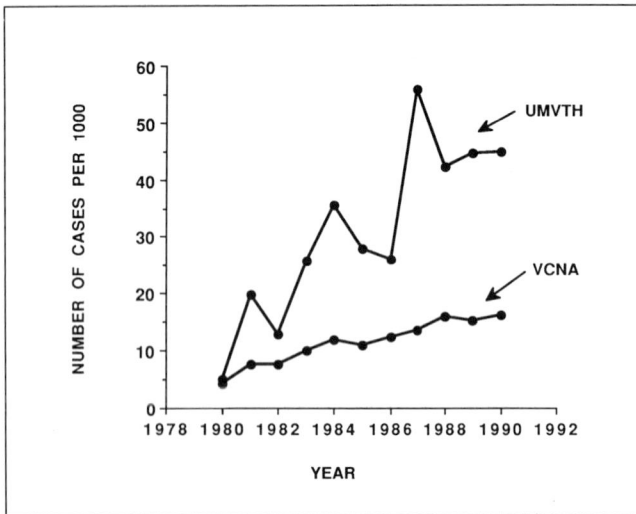

Figure 1—Yearly prevalence of renal failure in cats based on 189,371 case records from 23 veterinary colleges in North America as entered into the Veterinary Medical Data Base at Purdue University. *UMVTH* = University of Minnesota Veterinary Teaching Hospital; *VCNA* = veterinary colleges of North America.

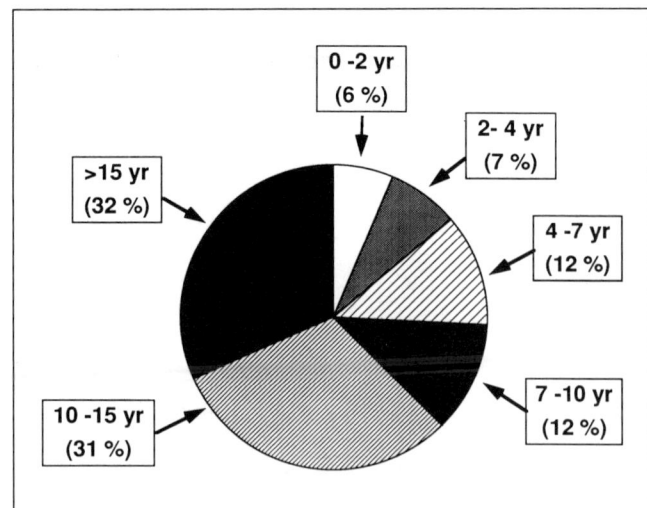

Figure 2—From 1980 through 1990, distribution of renal failure in cats of different ages based on 2228 case records from patients diagnosed at 23 veterinary colleges in North America as entered into the Veterinary Medical Data Base at Purdue University. In 87 cases, age of the cat was not determined.

increased to 45 per 1000. The prevalence of renal failure was highest in cats older than 15 years of age; for every 1000 cats examined, almost one third (310) was affected (Figure 3).

WHAT ARE THE CLINICAL, BIOCHEMICAL, AND MORPHOLOGIC CHARACTERISTICS OF RENAL FAILURE IN CATS?

In recent years, improved knowledge of the pathophysiology of uremia in humans and dogs has resulted in significant advancements in specific, supportive, and symptomatic treatment of renal failure in these species. In contrast to humans and dogs, the causes, metabolic consequences, and biologic behavior of renal failure in cats have been less well characterized.

To EVALUATE clinical and laboratory features of feline renal failure, the medical records of 132 cats with renal failure diagnosed at the University of Minnesota were reviewed. Cats were admitted between January 1968 and July 1986. In each case, the diagnosis of renal failure was defined as concurrent azotemia (serum creatinine concentration > 1.9 mg/dl and/or serum urea nitrogen concentration > 35 mg/dl) and inappropriate urine concentrating ability (specific gravity < 1.035). Blood and urine values represent data obtained at the time of initial diagnosis and before any form of treatment. Results from microscopic evaluation of renal tissue were obtained from samples collected from cats within 90 days of a diagnosis of renal failure.

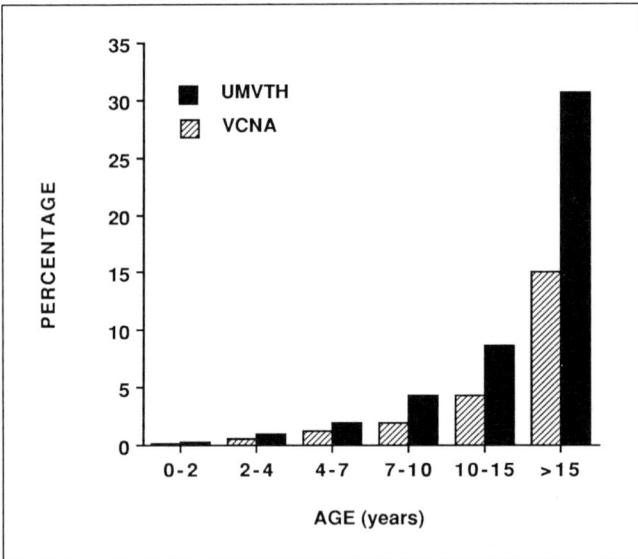

Figure 3—From 1980 through 1990, prevalence of renal failure in cats of different ages based on 8928 case records from the University of Minnesota College of Veterinary Medicine and 89,371 case records from 23 veterinary colleges in North America as entered into the Veterinary Medical Data Base at Purdue University. *UMVTH* = University of Minnesota Veterinary Teaching Hospital; *VCNA* = veterinary colleges of North America.

Signalment

Of 132 cats, 10 breeds of cats were represented. Short-haired varieties accounted for 68% (90) of affected cats; 29% (38) were long-haired breeds. The breed of four cats was not recorded. Fifty-eight percent (77) of cats with renal failure were male, and 42% (55) were female. A majority (55%) of cats were middle-aged or older; 28% (37) were between 10 and 15 years of age, while 27% (36) were older than 15 years of age. The percentages of cats in other age groups were 17% (22) between 7 and 10 years of age, 12% (16) between age 4 and 7 years, 7% (9) between 2 and 4 years of age, and 9% (12) younger than 2 years.

History

Anorexia was observed by owners in 80% (100 of 125) of cats with renal failure (Table III). Other nonlocalizing signs commonly reported were weight loss (72%), depression (68%), and weakness (47%). Polyuria and polydipsia were observed in only 40% of affected cats. Clinical signs referable to gastrointestinal dysfunction included vomiting (63 of 121; 52%), constipation (28 of 118; 24%), and diarrhea (4 of 118; 3%). Signs consistent with lower urinary tract disease (inappropriate urination and dysuria) were reported in less than 10% of the cats (Table III).

Physical Examination

Dehydration was detected in 70% (90 of 128) of cats with renal failure (Table IV). Fifty eight percent of cats were underweight. Kidney size, which was assessed by palpation in 107 cats, was abnormal in 44 cats; 27 (25%) had at least one kidney too large, and 17 (16%) had at least one kidney too small. Hypothermia (temperature lower than 99°F) was detected in 10 of 115 cats, while hyperthermia (temperature higher than 103.5°F) was detected in 6 of 115. Gingivitis (18%), halitosis (15%), and oral ulcers (2%) were uncommonly recognized.

TABLE III
Clinical Signs Identified by Owners of 132 Cats Admitted with Renal Failure to the University of Minnesota Veterinary Teaching Hospital

	Affected Cats	
Abnormality	*%*	*No.*
Anorexia	80	100 of 125
Weight loss	72	84 of 116
Depression	68	85 of 125
Vomition	52	63 of 121
Weakness	47	52 of 110
Polydipsia	40	46 of 114
Polyuria	40	44 of 110
Constipation	24	28 of 118
Inappropriate urination	9	10 of 109
Hematuria	8	9 of 111
Dysuria	6	7 of 110
Diarrhea	3	4 of 118

TABLE IV
Physical Examination Findings Identified in 132 Cats Admitted with Renal Failure to the University of Minnesota Veterinary Teaching Hospital

	Affected Cats	
Abnormality	*%*	*No.*
Dehydration	70	90 of 128
Underweight	58	67 of 116
Large kidneys (Figure 5)	25	27 of 107
Small kidneys (Figure 4)	16	17 of 107
Gingivitis	18	23 of 12
Halitosis	15	18 of 120
Oral ulcers	2	3 of 120
Hypothermia (temperature lower than 99°F)	9	10 of 115
Hyperthermia (temperature higher than 103.5°F)	5	6 of 115

TABLE V
Hematologic Abnormalities Identified in 132 Cats Admitted with Renal Failure to the University of Minnesota Veterinary Teaching Hospital

	Affected Cats			
Abnormality	*%*	*No.*	*Mean*	*Range*
Anemia (hematocrit <27%)	35	44 of 126	19.4	10.6 to 26.5
Polycythemia (hematocrit >50%)	1	1 of 126	52	52
Leukocytosis (>19,000 leukocytes/μl)	28	35 of 126	30,720	19,600 to 64,200
Leukopenia (<3800 leukocytes/μl)	0	0 of 126	0	0

TABLE VI
Serum Biochemical Abnormalities Identified in 132 Cats Admitted with Renal Failure to the University of Minnesota Veterinary Teaching Hospital

Abnormality	Affected Cats		Mean	Range
	%	No.		
Azotemia				
Urea nitrogen (>35 mg/dl)	100	132 of 132	120	36 to 375
Creatinine (>1.9 mg/dl)	97	115 of 119	6.35	2 to 25.6
pH (>7.44)	0	0 of 41	NA	NA
pH (<7.30)	88	36 of 41	7.16	6.87 to 7.29
pH (<7.20)	49	20 of 41	7.09	6.87 to 7.19
Bicarbonate (>24 mEq/L)	2	1 of 41	26.3	26.3
Bicarbonate (<17 mEq/L)	80	33 of 41	12.5	5.2 to 16.8
Hyperphosphatemia (>7.0 mg/dl)	63	72 of 115	12.82	7.1 to 45
Hyperphosphatemia (>6.0 mg/dl)	68	78 of 115	12.35	6.3 to 45
CO_2 content (>25 mEq/L)	2	1 of 42	27.5	27.5
CO_2 content (<17 mEq/L)	67	28 of 42	12.7	5.8 to 16.6
Anion gap (>25)	52	22 of 42	33.2	26 to 59.2
Hypophosphatemia (<3.0 mg/dl)	2	2 of 115	2.75	2.6 to 2.9
Hyperproteinemia (>8.8 g/dl)	9	6 of 55	9.3	9.0 to 9.8
Hyperproteinemia (>8.0 g/dl)	33	18 of 55	8.7	8.1 to 9.8
Hypoproteinemia (<6.1 g/dl)	9	6 of 55	5.2	4.2 to 6.0
Hyperglycemia (>160 mg/dl)	33	16 of 48	238	163 to 421
Hypoglycemia (<75 mg/dl)	4	2 of 48	60.5	55 to 66
Hyperamylasemia (>1590 U/L)	31	10 of 32	2598	1765 to 4615
Hyperkalemia (>5.3 mEq/L)	13	15 of 116	6.71	5.4 to 9.4
Hypokalemia (<3.5 mEq/L)	19	22 of 116	3.0	2.2 to 3.4
Hypokalemia (<3.1 mEq/L)	11	13 of 116	2.79	2.2 to 3.0
Hyperchloremia (>129 mEq/L)	5	6 of 112	134.5	130 to 146
Hypochloremia (<113 mEq/L)	18	20 of 112	104	82 to 112
Hypochloremia (<105 mEq/L)	8	9 of 112	98.6	82 to 104
Hypernatremia (>159 mEq/L)	17	20 of 116	164.2	160 to 175
Hyponatremia (<145 mEq/L)	6	7 of 116	131	108 to 144
Hypercalcemia (>11.0 mg/dl)	10	12 of 118	11.8	11.1 to 12.9
Hypocalcemia (<8.5 mg/dl)	13	15 of 118	7.6	4.2 to 8.4
Hyperalbuminemia (>4.0 g/dl)	4	4 of 115	4.3	4.1 to 4.7
Hypoalbuminemia (<2.5 g/dl)	13	15 of 115	2.1	1.2 to 2.4

Hemogram

Hemograms were evaluated in 126 cats (Table V). Anemia occurred in 35% (44 cats) with renal failure; polycythemia was detected in one cat. Because 70% of the cats were dehydrated, it is probable that anemia occurred with greater frequency than detected by the design of our clinical study.

In contrast to a decreased number of red blood cells, leu-

TABLE VII
Abnormalities Detected by Urinalysis in 132 Cats Admitted with Renal Failure to the University of Minnesota Veterinary Teaching Hospital

| | Affected Cats | |
Abnormality	*%*	*No.*
Proteinuria (dipstick dye test 1+ to 4+)	63	82 of 130
Specific gravity (1.012 to 1.035)	60	79 of 132
Specific gravity (1.008 to 1.012)	37	49 to 132
Specific gravity (<1.008)	3	4 of 32
Erythrocyturia (>5 red blood cells per high-power field; 450×)	26	33 of 129
Microburia (sediment analysis)	19	25 of 129
Leukocyturia (>5 white blood cells per high-power field; 450×)	15	19 of 129

kocytosis was detected in 28% of cats. Leukopenia was not observed.

Serum Biochemical Profile

By definition, all cats were azotemic; however, the occurrence of other serum biochemical abnormalities was variable (Table VI). For example, only 68% were hyperphosphatemic while 88% were acidemic, 31% were hyperamylasemic, and 19% were hypokalemic.

THE UNEXPECTED prevalence of acidemia identified in this retrospective study raises several questions. Was it associated with sampling technique, factors specifically related to feline renal failure, or species differences in acid-base homeostasis?

Urinalysis

The distribution of urine specific gravity values were 3% less than 1.008, 37% between 1.008 and 1.012, and 60% between 1.013 and 1.034. Proteinuria (1+ to 4+ by dipstick dye test) was detected in 63% of cats with renal failure (Table VII). Microscopic sediment analysis was performed in 129 urine samples. Clinically significant erythrocyturia was detected in 33, and clinically significant leukocyturia was detected in 19; bacteria or yeast was identified in 25. Nineteen of 25 urine samples with microburia were cultured for aerobic bacteria; growth was observed in only 12. An additional 15 urine samples without microburia also were aerobically cultured; bacteria were identified in five samples. *Escherichia coli* was isolated from the urine of 13 of 17 renal failure cats. *Staphylococcus* was retrieved from the urine of two cats, *Streptococcus*

TABLE VIII
Renal Size and Associated Morphologic Diagnosis of Kidneys Identified in 88 Cats Admitted with Renal Failure to the University of Minnesota Veterinary Teaching Hospital

Microrenale (<2.3 times the length of L2, Figure 4)	
Chronic generalized nephritis	5
Glomerular sclerosis	2
Tubular necrosis	1
Metastatic pulmonary carcinoma	1
Morphology unavailable	20
Total	29
Normal size (2.3 to 3.2 times the length of L2)	
Tubular necrosis	6
Chronic generalized nephritis	3
Lymphosarcoma	2
Amyloidosis	2
Hydronephrosis	1
Renal cell carcinoma	1
Morphology unavailable	20
Total	35
Macrorenale (>3.2 times the length of L2, Figure 5)	
Polycystic kidney disease	12
Lymphosarcoma	5
Pyelonephritis	1
Vasculitis	1
Membranoproliferative glomerulonephropathy	1
Tubular necrosis	1
Chronic generalized nephritis	1
Morphology unavailable	2
Total	24

from one cat, and *Proteus* from one cat. *Candida* was isolated from the urine of a cat with yeast pyelonephritis. These data indicate the need for a prospective study of the prevalence of bacterial urinary tract infection in cats with renal failure.

Radiography

Renal size was determined by survey abdominal radiography in 88 cats (Table VIII). Twenty-nine (33%) had small kidneys (Figure 4), 35 (40%) had normal kidneys, and 24 (27%) had larger than normal kidneys (Figures 5, 6, and 7). Unfortunately, attempts to correlate renal size with morphologic diagnosis were hindered by the large percentage of cats in which biopsies or necropsies were unavailable. With the possible exception of macrorenale, further studies are warranted to determine whether changes in renal size are indicative of specific types of underlying renal disease.

Morphology

Renal tissue was obtained from 68 cats for microscopic evaluation (Table IX). The most common morphologic findings were chronic generalized nephritis (20; 29%),

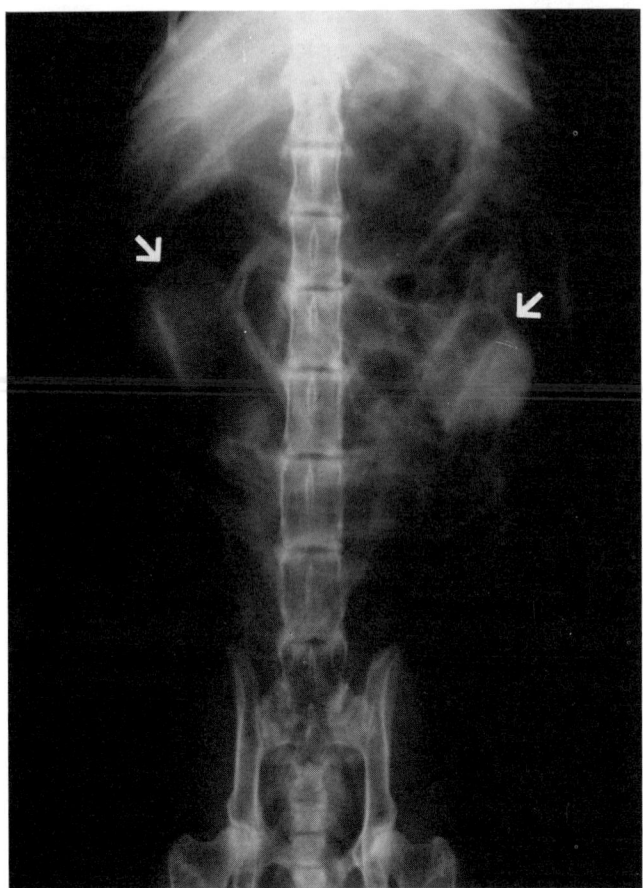

Figure 4—Ventrodorsal radiograph obtained five minutes after intravenous injection of a radiopaque contrast agent into a 14-year-old female Siamese cat with chronic generalized nephritis. Both kidneys are small and have an irregular contour (*arrows*).

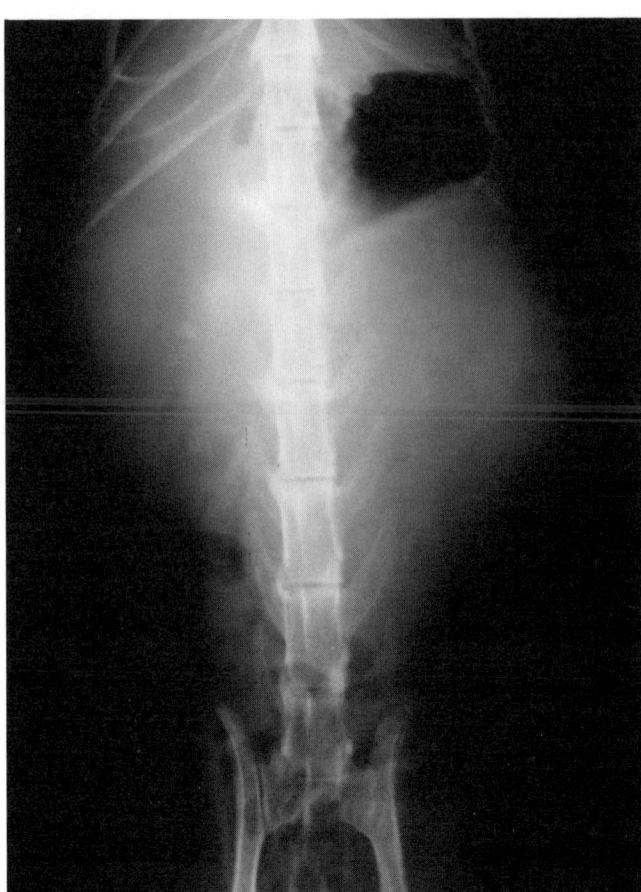

Figure 5—This ventrodorsal survey abdominal radiograph of a uremic cat illustrates bilateral renal enlargement caused by polycystic kidney disease (see Figure 6).

polycystic kidney disease (12; 18%), tubular necrosis (11; 16%), and lymphosarcoma (11; 16%).

HOW CAN THE DIAGNOSIS, PROGNOSIS, THERAPY, AND MONITORING OF FELINE RENAL FAILURE BE IMPROVED?

The following sections address questions pertaining to the diagnosis and treatment of renal failure in cats. Information derived from our retrospective study of renal failure in cats was used to help answer these questions.

How Can the Diagnosis Be Improved?
Redefining Failure

Most veterinary nephrologists define renal failure as loss of sufficient functional nephrons (usually ³/₄ or more) to impair homeostasis.[2] A diagnosis of primary renal failure (rather than prerenal or postrenal azotemia) is usually confirmed by detection of concurrent azotemia and impaired urine-concentrating capacity.

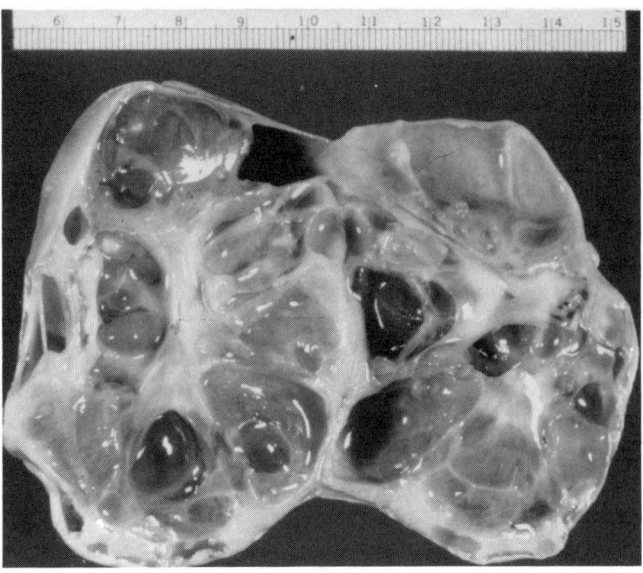

Figure 6—Photograph of a sagittally sectioned polycystic kidney from an 11-year-old male Domestic Longhair cat. Multiple cysts have displaced the functional renal parenchyma.

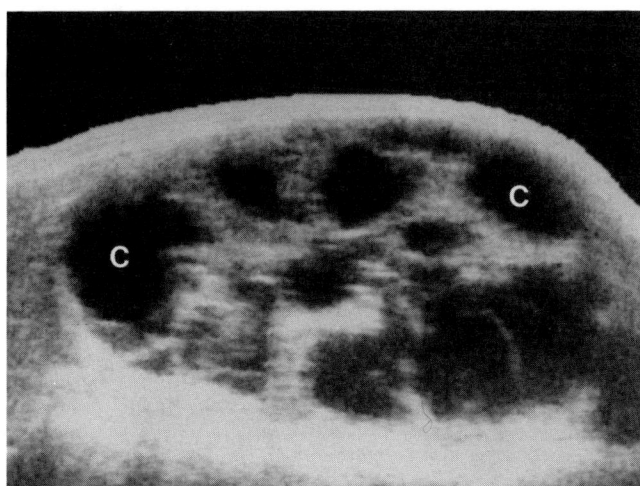

Figure 7—Sagittal static-B sonogram of the polycystic kidney illustrated in Figure 6. The multiple anechoic areas represent cysts (c).

TABLE IX
Morphologic Findings[a] in 68 Cats Admitted with Renal Failure to the University of Minnesota Veterinary Teaching Hospital[a]

Classification	No.
Glomerular	
Glomerulonephropathy (Figures 9 through 11)	
Membranoproliferative	2
Glomerulosclerosis	4
Metastatic pulmonary carcinoma	1
Tubular	
Polycystic kidney disease	12
Tubular necrosis	11
Hydronephrosis	1
Renal cell carcinoma	1
Interstitial	
Lymphosarcoma	11
Vascular	
Vasculitis/thrombosis	1
Glomerulointerstitial	
Amyloidosis	2
Tubulointerstitial	
Chronic generalized nephritis	20
Pyelonephritis	
Bacterial	1
Fungal	1

[a]Morphologic lesions identified by renal biopsy and/or necropsy.

THE ABILITY of cats to concentrate urine to a specific gravity of 1.035 or greater is generally accepted as evidence of adequate renal function to prevent the clinical signs of primary renal failure.[2] This value was extrapolated from data pertaining to urine-concentrating ability from other species (primarily humans and dogs) with renal failure and from uncontrolled clinical observations of azotemic cats. Results of studies of induced renal failure, however, suggest that the urine specific gravity end point of 1.035 may be too low.[3,4] For example, in one study, 5/6 reduction of renal mass (renal ligation and contralateral nephrectomy) resulted in mean urine specific gravity values of 1.038 ± 0.013 in seven cats fed a 51.7% protein diet and 1.050 ± 0.015 in seven cats fed a 27.6% protein diet.[3] Observations reported from another study were similar; urine specific gravity values were greater than 1.035 after surgical ablation of more than three quarters of the renal mass.[4] These findings in cats suggest that a urine specific gravity value of 1.040 or greater may be a more suitable end point of an adequate population of functional nephrons to prevent the clinical signs associated with naturally occurring primary renal failure. Stated in another way, urine specific gravity values between 1.006 and 1.040 in cats with clinical dehydration and/or azotemia are highly suggestive of primary renal failure (Figure 8). If this premise is valid, the prevalence of renal failure in cats was higher than that reported by the UMVTH and other North American veterinary colleges. Studies are in progress to clarify this important information.

Screening Patients

Detection of renal failure in the absence of laboratory data is difficult because mild forms of renal failure typically remain subclinical. In addition, many clinical findings associated with renal failure are not specifically referable to the urinary tract (Tables IV and V). In clinical terms, the signs do not allow localization of the underlying disease to the urinary tract; however, some trends that may help in the selection of patients likely to benefit from further evaluation have been identified.

For example, cats between 10 and 15 years of age were five times more likely to have renal failure than cats of other age groups while cats older than 15 years of age were 20 times more likely to have renal failure (Table X). Likewise, the Siamese, Abyssinian, Maine Coon, and Burmese breeds were two times more likely than other breeds to be diagnosed with renal failure (Table II). We emphasize, however, that the best predictor of future major disease is detection of existing minor disease. The aforementioned risk factors are not collectively as strong a predictor of renal failure as are laboratory findings of early renal dysfunction. Therefore, we recommend that older cats, especially those breeds at risk, be periodically screened for

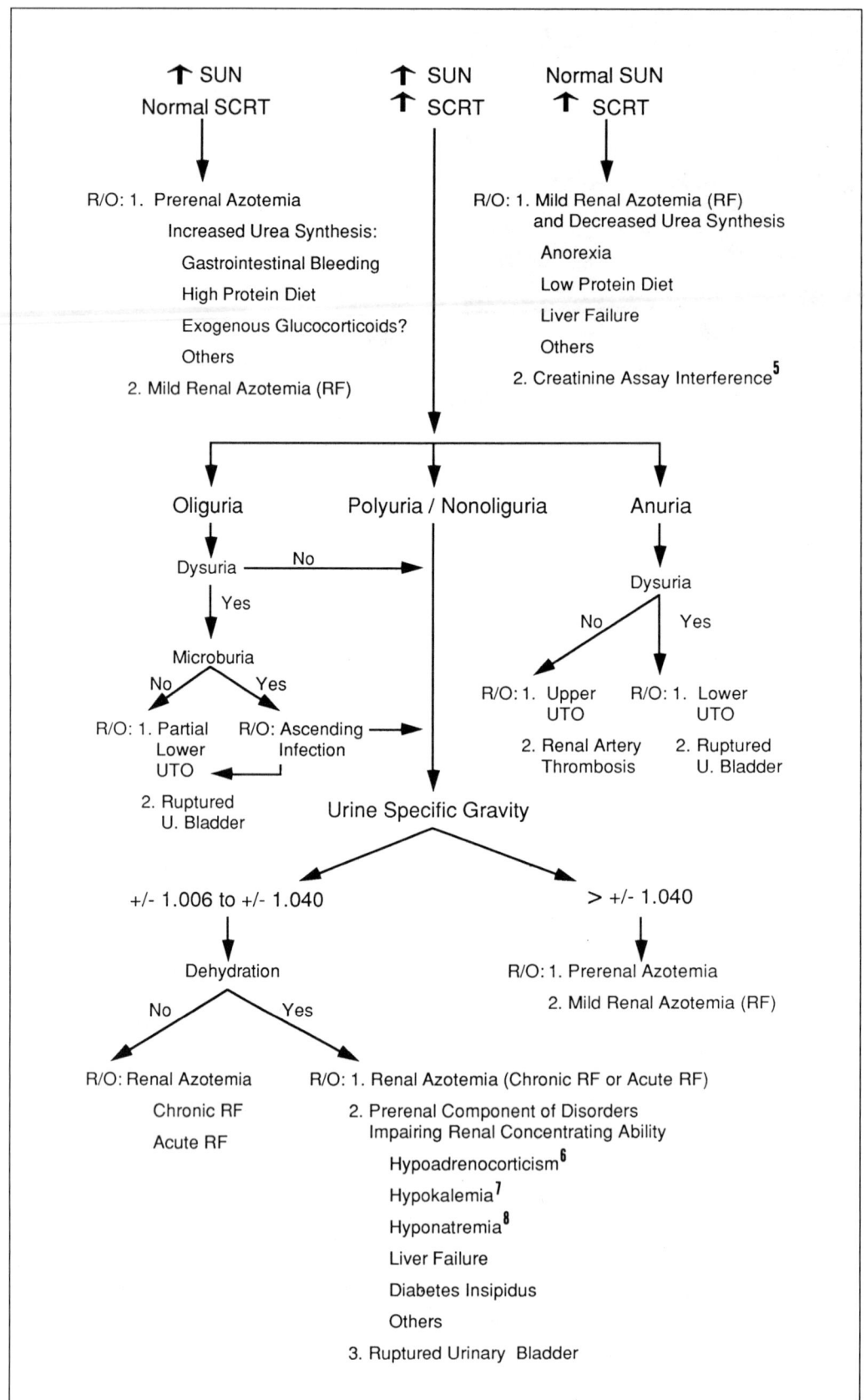

Figure 8—Localizing feline azotemia. *RF* = renal failure; *SCRT* = serum creatinine; *SUN* = serum urea nitrogen; *UTO* = urinary tract obstruction.

TABLE X
Risk of Renal Failure in Cats of Different Ages[a]

Age (years)	Risk		Number	
	Odd's Ratio	95% CI[b]	Affected	Total
0–2	0.05:1[c]	0.04 to 0.06	134	99,589
2–4	0.45:1[c]	0.38 to 0.54	158	26,343
4–7	1.11:1	0.97 to 1.27	258	19,533
7–10	1.77:1[c]	1.55 to 2.03	247	12,279
10–15	4.89:1[c]	4.45 to 5.37	662	15,377
>15	20.88:1[c]	17.94 to 23.02	682	4,525

[a]189,371 case records from 23 veterinary colleges in North America entered into the Veterinary Medical Data Base, Purdue University. In 11,725 cases, age of the cat was not determined.
[b]CI = Confidence interval.
[c]p = value < 0.05.

renal failure even in absence of clinical signs (Table XI). Even though not specifically related to the urinary system, renal failure should be considered in cats with anorexia, weight loss, dehydration, depression, vomiting, polyuria, or constipation. The index of suspicion of renal failure should be especially high when these signs occur in combination.

How Can the Prognosis Be Improved?
Overview

Forecasts of the probable future course of renal failure must be based on recognition of the pathogenesis of underlying cause, knowledge of the potential reversibility of renal lesions, and evaluation of the severity of renal dysfunction. The prognosis for each patient with renal failure should be subcategorized according to the probability of immediate recovery (short-term prognosis) and the probability of resolution of underlying morphologic and functional abnormalities (long-term prognosis). Because no two patients with renal failure caused by the same agent have identical degrees of functional and morphologic impairment, prognosis of renal failure should not be based on limited observations of the history and physical examination or on the results of laboratory tests performed only once. The clinical dogma that renal failure patients with serum creatinine concentrations of 5 mg/dl or greater had terminal disease is fiction, not fact.

Recognizing the Underlying Causes

Because patients with prerenal or postrenal azotemia have structurally normal kidneys that are initially capable of quantitatively normal function, rapid correction of the underlying cause is usually associated with complete restoration of renal function. The overall prognosis depends on the biologic behavior of the primary disease that precipi-

tated renal failure, unless secondary lesions of renal parenchyma have developed.

The prognosis for primary renal failure is variable, being dependent on the biologic behavior of the underlying cause (Table XII). For example, early recognition and appropriate treatment of aminoglycoside-induced acute tubular necrosis often prevent progression to chronic generalized nephritis. Although the short-term prognosis is poor to fair depending on the severity of disease, the long-term prognosis after recovery may be good to excellent. In contrast, renal amyloidosis is a progressive irreversible renal disease that ultimately results in death from renal failure.[9] Patients with early stages of renal amyloidosis typically have a good short-term prognosis but a poor long-term prognosis. In some instances, renal biopsy may be needed to establish the underlying cause (Figures 9, 10, and 11) (see How Can Therapy Be Improved?).

Knowledge of Disease Reversibility

Many causes of azotemia in cats are potentially reversible (Table XII). Reversibility of renal disease depends on the nature, location, and extent of lesions and on the rapidity and efficacy with which the underlying cause is eliminated. Evaluation of renal biopsies provides the only method of evaluating the morphologic nature of renal lesions in the living patient.

The degree of reversibility and functional compensation that occurs after injury to the kidneys varies with the disease and the patient. For example, in a study of cats (n = 18) with membranous glomerulopathy, the type, location, and severity of immune complex deposition were useful prognostic indicators.[10] Long-term survivors (2.5 to 6 years in eight cats) typically had only immunoglobulin G (IgG) and complement 3 (C3) deposits in glomerular capillary walls. In contrast, IgM or IgA deposition in addition to IgG or C3 deposition in glomerular capillary walls were observed in cats experiencing only short-term remissions. Likewise, detection of intramembranous as well as subepithelial electron-dense deposits by transmission electron microscopy was associated with advanced disease and a less favorable long-term prognosis.

Light microscopic examination alone is not a reliable index of prognosis in every instance. Both function and morphology must be evaluated when an attempt is being made to assess the ability of the kidneys to repair injury and regain adequate function. In the study of cats with membranous glomerulopathy, functional evidence of uremia also correlated with a poor long-term prognosis regardless of light microscopic findings.[10]

Differentiating Acute from Chronic Renal Failure

Medical history and physical examination findings are helpful when differentiating acute from chronic renal failure; however, because acute renal failure and chronic renal

---

TABLE XI
Problem-Specific Data Base for Feline Renal Failure

Minimum Data Base
1. Medical History Checklist
   a. Age?
   b. Breed?
   c. Duration of illness?
   d. Previous illness or injury?
   e. Past history of renal disease? Recent evaluation indicating adequate renal function?
   f. Exposure to possible nephrotoxins?
   g. Recent trauma, surgery, or anesthesia?
   h. Diet: Type? Frequency of feeding? Supplements? Recent diet changes? Preferences?
   i. Water consumption: Increased, decreased, unknown, or no change? If change noted, when?
   j. Micturition
      Frequency? Quantity? Color? Odor? Changes?
      Urinary incontinence?
      Micturition in abnormal locations?
   k. Detection of signs not directly referable to the urinary tract
      Anorexia?   Weight loss?
      Vomiting?   Constipation?
      Diarrhea?   Others?
   l. Are clinical signs increasing in severity, decreasing in severity, or remaining the same?
   m. Medication history: Medications given? When given? Dose? Response? Tolerance?

2. Physical Examination Checklist
   a. Temperature, pulse, and respiratory rate?
   b. Hydration status (skin pliability, xerostoma, etc.)?
   c. Body weight?
   d. Mouth: Mucosal ulcers? Discoloration of tongue? Pallor of mucous membranes? Loose or missing teeth? Enlargement of maxillary tissue?
   e. Cardiovascular system: Pulse rate and character? Mucous membrane color? Capillary refill time? Heart sounds? Venous distention? Arterial blood pressure (if available)?

   f. Kidneys: Both palpable? Bilaterally symmetric? Position? Size? Shape? Consistency? Contour? Pain?
   g. Urinary bladder: Size (before and after micturition)? Shape? Consistency? Position? Pain? Wall thickness? Intraluminal masses? (Consistency? Attached? Grating sensation?)
   h. Urethra (if possible?): Position? Size? Shape? Consistency? Intraluminal masses? (Consistency? Attached? Grating sensation?)
   i. Penis, prepuce, vulva: Shape? Consistency? Discharge? Pain?
   j. Ophthalmoscopic examination of fundus for evidence of hypertension: Retinal detachment? Hemorrhage? Others?

3. Laboratory Data Checklist
   a. Urinalysis, including urine sediment
   b. Kidney function tests (serum creatinine and urea nitrogen)
   c. Hematocrit, total plasma protein concentration (CBC?)

Further Diagnostic Consideration
1. Serum Biochemical Profile (Na, Cl, K, P, TCO_2, Ca, albumin, others to identify associated complications and extrarenal causes of azotemia [i.e., hypoadrenocorticism, hyponatremia, others])
2. Urine Culture (especially if microburia, dysuria, or hematuria is detected)
3. Survey Abdominal Radiography (to verify kidney number, size, shape, and position)
4. Urine Protein-to-Creatinine Ratio (to quantify protein loss in patients with proteinuria)
5. Intravenous Urography
6. Renal Ultrasonography
7. Renal Biopsy

---

failure have many similarities and can occur simultaneously (chronic renal failure is a recognized predisposition for acute renal failure[11]), frequent serial determinations of serum creatinine concentration in addition to results from other laboratory tests may be needed to distinguish accurately between them. For example, in cats with acute renal failure, serum creatinine concentrations progressively rise over several days while serum creatinine concentrations are usually stable in cats with chronic renal failure during this period. Likewise, reduced kidney size (Figure 4) and renal osteodystrophy are indicative of long-term functional impairment and are evidence of chronic renal failure.

Distinction between acute and chronic renal failure is of value in predicting reversible from irreversible disease. Greater potential usually exists for reversibility of morphologic and functional renal impairment in patients with acute primary renal failure than in patients with chronic primary renal failure. In cases of acute failure, parenchymal regeneration typically has not had an opportunity to occur and compensatory and adaptive mechanisms of viable nephrons have not been expended. If the patient is kept alive by supportive therapy for a sufficient period for these processes to occur, the kidneys may regain an adequate quantity of function to maintain homeostasis.

In cases of chronic renal failure, however, compensatory and adaptive nephron changes are unlikely to occur. It may be assumed that additional parenchymal regeneration has had an opportunity to occur. The fact that signs of renal failure are present indicates the inadequacy of regenerative and compensatory processes.

Nonetheless, chronic renal failure does not always imply irreversibility of associated clinical signs and biochemical

<table>
<tr><td colspan="1">

TABLE XII
Some Potentially Reversible
Causes of Azotemia in Feline
Patients with Primary Renal Failure

Prerenal Causes
  Decreased Renal Perfusion
    Dehydration
    Cardiovascular dysfunction
    Severe hypoalbuminemia
    Hypoadrenocorticism
  Increased Urea Metabolism
    Gastrointestinal hemorrhage
    Extensive tissue necrosis
    High-protein diet
    Catabolic drugs
      Glucocorticoids
      Antineoplastic agents
      Tetracyclines (antianabolic?)
      Excessive thyroid supplementation

Primary Renal Causes
  Acute Tubular Necrosis
    Ischemia
      Prolonged hypovolemia
      Nonsteroidal antiinflammatory toxicity
      Thromboembolic disorders
    Nephrotoxins, including
      Aminoglycoside antibiotics
      Ethylene glycol
      Heme pigments
      Amphotericin B
      Cis-platinum
  Hypercalcemic Nephropathy
  Bacterial and Fungal Urinary Tract Infection
  Some Glomerulonephropathies
  Immune Disorders
  Adverse Drug Reactions
  Heat Stroke

Postrenal Causes
  Rent in Excretory Pathway
  Urinary Tract Obstruction
    Uroliths
    Operable neoplasms
    Herniated urinary bladder
    Blood clots
    Spay granuloma
    Others

</td></tr>
</table>

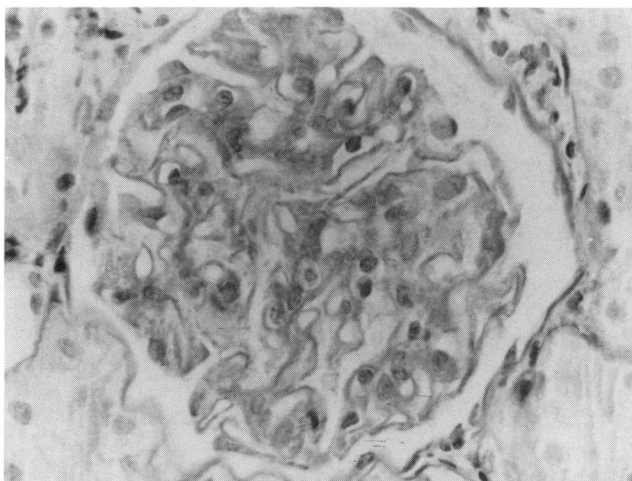

Figure 9—Photomicrograph of a kidney biopsy sample obtained from a nephrotic two-year-old Domestic Shorthair cat with membranous glomerulonephropathy associated with feline leukemia. Note the generalized thickening of glomerular capillary walls. (4-μm section, H&E stain, ×160 original magnification)

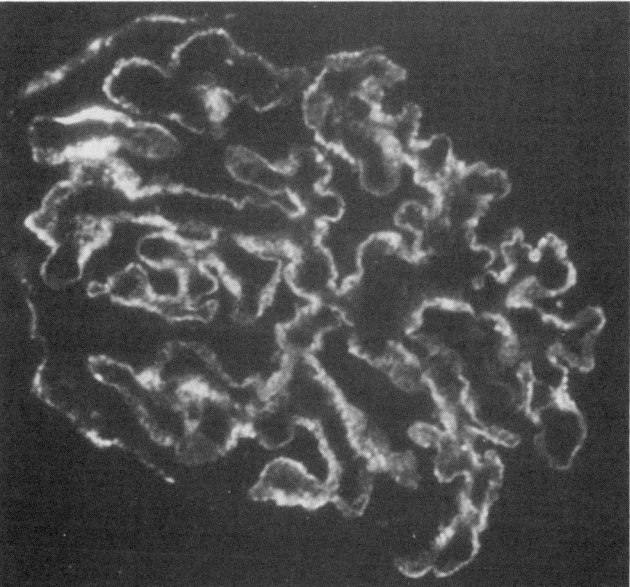

Figure 10—Immunofluorescent micrograph of the kidney biopsy sample shown in Figure 9. Fluorescein-labeled antibody with specific activity for feline γ-globulin (IgG) is localized in an interrupted granular pattern in glomerular capillary walls. (×160 original magnification)

abnormalities. Therapy designed to minimize abnormalities in fluid, acid-base, electrolyte, endocrine, and caloric balance (Tables XIII and XIV) may permit the patient to regain a comfortable state of existence for a period of months or years despite progressive loss of nephrons.

Determining the Severity of Renal Dysfunction

The chances for recovery decrease as renal functional capacity decreases and improve as functional capacity improves. Although estimation of the degree of renal dysfunction is initially of value in formulating prognosis, knowledge limited to early assessment of the functional state of the kidneys provides no information about the underlying cause and no information about potential reversibility of morphologic and functional impairment. Serial

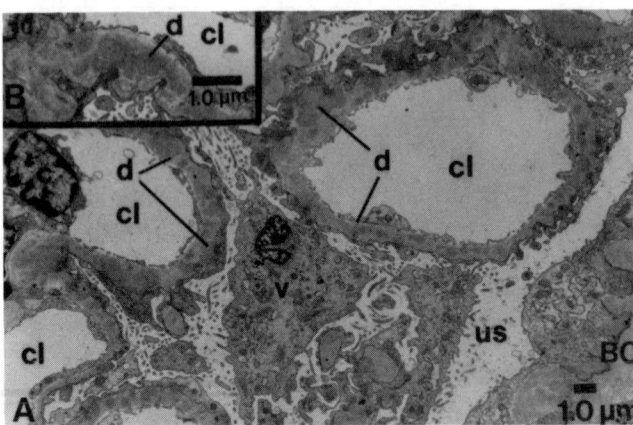

Figure 11—Electron micrograph of the kidney biopsy sample shown in Figure 9. (*A*) Low magnification of glomerular capillaries illustrating numerous electron-dense deposits (*d*) in glomerular basement membranes. There is generalized loss of foot processes because of swelling of visceral epithelial cell cytoplasm. *v* = visceral epithelial cell; *us* = urinary space; *cl* = capillary lumens; *BC* = Bowman's capsule. (*B*) Higher magnification of glomerular capillary wall containing numerous electron-dense deposits.

evaluation of renal function tests usually provides information of greater prognostic significance, as patient response to therapy and renal compensatory and regenerative processes can be judged by comparison of results of tests performed at different times.

How Can Therapy Be Improved?
Overview

One decade ago, we made the following statements regarding the treatment of renal failure in cats: "Many of the following recommendations are based on the therapy of renal failure in humans and dogs and on logic rather than results of controlled experimental and clinical trials. Therefore, their validity should be viewed as tentative pending further studies. Individualization of therapy within the guidelines outlined herein is essential. Therapeutic efficacy should be assessed by frequent reevaluation of the patient's physical condition and metabolic status."[19] Ironically these statements still apply today. We reiterate the need for properly controlled clinical trials to study various types of treatment advocated for cats with various types of renal failure.

Goals

Perhaps the most important conceptual goal in the treatment of feline renal failure is to strive to manage patients as we would ourselves. Specific goals for the treatment of renal failure are to (1) eliminate or minimize associated clinical signs; (2) correct deficits and excesses in fluid, acid-base, and electrolyte balance caused by renal failure

and minimize accumulation of metabolic wastes; (3) maintain adequate nutrition; and (4) stop or at least minimize the progression of further loss of renal function. Once renal failure has developed, no treatment will eliminate renal lesions. Although precipitating causes must be eliminated if further renal damage is to be prevented, the renal damage that has occurred must heal spontaneously over a period of days to weeks and/or the remaining viable nephrons must undergo compensatory adaptation if survival is to occur (Tables XV and XVI).

WITH INDIVIDUALIZED therapy designed and adjusted on the basis of patient evaluation, the quantity of renal function required to maintain homeostasis will be reduced. Some cats will regain sufficient renal function to maintain homeostasis without the need for long-term management (Table XII). In contrast, subclinical renal failure may remain undetected in many cats until it has progressed to an irreversible stage. For these patients, minimizing the adverse consequences of reduced renal function and their associated overtreatment are often adequate to maintain a satisfactory quality of life for months and sometimes years.

Correcting the Underlying Causes

Primary renal failure may be caused by a number of disease processes (i.e., anomalies and metabolic, neoplastic, nutritional, infectious, immune-mediated, ischemic, iatrogenic, toxic, traumatic, and obstructive processes) that have in common the destruction of greater than approximately three quarters of the parenchyma of both kidneys. By identifying the underlying causes, specific therapy can be formulated to stop further development of renal lesions by altering the underlying pathologic processes. Depending on the biologic behavior of disease, some forms of renal failure may be reversible (Table XII). For example, administration of antibiotics halts renal damage associated with bacterial infection; alleviation of obstructive uropathy mitigates parenchymal damage that could result in hydronephrosis; and correction of hypercalcemia minimizes the development of calcium-induced nephropathy. At the least, progression of renal lesions, and thus progression of failure, may be slowed or stopped by therapy designed to eliminate underlying causes. Therefore, diagnostic efforts directed especially at detecting reversible renal disease should be performed before formulating plans for conservative medical management.

Renal biopsy should be considered when knowledge of morphologic alterations in renal structure is likely to result in improved patient management. For example, detection of renal lesions secondary to polysystemic disease indicates the need for treatment of extrarenal disorders (Figures 9, 10, and 11). Retrospective analysis of morphologic renal lesions of 68 cats in our study revealed that 17 (25%)

TABLE XIII
Therapeutic Options for the Management of Renal Failure in Cats

Treatable Abnormality	*Clinical Correlates*	*Therapeutic Options*[a]
Negative fluid balance	Dehydration Vomiting/diarrhea Polyuria/nocturia Adipsia Hypernatremia Hyperproteinemia	Unlimited access to water If vomiting or unwilling to drink, consider parenteral fluid administration
Undernutrition	Weight loss attributable to tissue loss Hypoalbuminemia Proteinuria Leukopenia	Provide balanced diet to minimize deficits and excesses in fluid, acid-base, electrolyte, calorie, and endocrine balance and to minimize production of metabolic wastes Minimize anorexia (TABLE XIV)

Metabolic acidosis	Reduced serum concentrations of total CO_2 or HCO_3
	Decreased blood pH
		Dietary protein reduction
		  Prescription Diet® Feline k/d® (Hill's)
		  Homemade diets
		Avoid diets producing acidic urine
		Sodium bicarbonate (10 mg/kg every 8–12 hr)[b]
		Potassium citrate (40–60 mg/kg every 12 hr)[b]
		  (Caution: may enhance intestinal absorption of aluminum resulting in toxicity)

Hyperphosphatemia	Elevated serum phosphorus concentration
	Extraosseous mineralization
	Increased serum parathyroid hormone concentration
	Increased urinary fractional excretion of phosphorus
	Renal osteodystrophy
		Correct dehydration
		Dietary protein reduction
		  Prescription Diet® Feline k/d® (Hill's)
		  Homemade diets
		Intestinal phosphate binding agents
		  Aluminum hydroxide (30–90 mg/kg/day)[b] (Caution: use with citrate salts may enhance intestinal absorption of aluminum resulting in toxicity)
		  Calcium carbonate (100 mg/kg/day)[b]
		  Others

Hypoproliferative anemia	Typically normocytic, normochromic anemia
	Pale mucous membranes
	Anorexia
	Weakness
	Depression
		Minimize blood sampling
		Erythropoietin replacement[12]
		  Consider if hematocrit below ± 18%
		  Epogen (50–100 U/kg 3 times a wk); increase dose interval when hematocrit > ± 35%
		Androgen therapy (?)
		  Decanandrolin (1–1.5 mg/kg/wk); double dose if no response in 3 mth

Systemic hypertension	Increased arterial blood pressure Retinal lesions (hemorrhage, detachment, others)	Gradual dietary sodium reduction Enalapril (0.5 to 1 mg/kg every 12–24 hr)[b] Diltiazem (7.5 mg every 8–12 hr)[b] Propranolol (0.3 to 1.0 mg/kg every 8–12 hr)[b] Others Combinations

Hypokalemic	Muscle weakness
	Ventral neck flexion
	Decreased serum potassium concentration
		Oral potassium supplementation
		  Potassium gluconate (2–4 mEq every 8–12 hr)[b]
		  Potassium citrate (40–60 mg/kg every 12 hr)[b]
		Parenteral potassium supplementation[13]

Hypernatremia	Elevated serum sodium concentration Dehydration Depression	Correct dehydration Proper use of sodium-containing medications

TABLE XIII (Continued)

Treatable Abnormality	Clinical Correlates	Therapeutic Options[a]

Hyperkalemia	Oliguria/anuria
	Weakness
	Muscle trembling
	Electrocardiographic abnormalities
	   Spiked T waves
	   Reduced P waves
	   Bradycardia
	   Prolonged PR interval
		Correct dehydration with polyionic fluids containing
		   reduced quantities of potassium[14]
		Promote polyuria[11]
		Avoid potassium supplementation

Hypocalcemia	Decreased serum calcium concentration Muscle twitching	Verify absolute hypocalcemia[15] First correct hyperphosphatemia Oral calcium supplementation[b] Vitamin D therapy[16] Calcitriol (1.5–3.5 ng/kg/day)[b]
Hypercalcemia	Increased serum calcium concentration Polydipsia/polyuria Weakness Anorexia	Correct dehyration Correct hyperphosphatemia Others

Urinary tract infection	Microburia
	Pyuria, hematuria, proteinuria
	Positive urine culture
		Appropriate antimicrobial therapy
		Avoid nephrotoxic drugs (i.e., aminoglycosides,
		   amphotericin B)
		Adjust dose according to route of elimination and
		   degree of renal dysfunction

Progression of renal failure	Progressive decrease in creatinine
	   clearance
	Progressive increase in serum creatinine
	   concentration
	Progressive increase in the magnitude of
	   proteinuria
		Eliminate underlying causes of renal failure
		Correct reversible components of renal failure
		   Prerenal azotemia (TABLE XII)
		   Postrenal azotemia (TABLE XII)
		Minimize iatrogenic renal damage
		   Avoid nephrotoxic drugs
		   Avoid unnecessary urinary catheterization
		   Avoid unnecessary surgery of urinary system
		   Avoid unnecessary contrast radiographic procedures
		Dietary modification[17]
		   Provide only necessary quantities of high biologic
		     value protein
		   Minimize phosphorus
		   Gradual calorie reduction
		   Avoid saturated lipids
		   Others
		Avoid diets producing acidic urine
		Minimize hypokalemia
		Control hypertension

[a]Management options should be instituted sequentially and only if necessary.[18]
[b]Values represent starting dose, which should be adjusted on the basis of laboratory and clinical response

would likely have benefited from this additional information (Table IX). Specific therapy may have improved the quality of life for 11 cats with renal lymphosarcoma. Likewise, a morphologic diagnosis in six cats (two with glomerulonephritis, two with amyloidosis, one with metastatic pulmonary carcinoma, and one with thrombosis) may have prompted consideration of extrarenal causes for renal failure. For a majority of cats with a diagnosis of chronic gen-eralized nephritis, glomerulosclerosis, tubular necrosis, and polycystic kidney disease, however, biopsy results probably would not have altered management decisions substantially.

The role of renal biopsy in management of early renal disease and renal failure must be evaluated by prospective clinical trials before more specific generalities can be formulated. It is probable that early recognition of the under-

---

TABLE XIV
Checklist of Factors That May Minimize Nonemetic Uremic Anorexia

1. **Correct Underlying Abnormalities**
   (Minimize Deficits and Excesses in) Hydration
     Status
   Serum Concentrations of Nitrogenous Wastes
   Serum Electrolyte Concentrations
     Potassium
     Sodium
     Calcium
     Phosphorus
   Serum Hydrogen Ion Concentration
   Serum Concentrations of Hormones
     Parathyroid hormone
     Erythropoietin
     Vitamin D
     Angiotensin
     Renin
     Others

2. **Enhance Palatability of Diet**
   When Changing Diet
     Switch foods gradually
     Maintain texture and flavor similar to usual diet
   Try Flavoring Agents
     Clam juice
     Tuna juice
     Chicken broth
     Water
     Liquid elemental diets
       Feline RenalCare™ (Pet-Ag)
       Impact™ (Sandoz Nutrition) with taurine
         added
       Ensure® (Ross Laboratories) with taurine
         added
     Others
   Warm to Body Temperature

3. **Modify Feeding Patterns**
   Emphasize Frequent Small Meals
   Offer Rewards
     Favorite foods
     Maintenance foods
   Hand Feed
   Avoid Adverse Associations with Eating
     Medications
     Injections
     Others
   Prevent Food Aversion
     Do not offer diets designed for long-term
       management of renal failure during periods
       of nausea and vomiting

4. **Minimize Vomiting**
   Correct Underlying Abnormalities (see Number 1)
   Pharmacologic Antiemetics
     Metoclopramide (0.2–0.5 mg/kg every 12 hr)
     Cimetidine (2.5–5 mg/kg every 12 hr)

5. **Implement Pharmacologic Appetite Stimulation**
   Diazepam (0.2–0.3 mg/kg every 12 hr)
   Oxazepam (0.2–0.4 mg/kg every 24 hr)
   Cyproheptadine? (2–4 mg/kg every 24 hr)
   B Vitamins
   Anabolic Agents?

6. **Enteral Feeding**
   Hand Feeding
   Nasogastric Tube Feeding
   Gastrotomy Tube Feeding?

---

lying causes and pathophysiologic events leading to chronic generalized nephropathy so common in older cats may improve more effective treatment of them.

Differentiating Oliguric from Nonoliguric Renal Failure

Optimum therapy for feline renal failure should include both specific therapy directed at correcting underlying causes and supportive and symptomatic therapy designed to correct deficits and excesses in fluid balance, electrolyte balance, acid-base balance, nutritional balance, and accumulation of metabolic wastes. The primary goal of supportive and symptomatic therapy is to keep the patient alive until the processes of regeneration, repair, and compensatory adaptation allow the kidneys to regain sufficient function to maintain homeostasis. An effective form of specific therapy may be ineffective if not combined with appropriate supportive and symptomatic treatment. For patients with generalized irreversible renal disease, supportive and symptomatic treatment are designed to reestablish and maintain biochemical homeostasis despite ongoing renal dysfunction.

The primary reason for differentiating oliguric from nonoliguric primary renal failure is that they are associated with substantial differences in the type and magnitude of excesses and deficits of fluids and electrolytes. Patients with oliguric renal failure have a tendency to develop excesses of body fluids and several electrolytes. For example, in our study, 10 cats with oliguric renal failure (generally accepted as urine formation of < 0.5 ml/kg/hr) had marked excesses in serum concentrations of phosphorus, hydrogen ion, and potassium (Table XVII). Such data emphasize the potential for adverse reactions attributable to overzealous fluid and electrolyte therapy in patients with

TABLE XV
Seven Principles Guiding Treatment of Renal Failure in Cats

1. No therapy will eliminate renal lesions; renal lesions must heal spontaneously. The polysystemic metabolic and biochemical disorders caused by generalized renal lesions, however, may be modified or eliminated by appropriate therapy.
2. Detect and eliminate reversible nonrenal disorders that may have precipitated or aggravated a uremic crisis.
3. Evaluate the potential reversibility of renal disease and renal dysfunction with the knowledge that adequate renal function is not synonymous with total renal function.
4. Formulate specific therapy to eliminate or control underlying causes with the objective of preventing further renal destruction.
5. Formulate supportive and symptomatic therapy that minimize alterations in fluid, electrolyte, acid-base, endocrine, and nutrient balance and, therefore, sustain life until the processes of regeneration, repair, and compensatory adaptation allow the kidneys to regain adequate function to reestablish homeostasis. Formulate supportive and symptomatic therapy according to whether the patient has oliguric or nonoliguric primary renal failure.
6. Administer drugs to patients with renal failure only after consideration of their routes and rates of metabolism and elimination and their potential to induce adverse reactions in the uremic environment (TABLE XVI).
7. Avoid overtreatment.

TABLE XVI
Some Common Drugs That Should Generally Be Avoided in Cats with Renal Failure

1. Prophylactic Antibiotics (unless there is need for urinary tract catheterization)

2. Catabolic Drugs
   Glucocorticoids
   Antineoplastic agents
   Tetracycline (?)

3. Nonsteroidal Antiinflammatory Agents

4. Urine Acidifiers
   Ammonium chloride
   Methionine

5. Urinary Antiseptics
   Methenamine mandelate
   Nalidixic acid

6. Magnesium and Phosphorus-Containing Antacids

7. Nephrotoxic Drugs
   Aminoglycoside antibiotics
   Amphotericin B
   Cis-platinum

TABLE XVII
Serum Biochemical Abnormalities Identified in 10 Cats Admitted with Oliguric Renal Failure to the University of Minnesota Veterinary Teaching Hospital

Abnormality	Affected Cats		Mean	Range
	%	No.		
Azotemia				
Urea nitrogen (>35 mg/dl)	100	10 of 10	207.8	92 to 375
Creatinine (>1.9 mg/dl)	100	7 of 7	14.8	4.7 to 25.6
Hyperphosphatemia (>7.0 mg/dl)	100	7 of 7	16.4	8.3 to 45
pH (<7.30)	80	4 of 5	7.04	6.87 to 7.09
pH (<7.20)	80	4 of 5	7.04	6.87 to 7.09
Anion gap (>25)	71	5 of 7	37.02	25.3 to 59.2
Hyperkalemia (>5.3 mEq/L)	50	5 of 10	7.24	5.4 to 9.4
Hypokalemia (<3.5 mEq/L)	10	1 of 10	3.2	3.2
Hypercalcemia (>11.0 mg/dl)	22	2 of 9	12.6	12.3 to 12.8
Hypocalcemia (<8.5 mg/dl)	33	3 of 9	8.1	8.0 to 8.2
Hypernatremia (>159 mEq/L)	20	2 of 10	163	160 to 166
Hyponatremia (<145 mEq/L)	20	2 of 10	140.5	139 to 142

pathologic (not physiologic) oliguria. Once fluid and electrolyte deficits have been corrected, additional fluid therapy should be designed to replace continuing fluid losses from the urinary tract, contemporary losses from the gastrointestinal tract (vomiting and diarrhea), and insensible losses from the respiratory tract. Urinary and contemporary losses should be carefully replaced with a proper balance of rehydration and maintenance fluids. In the nonoliguric state, insensible losses have been estimated to be about 20 to 25 ml/kg/day but may vary with body temperature, air temperature, and humidity.[11] Appropriate adjustments of these values must be considered in patients with pathologic oliguria. Insensible fluid losses can be replaced with 5% dextrose in sterile water. Generally, parenteral fluids given to oliguric patients should contain little or no potassium but should contain sufficient quantities of other electrolytes to replace deficits and to provide daily requirements. The quantity of fluids administered should be adjusted so that body weight remains stable; in instances in which the patient is not receiving oral or parenteral calories, a slight but continuous loss of body weight occurs because of tissue catabolism. Significant increases in body weight usually reflect overhydration.

UNLIKE PRIMARY oliguric renal failure, primary polyuric renal failure is typically associated with excessive losses of fluid and several electrolytes (i.e., sodium, potassium, bicarbonate, and water-soluble vitamins). Supportive treatment of nonuremic polyuric patients that do not require parenteral forms of therapy should consist of conservative medical management (Table XIII). In general, this form of therapy is designed to maintain fluid, electrolyte, acid-base, and caloric balance by providing unlimited access to water, reducing the quantity of metabolic waste products to be excreted by the kidneys, and providing essential metabolites (electrolytes and vitamins) that the kidneys cannot efficiently conserve or that are affected by anorexia. Because uremic crises are complicated by anorexia and vomiting, parenteral forms of therapy are initially required to correct dehydration, hyperkalemia or hypokalemia, severe metabolic acidosis (serum total CO_2 concentrations < 10 to 12 mEq/L), and hypertension. Intensive management of uremic cats has been evaluated elsewhere.[14,20]

Modifying Therapy for Patients with Protein-Losing Glomerulonephropathy

A variety of recommendations for treating patients with glomerular proteinuria have been made. Some recommendations have been based on results of controlled studies, more have been based solely on logic, while many appear to have been based on the illogical concept that some form of therapy is better than none. Pending further studies, we

---

TABLE XVIII
Management of Protein-Losing Glomerulonephropathy

1. Strive to detect and eliminate underlying causes.

2. Consider dietary protein restriction.
   a. Goal is to minimize glomerular hyperfiltration.
   b. Consider initial intake similar to recommendations for renal failure.
   c. If needed, increase dietary protein gradually while monitoring serum albumin and urine protein-to-creatinine ratios.

3. Consider angiotensin-converting enzyme inhibitors.
   a. Goal is to minimize glomerular hyperfiltration.
   b. Consider enalapril at initial dosage of 0.5 to 1.0 mg/kg every 12–24 hr.
   c. In patients with decreased glomerular filtration (renal failure), dose may need to be reduced.
   d. Consider titrating dose according to blood pressure (< 180/95).

4. Avoid routine use of corticosteroids, as they may aggravate the magnitude of glomerular proteinuria.

5. Avoid routine use of nonsteroidal antiinflammatory agents.
   a. They may result in reductions in glomerular filtration, (especially in hypovolemic, hypoalbuminemic patients).
   b. Because of protein binding, accurate dosing may be difficult.

6. Avoid additional immunogenic stresses.
   a. Plasma or blood administration may potentiate immune-mediated glomerular disease.
   b. Immunogenic drugs (trimethoprim-sulfa, routine vaccinations, nonsteroidal agents, etc.) may augment immune-mediated phenomena.

7. Avoid diuretics only for cosmetic control of edema.

8. When giving drugs to patients with hypoalbuminemia, consider whether reduced protein binding of the drug will affect dose (e.g., aspirin).

9. Monitor response to therapy (TABLE XIX).

---

recommend a conservative approach to management of feline protein-losing glomerulonephropathy. As with all patients with renal failure, it is best to initiate therapy in a stepwise fashion, beginning with procedures likely to be beneficial and unlikely to be harmful (Table XVIII).

How Can Monitoring Be Improved?

If laboratory evaluation of renal function is the gold standard for diagnosis of renal failure, serial assessment of the patient's response is the silver bullet of therapy (Table XIX). The most common problem identified in feline renal failure patients referred to the University of Minnesota and in patients discussed during telephone consultations with

---

TABLE XIX
Therapeutic-Specific Data Base for Monitoring Renal Failure in Cats

Minimum Follow-Up Data
1. History Checklist
   a. Diet: Type? Compliance? Frequency of feeding? Willingness to eat? Quantity consumed? Supplements?
   b. Water consumption: Increased? Decreased? No change? Unknown?
   c. Micturition: Frequency? Quantity? Color? Odor?
   d. Amelioration of polysystemic signs
      Anorexia?   Weight loss?
      Vomiting?   Constipation?
      Diarrhea?   Others?
   e. Medication history: Medications given? When given? Dose? Compliance? Response?
2. Physical Examination Checklist
   a. Temperature, pulse, respiratory rate, and body weight?
   b. Amelioration of clinical signs
      Dehydration?
      Gastrointestinal signs?
        Mucosal ulcers? Discoloration of tongue?
      Cardiovascular signs
        Pale mucous membrane color?
        Abnormal pulse rate and character?
        Delayed capillary refill time?
        Venous distention?
        Elevated arterial blood pressure?
      Abnormal kidney size, shape, consistency, contour, pain?
3. Laboratory Data Checklist
   a. Urinalysis
   b. Kidney function tests (serum creatinine and urea nitrogen)
   c. Hematocrit, total plasma protein concentration (CBC?)

Problem-Specific Considerations
1. Urinary Tract Infection
   Quantitative urine culture
2. Protein-Losing Glomerulonephropathy
   Urine protein-to-creatinine ratio
   Serum albumin concentration
3. Obstructive Uropathy
   Ultrasonography or contrast radiography (intravenous urography, cystography, etc.) to verify continued patency of urinary tract
4. Divalent Ion Disorders
   Serum concentrations of phosphorus, calcium, parathyroid hormone (?), and 1,25 vitamin D (?)
   Evaluate for signs of osteodystrophy
     Loose or missing teeth?
     Enlargement of maxillary tissue?
     "Rubber jaw"?
5. Acidosis
   Serum concentrations of total CO_2, HCO_3, hydrogen ion (pH), and potassium (K)
6. Anemia
   Hematocrit
   Total plasma protein concentration
7. Hypertension
   Arterial blood pressure
   Ophthalmoscopic examination for retinopathies
     Detachment? Hemorrhage? Others?
8. Potassium Disorders
   Serum concentration of potassium
   Evaluate for signs of hypokalemia
     Muscle weakness
     Renal concentration
   Evaluate for signs of hyperkalemia
     Auscultate heart rate and rhythm
     Electrocardiogram

---

colleagues is related to the consequences of poorly controlled stereotyped treatment. At this time, it is our impression that the single most important factor that can aid most veterinarians in improving management of cats with renal failure is use of prospectively designed protocols to assess patient response to therapy. Because of the variable course of many cats with renal failure, treatment must be monitored and adjusted to meet changing needs. Cats with severe metabolic disturbances (i.e., marked dehydration, hyperkalemia, severe metabolic acidosis) may require frequent laboratory and clinical evaluation, whereas patients with less severe disturbances (i.e., minimal weight loss, mild anemia, mild hyperkalemia) generally require less frequent monitoring. The frequency of monitoring should be adjusted according to the trends observed and the clinical condition of each patient.

Use of a therapeutic-specific data base (Table XIX) allows early detection of complications (malnutrition and over- or undercorrection of deficits and excesses in fluid, electrolyte, and acid-base balance). The data base also allows assessment of, and likely improvement in, client and patient compliance with management protocols.

EPILOGUE

The major goals of this review are to increase awareness of the prevalence of renal failure in cats, especially with advancing age; identify risk factors that may aid in the diagnosis, prognosis, and treatment of renal failure; and identify questions deserving of future study. What is a reliable and reproducible clinical detector of renal failure that will aid in its early detection? Why do some breeds of cats appear to be more predisposed than others to renal failure? How can the relatively high prevalence of renal failure in aged cats be reduced? What are the underlying causes of chronic generalized renal disease in cats? When do the benefits of renal biopsy outweigh the risks? How can answers to these questions improve the veterinarian's ability to reverse or at least minimize the morbidity and mortality that are associated with most feline patients with this disorder? The answers to these and other questions can only be obtained by further study. We sincerely hope that all will support the efforts of those who have declared war on renal failure—feline enemy number 1.

About the Authors

Drs. Lulich, Osborne, and Polzin are associated with the Department of Small Animal Clinical Sciences and Dr. O'Brien with the Department of Veterinary Pathobiology at the College of Veterinary Medicine, University of Minnesota, Saint Paul, Minnesota. Drs. Lulich, Osborne, and Polzin are Diplomates of the American College of Veterinary Internal Medicine; and Dr. O'Brien is a Diplomate of the American College of Veterinary Pathologists.

REFERENCES

1. Fletcher RN, Fletcher SW, Wagner EN: *Clinical Epidemiology: The Essentials*, ed 2. Baltimore, Williams & Wilkins, 1988, p 77.
2. Osborne CA, Polzin DJ: Azotemia: A review of what's old and what's new. Part 1. Definition of terms and concepts. *Compend Contin Educ Pract Vet* 5:497–510, 1983.
3. Adams LG: Effects of reduced dietary protein in normal cats and cats with chronic renal failure. PhD Thesis. College of Veterinary Medicine, University of Minnesota, Saint Paul, Minnesota, 1991.
4. Ross LA, Finco DR: Relationship of selected clinical renal function tests to glomerular filtration rate and renal blood flow in cats. *Am J Vet Res* 42:1704–1710, 1981.
5. Brezis M, Rosen S, Epstein FH: Acute renal failure, in Brerner BM, Rector FC (eds): *The Kidney*, ed 4. Philadelphia, WB Saunders Co, 1991, p 1019.
6. Peterson ME, Greco DS, Orth DN: Primary hypoadrenocorticism in ten cats. *J Vet Int Med* 3:55–58, 1989.
7. Dow SW, Fettman MJ, LeCouteur RA, Narnar DW: Potassium depletion in cats: Renal and dietary influences. *JAVMA* 191:1569–1575, 1987.
8. Tyler RD, Quails CW, Neaid RD, et al: Renal concentration ability in dehydrated hyponatremic dogs. *JAVMA* 191:1095–1100, 1987.
9. Chew DJ, DiBartola SP, Boyce JT, Gasper PW: Renal amyloidosis in related abyssinian cats. *JAVMA* 181:139–142, 1982.
10. Arther JE, Lucke VM, Newby TJ, Bourne FJ: The long-term prognosis of feline idiopathic membranous glomerulonephropathy. *JAAHA* 22:731–737, 1986.
11. Polzin DJ, Osborne CA, O'Brien TD: Diseases of the kidneys and ureters, in Ettinger SJ (ed): *Textbook of Veterinary Internal Medicine: Diseases of the Dog and Cat*, ed 3. Philadelphia, WB Saunders Co, 1989, pp 1962–2046.
12. Cowgill LD: Clinical experience and use of recombinant human erythropoietin in uremic dogs and cats—Proceedings of the ninth annual veterinary medical forum. *Am Col Vet Med*:147–149, 1991.
13. Willard MD: Disorders of potassium homeostasis. *Vet Clin North Am [Small Anim Pract]* 19:241–259, 1989.
14. Cornelius LM: Fluid therapy in the uremic patient, in Kirk RW (ed): *Current Veterinary Therapy VIII [Small Anim Pract]*. Philadelphia, WB Saunders Co, 1983, pp 989–994.
15. Meuten DJ, Armstrong PJ: Parathyroid disease and calcium metabolism, in Ettinger SJ (ed): *Textbook of Veterinary Internal Medicine: Diseases of the Dog and Cat*, ed 3. Philadelphia, WB Saunders Co, 1989, p 1621.
16. Nagode LA, Chew DJ: The use of calcitriol in the treatment of renal disease of the dog and cat, in *Proceedings of Purina International Nutrition Symposium*. St. Louis, MO, Ralston Purina Co, 1991, pp 39–49.
17. Polzin DJ, Osborne CA, Adams LD, Lulich JP: Medical management of chronic renal failure—New concepts. *Proc XVI World Small Anim Vet Assoc*:477–481, 1991.
18. Polzin DJ, Osborne CA: Update—Conservative medical management of chronic renal failure, in Kirk RW (ed): *Current Veterinary Therapy IX [Small Anim Pract]*. Philadelphia, WB Saunders Co, 1986, pp 1167–1173.
19. Osborne CA, Polzin DJ: Conservative medical management of feline chronic polyuric renal failure, in Kirk RW (ed): *Current Veterinary Therapy VIII [Small Anim Pract]*. Philadelphia, WB Saunders Co, 1983, pp 1008–1019.
20. Low DC, Cowgill LD: Emergency management of the acute uremic crisis, in Kirk RW (ed): *Current Veterinary Therapy VIII [Small Anim Pract]*. Philadelphia, WB Saunders Co, 1983, pp 981–989.
21. Lulich JP, Osborne CA: Interpretation of urine protein-creatinine ratios in dogs with glomerular and nonglomerular disorders. *Compend Contin Educ Pract Vet* 12:59–72, 1990.

Control of Parathyroid Hormone in Chronic Renal Failure

KEY FACTS

- Supranormal levels of parathyroid hormone (a devastating uremic toxin) are present at the initiation of chronic renal failure before azotemia, hypocalcemia, and hyperphosphatemia are evident.
- In chronic renal failure, increased fractional excretion of phosphorus indirectly reflects elevated plasma parathyroid hormone levels.
- Early detection of excessive phosphate excretion and early medical intervention can prevent or slow the progression of secondary hyperparathyroidism.
- Medical management of hyperphosphatemia is based on modifying diet and giving oral phosphate binders.

University of Missouri-Columbia

Marilyn G. Mikiciuk, DVM

Veterinary Internal Medicine Center
Barrington, Illinois

Jerry A. Thornhill, DVM

Dogs AND CATS with chronic renal failure (CRF) can be medically managed. Early recognition and diagnosis, before signs of secondary hyperparathyroidism become clinically apparent, are necessary for long-term management of such patients. The goal of medical management is to control the uremic toxins that contribute to the syndrome of chronic renal failure.

Although there are many uremic toxins, parathyroid hormone apparently is the one with the most widespread and devastating effects. Extensive research in human medicine has documented that supranormal levels of parathyroid hormone are responsible for elevated calcium and phosphorus product, acidosis, neuropathies, electroencephalographic abnormalities, immunodeficiencies, uremic pruritus, bone pain, glucose intolerance, anemia, parathyroid hormone–induced skeletal resistance to vitamin D, and fibrosis of the kidneys. These features characterize chronic renal failure syndrome.[1–5]

Early renal failure in dogs and cats can be recognized by means of specific diagnostic procedures. Medical intervention before clinical signs of uremia are evident contributes to a higher quality, longer life for animals with the condition.

PHYSIOLOGY

Parathyroid hormone facilitates calcium and phosphorus absorption from the intestinal tract, calcium and phosphorus resorption from bone, renal calcium resorption and phosphorus excretion, and conversion of 25-hydroxycholecalciferol to 1,25-dihydroxycholecalciferol.[6] When renal function is normal, parathyroid hormone is primarily responsible for calcium absorption and phosphorus excretion. All except a small quantity of the blood calcium in the glomerular filtrate is reabsorbed in the proximal tubules and in the ascending Henle's loops.[6,7] In the distal tubules and the collecting duct, further reabsorption of the remaining calcium depends on the plasma calcium ion concentration.[6,7] The fraction of filtered calcium excreted daily ranges from 1.0% to 1.5%.[7]

Phosphorus, unlike calcium, is a threshold substance. When the serum concentration is below a critical level (approximately 1 mmol/L), phosphorus is not lost in urine.[6] With additional increases in the filtered load, however, proportional amounts of phosphorus are excreted.[6,8] When renal function is normal, phosphate intake equals output.[8] Sixty-five percent of phosphate is excreted by the kidneys; the remainder is excreted in the feces.[8] Fractional phosphorus excretion in dogs and cats ranges from 0.1 to 0.33 (10% to 33%).[9,10]

Vitamin D has a potent effect on increasing calcium reabsorption from the intestinal tract and plays an important role in bone deposition and resorption.[11] Before vitamin D can exert these actions, however, it must be converted (through successive reactions in the liver and kidneys) to the active product 1,25-dihydroxycholecalciferol. The rate-limiting step is controlled by parathyroid hormone, which stimulates the enzyme 1-α-hydroxylase in the kidneys.[11]

The rate of secretion of parathyroid hormone is controlled almost entirely by the plasma calcium ion concentration. Elevated plasma calcium ion concentrations thus reduce plasma concentrations of parathyroid hormone and 1,25-dihydroxycholecalciferol; reduced plasma calcium concentration results.[7,11]

IN CASES OF chronic renal failure, the glomerular filtration rate (GFR) decreases. Early stages of chronic renal failure are subclinical, and early decreases in the glomerular filtration rate are not evident in serum chemistry profiles.[12] Elevations in the serum urea nitrogen (SUN) are not recognized until approximately 75% of the renal mass is nonfunctional.[12,13] As the glomerular filtration rate decreases, serum phosphorus increases with a compensatory decrease in calcium. These changes cause an increase in parathyroid hormone as the metabolism attempts to restore serum calcium and phosphorus concentrations to normal.[9,14]

The progression of renal failure is concurrent with a decrease in the formation of 1,25-dihydroxycholecalciferol caused by decreased renal mass and by inhibition of 1-α-hydroxylase because of the increase in plasma phosphorus.[11,15,16] The decrease in 1,25-dihydroxycholecalciferol leads to decreased intestinal calcium absorption and decreased calcium resorption from bone.

The lowered serum calcium concentration further stimulates parathyroid hormone production, decreases calcitonin secretion, and increases 1-α-hydroxylase activity. This increase in plasma parathyroid hormone production promotes vitamin D–dependent calcium absorption in the intestines, stimulates calcium and phosphorus resorption from bone, stimulates 1-α-hydroxylase activity in the distal renal tubules, and inhibits phosphorus resorption in the proximal renal tubules.

Elevated plasma parathyroid hormone concentrations initiate phosphaturia; the metabolism of calcium, phosphorus, and vitamin D then returns to balance. In a progressive decrease in the glomerular filtration rate, these events are repeated; a new balance for calcium, phosphorus, and vitamin D is maintained at the expense of sustained supranormal parathyroid hormone levels.[12,14,16–18]

As renal function deteriorates, the amount of functional tissue mass and the glomerular filtration rate decrease. Plasma phosphorus concentrations do not return to normal. The insufficient 1,25-dihydroxycholecalciferol produced for calcium absorption leads to chronic mild hypocalcemia, hyperphosphatemia, and clinically advanced secondary hyperparathyroidism.

CLINICAL SIGNIFICANCE

In humans, dogs, and cats, supranormal concentrations of parathyroid hormone are directly and indirectly associated with the clinical signs of secondary hyperparathyroidism characteristic of chronic renal failure.[1–5,13,19] Early recognition of the condition enables the practitioner to initiate medical management before advanced disease stages are evident and to slow the rate of disease progression.[20–23]

DIAGNOSIS

Although detection of elevated plasma parathyroid hormone levels is possible, it is not routinely performed because of special handling requirements and laboratory availability. In a well-controlled research experiment in dogs,[14] Slatopolsky demonstrated that plasma parathyroid hormone levels increase as glomerular filtration rate decreases.

Glomerular filtration rate is determined by an endogenous or exogenous creatinine clearance test[24,25] (Figure 1). Normal creatinine clearance in dogs ranges from 2.0 to 4.0 ml/kg/min.[25] In cats, the range is 1.6 to 3.8 ml/kg/min.[25]

Fractional excretion of phosphorus (Fe_p) indirectly reflects elevated plasma parathyroid hormone levels. In cases of renal failure, fractional excretion of phosphorus is elevated earlier than serum phosphorus is.[10] To assess fractional excretion of phosphorus, serum and urine samples from fasted dogs or cats are required (Table I). In normal dogs and cats, the fractional excretion of phosphorus is usually 0.1 (10%) or less.[9] Values less than 0.3 (30%) are considered to demonstrate adequate phosphorus restriction,[9,10] but we strive for 10%.

MEDICAL MANAGEMENT

Medical management of secondary hyperparathyroidism entails restriction of dietary phosphorus and prevention of phosphorus absorption. We institute phosphorus restriction when the fractional excretion of phosphorus is increased; serum urea nitrogen and phosphorus might remain normal. Initially, a restricted-protein diet is instituted. Increases in metabolizable protein are proportional to increases in protein in the diet.[26] There are commercially prepared veterinary diets that restrict protein and phosphorus. Prescription Diet® Canine k/d® and g/d® and Feline k/d® (Hill's Pet Products) meet these requirements. Homemade recipes are also available.[26]

The fractional excretion of phosphorus is monitored to assess therapeutic results. Evaluated dogs and cats are handled as outpatients. If the fractional excretion of phosphorus remains elevated, phosphate binders can be instituted. Patients that refuse low-protein diets can be maintained with regular pet food and increased amounts of phosphate binders.

PHOSPHATE BINDERS in the form of aluminum hydroxide gel (Amphojel®—Wyeth Laboratories) or aluminum carbonate gel (Basaljel®—Wyeth Laboratories) are administered orally, preferably with meals. In dogs, aluminum hydroxide is given to effect. The recommended dos-

Serum creatinine$_1$ (mg/dl) _____

Serum creatinine$_2$* (mg/dl) _____

Urine creatinine (mg/dl) _____

Urine volume (ml) _____

Urine collection time (min) _____

Body weight (kg) _____

$$\text{Creatinine clearance} \ = \ \frac{\text{Urine creatinine}}{\text{Serum creatinine}} \ \times \ \text{Urine volume/min/kg}$$

$$\text{Fractional excretion of phosphorus} \ = \ \frac{\text{Urine phosphorus}}{\text{Serum phosphorus}} \ \times \ \frac{\text{Serum creatinine}}{\text{Urine creatinine}} \ \times \ 100$$

*Average of serum creatinine at initiation and completion.

Figure 1—Formulas for endogenous creatinine clearance and fractional excretion of phosphorus.

TABLE I
Signalment, Creatinine Clearance, and Fractional Phosphate Excretion Before and After Aluminum Hydroxide Therapy[a]

Signalment	Case			
	1	*2*	*3*	*4*
Breed	Chihuahua	Golden retriever	Mixed-breed dog	Domestic Longhair cat
Sex	Castrated male	Spayed female	Spayed female	Castrated male
Weight (kg)	6.3	32.7	24.0	4.2
Age (yr)	9.0	7.0	8.0	8.0
Creatinine clearance (% normal)	9.7	18.3	27.4	11.4
Laboratory Parameters	*Before/After*	*Before/After*	*Before/After*	*Before/After*
Serum creatinine (mg/dl)	5.7/4.9	1.9/1.8	1.0/1.2	6.8/6.1
Urine creatinine (mg/dl)	98.7/89.2	88.2/98.6	112/105	190.6/138.2
Serum phosphorus (mg/dl)	16.9/7.6	6.8/6.4	4.6/4.2	6.2/5.8
Urine phosphorus (mg/dl)	158/48.6	94.3/48.6	92.8/53.6	94.2/47.6
Fractional phosphate excretion (%)	53/35	28.4/13.8	18.8/14.6	54/36

[a]See text for dosages.

age to control hyperphosphatemia is 300 to 600 mg (5 to 10 ml) orally three times daily.[27] In cats, the recommended regimen is 30 to 90 mg/kg/day in divided doses.[13] Drawbacks include constipation and poor palatability.[9,13] Compounds that contain magnesium are avoided because magnesium excretion is believed to be altered in renal dysfunction.[13]

Aluminum toxicity has been reported in humans.[16,28-30] Clinical signs are bone pain, osteomalacia, microcytic anemia, and encephalopathy. Most patients depend on dialysis, however, and require a high concentration of aluminum in the dialysate bath. With dogs and cats, we have not found evidence of similar clinical signs of aluminum toxicity secondary to giving phosphate binders.

HYPOPHOSPHATEMIA must be avoided. Although acute hypophosphatemia does not usually produce clinical signs, prolonged hypophosphatemia does deplete total body stores of phosphorus. This depletion contributes to red cell lysis, deficient phagocytic and bactericidal capabilities of white blood cells, central nervous system abnormalities, and severe muscle disease.[31] One researcher observed a dog and a cat with acute hemolytic episodes that apparently resulted from hypophosphatemia; in another dog, central nervous system dysfunction was believed to be partially caused by hypophosphatemia.[31] Monitoring the serum phosphorus and fractional excretion of phosphorus and adjusting the dose of the phosphate binder accordingly are recommended.

Table I outlines the medical management of four cases of chronic renal failure. The three dogs (Cases 1 through 3) had been eating restricted-phosphorus diets for six months to one year before referral for renal failure. The cat (Case 4) had been eating a restricted-phosphorus diet mixed with a brand name cat food for one month before referral. Confirmation of chronic renal failure was based on serum creatinine values, hyposthenuria, and subnormal endogenous creatinine clearances as well as on radiographic and ultrasonographic evidence of kidneys that were small and fibrotic.

Aluminum hydroxide gel was administered with meals. Patient 1 received 300 mg (5 ml) twice daily; Patients 2 and 3 received 600 mg (10 ml) twice daily. The cat received 120 mg (2 ml) twice daily. The fractional excretion of phosphorus was again measured in three weeks. In Patient 1, the fractional excretion of phosphorus decreased from 53% to 35% while serum phosphorus decreased considerably (from 16.9 to 7.6 mg/dl). The dosage of aluminum hydroxide gel was increased to 420 mg (7 ml) twice daily; the dog was maintained on an ongoing basis at a fractional excretion of phosphorus level of 18%. In the cat, the dosage of aluminum hydroxide gel was increased to 150 mg (2.5 ml) twice daily.

ADDITIONAL MEDICATIONS

Other medications for controlling phosphorus absorption are used in humans with chronic renal failure. Calcium carbonate has been substituted for products that contain aluminum.[16,32,33] Various forms of vitamin D therapy are applied to humans with the disease.[15,26,34,35] Both of these therapeutic modes require further investigation in dogs and cats.

Another oral preparation used for its phosphate-binding properties is sucralfate (Carafate® Tablets—Marion Laboratories), a complex polyaluminum hydroxide salt of sulfate. Sucralfate's primary use is for peptic ulcers.[36] The agent is a suitable medication for intermittent chronic human dialysis patients because it normalizes serum phosphorus and thus corrects secondary hyperparathyroidism. The use of this drug in veterinary medicine needs more research.

Cimetidine (Tagamet®—Smith Kline & French), a histamine H_2-receptor antagonist, directly decreases parathyroid hormone secretion in dogs with experimentally induced uremia.[37] At therapeutic doses, cimetidine suppresses supranormal plasma levels of parathyroid hormone by a mechanism that is not fully understood.[38] Data suggest that the mode of action might be to impair synthesis or release of parathyroid hormone from the parathyroid glands or to decrease the total mass of the glands. Such data imply that there are histamine receptors in the parathyroid glands.[38] A study in dogs confirmed the direct decrease in parathyroid hormone secretion with cimetidine; this decrease led to diminished phosphorus loss from bone, increased 1-α-hydroxylase activity, increased 1,25-dihydroxycholecalciferol, and a positive calcium balance.[37]

Cimetidine also decreases the hypergastrinemia and gastric hyperacidity associated with chronic renal failure in dogs.[39] Studies in humans and dogs demonstrate that the major site of gastrin degradation is the kidneys; reduced gastrin clearance is thus apparent with chronic renal failure.[40-42]

As renal failure progresses, medical management fails to control secondary hyperparathyroidism. In humans, the parathyroid glands become autonomous and secrete parathyroid hormone uncontrollably.[43] Subtotal parathyroidectomy and renal transplantation are further forms of therapy in humans.[43-45] Renal transplantation might become available in veterinary medicine, but the procedure is unsuccessful in dogs with chronic renal failure.[46,47]

About the Authors

Dr. Mikiciuk, a Diplomate of the American Board of Veterinary Practitioners, is currently affiliated with the Angell Memorial Hospital, Boston, Massachusetts. When this article was submitted for publication, she was with the Department of Small Animal Medicine and Surgery, College of Veterinary Medicine, University of Missouri, Columbia, Missouri. Dr. Thornhill, a Diplomate of the American College of Veterinary Internal Medicine, is affiliated with the Veterinary Internal Medicine Center, Barrington, Illinois.

REFERENCES

1. Chesney RW, Mehls O, Anast CS, et al: Renal osteodystrophy in children: The role of vitamin D, phosphorus, and parathyroid hormone. *Am J Kidney Dis* 2(4):275–284, 1986.

2. Massry SG: Toxic effects of parathyroid hormone in uremia. *Semin Nephrol* 3(4):306–328, 1983.

3. Brickman A, Coburn JW, Norman AW: Action of 1,25-dihydroxy-cholecalciferol, a potent, kidney-produced metabolite of vitamin D, in uremic man. *N Engl J Med* 287(18):891–895, 1972.

4. Akmal M, Telzer N, Ansari A, et al: Erythrocyte survival in chronic renal failure. *J Clin Invest* 76:1695–1698, 1985.

5. Goldstein D, Chui L, Massry S: Effect of parathyroid hormone and uremia on peripheral nerve calcium and motor nerve conduction velocity. *J Clin Invest* 62:88–93, 1978.

6. Guyton AC: *Textbook of Medical Physiology*, ed 6. Philadelphia, WB Saunders Co, 1981, pp 973–986.

7. Agus ZS, Goldfarb S: Renal regulation of calcium balance, in Seldin DW, Giebisch G (eds): *The Kidney: Physiology and Pathophysiology.* New York, Raven Press, 1985, pp 1323–1333.

8. Knox FG, Haramati A: Renal regulation of phosphate excretion, in Seldin DW, Giebisch G (eds): *The Kidney: Physiology and Pathophysiology.* New York, Raven Press, 1985, pp 1381–1392.

9. Finco DR: The role of phosphorus restriction in the management of chronic renal failure of the dog and cat. *Proc 7th Kal Kan Symp*:131–133, 1983.

10. Krawiec D: Renal failure in immature dogs. *JAAHA* 23(1):101–107, 1987.

11. Ganong WF: *Review of Medical Physiology*, ed 12. Los Altos, CA, Lange Medical Publications, 1983, pp 318–328.

12. Bricker NS: On the pathogenesis of the uremic state. *N Engl J Med* 286(20):1093–1099, 1972.

13. Ross L: Feline renal failure, in Breitschwerdt EB (ed): *Contemporary Issues in Small Animal Practice*, vol 4. New York, Churchill Livingstone, 1986, pp 109–135.

14. Slatopolsky E, Calgar S, Pennell JP, et al: On the pathogenesis of hyperparathyroidism in chronic experimental renal insufficiency in the dog. *J Clin Invest* 50:492–499, 1971.

15. Korkor AB: Reduced binding of [³H] 1,25-dihydroxyvitamin D3 in the parathyroid glands of patients with renal failure. *N Engl J Med* 316(25):1573–1577, 1987.

16. Slatopolsky E, Weerts C, Lopez-Hilker S, et al: Calcium carbonate as a phosphate binder in patients with chronic renal failure undergoing dialysis. *N Engl J Med* 315(3):157–161, 1986.

17. Slatopolsky E, Bricker N: The role of phosphorus restriction in the prevention of secondary hyperparathyroidism in chronic renal disease. *Kidney Int* 4:141–145, 1973.

18. Arnaud C: Hyperparathyroidism and renal failure. *Kidney Int* 4:89–95, 1973.

19. Rutherford WE, Bordier P, Marie P, et al: Phosphate control and 25-hydroxycholecalciferol administration in preventing experimental renal osteodystrophy in the dog. *J Clin Invest* 60:332–341, 1977.

20. Polzin DJ, Osborne CA, Hayden DW, et al: Influence of reduced protein diets on morbidity, mortality, and renal function in dogs with induced chronic renal failure. *Am J Vet Res* 45(3):506–517, 1984.

21. Acchiardo SR, Moore LW, Cockrell S: Does low protein diet halt the progression of renal insufficiency? *Clin Nephrol* 25(6):289–294, 1986.

22. Slatopolsky E, Rutherford E, Hruska K, et al: How important is phosphate in the pathogenesis of renal osteodystrophy? *Arch Intern Med* 138:848–852, 1978.

23. Bricker NS, Fine LG: The trade-off hypothesis: Current status. *Kidney Int* 13:S5–S8, 1978.

24. Bovee KC: Glomerular filtration and the clearance concept, in Bovee KC (ed): *Canine Nephrology*. New York, Harwal Publishing Co, 1984, pp 76–79.

25. Ross LA: Assessment of renal function in the dog and cat, in Kirk RW (ed): *Current Veterinary Therapy. IX*. Philadelphia, WB Saunders Co, 1986, pp 1103–1107.

26. Lewis L, Morris M, Hand M: *Small Animal Clinical Nutrition. III*. Topeka, KS, Mark Morris Associates, 1987, pp 8-38–8-45.

27. Bovee KC: Conservative management of chronic renal failure, in Bovee KC (ed): *Canine Nephrology*. New York, Harwal Publishing Co, 1984, p 634.

28. Alfrey AC, Mishell JM, Burks J, et al: Syndrome of dyspraxia and multifocal seizures associated with chronic hemodialysis. *Trans Am Soc Artif Intern Organs* 18:257–261, 1972.

29. Pierdes AM, Edwards WG, Cullum UX, et al: Hemodialysis encephalopathy with osteomalacic fractures and muscle weakness. *Kidney Int* 18:115–124, 1980.

30. Short AI, Winney RJ, Robson JS: Reversible microcytic hypochromic anemia in dialysis patients due to aluminum intoxication. *Proc Eur Dial Transplant Assoc* 17:226–233, 1980.

31. Willard MD: Severe hypophosphatemia: Significance and treatment. *Proc 5th Annu Vet Med Forum ACVIM*:141–143, 1987.

32. Lerner A, Kramer M, Goldstein S, et al: Calcium carbonate—A better phosphate binder than aluminum hydroxide. *Trans Am Soc Artif Intern Organs* 32:315–318, 1986.

33. Taber T, Hegeman T, York S: Calcium carbonate as a phosphate binder in hemodialysis patients. *Trans Am Soc Artif Intern Organs* 32:127–129, 1986.

34. Buccianti G, Valenti G, Miradoli R, et al: Treatment of uremic osteodystrophy: A clinical trial with calcitonin, 25-hydroxycholecalciferol and 1,25-dihydroxycholecalciferol. *Dial Transpl* 10(6):523–526, 1981.

35. Slatopolsky E, Weerts C, Thielan J, et al: Marked suppression of secondary hyperparathyroidism by IV 1,25 (OH₂) D3 in uremic patients. *Kidney Int* 23:162, 1983.

36. Vucelic B, Hadzic N, Gragas J, et al: Changes in the serum phosphorus, calcium and alkaline phosphatase due to sucralfate. *Int J Clin Pharmacol Ther Toxicol* 24(2):93–96, 1986.

37. Jacob AI, Lambert PW, Canterbury JM, et al: Further studies with cimetidine in uremic dogs. *Kidney Int [Suppl]* 19:111, 1981.

38. Jacob AI, Lanier D, Canterbury J, et al: Reduction by cimetidine of serum parathyroid hormone levels in uremic patients. *N Engl J Med* 302:671–674, 1980.

39. Thornhill JA: Control of vomiting in the uremic patient, in Kirk RW (ed): *Current Veterinary Therapy. VIII*. Philadelphia, WB Saunders Co, 1983, pp 1022–1025.

40. Booth RA, Reeder DD, Hjelmquist U, et al: Renal inactivation of endogenous gastrin in dogs. *Arch Surg* 106:851–853, 1973.

41. Hallgren R, Karlsson FA, Lundqvist G: Serum levels of immunoreactive gastrin: Influence of kidney function. *Gut* 19:207–213, 1978.

42. Clendinnen BG, Reeder DD, Brandt EN, et al: Effect of nephrectomy on the rate and pattern of the disappearance of exogenous gastrin in dogs. *Gut* 14:462–467, 1973.

43. Fujimoto Y, Obara T, Ito Y, et al: Surgical treatment of secondary hyperparathyroidism in patients with chronic renal failure: Reevaluation of indications for parathyroidectomy. *Endocrinol Jpn* 32(6):863–874, 1985.

44. White KS, Wilkinson MD, Nixon WP, Almkuist WP: Total parathyroidectomy and forearm autotransplantation for chronic renal failure: A useful tool for the general surgeon in private practice. *South Med J* 79(7):844–846, 1986.

45. Sitges-Serra A, Gores P, Hesse U, et al: Serum calcium as an early indicator for surgical treatment of hyperparathyroidism after renal transplantation. *World J Surg* 10:661–667, 1986.

46. Finco DR, Barsanti JE: Organ transplantation in dogs: Present and future, in Kirk RW (ed): *Current Veterinary Therapy. IX*. Philadelphia, WB Saunders Co, 1986, pp 114–117.

47. Gregory CR, Gourley IM, Taylor NJ, et al: Preliminary results of clinical renal allograft transplantation in the dog and cat. *J Vet Intern Med* 1:53–60, 1987.

UPDATE

Adjunct control of parathyroid hormone oversecretion (which facilitates control of secondary hyperparathyroidism) has been accomplished with the application of low-dose calcitriol. Dosage range used in our clinic application has been 4 to 6 ng/kg body weight per day divided into two daily doses. Because the lowest strength calcitriol available, however, is the 0.25 µg capsule, it is necessary to fractionate the dosage from this capsule source. Calcitriol is an oil, and each capsule can be evacuated using a tuberculin syringe and proper dosage adjustment calculated at 1 µg = 1,000 ng.

In our experience, application of low-dose calcitriol has appeared to control secondary hyperparathyroidism in a majority of canine and feline patients. Fractional phosphate and fractional calcium excretion studies performed before and after the therapeutic management protocol have supported the efficacy of calcitriol administration.

Drug Metabolism in Renal Failure

Alexander Stern, Dr Med Vet*
Department of Veterinary
Medicine and Surgery
College of Veterinary Medicine
University of Missouri
Columbia, Missouri

Patients in renal failure (loss of greater than 70% of their functional renal nephrons) are often treated with a variety of drugs for both renal dysfunction and concurrent acute or chronic illnesses that may develop. These patients may have abnormal or unpredictable drug-induced reactions when normal drug doses or dosage intervals are used. Frequently these reactions are confused with the clinical signs of uremia and are not identified as being drug related.[1] The incidence of these toxic manifestations is probably underestimated because the symptoms are nonspecific. The disappearance of clinical signs following withdrawal of therapy is indicative of drug toxicity. Drug toxicity in patients with chronic renal failure results from the accumulation of a drug or its metabolites that normally would be partly or primarily excreted by the kidneys. The drug or its metabolites may also exacerbate kidney damage.[2,3]

This article provides a basic understanding of the mechanisms involved in adverse drug reactions induced by the altered pharmacokinetics in renal failure. Some practical guidelines for drug use in renal failure are also presented. Although most of the available information pertains to humans, adequate precautions should be taken when administering drugs to dogs and cats with kidney disorders until drug metabolism in these animals is better understood. The basic principles covered here apply to domestic animals, but some species variations may be observed.

Pharmacokinetic Principles

The onset, intensity, and duration of a drug's pharmacologic action are largely related to its plasma concentration. Pharmacokinetics are defined as factors that influence drug concentration in the plasma. These factors include drug absorption or bioavailability, distribution in the body fluids, biotransformation, and elimination (Figure 1).[3,4]

Absorption

Bioavailability is defined as the rate and extent of drug absorption into the systemic circulation. This determination is made by measuring the appearance rate and the peak plasma level of a drug after a single parenteral or oral dose.[3,4] The factors that influence the drug's bioavailability are blood flow, contact time, surface area of the absorption site, drug interactions, molecular size, nature of the drug formulation, dissociation constant (pK_a), and lipid solubility.[3,4] The intestinal membranes play a major role in determining bioavailability because more than 80%

*Dr. Stern's current address is Santa Anita Small Animal Hospital, Monrovia, CA.

Originally published in Volume 5, Number 11, November 1983

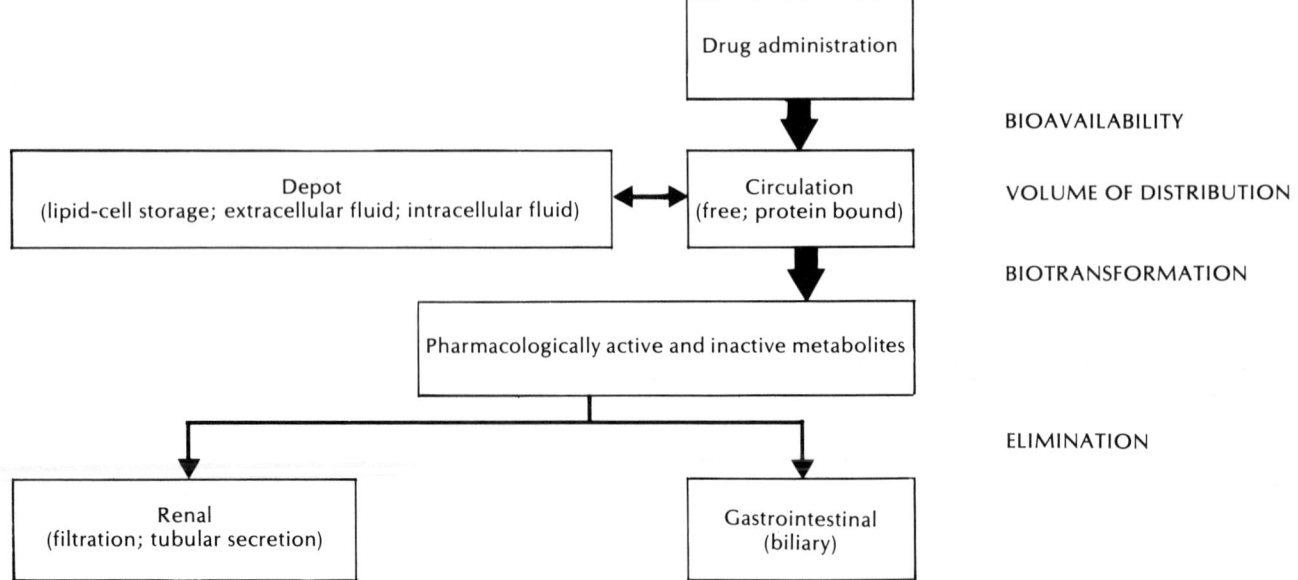

Figure 1—Schema of pharmacokinetics.

of drugs are given orally.[5] This intestinal barrier is semipermeable; it allows the absorption of some products but retards the absorption of others. Absorption may be either passive or active. Most drugs, especially those of small molecular size and high lipid solubility, are absorbed passively. Passive absorption requires no energy and is not retarded by metabolic inhibitors. Drugs may also be transported across the intestinal wall by specific carriers in the lipoprotein membranes of intestinal cells. These carriers can be competitively inhibited, and they use energy for transport. The number of carriers available for any given drug is limited, so there is a maximum rate of absorption.[6] Little information is available on the effects of chronic renal failure on drug bioavailability and on the numerous physiologic abnormalities that may alter the characteristics of the gastrointestinal absorption of drugs given orally. A decreased diuretic effect of oral as compared with intravenous furosemide occurs in uremia, for example, but the cause of this decreased bioavailability is unknown. Gastrointestinal "edema" in uremic patients may be responsible.[7]

Volume of Distribution

Once absorbed, a drug is distributed from the blood to the extravascular fluid space in a reversible process that continues until the drug concentration in the plasma and tissue is equal. The volume of distribution is primarily determined by a drug's lipid solubility (its ability to penetrate tissues) and its plasma-protein-binding characteristics. Lipid-soluble drugs have a large volume of distribution and penetrate cells more easily. Other drugs, such as penicillin, are highly protein bound, are often restricted to the extravascular com-

partment, and thus have low volumes of distribution. Protein binding acts as a depot for a drug and prevents large fluctuations in the concentration of the unbound, active drug in body fluids. Impaired protein binding in patients with renal disease results from (1) a decrease in serum albumin combined with a decrease in the binding capacity of the albumin site because of a change in molecular configuration, or (2) from an accumulation of endogenous inhibitors.[5] These endogenous inhibitors are thought to be small molecules that are retained in uremia and competitively displace drugs from their normal binding sites.[8]

The frequency of adverse drug reactions often increases in patients with impaired protein binding or hypoalbuminemia.[9] An abnormal amino acid composition of albumin in uremic plasma has been identified,[10] but this finding alone does not explain impaired binding ability. In the nephrotic syndrome without uremia, a decreased plasma protein binding of phenytoin and clofibrate is observed with hypoalbuminemia.[11] In addition, a correlation exists between side effects resulting from prednisone and a serum albumin concentration of <2.5 g/dl.[12] Most of the drugs that demonstrate abnormal protein binding in the presence of renal failure are organic acids. Organic bases usually display normal protein binding (Table I). Investigators have suggested that the diminished protein binding of organic acids is related to their tendency to bind to a single site on serum albumin, whereas organic bases usually bind albumin at more than one site.[8] The peak concentration of a drug is higher in patients with impaired binding. An increase in the free fraction of the drug in the plasma will cause more severe drug-related side effects by increasing the intensity of the pharmacologic effect.[13]

TABLE I

PLASMA PROTEIN BINDING OF
SELECTED DRUGS IN UREMIA[4,8,21]

Decreased	*Unaffected*
Barbiturates (A)	Chloramphenicol (B)
Diazepam (B)	Dapsone (B)
Furosemide (A)	Indomethacin (A)
Morphine (B)	Quinidine (B)
Penicillin (A)	Propranolol (B)
Phenylbutazone (A)	Trimethoprim (B)
Sulfamethazine (A)	

A = organic acids
B = organic bases

The factors that influence intrarenal antibiotic distribution are the state of hydration, the significance of antibiotic binding to renal tissue, drug pK_a, and the role of urinary pH. In general, it is difficult to predict the intrarenal distribution of an antibiotic because factors other than plasma concentration and renal clearance seem to exert significant influences on drug accumulation in the various renal regions. The hydropenic state enhances the corticopapillary gradient of several antibiotics—in particular the penicillins, cephalothin, and, to a lesser degree, the sulfonamides. The drug concentrations follow this sequence: penicillin G > carbenicillin > ampicillin = cephalothin. The hydrated state will markedly reduce the urinary concentration of all antibiotics. Penicillins, cephalothin, kanamycin, oxytetracycline, and the sulfonamides are reduced or washed out from the renal parenchyma during water diuresis. As urine pH increases, the ionized fraction of weak acids increases, reabsorption decreases, and renal clearance increases. For weak bases, the ionized fraction and renal excretion increase as the urine pH decreases. Alkaline urine increases ampicillin concentrations in the renal medulla and papilla. Acid urine increases sulfasoxazole in the papilla. The presence of severe renal disease significantly changes the intrarenal pharmacokinetics of antibiotics and is associated with reduced tissue concentrations of all drugs.[14]

Biotransformation

The majority of drugs are not excreted unchanged. Rather, they are biotransformed to metabolites, which are then excreted. Renal failure may alter the biotransformation rate of drugs and slow the excretion rate of the final metabolites. However, the elimination rate of most drugs metabolized by microsomal oxidations is normal in most patients with renal failure.[15] The biotransformation of drugs occurs in two phases (Figure 2). Most oxidative biotransformation reactions occur in hepatic cells by enzymes found in the smooth endoplasmic reticulum. The result is the formation of more polar and less lipid-soluble metabolites that are more easily excreted than the parent drug.[16] Metabolites of drugs may be pharmacologically active or inactive. Additionally, the kidney may also contain active enzyme systems capable of metabolically activating drugs. The kidney is a primary site of drug exposure because it receives 25% of the cardiac output and contains specialized transport processes for concentrating and secreting drugs.[17] This metabolic activation may be involved in the pathogenesis of several drug-induced renal disorders. Small doses of cephalosporins, for example, cause alterations in the proximal tubular brush border and larger doses cause massive tubular necrosis.

The major renal metabolic pathway of oxidation followed by conjugation is normal in humans with renal failure but is slowed in uremic animals.[18-20] Conjugations with glucuronic acid, sulfate, and glycine seem normal but acetylations are often slow. Additionally, hydrolysis seems slowed.[21] The effects of renal failure on the biotransformation and elimination of selected drugs are shown in Table II. If the clinician is familiar with the major pathway of metabolism and elimination, it is possible to predict the probable effect of uremia or chronic renal failure on a drug's rate of elimination.

Elimination

Drugs are divided into three classifications according to their route of elimination. The first group of drugs is those primarily eliminated via the kidneys (Table III). The half-lives of these drugs increase with the successive fall in the glomerular filtration rate. A second group of

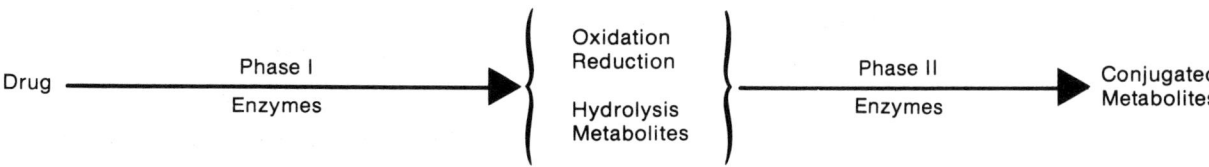

Figure 2—Schema of biotransformation.

TABLE II

EFFECTS OF RENAL FAILURE ON THE ELIMINATION
OF METABOLIZED DRUGS[21]

Drug	Reaction	Elimination Rate
Digitoxin		Normal to rapid
Lidocaine		Normal to rapid
Meperidine	Oxidation	Normal
Barbiturates		Normal
Phenytoin		Rapid
Propranolol		Normal to rapid
Cortisol	Reduction	Slowed
Chloramphenicol		Normal
Sulfasoxazole	Synthesis	Slowed
Salicylate		Normal
Glucagon		Slowed
Insulin	Hydrolysis	Slowed
Cephalothin		Slowed

drugs is those eliminated partly by the kidneys and partly by metabolism. The half-lives of these drugs are prolonged, but not to the extent of drugs eliminated primarily by the kidneys. The third classification is drugs eliminated by biochemical pathways. The half-lives of these drugs remain unchanged despite any changes in the glomerular filtration rate.[22] The risk of retention concerns only those substances that are excreted primarily by the kidneys.

The rate of renal elimination is based on extrarenal and renal considerations. The extrarenal influences are (1) the percent of protein-bound drug (protein-bound drugs are not filtered at the glomerulus unless there is a protein-losing nephropathy); (2) the volume distribution (drugs with large volume distributions are not available for renal elimination); and (3) the rate of biotransformation (rapid drug metabolism reduces significant renal excretion of the unchanged drug).[3] Renal influences on drug clearance depend on (1) the renal blood flow, which determines the delivery of the drug to the kidneys; (2) the glomerular filtration rate, which determines the entry of the drug into the tubular fluid and is unidirectional; and (3) tubular transport, which involves active and passive secretion and reabsorption.[3,23]

Two tubular transport systems that show some degree of structural specificity are present—one for organic acids and one for organic bases. These systems are highly dependent on renal blood flow, yet are not significantly affected by the degree of protein binding. Tubular secretion can be competitively inhibited by drugs with similar structures that use the same transport mechanisms. Probenecid, for example, inhibits the tubular secretion of penicillin and cimetidine, and trimethoprim inhibition of serum creatinine secretion results in an increased serum creatinine and a decreased creatinine clearance.[24,25]

Mechanisms of Drug Toxicity

Drug metabolism pathways have been considered "detoxification" mechanisms in the past. This term implied that the products of biotransformation have no pharmacologic activity. Although this may be true of many drug metabolites, others do have pharmacologic activity. The causes of drug toxicity resulting from renal failure relate only to those drugs that are eliminated by renal pathways. These factors include nephrotoxicity of the parent drug or its metabolite, altered sensitivity, and the metabolic load of the drug.

Numerous drugs have an affinity for serum proteins that allows them to participate in the proximal tubular transport system. The result is an increased intracellular or intraluminal concentration of the drug in the proximal segments of the nephron. Mechanisms of drug-mediated cellular injury or death may occur through the uncoupling of the mitochondrial respiratory chain or by modifying enzymatic activity sufficiently to disrupt cellular metabolism. Lipophilic drugs can interact directly with the plasma membrane, leading to permeability changes that can impair osmoregulation and result in cell swelling and death. Hydrophilic drugs either interact with membrane carrier systems or passively diffuse through pores and cause cellular injury or death.[2,26] Researchers have postulated that the action of the countercurrent multiplier may account for the accumulation of abnormally high concentrations of analgesics, which may be responsible for papillary necrosis.[27] Whatever the mechanism involved, the end result is the acute exacerbation of an already compromised renal function. Clinicians must remember that kidneys suffering from nephropathy have an increased sensitivity to nephrotoxic drugs. The factors that predispose the kidneys to nephrotoxic injury are summarized in Table IV.

Patients with chronic renal failure have an increased

TABLE III

SELECTED DRUGS WITH
PRIMARY RENAL EXCRETION[4,15,21]

Ampicillin	Kanamycin
Carbenicillin	Methotrexate
Cephalothin	Procainamide
Digoxin	Streptomycin
5-fluorocytosine	Tetracycline
Gentamicin	Tobramycin

TABLE IV

FACTORS PREDISPOSING KIDNEYS
TO NEPHROTOXICITY[26]

Large endothelial surface

Large filtration area

Large negative charge

Organic acid or base transport systems

Medullary countercurrent multiplier

Distal tubule acidification

systemic sensitivity to the undesirable side effects of drugs that cannot be explained by altered biotransformation or reduced elimination alone. Factors incriminated in this increased sensitivity are (1) a functional or morphologic modification of drug receptors; (2) an increase in permeability in the blood–brain barrier, which probably contributes to the drug sensitivities seen in uremic patients; and (3) the possible enzyme activity disturbances found in renal failure, such as the deficiency of acetylcoenzyme A.[28]

Metabolic Load

Certain drugs may result in substantial metabolic loads in patients with chronic renal failure or uremia (Table V). These effects are deleterious in a patient with an already precarious fluid or electrolyte status.

Principles of Drug Use in Renal Failure

Some simple guidelines can reduce the number of adverse drug reactions in renal patients:

1. A drug should be used only when specific indications exist.
2. The clinician must become familiar with the pharmacologic and potential toxic side effects of drugs used.
3. Creatinine clearances, when available, or serum creatinine levels can be used for dosage modification.
4. Modified dosage schedules that have been previously established in renal patients can be used if such schedules are available.
5. A clinician *must* monitor the pharmacologic effects of any drugs used.

TABLE V

METABOLIC LOADS OF SELECTED DRUGS[3]

Sodium	Ampicillin	3.0 mEq/g
	Cephalothin	2.5 mEq/g
	Carbenicillin	4.7 mEq/g
	Penicillin G	1.7 mEq/10^6 IU
Potassium	Penicillin G	1.7 mEq/10^6 IU
	Spironolactone	
	Triamterene	
Acidosis	Carbenicillin	
	Methenamine mandelate	
	Nitrofurantoin	
	Ammonium chloride	
	Acetazolamide	
Alkalosis	Carbenicillin (large dose)	
	Penicillin G (large dose)	
	Viomycin	
Increased blood urea nitrogen	Androgenic steroids	
	Glucocorticoids	
	Tetracyclines	
Fluid retention	Cyclophosphamide	
	Phenylbutazone	
	Vincristine	

Modification of Dosage

If drug accumulation and toxicity are to be avoided in the patient with reduced renal function, dosage modifications are necessary. Most dosage adjustments involve decreasing the amount or the frequency of the maintenance schedule. Failure to make the appropriate adjustments results in a buildup of drug (Figure 3).

Drugs that are excreted 100% unchanged via the kidneys can be altered according to the following formula:

> Dose interval for
> renal failure patient = normal dose interval
>   × normal creatinine clearance/
>   patient creatinine clearance.

An alternative is to reduce the dose and keep the interval the same:

> Dose for
> renal failure patient = normal dose
>   × patient creatinine clearance/
>   normal creatinine clearance.

It is unclear which method is best. For drugs with a wide therapeutic index, either method is probably satisfactory. Lengthening the dosing interval causes large fluctuations in the plasma levels and results in periods of potential toxicity and periods of subtherapeutic levels (Figure 4A). Bacteriostatic antibiotics with longer half-lives are best given by this method. Wide ranges in plasma drug levels may be reduced by using a smaller maintenance dose than normal and the normal dosing interval (Figure 4B). The advantage of this method is the safety afforded by a more constant plasma concentration, but it often results in subtherapeutic levels. Bactericidal antibiotics with short half-lives can be given according to this type of dosage schedule.[4]

Most drugs are not excreted in an unchanged form by the kidneys; metabolism plays a major role in their

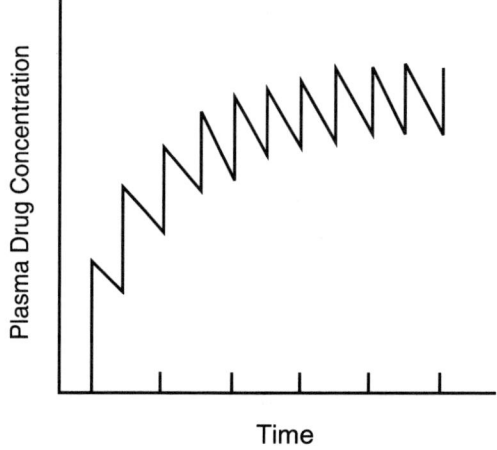

Figure 3—Multiple doses of a drug result in an accumulation rate equal to the half-life.

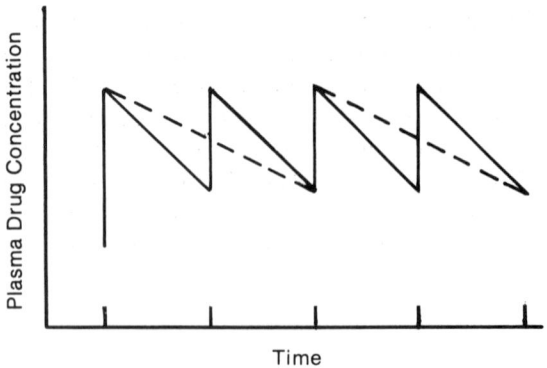

Figure 4A

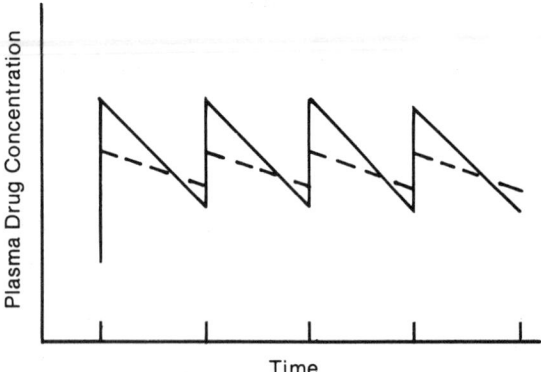

Figure 4B

Figure 4—Plasma drug concentration in normal (*solid line*) versus uremic patients (*broken line*). (**A**) Results of drug interval adjustment. (**B**) Results of drug dosage adjustment.

elimination. In these cases, reduction of renal function will cause an increase in the half-life, but not to the extent of that seen with drugs excreted totally by the kidneys. The following formulas may be used to calculate dosage adjustment:

Dose interval for
renal failure patient = normal dose interval
$$\times\ 1/f(Kf-1)+1$$

Dose for
renal failure patient = normal dose
$$\times\ f(Kf-1)+1/1$$

where

f = the fraction of the absorbed dose normally eliminated in an unchanged form by the kidneys and

Kf = a measure of the patient's renal function divided by the normal creatinine clearance.

To make use of the latter two formulas, the fraction of the drug excreted unchanged by the kidneys must be known. Unfortunately, this information is not readily available in clinical veterinary medicine.

In view of the fact that renal disease represents a dynamic state, serial creatinine clearances are necessary to determine the progression or regression of the dys-

function. These determinations are time consuming and reflect only the renal function at given periods of time. Estimations of the clearance rate vary with the methodology used, and a standardization of the method and the normal values needs to be established.[29]

An alternative is to use serum creatinine concentrations, which are more easily obtained, to modify drug dosages. The following formula can be used as a guide for calculating the drug dosage:

Dose interval for
renal failure patient = normal dosage interval
$$\times\ \text{serum creatinine}$$
$$\text{concentration.}$$

The interval adjustment becomes necessary only when the serum creatinine concentration is >2.5 to 3.0 mg/dl.[23] A linear relationship probably exists between serum creatinine and the endogenous creatinine clearance in animals with stable renal function, but this has not yet been established for the various degrees of renal dysfunction in veterinary medicine.

Many of the methods available for monitoring drug levels in humans are not yet feasible in veterinary medicine. Direct assay of the plasma drug concentration is often expensive and not readily available. In addition, reference ranges of drugs being assayed are needed for animals. Drugs that can be assayed include digoxin, thyroid hormone, and phenobarbital. Drug elimination rates are not always known in veterinary medicine, especially in cases of renal dysfunction. Additionally, various nomograms have been established for use in patients with renal disease,[30-34] but their application to veterinary medicine has not been reported. The use of drugs in humans with chronic renal failure has been widely studied.[35-37]

Conclusion

When treating patients with renal failure, the clinician should use drugs that are not influenced by renal dysfunction, if possible. In cases where nephrotoxic drugs or drugs excreted by the kidneys must be used, dosages or intervals should be modified based on endogenous creatinine clearances or serum creatinine levels. The patient should also be monitored for any possible undesirable side effects.

REFERENCES

1. Smith JW, Seidle LG, Cluff LE: Studies on the epidemiology of adverse drug reactions. V. *Ann Int Med* 65:629-640, 1966.
2. Drayer DE: Active drug metabolites and renal failure. *Am J Med* 62:486-489, 1977.
3. Henrich WL, Anderson RJ: Drug use in renal failure. *Post Grad Med* 64(5):153-163, 1978.
4. Muther RS, Bennett WM: Drug metabolism in renal failure, in Brenner B, Stein J (eds): *Contemporary Issues in Nephrology VII: Chronic Renal Failure.* New York, Churchill, 1981, pp 287-323.
5. Gibaldi M: Drug distribution in renal failure. *Am J Med* 62:471-474, 1977.

6. Rowland M: Drug absorption, in Melmon KL, Morelli HF (eds): *Clinical Pharmacology: Basic Principles in Therapeutics.* Toronto, Macmillan Co, 1978, p 48.

7. Huang CM, Atkinson AJ, Levin N, et al: Pharmacokinetics of furosemide in advanced renal failure. *Clin Pharmacol Ther* 16:659-666, 1977.

8. Reidenberg MM: The binding of drugs to plasma proteins and the interpretation of measurements of plasma concentrations of drugs in patients with poor renal function. *Am J Med* 62:466-470, 1977.

9. Boston collaborative drug surveillance program. Diphenylhydantoin side effects and serum albumin levels. *Clin Pharmacol Ther* 14:529-532, 1973.

10. Boobis SW: The alteration of plasma albumin in relation to decreased drug binding in uremia. *Clin Pharmacol Ther* 22:147-153, 1977.

11. Gugler R, Shoeman DW, Huffman DH, et al: Pharmacokinetics of drugs in patients with the nephrotic syndrome. *J Clin Invest* 55:1182-1189, 1975.

12. Lewis GP, Jusko WJ, Burke CW, et al: Prednisolone side effects and serum protein levels. *Lancet* 2:778-780, 1971.

13. Levy G: Effect of plasma protein binding of drugs on duration and intensity of pharmacologic activity. *J Pharm Sci* 65:1264-1265, 1976.

14. Whelton A, Walker WG: Intrarenal antibiotic distribution in health and disease. *Kidney Intl* 6:131-137, 1974.

15. Reidenberg MM: The biotransformation of drugs in renal failure. *Am J Med* 62:482-485, 1977.

16. Mandel HG: Pathways of drug biotransformation, in LaDu BN, Mandel HG, Way EL (eds): *Fundamentals of Drug Metabolism and Drug Disposition.* Baltimore, The Williams & Wilkins Co, 1971, pp 131-145.

17. Mitchell JR, McMurtry RJ, et al: Molecular basis for several drug-induced nephropathies. *Am J Med* 62:518-526, 1977.

18. Lichter M, Black M, Arias IM: The metabolism of antipyrine in patients with chronic renal failure. *J Pharmacol Exp* 187:612-619, 1973.

19. Dundee JW, Annis D: Barbiturate narcosis in uremia. *Br J Anaesth* 27:114-123, 1955.

20. Leber HW, Schutterle E: Oxidative metabolism in liver microsomes from uremic rats. *Kidney Intl* 2:152-158, 1972.

21. Reidenberg MM, Drayer DE: Drug therapy in renal failure. *Ann Rev Pharmacol Toxicol* 20:45-54, 1980.

22. Dettli L: Individualization of drug dosage in patients with renal disease. *Med Clin North Am* 58:977-985, 1974.

23. Senoir DF: Drug therapy in renal failure. *Vet Clin North Am* 9(4):805-817, 1979.

24. Burgess E, Cutler RE, Blair AD: Cimetidine pharmacokinetics in hemodialysis patients and inhibition of creatinine secretion in healthy subjects. *Clin Pharmacol Ther* 27:247, 1980.

25. Berglund F, Killander J, Pompeuis R: The effect of trimethoprim-sulfamethoxazole on renal excretion of creatinine in man. *J Urol* 114:802-808, 1975.

26. Porter GA, Bennett WM: Nephrotoxin-induced acute renal failure, in Brenner BM, Stein JH (eds): *Contemporary Issues in Nephrology VI: Acute Renal Failure.* New York, Churchill, 1980, pp 123-162.

27. Kincaid-Smith P: Pathogenesis of the renal lesion associated with the abuse of analgesics. *Lancet* 1:859-862, 1967.

28. Fabre J, Balant L: Renal failure, drug pharmacokinetics and drug action. *Clin Pharmacokin* 1:99-120, 1976.

29. Bovee KC, Joyce T: Clinical evaluation of glomerular function: 24 hour creatinine clearance in dogs. *JAVMA* 174:488-492, 1979.

30. Bryan CS, Stone WJ: Antimicrobial dosage in renal failure: A unifying nomogram. *Clin Nephrol* 7:81-84, 1977.

31. Dettli L: Drug dosage in renal disease. *Clin Pharmacokin* 1:126-134, 1976.

32. Dettli L, Spring P, Habersang R: Drug dosage in patients with impaired renal function. *Post Grad Med* 46:32-35, 1970.

33. Spring P: Calculation of drug dosage regimens in patients with renal disease: A new nomographic method. *Int J Clin Pharmacol* 11(1):76-80, 1975.

34. Tozer TN: Nomogram for modification of dosage regimens in patients with chronic renal function impairment. *J Pharmacokin Biopharm* 2:13-28, 1974.

35. Bennett WM, Singer I, Golper T, et al: Guidelines for drug therapy in renal failure. *Ann Int Med* 86:754-783, 1977.

36. Bennett WM, Muther RS, Parker RA, et al: Drug therapy in renal failure: Dosing guidelines for adults. Part I: Antimicrobial agents, analgesics. *Ann Int Med* 93:62-89, 1980.

37. Bennett WM, Muther RS, Parker RA: Drug therapy in renal failure: Dosing guidelines for adults. Part II: Sedatives, hypnotics and tranquilizers; cardiovascular, antihypertensive and diuretic agents; miscellaneous agents. *Ann Int Med* 93:286-325, 1980.

Developmental Aspects of Fluid and Electrolyte Metabolism and Renal Function in Neonates

KEY FACTS

- The ability to excrete a solute load is impaired early in life.
- In comparison with adults, neonates consume more energy and require more water relative to their body mass.
- Increased body temperature imposes a proportionately greater burden on water balance in neonates, which have relatively greater surface losses than do adults.
- The greater body water content and extracellular fluid compartment size and lower body fat content and circulating plasma protein levels in neonates affect the volumes of distribution of many drugs.
- Because of renal immaturity, the elimination of many drugs or drug metabolites is limited in neonates.
- Because of their uniquely mature renal clearance and excretory functions, neonatal calves benefit from large-volume, high-solute fluid replacement.

Colorado State University
Martin J. Fettman, DVM, MS, PhD

Mark Morris Associates
Topeka, Kansas
Timothy A. Allen, DVM

NEONATAL animals are, in general, more susceptible to derangements in fluid and electrolyte metabolism than are adults of the same species. This is particularly true of diseases of the gastrointestinal tract, whether they result from infectious, nutritional, or metabolic causes. Comparative limitations in renal clearance and resorptive functions in neonates may contribute to progressive fluid dyshomeostasis and complicate treatment. Species differences in the development of renal function may further complicate the accurate estimation and replacement of fluid and electrolyte deficits in newborns.

The purpose of this review is to characterize differences in renal function between neonates and adults and to demonstrate the application of such knowledge to practical fluid therapy. Species differences are emphasized where appropriate.

PERINATAL DEVELOPMENT OF THE KIDNEY

The mammalian urinary system develops through three phases, beginning with the pronephros, a transitory structure located cranially in the body of the embryo.[1-3] The mesonephros is larger, develops caudad to the pronephros, and actually attains some function through the first few weeks of fetal life.[2] The final developmental stage, the metanephros, arises in part from the mesonephros and in part from undifferentiated intermediate mesoderm (metanephric blastema).[1-3] The former gives rise to the ureteral bud, which later develops into the system of drainage ducts, including the ureter, papillary ducts, straight collecting tubules, and (in appropriate species) the pelvis or calyxes. The nephron develops from the calyxes. Simultaneous to the development of the metanephric tubules, a renal artery grows from the aorta, giving rise to numerous branches that form the afferent arterioles, glomerular capillary tufts, efferent arterioles, and peritubular capillary system and ultimately drain into the renal venules and vein.[1]

The metanephros undergoes three phases of growth and development.[3] During the first, the nephrogenic phase, metanephric tubules undergo differentiation, giving rise to the nephrons that will serve the individual throughout adult life. This period ceases by term in humans, lambs, and guinea pigs.[3-5] By contrast, nephrogenesis continues beyond birth for approximately three weeks in dogs and pigs and four to six weeks in rats.[3,6-8]

The next period of renal development is the phase of histologic and functional development, during which renal blood flow, glomerular filtration rate, and tubule function mature. In calves, this process is close to completion at birth,[9] whereas several weeks to months may be required in other species and as much as one year in human infants before mature function is attained.[7] In the final phase of development, growth takes place without further histologic or biochemical maturation, although differences in growth rate among the segments of each nephron may alter final function significantly.[3,10,11]

NEPHRON DEVELOPMENT and growth starts in the juxtamedullary region and proceeds centrifugally toward the outer cortex of the kidneys.[5,6] Thus, deep nephrons are the first to reach maturity; the nephrons in the outer cortex are progressively less mature. Although all nephrons undergo the same three metanephric phases of maturation, significant differences exist in regional renal function, thus resulting in developmental heterogeneity.

RENAL BLOOD FLOW AND GLOMERULAR FILTRATION

Renal blood flow increases immediately after the umbilical cord is severed; that is, when the newborn's kidneys must assume the excretory functions previously performed by the placenta. The greater the placental blood transfusion, the more replete is the neonate's circulatory volume and hence the greater is initial renal blood flow.[12] Thereafter, the development of renal blood flow depends on cardiac output and the fraction perfusing the kidneys.[7] Kidney perfusion depends, in turn, on renal vascular resistance relative to systemic arterial pressure.

In piglets, cardiac output increases approximately sevenfold during the first seven weeks of life.[7] Combined with an 86% decrease in renal vascular resistance, renal blood flow may increase as much as 18-fold.[7] In puppies, renal blood flow reportedly almost triples between one day and one month of age (0.70 to 1.80 ml/min/g of kidney weight) and triples again between 6 and 16 weeks of age (1.2 to 3.5 ml/min/g of kidney weight).[8,13] In infants, fully one year may pass before renal blood flow reaches adult values (relative to body mass).[7] Changes in renal vascular resistance must contribute significantly to the increase in renal blood flow. Turgid regulatory cells of the juxtaglomerular apparatus in the afferent arterioles reportedly obstruct glomerular blood flow immediately after birth.[14] As these cells disappear, afferent blood flow increases. In addition, as the

renal vasculature grows, the arterial lumina increase in diameter, thus contributing to a decrease in renal vascular resistance.[15]

Owing to the centrifugal development of nephrons in neonatal kidneys, inner cortical blood flow is much higher at birth than is outer cortical flow because of the higher number of mature nephrons and higher blood flow in individual nephrons.[6,10] With maturation, a gradient of increased blood flow from the juxtamedullary region to the outer cortex develops. Although the increases in glomerular perfusion may match those in cardiac output initially, the development of outer cortical perfusion eventually overtakes that of cardiac output, so that by two to three months in lambs,[4] one to two months in dogs and guinea pigs,[5,10,11] and one month in rats,[8] a mature pattern of distribution of intrarenal blood flow is achieved.

In puppies, for example, total renal blood flow may increase fivefold between the first and second weeks of life.[11,16] During the first week of life, the cortex is perfused homogeneously; but during the second week, a narrow band consisting of 15% of cortical mass develops, receiving about 20% of total renal blood flow.[11,16] Outer cortical flow continues to increase and reaches adult values at 6 to 10 weeks, when this highly perfused area consisting of 40% of cortical mass receives approximately 3.4 times the blood flow as the inner cortex or as much flow as the inner cortex and medulla combined.[11,16,17]

Increases in glomerular filtration with maturation depend, in turn, on changes in renal blood flow, systemic blood pressure, and development of intrinsic morphologic and functional properties of the glomeruli themselves. Increases in the number of glomeruli, capillary surface area, permeability, and perfusion pressure all contribute to increases in the total glomerular filtration rate of the kidney; these increases exceed the increases in cardiac output and mean arterial pressure.[6-8,10-17] Postnatal nephrogenesis contributes to the increase in glomerular filtration rate in piglets, rats, or puppies but not in species with a complete set of glomeruli at birth. Although the total potential glomerular filtration area of all nephrons combined increases with age relative to kidney or body mass, the diameter of the neonatal glomerulus may be fully one third greater than is that of the adult.[6,7,18] Thus, the volume of individual glomeruli is not a likely contributor.

INTRINSIC CHANGES in glomerular permeability and autoregulation of transglomerular capillary pressure contribute to the maturation of glomerular filtration in neonates.[7] In guinea pigs, mean arterial pressure increases by 50% during the first seven weeks of life whereas glomerular capillary pressure more than doubles.[19] Intratubular hydrostatic pressure and intracapillary colloid osmotic pressure double as well, but the difference in their absolute values leads to a two- to threefold increase in effective filtration pressure (5.3 to 12.6 mm Hg) over this period. This increase in filtration pressure is, however, coupled with a 20-fold increase in glomerular filtration rate.[19] Although changes in the permeability coefficient (K_f) have not been directly determined, a significant change in glomerular permeability probably accompanies these other factors.

Just as nephron development and intrarenal blood flow mature in a centrifugal pattern, so does single-nephron glomerular filtration rate (SNGFR). Between two hours and 38 days of age, the glomerular filtration rate of the entire kidney in guinea pigs increases from 0.19 to 1.31 ml/min, whereas the glomerular filtration rate of superficial nephrons increases from 0.92 to 19.32 ml/min.[5] During the first 15 days of life, the average increase in the single-nephron glomerular filtration rate was 0.48 ml/min/day in comparison with 0.21 ml/min/day for superficial nephrons.[5] During the remainder of the first month, however, the glomerular filtration rate of single, superficial nephrons increased 0.97 ml/min/day in comparison with 0.71 ml/min/day for the entire kidney.[5] Thus, deep nephrons assume most of the function of the kidneys shortly after birth and are soon thereafter replaced by accelerating maturation of superficial nephrons. Interestingly, this increase in the glomerular filtration rate of superficial nephrons correlates well with increases in the length and function of proximal tubules.[5] The significance of this increase to changes in glomerulotubular balance may be important.

During the early neonatal period, autoregulation of renal blood flow in response to acute changes in systemic arterial pressure is not as efficient as it is in adults.[13,20] There is a good correlation between developmental increases in arterial pressure and renal blood flow; however, the rate of perinatal growth and changes in intrinsic glomerular function apparently are more important in determining renal blood flow.[8,20] In other words, renal perfusion is directly responsive to increases in arterial blood pressure but this responsiveness may be related to immaturity of the autoregulatory reflexes.[13]

Glomerulotubular balance, the match between solute filtration and tubular modification of filtrate, is not present at birth for selected solutes in different species.[5,21] Traditionally, this phenomenon in neonates has been attributed to preponderance of glomeruli in relation to tubule development.[3,7,21] Just as there is a centrifugal gradient of nephron development, renal blood flow, and glomerular function, there is a gradient for morphologic and functional maturation of the renal tubules. As described, increases in the glomerular filtration rate of superficial nephrons may be directly related (either through cause or effect) to growth in length and functional development of proximal tubules.[5,7,15,22] One hypothesis states that immature function of proximal tubules in neonates leads to less resorption of filtered solute than in adults and a greater solute load in the distal tubule.[5]

Despite lower autoregulatory sensitivity, this osmotic burden then activates the macula densa, thus leading to increased renin secretion by the juxtaglomerular apparatus. The increased rate of renin release would lead to more angiotensin II production, which in turn would mediate afferent arteriolar constriction, thus restricting glomerular perfusion pressure and filtration rate. Glomerulotubular balance may therefore mediate in part the high intrarenal vascular resistance characteristic of neonates. Angiotensin II produced as a result of this imbalance may directly effect mesangial cell contraction as well as changes in glomerular surface area and permeability for filtration.

PROXIMAL TUBULE FUNCTION

A major function of the epithelium of proximal renal tubules is extraction of organic compounds from the peritubular capillary blood for secretion into the urine. This function is the basis for the estimation of effective renal blood flow by the rate of clearance of such organic acids as *p*-aminohippuric acid (PAHA) or such organic bases as tetraethylammonium bromide (TEA).[23] If extraction by the proximal tubules approaches 100%, the clearance of these solutes represents an estimate of effective perfusion of the tubules. Large discrepancies between actual measured renal blood flow and effective renal blood flow have, however, been noted in neonates of some species and attributed to decreased solute extraction by the tubules.[23-25]

In dogs, tetraethylammonium bromide extraction is extremely low at birth and progressively increases to adult values by nine weeks of life.[23] Extraction of *p*-aminohippuric acid, by contrast, is more efficient at birth. In pigs, extraction of tetraethylammonium bromide and *p*-aminohippuric acid is low during the first two weeks of life and increases progressively for the following six weeks.[23] As expected, centrifugal development of these functions is noted as well, with inner cortical function exceeding outer cortical until four weeks of age.[23]

BETWEEN THREE days and three weeks after birth in rats, the clearance of inulin (glomerular filtration rate) increases sevenfold whereas the clearance of *p*-aminohippuric acid triples.[24] The extraction efficiency of *p*-aminohippuric acid simultaneously increases threefold.[24] Because renal plasma flow changes comparatively little relative to kidney weight while glomerular filtration rate increases markedly, filtration fraction increases. Similarly, in puppies, *p*-aminohippuric acid extraction has been reported to increase from between 40% and 50% at six weeks to between 75% and 85% at 14 weeks, which is comparable to that of an adult.[25] Because there are significant differences in postnatal nephrogenesis between these species, any generalized interpretations of maturational changes in tubule function are difficult.

In infants less than 34 weeks gestational age at birth, creatinine clearance is 0.45 ml/min, increasing to 1.01 ml/min between 34 and 37 weeks gestational age and 2.24 ml/min from 38 to 41 weeks gestational age.[26] During these time periods, fractional resorption of glucose progressively increases from 92.5% to 99.2% and 99.4%, respectively.[26] Alpha amino nitrogen (free amino acid) clearance similarly decreases by approximately 50% between 34 and 41 weeks of age.[26] In puppies between 18 hours and 40 days of age, however, glomerular filtration rate increases significantly while the ratio of maximum tubular resorption of glucose to inulin clearance actually decreases significantly from 4.22 to approximately 3.0 (adult levels).[21] This finding implies that glucose resorption, which is a tubule function, matures before glomerular filtration. The finding may, however, reflect increased utilization of glucose by the tubule epithelium and does not necessarily reflect functional maturation of tubular transport processes.

PUPPIES up to three weeks of age may develop a much greater osmotic diuresis in response to the same solute concentration than do adult dogs.[27] This finding has been attributed to the inability of puppies to generate and sustain a significant transtubular sodium gradient to counter the gradient produced within the tubules by the diuretic solute.[27] In addition, less-tight intercellular junctions in the epithelium of the proximal tubules of neonatal kidneys contribute to significant back-leakage, thus further impairing generation of a transtubular sodium gradient.[28,29] The enhanced diuretic effect declines during the first few weeks of life as the length of the proximal tubules and the activity of sodium-potassium-adenosinetriphosphatase increase toward levels observed in adults.[27]

Immature function of distal nephrons and lower circulating aldosterone levels contribute to the neonate's relative inability to conserve sodium.[30] Fractional excretion of sodium decreases significantly from 14.3% in 100- to 125-day-old lamb fetuses to 0.73% in the three- to eight-day-old lambs, thus corresponding to increases in the length and function of the loops of Henle, plasma renin activity, circulating aldosterone concentrations, and enhanced responsivity of distal tubules to mineralocorticoid modulation.[30]

The physiologic acidosis present in neonates of some species results, in part, from a lower renal bicarbonate threshold than is present in adults.[31] In infants, the threshold may be as low as 21.5 mmol/L. The maximum rate of bicarbonate resorption (2.6 to 2.9 mmol/dl of glomerular filtrate) is identical to that of adults, thereby implying normal transport capacity with an immature setpoint.[31]

In one study, resorption of phosphate by proximal tubules of infants 0.5 to 12 months of age was compared with that of children 1 to 15 years of age.[32] The infants consistently demonstrated higher plasma phosphate concentrations, urinary phosphate excretion, and endogenous phosphate clearance than did the older children. Higher plasma phosphate concentrations had previously been attributed to increased growth rates, transient hypoparathyroidism, or the higher phosphorus content of cow's milk in comparison with human milk.[32] Rates of tubular phosphate resorption in infants were approximately 60% of those in children.[32] Plasma phosphate and fractional phosphate resorption in both groups, however, were closely correlated.[32]

This relationship indicates that although children have a higher phosphate resorption capacity than infants have, lower rates of glomerular filtration in infants maintain higher plasma phosphate concentrations. In other words, infants have mature tubule function with regard to phosphate transport but (because of reduced glomerular filtration rates) maintain a higher plasma phosphate concentration.[32] This phenomenon may not occur in other species because urinary acidification studies in dogs have demonstrated significantly lower urinary phosphate excretion in neonates than in adults.

ACID-BASE REGULATION

Excretion of hydrogen ions by the kidneys occurs by three mechanisms.[33] The first is proton secretion and subsequent neutralization by tubule fluid bicarbonate, thus resulting in carbon dioxide formation; uptake by tubule epithelial cells; and regeneration of bicarbonate for resorption. The second is through the excretion of secreted protons in combination with bases present in the filtrate, such as phosphate and sulfate. This combination is titratable acid and is limited by the quantity of filtered base delivered to the site of proton secretion in the distal tubules.

The final process involves trapping of secreted protons by combination with ammonia (NH_3) in the tubular fluid. The ammonium (NH_4^+) thus formed is trapped in tubule fluid and secreted as a salt (e.g., ammonium chloride [NH_4Cl]). Because bicarbonate reclamation in the proximal tubules occurs by isohydric proton transport, no net gradient may be established. Similarly, because titratable acidity is limited by rates of conjugate anion clearance, net acid secretion by the kidneys is regulated chiefly through their capacity for ammoniagenesis in response to acidosis.[33] Thus, studies comparing neonatal and adult renal acidification capacity rely heavily on changes in rates of renal ammoniagenesis as well as urine pH and titratable acidity.

NUMEROUS in vitro studies have demonstrated significant differences in renal ammoniagenesis between neonates and adults. Kidney slices from 5- to 13-day-old rats were shown in vitro to consume less oxygen and produce less ammonia in response to an acidic medium pH than their 6- to 12-month-old adult counterparts.[34] Similar in vitro studies revealed impaired ammoniagenesis in kidney slices from puppies up to two weeks of age compared with those from adult dogs. Little difference between kittens and adult cats was observed in this study.[34]

In vivo studies conducted by administering an ammonium chloride or ammonium sulfate bolus to dogs and puppies showed that neonates developed a more severe systemic acidosis and were less able to increase renal ammoniagenesis, secrete protons, or acidify urine.[35] Administration of 0.16-M ammonium chloride or 0.08-M ammonium sulfate $(NH_4)_2SO_4$ as an aqueous solution at 2% of body weight along with water at 3% of body weight resulted in a significant decrease in blood pH within 30 minutes in neonates and adult dogs. In adults, blood pH declined to 7.10 and returned to 7.40 (baseline value) within six hours; whereas the puppies' blood pH decreased to 7.00 and increased to no more than 7.20 (in comparison with 7.40 before acidification). Urinary pH in adults started at 5.50, decreased to 4.50 within one hour, and returned to 5.00 within 1.5 hours of ammonium chloride administration. In puppies, urine pH also started at 5.50, did not decrease to 4.50 for four hours, and returned to 5.00 at five hours, thereby demonstrating a delay in onset of acid excretion and the limited quantity of acid that could be voided.

Urinary phosphate excretion, which reflects titratable acidity, increased over six hours in the adult dogs from 0.4 to 0.5 mmol/kg/hr while changing only from 0.03 to 0.05 mmol/kg/hr in the puppies. Urinary ammonia excretion similarly changed more dramatically in adults (0.5 to 0.6 mEq/kg/hr) than in the puppies (0.03 to 0.05 mEq/kg/hr). After six hours, adult dogs had excreted 61.2% of their acid equivalents from ammonium chloride and 79.8% from ammonium sulfate whereas puppies had excreted only 1% of that amount. Puppies were able to excrete only about 40% of the administered fluid volume in comparison with 80% in adult dogs.[35]

ACIDIFICATION tolerance tests of pigs with an oral ammonium chloride challenge similarly demonstrated a defect in renal ammoniagenesis and capacity to secrete hydrogen in urine in one- to two-day-old piglets in comparison with those 10 to 12 weeks of age.[36] After eight hours, newborn piglets excreted only 5.3% of the acid load as urinary ammonium whereas adults were able to excrete 13.5% as ammonium. Neonates were also unable to excrete more than 14.7% of the chloride load in eight hours in comparison with 50.7% in mature animals.

DISTAL NEPHRON FUNCTION
Renal Concentration Capacity

Although most neonates are born with the capacity to concentrate or dilute urine and respond appropriately to solute or volume loading, these responses are far less capable than in adults. In 10-day-old rats, medullary interstitial intercellular material is more abundant, renal tubule epithelium is cuboidal with fewer basal in-foldings and less functional surface area, the Henle's loops have not completely descended into the medulla, specialized fornices of the renal pelvis are just appearing, and outer medullary vasa recta bundles are less well developed than in adults.[37] As a result of this morphologic immaturity, neonates are unable to dilute distal nephron fluid maximally; this incapacity limits the ability to generate hypotonic urine and to accumulate solute in the medulla. The latter limits the degree to which urine may be concentrated.

TEN-DAY-OLD rats are virtually incapable of accumulating additional urea in the medulla in response to an exogenous urea load.[37] By 20 days of age, rats can respond to urea loading; and increased papillary solute concentrations allow them to concentrate urine to at least 1400 mOsm/L, in comparison with only 900 mOsm/L at 10 days of age.[37] In all, sodium accumulation in the medulla increases 1.4-fold and urea accumulation 1.7-fold.[37] Urine-to-plasma osmolality ratios increase in this 10-day span from 3.0 to 4.8.[37] In dogs between 2 and 77 days of age, the urine-to-plasma osmolality ratio may increase from 2.0 to 7.0 and is associated with increased urea retention, more efficient sodium resorption, and descent of Henle's loops into the medulla.[15]

Response to Volume or Solute Loading

The ability to excrete a solute load is also impaired early in life. Up to approximately three weeks of age, puppies are able to excrete only 10% of an isotonic saline load within two hours of administration in comparison with up to 50% in adult dogs.[38,39] Despite reduced sodium resorption capacity in the proximal tubules, puppies are unable to decrease fractional sodium resorption by the whole nephron below 98%.[38] In adults, fractional sodium absorption may decrease to 94% in response to a saline load.[39]

In dogs 1 to 23 days of age, the contribution of the proximal and distal tubules to this functional change was studied through distal nephron blockade induced by ethacrynic acid (a loop diuretic) and chlorothiazide (a distal-tubule diuretic).[39] One and a half hours after an intravenous saline load, fractional sodium resorption in normal puppies was 98.5%. With distal blockade, resorption was reduced to approximately 50%. During distal blockade, changes in filtered sodium load produced by varying glomerular filtration rate demonstrated a close correlation between filtered and resorbed sodium, thus indicating that the neonatal distal tubule is normally incapable of rejecting an increased sodium load.[39,40] The inability of neonatal kidneys to respond appropriately to saline loading provides another example of immature glomerulotubular balance.

INAPPROPRIATELY high circulating plasma renin activity is observed during isotonic volume expansion in some neonates.[40] Increased plasma renin activity may contribute, through increased production of angiotensin II and aldosterone, to inappropriately high resorption of sodium ions in the distal tubules of neonates. The high plasma renin activity and nonresponsive sodium-transport mechanism in the distal tubules may be a consequence of immaturity of the macula densa.[40]

Development of the neonatal natriuretic response can be accelerated by several factors, including high dietary salt and artificially increased rate of perinatal growth. Neonates fed a high-salt diet apparently develop a more responsive excretory mechanism for sodium ions more rapidly than did those fed a low- or normal-sodium diet, although this mechanism was still not as efficient as in adults.[38]

Rats 14 to 50 days of age were used to demonstrate the effect of increased growth rate on the rate of development of the sodium-ion excretory response. When raised in reduced litters, rat pups gained 30% more weight by 50 days of age than did those from intact litters. Although there was no major effect of faster growth rate on development of glomerular filtration, natriuretic efficiency in response to blood volume expansion by autologous transfusion was significantly higher in fast-growing rats (98.2% in comparison with 92.2%).[41] Maturation of natriuretic response was not related to blood pressure, chronologic age, or body weight but rather to some function of rate of growth.

UNLIKE that observed in rats, puppies, and infants, the renal response to salt challenge in piglets 14 to 40 days of age appears to be more similar to that in adults,[42] although glomerular filtration rates are still immature. This finding also probably reflects differences in the rates of maturation of distal tubules.

RENAL FUNCTION IN NEONATAL CALVES

Newborn calves are unusual in that renal function approaches that of adult cattle at or within two to three days of birth.[9] Inulin and thiosulfate clearances in calves as young as two days are approximately 130 ml/min/1.73 m^2, which is comparable with that measured in adults.[9] Likewise, *p*-aminohippuric acid clearance is about 590 ml/min/1.73 m^2, which is eight times that of a human infant and similar to that observed in adult cattle.[9] Filtration fraction (22%) is thus comparable with mature levels.

Urea clearance in calves is approximately 65 ml/min/1.73 m^2, which is three times that of infants and similar to that reported for adult humans and dogs.[43] When expressed relative to body weight, urea clearance in calves (1.20 ml/min/kg) is greater than that for adult cows (0.88 ml/min/kg).[43] When expressed relative to body surface area or metabolic body size, however, values for calves (65 ml/min/1.73 m^2) are less than those for adult cows (156 ml/min/1.73 m^2).[43]

The ratio of surface area to weight in calves (1:4.6) is much greater than that for adult cows (1:15).[43] It has been proposed that in taking account of this surface area–mass bias, comparisons made between calves and other species of similar body size and weight may lead to accurate estimation of the relative maturity of renal function in neonatal calves. This exceptional relationship may hold for other large animals, such as horses.

IN RESPONSE to starvation and water deprivation, 2- to 20-day-old calves are able to concentrate their urine significantly, thereby conserving water much like an adult animal.[44] After 24 hours of starvation, the neonatal calf may lose approximately 5% of its body weight, progressing to a 14% loss after 96 hours. During this time, urine output may be reduced from 2350 ml/day to as little as 268 ml/day and urine osmolality may be markedly increased (from 257 to 1323 mOsm/L). Whereas a human infant requires an estimated 2.5 liters of water to excrete 1000 mOsm of urinary solute, an adult human or neonatal calf may do so with less than one liter of water.[44] In neonatal calves, hematocrit and blood urea nitrogen did not increase significantly until the third day of starvation or water deprivation.[44]

Unlike other neonatal animals, calves are also able to dilute urine and excrete large volume loads as efficiently as adults.[45] After loading with milk, water, or hypotonic saline, calves were able to increase urine output up to tenfold.[45] Neonatal rats given a water load of 4.5% of body weight might show no change in urine output within five hours; whereas calves achieved maximum urine output within 60 to 90 minutes of loading with water, milk, or hypotonic saline and had excreted 70% to 100% of the volume load by the end of four hours.[45] This response is possible because of a mature glomerular filtration rate and the ability of calves to rapidly dilute their urine to as little as 35 mOsm/L after water loading. The diuretic response of calves is, in fact, more similar to that of adult monogastric animals than to that of an adult cow, whose time to onset of diuresis (45 minutes), time to peak diuresis (150 minutes), and long-lived response (six hours) far exceed those observed in calves, adult humans, or dogs.[45]

The response of neonatal calves to short-term and long-term loading with ammonium chloride is also surprisingly mature for a newborn.[46] This mature response has been attributed to calves' unique ability to increase renal ammoniagenesis.[46] This ability may be induced by diet because of the high total acid load and titratable acidity of cow's milk.[46] In one study, 10- to 20-day-old calves were able to increase urinary ammonia excretion fivefold in long-duration ammonium chloride tolerance tests and by sevenfold in short-term tests.[46] Although plasma pH and bicarbonate concentrations were lowered significantly during these tests, calves were able to compensate much more rapidly and efficiently than were neonatal puppies, piglets, or infants in similar studies. Finally, neonatal calves do not experience physiologic acidosis, thus indicating that the bicarbonate threshold of their proximal tubules resembles that of adults.[46]

The unique renal functional maturity of neonatal calves may explain their favorable response to fluid and electrolyte resuscitation schedules that would harm neonates of other species.[47,48] In diarrheic infants, hypertonic hypernatremic hypervolemia is a frequent response to hypertonic oral or intravenous fluid replacement therapy.[49-51] Neonatal calves, however, have mature renal clearance and excretory functions; calves therefore can benefit from large-volume, high-solute replacement without incurring the potential deleterious effects of such extreme therapy.[47,48]

FLUID COMPARTMENTS AND METABOLIC SIZE

Neonatal animals differ considerably from adults in the size of their fluid compartments and the percentage and distribution of water within the body.[52,53] For example, total body water in the infant at birth is approximately 80% of the body weight, declining rapidly within the first year of life to approximately 60%.[52,53] The fraction of this water within the extracellular fluid compartment decreases from slightly more than one half at birth (40% of body weight) to one third to one half of total body water (25% of body weight) in adulthood.[54]

IN ADULTS, about 50% of the total body water is in the musculature but only one fifth is extracellular. In newborn infants, approximately 30% of total body water is found in muscle tissue; one third of this 30% is extracellular.[52] In cases of hypertonic dehydration, the intracellular compartment loses more water than the extracellular compartment in order to replete the latter's volume deficit and share the osmotic imbalance.[55] Neonates, however, have a smaller reserve of intracellular fluid. On the other hand, loss of an equivalent percentage of body weight as water through isotonic dehydration does not represent nearly as great a relative loss of extracellular fluid volume as it would in an adult.

The absolute amount of water and calories required by neonates is lower than that required by adults; but because of their higher ratio of body surface area to body weight,

neonates have higher relative requirements. Water and energy requirements relative to body mass are significantly greater in neonates.[56,57]

The smaller an individual is, the greater is its body surface area relative to weight. Heat dissipation from the body is a function of convection, conduction, radiation, and evaporative surface losses. With a greater relative surface area, neonates lose more body heat by radiation. Similarly, there is a larger surface relative to body mass from which evaporative losses may occur. To balance these larger, insensible losses of heat and water, neonates must generate a larger quantity of heat and consume a greater amount of water relative to body mass.

The larger metabolic body size of neonates helps account for their higher basal metabolic rate and higher relative calorie requirements. The greater insensible water loss associated with their metabolic body size, in combination with higher obligatory urinary water losses attributable to an immature renal concentration capacity, accounts for higher relative water requirements in neonates.[54,57] Increased body temperature resulting from fever or heat stress imposes a proportionately greater burden on water balance in neonates, whose surface losses are relatively greater.

PHARMACOKINETICS

A drug's disposition is influenced by its relative distribution among the body's fluid compartments, the activity of drug-metabolizing enzyme systems, and the rates of renal clearance.[58] In neonates, the greater body water content and extracellular fluid compartment size relative to body mass affect the volumes of distribution of certain drugs.[59,60] Conversely, lower fat content in neonates also affects the distribution of fat-soluble compounds.[59,60] Neonates therefore have a relatively larger volume of distribution for water-soluble drugs but a smaller reserve of lipid-soluble drugs. Because of lower plasma protein concentrations, neonates also have less protein-binding and plasma compartment restriction.[58-61] Thus, the circulating protein-bound reserve of a given drug may be limited and its rate of extraction for metabolism or elimination may be enhanced.

In neonates, hepatic biotransformation pathways responsible for oxidation, reduction, hydroxylation, sulfation, and glucuronoside conjugation are underdeveloped.[58,59,61] Deficiencies in glucuronoside conjugation are, in particular, responsible for the prolonged half-lives and increased toxicity of various clinically useful drugs, including barbiturates, antiepileptics, nonsteroidal antiinflammatory drugs, and certain classes of antibiotics (e.g., sulfonamides and chloramphenicol).[61,62]

Because of renal immaturity at birth, the elimination rate of parent compounds or biologically transformed daughter metabolites of many drugs may be limited in neonates. Lower rates of renal blood flow and glomerular filtration can limit the clearance of compounds of low molecular weight; such compounds may pass through the glomerulus.[58,59] Limited organic acid–transport mechanisms in immature proximal convoluted tubules may restrict the rate of extraction of drug and drug metabolites cleared by active secretion into the urine.[58,59] In addition, reduced urinary acidification capacity may affect the elimination of alkaline drugs by ionic diffusion trapping.[58,59]

Because of immaturity of proximal convoluted tubules, neonatal kidneys may not accumulate critical quantities of otherwise nephrotoxic drugs (e.g., aminoglycoside antibiotics).[63,64] In addition, the comparative insensitivity of tubule epithelium in neonates may afford additional protection against certain nephrotoxins. For example, such heavy metals as inorganic mercury are apparently less toxic in neonates than in adults.[65,66] This lower sensitivity may be a function of lower renal blood flow and glomerular filtration rate in neonates, whose kidneys thereby receive a smaller fractional burden of the toxic element.[65,66] Alternatively, higher metallothionein content in the tubule epithelium in neonates may afford greater protection against functional proteins and enzymes by preferential binding of the elements.[67] As has been demonstrated in adult animals subjected to repetitive or increasing doses of mercuric chloride, high turnover rates of epithelial cells in proximal tubules may enhance elimination of metal-laden cells and result in a predominant population of younger, more resistant cells.[68]

EXCEPT in newborn calves, the capacity for renal elimination of drugs and drug metabolites is directly related to the rate of development of the particular renal function (glomerular filtration, tubular secretion, ionic/nonionic diffusion disequilibrium) in the species. Renal toxicity of certain substances is likewise affected by the rate of development of transport or detoxification pathways.

THERAPEUTIC CONSIDERATIONS

Because neonates are less able to concentrate urine maximally while maintaining solute excretion and because their insensible water losses (by surface evaporation) are relatively greater, neonates are much more prone to dehydration after water restriction than are adults. Although neonates have relatively greater requirements for water and calories, they cannot accommodate large volumes over short periods. Limited cardiovascular function and immature renal response to volume and solute loading make fluid and electrolyte replacement in most neonates a delicate, if not precarious, operation. Successful fluid resuscitation requires an appreciation of the limited functional development of the kidneys and the differences in fluid compartment sizes in the newborn. Because neonates are

predisposed to water and solute loss and because clinical signs of imbalance may become apparent rapidly, clinicians must temper their enthusiasm for deficit replacement to avoid problems of overhydration or solute overloading. Frequent reevaluation of neonatal patients and frequent smaller volumes of replacement fluids administered at more conservative rates would certainly meet with greater success.

Consideration of species differences in neonatal renal function may allow the clinician to individualize therapy for a species. For example, hypertonic fluids can be administered to diarrheic neonatal calves; or the clinician can take advantage of a mature glucose threshold in the renal tubules in replacing caloric deficits in puppies. Conversely, it would be ill-advised to replace the entire calculated fluid deficit in a dehydrated puppy without allowing for a delayed renal adaptive response to isotonic fluid loading.

CLINICAL SIGNS and cardiovascular indexes of volume repletion, with the aid of ancillary laboratory parameters indicative of renal clearance (e.g., blood urea nitrogen, urine osmolality, and fractional electrolyte excretion), should guide resuscitative therapy. In evaluating acid–base balance, the clinician must consider the possibility of a physiologic acidosis in order to calculate the true base deficit as well as to avoid excess solute loading and osmotic diuresis resulting from excessive alkalinizing salt therapy.

About the Authors

Dr. Fettman is a Diplomate of the American College of Veterinary Pathologists and an Associate Professor in the Comparative Nephrology Unit of the Department of Pathology, College of Veterinary Medicine and Biomedical Sciences, Colorado State University, Fort Collins, Colorado. Dr. Allen is a Diplomate of the American College of Veterinary Internal Medicine and is affiliated with Mark Morris Associates in Topeka, Kansas.

REFERENCES

1. Patten BM: *The Embryology of the Pig.* Philadelphia, P Blakiston's Son & Co, 1927, pp 188–198.
2. Arey LB: *Developmental Anatomy,* ed 7. Philadelphia, WB Saunders Co, 1974, pp 295–308.
3. Kleinman LI: Developmental renal physiology. *The Physiologist* 25:104–110, 1982.
4. Aperia A, Broberger O, Herin P: Maturational changes in glomerular perfusion rate and glomerular filtration rate in lambs. *Pediatr Res* 8:758–765, 1974.
5. Spitzer A, Brandis M: Functional and morphologic maturation of the superficial nephrons. *J Clin Invest* 53:279–287, 1974.
6. Horster M, Kemler BJ, Valtin H: Intracortical distribution of number and volume of glomeruli during postnatal maturation in the dog. *J Clin Invest* 50:796–800, 1971.
7. Gruskin AB, Edelmann CM, Yuan S: Maturational changes in renal blood flow in piglets. *Pediatr Res* 4:7–13, 1970.
8. Aperia A, Herin P: Development of glomerular perfusion rate and

nephron filtration rate in rats 17–60 days old. *Am J Physiol* 228:1319–1325, 1975.

9. Dalton RG: Renal function in neonatal calves: Inulin, thiosulphate, and paraaminohippuric acid clearance. *Br Vet J* 124:498–502, 1968.

10. Jose PA, Logan AG, Slotkoff LM, et al: Intrarenal blood flow distribution in canine puppies. *Pediatr Res* 5:335–344, 1971.

11. Aschinberg LC, Goldsmith DI, Olbing H, et al: Neonatal changes in renal blood flow distribution in puppies. *Am J Physiol* 228:1453–1461, 1975.

12. Guignard JP: Renal function in the newborn infant. *Pediatr Clin North Am* 29:777–790, 1982.

13. Kleinman LI, Lubbe RJ: Factors affecting the maturation of glomerular filtration rate and renal plasma flow in the newborn dog. *J Physiol* 223:395–409, 1972.

14. Jaykka S: The problem of dormant fetal organs: The kidneys, lungs, and the gut. *Biol Neonatol* 3:343–356, 1961.

15. Horster M, Valtin H: Postnatal development of renal function: Micropuncture and clearance studies in the dog. *J Clin Invest* 50:779–795, 1971.

16. Olbing H, Blaufox MD, Aschinberg LC, et al: Postnatal changes in renal glomerular blood flow distribution in puppies. *J Clin Invest* 52:2885–2895, 1973.

17. Kleinman LI, Reuter JH: Maturation of glomerular blood flow distribution in the new-born dog. *J Physiol* 228:91–103, 1973.

18. Fetterman GH, Shuplock NA, Phillip FJ, et al: The growth and maturation of human glomeruli and proximal convolutions from term to adulthood. Studies by microdissection. *Pediatrics* 35:601–619, 1965.

19. Spitzer A, Edelmann CM: Maturational changes in pressure gradients for glomerular filtration. *Am J Physiol* 221:1431–1435, 1971.

20. Buckley NM, Brazeau P, Frasier ID: Renal blood flow autoregulation in developing swine. *Am J Physiol* 245:H1–H6, 1983.

21. Arant WS, Edelmann CM, Nash MA: The renal reabsorption of glucose in the developing canine kidney: A study of glomerulotubular balance. *Pediatr Res* 8:638–646, 1974.

22. Vogh B, Cassin S: Stop flow analysis of renal functions in newborn and maturing swine. *Biol Neonatol* 10:153–165, 1966.

23. Rennick B, Hamilton B, Evans R: Development of renal tubular transports of TEA and PAH in the puppy and piglet. *Am J Physiol* 201:743–746, 1961.

24. Horster M, Lewy JE: Filtration fraction and extraction of PAH during neonatal period in the rat. *Am J Physiol* 219:1061–1065, 1970.

25. Kleinman LI, Lubbe RJ: Factors affecting the maturation of renal PAH extraction in the new-born dog. *J Physiol* 223:411–418, 1972.

26. Arant WS: Developmental patterns of renal functional maturation compared in the human neonate. *J Pediatr* 92:705–712, 1978.

27. Kleinman LI, Disney TA: Renal osmotic effect of mannitol in the neonatal and adult dog. *Am J Physiol* 247:F396–F402, 1984.

28. Larsson L: Ultrastructure and permeability of intercellular contacts of developing proximal tubules in the rat kidney. *J Ultrastruct Res* 52:100–113, 1975.

29. Horster M, Larsson L: Mechanisms of fluid absorption during proximal tubule development. *Kidney Intl* 10:348–363, 1976.

30. Robillard JE, Ramberg E, Sessions C, et al: Role of aldosterone on renal sodium and potassium excretion during fetal life and newborn period. *Dev Pharmacol Ther* 1:201–216, 1980.

31. Edelmann CM, Soriano JR, Boichis H, et al: Renal bicarbonate reabsorption and hydrogen ion excretion in normal infants. *J Clin Invest* 46:1309–1317, 1967.

32. Brodehl J, Gellissen K, Weber HP: Postnatal development of tubular phosphate reabsorption. *Clin Nephrol* 17:161–171, 1982.

33. Cohen JJ, Kassirer JP: Acid-base metabolism, in Maxwell MH, Kleeman CR (eds): *Clinical Disorders of Fluid and Electrolyte Metabolism*, ed 3. New York, McGraw-Hill Book Co, 1980, pp 181–232.

34. Robinson JR: Ammonia formation by surviving kidney slices without specific substrates. *J Physiol* 124:1–7, 1954.

35. Cort JH, McCance RA: The renal response of puppies to an acidosis. *J Physiol* 124:358–369, 1954.

36. Hatemi N, McCance RA: The response of piglets to ammonium chloride. *J Physiol* 157:603–610, 1961.

37. Trimble ME: Renal response to solute loading in infant rats: Relation to anatomical development. *Am J Physiol* 219:1089–1097, 1970.

38. Steichen JJ, Kleinman I: Influence of dietary sodium intake on renal maturation in unanesthetized canine puppies. *Proc Soc Exp Biol Med* 148:748–751, 1975.

39. Kleinman LI: Renal sodium reabsorption during saline loading and distal blockade in newborn dogs. *Am J Physiol* 228:1403–1408, 1975.

40. Goldsmith DI, Drukker A, Blaufox MD, et al: Hemodynamic and excretory response of the neonatal canine kidney to acute volume expansion. *Am J Physiol* 237:F392–F397, 1979.

41. Bengele HH, Solomon S: Development of the renal response to blood volume expansion in normal and fast-growing rats. *Am J Physiol* 231:832–836, 1976.

42. Kaskel FJ, Kleinman LI: Effect of diet on renal response to salt challenge in neonatal piglets. *Biol Neonatol* 29:306–314, 1976.

43. Dalton RG: Renal function in neonatal calves: Urea clearance. *Br Vet J* 124:451–459, 1968.

44. Dalton RG: The effect of starvation on the fluid and electrolyte metabolism of neonatal calves. *Br Vet J* 123:237–246, 1967.

45. Dalton RG: Renal function in neonatal calves. *Br Vet J* 124:371–381, 1968.

46. Dalton RG, Phillips GD: Renal function in neonatal calves: Response to acidosis. *Br Vet J* 125:367–378, 1969.

47. Jones R, Phillips RW, Cleek JL: Hyperosmotic oral replacement fluid for diarrheic calves. *JAVMA* 184:1501–1505, 1984.

48. Fettman MJ, Brooks PA, Burrows KP, Phillips RW: Comparative evaluation of commercial oral replacement formulae in healthy neonatal calves. *JAVMA* 188:397–401, 1986.

49. Gottlieb RP: Dehydration and fluid therapy. *Emerg Med Clin North Am* 1:113–123, 1983.

50. Nalin DR, Harland E, Ramlal A, et al: Comparison of low and high sodium and potassium content in oral rehydration solutions. *J Pediatr* 97:848–853, 1980.

51. Santosham M, Daum RS, Dillman L, et al: Oral rehydration therapy of infantile diarrhea. *N Engl J Med* 306:1070–1076, 1982.

52. Friis-Hansen B: Body water compartments in children: Changes during growth and related changes in body composition. *Pediatrics* 28:169–181, 1961.

53. Fomon SJ: Body composition of the male reference infant during the first year of life. *Pediatrics* 40:863–870, 1967.

54. Finberg L: Fluid, electrolyte, and acid–base abnormalities in pediatrics, in Maxwell MH, Kleeman CR (eds): *Clinical Disorders of Fluid and Electrolyte Metabolism*, ed 3. New York, McGraw-Hill Book Co, 1980, pp 1563–1580.

55. Holliday M, Egan TJ: Dehydration, salt depletion, and potassium loss. *Pediatr Clin North Am* 6:81–98, 1959.

56. Darrow DC: The significance of body size. *Am J Dis Child* 98:416–425, 1959.

57. Holliday MA, Segar WE: The maintenance need for water in parenteral fluid therapy. *Pediatrics* 19:823–832, 1957.

58. Baggot JD: Drug therapy in the neonatal animal, in *Principles of Drug Disposition in Domestic Animals*. Philadelphia, WB Saunders Co, 1976, pp 219–224.

59. Short CR: Drug disposition in neonatal animals. *JAVMA* 184:1161–1162, 1984.

60. Svendsen O: Pharmacokinetics of hexobarbital, sulphadimidine and chloramphenicol in neonatal and young pigs. *Acta Vet Scand* 17:1–14, 1976.

61. Davis LE, Westfall BE, Short CR: Biotransformation and pharmacokinetics of salicylate in newborn animals. *Am J Vet Res* 34:1105–1108, 1973.

62. Burrows GE, Barto PB, Martin B, et al: Comparative pharmacokinetics of antibiotics in newborn calves: Chloramphenicol, lincomycin, and tylosin. *Am J Vet Res* 44:1053–1057, 1983.

63. Riviere JE, Coppoc GL: Pharmacokinetics of gentamicin in the juvenile dog. *Am J Vet Res* 42:1621–1623, 1981.

64. Cowan RH, Jukkola AF, Arant WS: Pathophysiologic evidence of gentamicin nephrotoxicity in neonatal puppies. *Pediatr Res* 14:1204–1211, 1980.

65. Daston GP, Kavlock RI, Rogers EH, et al: Toxicity of mercuric chloride to the developing rat kidney. I. Postnatal ontogeny of renal sensitivity. *Toxicol Appl Pharmacol* 71:24–41, 1983.

66. Daston GP, Gray JA, Carver B, et al: Toxicity of mercuric chloride

to the developing rat kidney. II. Effect of increased dosages on renal function in suckling pups. *Toxicol Appl Pharmacol* 74:35–45, 1984.
67. Oh SH, Whanger PD: Biological function of metallothioneins. VII. Effect of age on its metabolism in rats. *Am J Physiol* 237:E18–E22, 1979.
68. Hall RL, Wilke WL, Fettman MJ: Renal resistance to mercuric chloride toxicity during prolonged exposure in rats. *Vet Hum Toxicol* 28:305–307, 1986.

UPDATE

Acute Renal Failure. Part I. *(continued from page 19)*

production of thromboxane A_2. The protective activity of eicosapentaenoic acid and docosahexaenoic acid supplementation was demonstrated in a study in which dogs were treated with fish oils prior to an ischemic insult.[10] The role of dietary lipids in the progression and management of chronic renal disease in dogs and cats is also being studied.

Cellular protectants under investigation include glycine infusions,[11] epidermal growth factor, and insulin-like growth factor. In rats, glycine attenuates the morphologic and functional damage associated with cisplatin administration and hypoxic injury.[12] Epidermal growth factor and insulin-like growth factors helped promote tissue repair in gentamicin-induced and ischemic acute renal failure in rat models.[13,14]

The efficacy of any of these strategies remains purely speculative in clinical practice. In veterinary medicine, efforts have focused on elucidating protocols and strategies for preventing nephrotoxicosis due to commonly used chemotherapeutic agents. Current recommendations for the administration of aminoglycosides, cisplatin, and amphotericin B have been reviewed.[15–17]

REFERENCES

1. Brown SA, Barsanti JA, Finco DR: Effects of vasoactive agents on kidney function, in Kirk RW, Bonagura JD (eds): *Current Veterinary Therapy XI: Small Animal Practice*. Philadelphia, WB Saunders, 1992, pp 832–833.
2. Longhofer SL, Dricsson GF, Cifelli S, Benitz AM: Renal function in heart failure dogs receiving furosemide and enalapril maleate. *Proceedings of 11th ACVIM Forum*, 1993, p 936 (abstract).
3. Forrester SD, Lees GE: Acute renal failure associated with systemic infectious disease, in Kirk RW, Bonagura JD (eds): *Current Veterinary Therapy XI: Small Animal Practice*. Philadelphia, WB Saunders, 1992, pp 829–831.
4. Taboada J, Palmer GH: Renal failure associated with bacterial endocarditis in the dog. *JAAHA* 25:243–251, 1989.
5. Cesare JF, Ligas JR, Hirvela ER: Enhancement of urine output and glomerular filtration in acutely oliguric patients using low-dose norepinephrine. *Circ Shock* 39:207–210, 1993.
6. Schaer GL, Fink MP, Parrillo JE: Norepinephrine alone versus norepinephrine plus low-dose dopamine: Enhanced renal blood flow with combination pressor therapy. *Crit Care Med* 13:492–496, 1985.
7. Mason J: The pathophysiology of ischaemic acute renal failure: A new hypothesis about the initiation phase. *Renal Physiol* 9:129–147, 1986.
8. Simonson MS: Endothelins: Multifunctional renal peptides. *Physiol Rev* 73:375–411, 1993.
9. Kon V, Yoshioka T, Fogo A, Ichikawa: Glomerular actions of endothelin in vivo. *J Clin Invest* 83:1762–1767, 1989.
10. Neumayer HH, Heinrich M, Schmissas M, et al: Amelioration of ischemic acute renal failure by dietary fish oil administration in conscious dogs. *J Am Soc Nephrol* 3:1312–1320, 1992.
11. Heyman SN, Rosen S, Silva P, et al: Protective action of glycine in cisplatin nephrotoxicity. *Kidney Int* 40:273–279, 1991.
12. Weinberg JM, Davis JA, Abarzua M, Raja T: Cytoprotective effects of glycine and glutathione against hypoxic injury to rat tubules. *J Clin Invest* 80:1446–1454, 1987.
13. Morin NJ, Laurent G, Nonclercq D, et al: Epidermal growth factor accelerates renal tissue repair in a model of gentamicin nephrotoxicity in rats. *Am J Physiol* 263:F806–F811, 1992.
14. Ding H, Kopple JD, Cohen A, Hirschberg R: Recombinant human insulin-like growth factor I accelerates recovery and reduces catabolism in rats with ischemic acute renal failure. *J Clin Invest* 91:2281–2287, 1993.
15. Forrester SD: Preventing nephrotoxic acute renal failure. *Proceedings of 10th ACVIM Forum*, 1992, pp 30–132.
16. Forrester SD, Jacobson JD, Fallin EA: Taking measures to prevent acute renal failure. *Vet Med* 89:231–236, 1994.
17. Ogilvie GK, Straw RC, Powers BE, et al: Prevalence of nephrotoxicosis associated with a short-term saline solution diuresis protocol for the administration of cisplatin to dogs with malignant tumors: 61 cases. *JAVMA* 199:613–616, 1991.

KEY FACTS
- For several reasons, the kidneys are exceptionally vulnerable to toxins.
- The high level of biochemical activity makes the proximal renal tubules the portion of the nephron that is most susceptible to toxic compounds.
- Supportive therapy is directed at improving renal blood flow and promoting diuresis.

Drug-Related Nephropathies Part I. Mechanisms, Diagnosis, and Management*

Scott Anthony Brown, DVM, PhD[†]
Department of Veterinary Physiology
  and Pharmacology

Jeffery A. Engelhardt, MS, DVM
Department of Microbiology, Pathology,
  and Public Health

School of Veterinary Medicine
Purdue University
West Lafayette, Indiana

Induction of renal disease is a serious side effect of treatment with some therapeutic agents. Although the exact underlying causes are poorly understood, a few general mechanisms of toxicity are known. This article discusses the mechanisms of the glomerular and tubular toxicity caused by commonly used drugs and outlines general principles for the diagnosis and management of drug-related nephropathies. The drugs mentioned in Part I of this series are presented as examples of specific nephrotoxic mechanisms and are limited to therapeutic agents (Table I). Classic nephrotoxic compounds, such as organic solvents, heavy metals, and mycotoxins, have been purposely omitted. Part II of this two-part series describes current understanding of the toxicities of specific therapeutic agents.

Mechanisms of Drug-Induced Nephrotoxicity

The kidneys are exceptionally vulnerable to toxins for several reasons. Although the kidneys constitute less than 1% of body weight in dogs and cats, renal blood flow accounts for 20% of cardiac output, with 90% of the blood entering the kidneys going to the renal cortex. When the extensive blood flow is coupled with the glomerular capillary system, the result is an extremely large potential for the presentation of toxic substances to a vast endothelial surface area in the renal cortex. In addition, because the kidney consumes oxygen at an extraordinary rate, it is very susceptible to substances that cause cellular hypoxia. Furthermore, the countercurrent mechanism of the kidney predisposes the medullary interstitium to toxicity by progressively increasing tissue concentrations of certain nephrotoxic substances.

The cortex and the medulla each has distinct biochemical activities that relate to the function and metabolism of pharmacologic agents and xenobiotics (Table II). The kidney possesses drug-metabolizing enzymes, which

*Published as Purdue University Agricultural Experiment Station Journal Paper Number 10,497.

[†]Dr. Brown's present address is Department of Veterinary Physiology and Pharmacology, College of Veterinary Medicine, Texas A&M University, College Station, Texas.

TABLE I
Therapeutic Drugs That May Cause Nephropathies

Antimicrobials	**Cardiovascular drugs**
Aminoglycosides	Captopril
Cephalosporins	Hydralazine
Isoniazid	Procainamide
Penicillins	
Sulfonamides	**Anticancer drugs**
Tetracyclines	Daunorubicin
	Methotrexate
Antifungals	
Amphotericin B	**Immunosuppressive agents**
	Azathioprine
Anthelmintics	Cyclophosphamide
Thiacetarsamide	Cyclosporins
Arsenicals	Penicillamine
Analgesics	**Miscellaneous therapeutic agents**
Acetaminophen	Probenecid
Ibuprofen	Protamine sulfate
Phenacetin	Puromycin
Phenylbutazone	
Salicylates	

TABLE II
Biochemical Activities of the Kidney[32,37]

Region	Activity
Cortex	Gluconeogenesis
	Fatty acid utilization
	Cytochrome P-450 enzyme system
	Deamination
Medulla	Glycolysis
	Lipogenesis
	Prostaglandin endoperoxide synthetase

not only detoxify chemicals but may also create metabolites that are more toxic. These actions combine to increase the susceptibility of the kidney to chemically induced damage. The adverse reaction may be a response to the parent compound, toxic metabolites, or both. Tubular secretion and reabsorption increase the tubular concentrations of these compounds to concentrations that are toxic to renal tubular epithelium, although the remainder of the body may be subjected to far lower concentrations.

Glomerulus
Anatomy and Physiology

The normal glomerulus, an exquisitely adapted dynamic sieve, forms an ultrafiltrate that is virtually devoid of blood cells and plasma proteins. The ultrafiltration membrane includes the fenestrated capillary endothelium, the glomerular basement membrane, and the visceral epithelial cells or podocytes. The entire glomerulus is enmeshed by the mesangial cells and their accompanying matrix. Drug-induced changes in these structures, either direct or immune mediated, affect several physiologic parameters that govern single-nephron glomerular filtration rate (GFR), i.e., transcapillary hydraulic pressure, glomerular plasma flow rate, glomerular filtration surface area, and the intrinsic permeability of the glomerular filtration barrier.[1]

The glomerular capillaries and the mesangium determine the functional surface area for ultrafiltration.[1] Alteration of a luminal factor at the loop of Henle is detected by the macula densa at the distal tubule. The exact luminal factor has not been precisely determined. Increased perfusion at the loop of Henle causes an increase in the intraluminal concentration of sodium, and the GFR decreases. The decreased GFR may be the result of a change in the salt concentration of the tubular fluid rather than in the flow rate. This change has been found to be correlated best with chlo-

ride ion concentrations, and blockade of chloride excretion by furosemide significantly decreases the GFR response.[2] The macula densa releases renin, which then activates angiotensin II.[3] Angiotensin II can constrict the afferent renal arterioles to decrease glomerular plasma flow. Angiotensin II also constricts the mesangium to decrease the filtration surface area of the glomerulus. Both of these changes effectively decrease the GFR. Therefore, any drug that either affects the renin–angiotensin system (e.g., captopril[4]) or alters renal blood flow (e.g., epinephrine) can alter the glomerular ultrastructure and, thus, the filtration surface area. In addition, the role of prostaglandins and natriuretic factor in this mechanism is the subject of intense investigation. Because of this tubuloglomerular feedback, tubular toxins can also cause dose-related glomerular alterations.[5] Specifically, aminoglycosides have been shown to decrease both the diameter and the density of the endothelial fenestrae, thereby decreasing the surface area available for ultrafiltration (Figure 1).[6,7] This phenomenon may be the result of a direct toxic effect of aminoglycosides, although this direct toxicity is not universally accepted.[8] Other tubular nephrotoxins may elicit similar glomerular changes.

Mesangial cells are also phagocytic cells derived from the monocyte–macrophage system. Administration of cytostatic drugs, such as azathioprine, penicillamine, and daunorubicin,[9] results in increased amounts of mesangial matrix and proliferation of mesangial cells.[10,11] These drugs may alter mesangial cell function, thereby allowing accumulation in the matrix of macromolecules that would normally be phagocytized by mesangial cells. As a result, feedback recruitment of additional phagocytic cells may occur, producing the histologic appearance of membranous glomerulonephritis.[12]

The plasma membranes of visceral epithelial cells are rich in anionic sialoglycoproteins, which not only act as an electrostatic barrier against negatively charged molecules but also serve to maintain normal separation of podocytic foot processes.[12] When the negative charge of podocytes is disrupted by highly cationic molecules, the podocytes become swollen, foot processes become blunted, cell junctions between foot processes are formed, and the slit diaphragms between adjacent foot processes are destroyed. Functionally, the barrier against negatively charged macromolecules, such as albumin, is disrupted, and the selectiv-

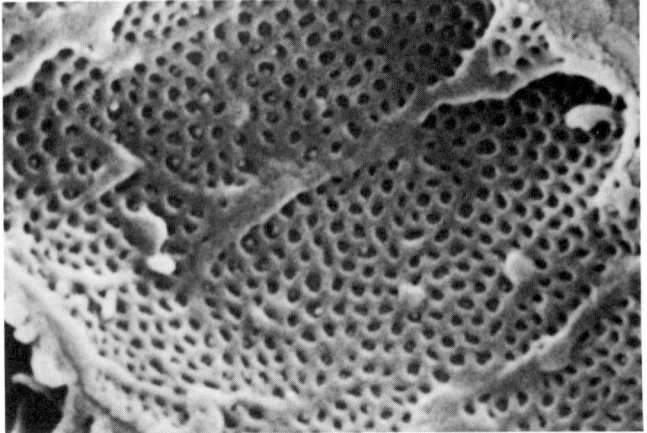

Figure 1A

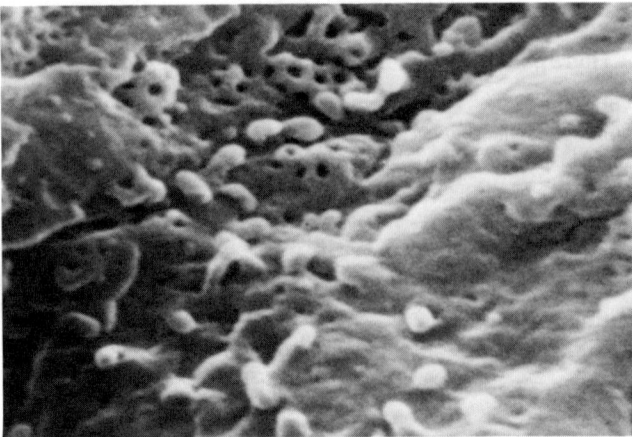

Figure 1B

Figure 1—Scanning electron micrographs of rat glomerular endothelial cells. (**A**) Normal rat endothelial cells with normal endothelial fenestrae. (**B**) Extensive loss and narrowing of endothelial fenestrae from a rat treated with gentamicin, 80 mg/kg/day for 15 days. (×25,000) (Courtesy of Dr. A. P. Evan, Indiana University School of Medicine)

ity of the ultrafiltration apparatus diminishes.[13] Decreases in the fixed negative charge of the visceral epithelial cells also cause accumulation of macromolecules in the mesangial matrix.[14] These electrostatic imbalances can be reversed by perfusion with heparin, a negatively charged glycoprotein.[12] Drugs that can cause loss of these anionic glycoproteins include the aminonucleoside puromycin,[13,15,16] daunorubicin,[9,14,17] Adriamycin,[18] probenecid,[14,19] and protamine sulfate.[20,21] Other organic acids may cause similar glomerular changes.

Most drug-related glomerulonephropathies are immune mediated. The drug may act as a hapten or as a full antigen to cause type III or, less frequently, type II hypersensitivity.[9] On the other hand, some drugs cause a systemic lupus erythematosus (SLE)-like syndrome, in which case the production of antinuclear or anti-DNA antibodies is stimulated by the drugs.[22] In these situations, immune complexes are deposited in the subepithelial layer, the glomerular basement membrane, or the mesangial matrix. The subsequent activation of complement then results in the liberation of cytotoxic free oxygen radicals from cells of the monocyte–macrophage system[23] and the recruitment of other inflammatory components.[24] Among the drugs that have been shown to precipitate immune complex lesions are penicillin,[25] penicillamine,[9,26] gold salts,[27,28] and sulfadiazine.[29] Drugs that produce SLE-like reactions in humans include procainamide,[30,31] probenecid,[32] hydralazine,[9] and isoniazid.[9] Although drug-induced SLE-like reactions of this type have not been documented in veterinary medicine, they may be revealed in further studies as the use of these drugs increases.

Tubular Network
Anatomy and Physiology
The renal tubular network of the nephron is composed of the proximal tubule, the loop of Henle, the distal tubule, and the collecting duct. The morphology, metabolic activity, and function of the tubular epithelial cells vary from

the proximal tubule to the collecting duct, as does the susceptibility of the cells to nephrotoxic compounds.

Proximal Tubules. The proximal tubule begins at the urinary pole of the renal corpuscle, with the tubular epithelium continuous with the epithelium of Bowman's capsule. The proximal tubule initially has a convoluted structure (pars convoluta) and then assumes a straight path (pars recta) as it continues. A single layer of cuboidal to columnar epithelial cells lines the proximal tubules. Numerous mitochondria and extensive endoplasmic reticulum impart a high degree of metabolic activity to these cells. The luminal border is lined by well-developed microvilli and an extensive membrane-bound enzyme system, which includes alkaline phosphatase, γ-glutamyl transpeptidase, and β-N-acetylglucosaminidase. Adenosine triphosphatases (ATPases) are present on both the luminal and the basolateral membranes, but predominantly on the latter.[33,34]

Functionally, the proximal tubule is responsible for the active reabsorption of glucose, proteins, amino acids, sodium, potassium, calcium, phosphate, and bicarbonate.[2] In addition, chloride, water, and urea are passively resorbed, and hydrogen ion is actively secreted.[2,35]

Loops of Henle. The loops of Henle, which are continuous with the proximal tubule, are lined by a single layer of low cuboidal to squamous epithelium. The length of the loop is related to the position of the nephron within the kidney, with longer loops in juxtamedullary nephrons and shorter loops in cortical nephrons.[33] The metabolic activity of the epithelial cells is much less than in other tubular segments. The loops of Henle function primarily to generate a gradient of solute concentration within the medullary interstitium in order to concentrate the urine.[35]

Distal Segments. The distal tubule is composed of (1) the straight portion (pars recta); (2) the portion adjacent to the renal corpuscle, containing the macula densa (pars maculata); and (3) the convoluted portion (pars convoluta). The cells in the single layer of tubular epithelial cells are cuboidal to columnar but generally lack apical microvilli. Mitochondria and other subcellular organelles are less abundant than in the proximal tubule.[33]

Functionally, the distal tubules actively reabsorb sodium, calcium, and bicarbonate and passively reabsorb chloride and water. Hydrogen ions, ammonium ions, and urea are actively secreted, whereas potassium is passively secreted.[35]

Collecting Ducts. The collecting ducts, which complete the renal tubular network, are lined by cuboidal to columnar epithelial cells. As the ducts progress distally, the epithelial cell height increases. Mitochondria are present in approximately the same concentration as in the distal tubule, supplying the energy necessary for active reabsorption of sodium and active secretion of hydrogen ions. Chloride and water are passively resorbed, and potassium is passively secreted.[35]

Mechanisms of Tubular Damage

If a nephrotoxin is not directly toxic to tubular epithelium, the mechanisms of the nephrotoxic tubular damage are similar to those of ischemic tubular necrosis.[14] Several theories have been presented to explain tubular necrosis. Historically, passive diffusion, leakage of tubular fluid into the interstitium, or mechanical obstruction resulting from intraluminal casts was believed to be the principal mechanism of tubular damage. These theories of backleak and tubular obstruction were based on morphologic studies in which intraluminal casts were consistently found in association with tubular necrosis and basement membrane disruption. Alterations in GFR could not be explained by obstruction or backflow of the filtrate, however, and these theories are no longer widely accepted.[36]

One current theory suggests that the initial nephrotoxic or ischemic insult produces hypoxic endothelial cell swelling in renal arterioles, apparently through ischemic impairment of the sodium pump. The endothelial swelling then leads to a decrease in glomerular permeability.[37] This theory has not been proven in the clinical situation.

The factor most widely accepted as the cause of nephrotoxic or ischemic alterations is the vasoconstriction that results from persistent vasomotor hyperactivity. The renin–angiotensin system may play an important role in this mechanism and is discussed further as it relates to renal papillary and interstitial toxicity. The resultant profound vasoconstriction decreases renal blood flow and, thus, GFR.[38]

Often, chemicals are directly toxic to renal tubular epithelium. Because of the heterogeneity of the cell types present within the renal tubules, the tubules have the capacity to perform many complex and diverse functions simultaneously. This high level of biochemical activity also makes the proximal renal tubules the portion of the nephron that is most susceptible to toxic compounds. Androgens also appear to influence the susceptibility of the renal tubules to various nephrotoxins.[39]

For most nephrotoxins, specific mechanisms of cellular or subcellular damage are not understood, but several general mechanisms are known. Compounds may directly affect tubular function by several mechanisms, including metabolic alterations affecting cellular respiration, interference with tubular transport systems, and damage to specific organelles.[40]

The mixed-function oxidase system is principally responsible for the oxidative biotransformation of many endogenous and exogenous compounds.[41,42] Cytochrome P-450 is a unique hemoprotein that functions as the terminal oxidase for the mixed-function oxidase system.[43] The distribution of this system within the kidney varies among species,[40] but the highest concentrations tend to be found in the pars recta of the proximal tubule.[44] With this high degree of metabolic activity and transport functions, the proximal tubule is probably the portion of the nephron that is most susceptible to nephrotoxicity.

Membrane Effects. Compounds that induce nephrotoxicity by altering the cell membrane do so via surface-active properties or interference with ATP-mediated transport activities. Polymyxins and amphotericin B exert their effects in part by disrupting the normal membrane sterol–lipid interactions, allowing the membranes to become more permeable to hydrogen ions and other ions (Figure 2).[45] Breakdown of the permeability barrier leads to osmotic disruption of the cell. Gentamicin and other aminoglycosides tend to affect the membrane by interfering with the Na^+, K^+–ATPase system.[46-48] This disruption, in turn, alters organic ion and bicarbonate transport, leading to tubular dysfunction (Figure 3).[49,50] Cephaloridine and cephalothin exert similar effects.[46] Cephaloridine also causes peroxidation of membrane lipids,[51] which interferes with ion transport, and depletion of glutathione, which contributes to membrane and subcellular alterations.[52] Effects on membranes tend to be most marked in the proximal tubule.[45] Sulfonamides, which precipitate in the tubules, bind to membrane proteins and interfere with ion transport and osmotic balance.[53]

Subcellular Metabolism. The creation of metabolites that are capable of covalent binding with cellular macromolecules is another general nephrotoxic mechanism.[54] Metabo-

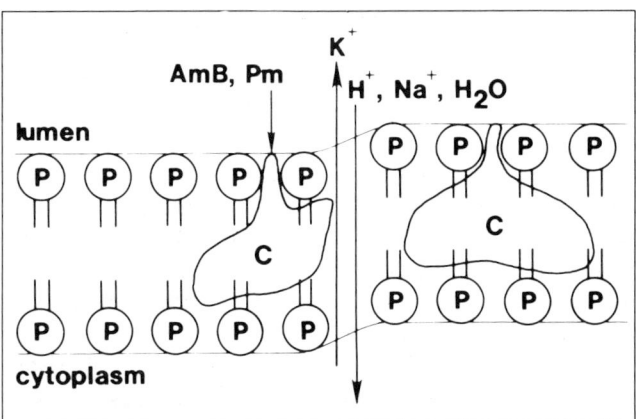

Figure 2—Disruption of the normal renal proximal tubular membrane cholesterol (*C*)–phospholipid (*P*) interaction by polymyxins (*Pm*) and amphotericin B (*AmB*), leading to leakage of K^+ out of the cell and H^+ into the cell.

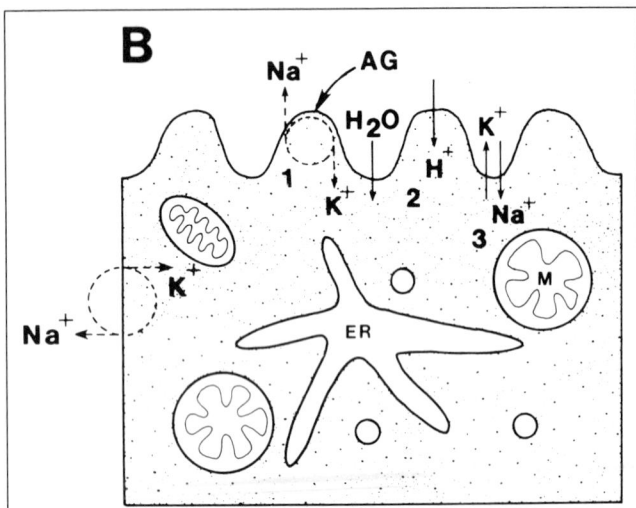

Figure 3—Aminoglycosides (*AG*) can cause (**1**) inhibition of the Na^+, K^+–ATPase transport system on the luminal and, predominantly, the basolateral membranes of renal proximal tubular cells, leading to (**2**) intracellular accumulation of H^+ and H_2O, with (**3**) subsequent loss of K^+ into the tubular lumen and accumulation of intracellular Na^+. As a result of these ionic alterations, mitochondria (*M*) and endoplasmic reticulum (*ER*) swell and lose functional capacity.

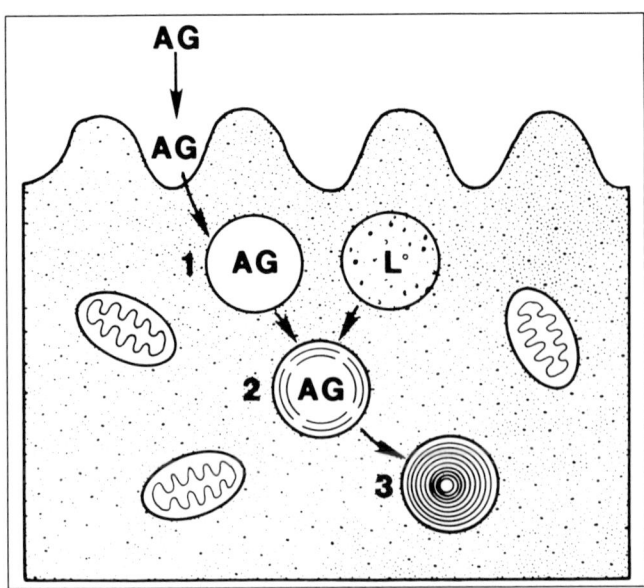

Figure 5—Aminoglycoside inhibition of phospholipases in the proximal tubular brush border membrane causes (**1**) accumulation of aminoglycosides (*AG*) in endocytic vesicles, (**2**) fusion of the endocytic vesicles with lysosomes (*L*) to form cytosegresomes, and (**3**) formation of myeloid figures as a result of phospholipid accumulation in the cytosegresomes.

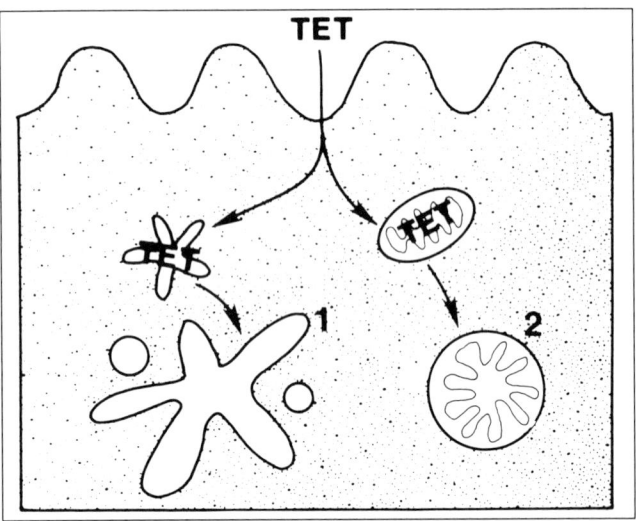

Figure 4—Accumulation of outdated tetracycline metabolites (*TET*) within (**1**) endoplasmic reticulum and (**2**) mitochondria, causing loss of function and architecture.

lites of acetaminophen[55] form covalent links with endoplasmic reticulum, leading to cell dysfunction through interruption of normal protein synthesis. Outdated tetracycline products cause a reversible Fanconi-like syndrome (glycosuria, aminoaciduria, and hyperphosphatemia), which is most likely related to the accumulation of metabolites within mitochondria; the result is disruption of cristae and inhibition of many of the oxidative enzymes involved in glycolysis, the Krebs cycle, the hexose monophosphate shunt, and β-oxidation of fatty acids (Figure 4). This effect, seen solely in the proximal tubule, leads to progressive nephropathy. Tetracycline products that are not out-

dated caused only slight functional impairment.[45,51] Another antibiotic, kanamycin, has been shown only to inhibit glycolysis,[56] although this activity is only part of the nephrotoxic mechanism for kanamycin. Interruption of the energy-producing machinery of the tubular cells begins the potential cascade leading from cell death to disruption of tubular function.

An early event in aminoglycoside nephrotoxicity is the accumulation of phospholipids and antibiotics within the lysosomes of proximal tubular epithelial cells. The accumulation of phospholipids results from aminoglycoside inhibition of phospholipases A and C,[57,58] which leads to renal phospholipidosis,[59] a proposed mechanism for the formation of intracellular myeloid figures or cytosegresomes (Figure 5).[60] The enzyme inhibition apparently results from binding of the aminoglycosides to phospholipids (e.g., phosphatidylinositol) and alteration of the substrate for phospholipases.[58] The physiologic significance of phospholipase inhibition remains unknown but may be related either to the role of phospholipases in prostaglandin synthesis and degradation[57] or to the induction of lysosomal instability.[59]

Renal Papilla and Interstitium

The pathophysiology of drug-related papillary and interstitial disease involves either hypersensitivity or inhibition of protective prostaglandins by nonsteroidal antiinflammatory drugs (NSAIDs). The hypersensitivity reactions generally arise from the penicillin class of antibiotics. Interstitial nephritis develops in only a small percentage of patients receiving penicillin or its derivatives; and the accompanying clinical signs are consistent with an immune mechanism. Clinical indices often include a high IgM titer and IgG antibodies directed against the penicilloyl moiety.[61,62] Cell-mediated immunity may also be operative in drug-related interstitial nephritis. The penicilloyl haptens may uniquely bind to renal proteins in certain patients. Alternatively, these patients may be uniquely capable of forming hapten–renal protein conjugates.[61]

Renal papillary necrosis resulting from medullary ischemia is presumed to be induced by the inhibition of prostaglandin synthetase; the decreased amounts of prostaglandin synthetase cause a decrease in the production of renal prostaglandins, with a concomitant increase in leukotriene production.[63] During systemic vasoconstriction, the formation of angiotensin II causes the localized production of vasodilatory renal prostaglandins to offset the vasoconstrictive action of angiotensin II.[64] In patients in which this scenario is manifested, large amounts of urinary prostaglandins are excreted. Treatment with NSAIDs decreases renal prostaglandin production, thereby allowing the vasoconstrictive action of angiotensin II to predominate in the renal vasculature. Further vasoconstriction is caused by the increased leukotriene production that results from blockade of cyclooxygenase and the consequent increase in the amount of substrate diverted through the lipoxygenase pathway, which is responsible for leukotriene production. The result is profound vasoconstriction, which causes decreased renal blood flow followed by ischemic necrosis of the renal papilla.[64] Phenylbutazone, the drug that has been incriminated most often in the horse as a cause of renal papillary necrosis,[65-67] apparently is able to cause medullary ischemia via prostaglandin inhibition.[68] Similar alterations also occur with phenacetin, aspirin, acetaminophen, and indomethacin.[63]

Diagnosis

Drug-related nephropathies appear clinically as typical renal diseases; therefore, documentation of drug-related nephrotoxicosis must include a history of administration of a nephrotoxic drug as well as demonstration of the clinical signs consistent with the nephrotoxic mechanisms of that drug (Table III). Definitive diagnosis usually requires renal biopsy.[69]

Although the GFR cannot be used to differentiate glomerular damage from tubular damage, it is a good indicator of overall renal function. Inulin clearance is the most accurate index of GFR, but endogenous or exogenous creatinine clearance is extremely well correlated with GFR.[70-72] Serum creatinine concentrations[73] are inversely related to GFR, but confounding variables[74] make this index only a crude approximation of GFR. Inability to concentrate urine occurs in patients with tubular and medullary damage, but this feature is not specific for renal insufficiency. Furthermore, for patients in which isosthenuria is the result of renal parenchymal disease, significant decreases in functional renal mass must occur before urine-concentrating ability is affected.

Differentiation between oliguria and polyuria is essential for determining a diagnosis and prognosis. Oliguria (in the dog, for example, production of less than 1 ml urine/kg/hr) denotes acutely disordered renal function. Acute renal failure, acute nephritis, urinary tract obstruction, and terminal chronic renal failure may all present as oliguric renal failure. The short-term prognosis for oliguric renal failure is very poor without emergency treatment or dialysis. Polyuria, on the other hand, is a classic sign of early chronic renal failure and of tubular resorption defects, although a plethora of other disorders may also cause polyuria. The short-term prognosis for polyuric renal failure is not as

TABLE III
Nephrotoxic Action of Some Drugs in Common Clinical Use

Renal Location	Effect	Drug
Glomerulus		
Endothelium	Decreased fenestral area	Aminoglycosides
Basement membrane	Immune complex deposition	Penicillins, cephalosporins
	SLE-like immune reaction	Hydralazine, procainamide
Podocytes	Decreased amounts of sialoglycoproteins, leading to foot process alteration	Puromycin, probenecid, Adriamycin
Proximal tubule	Membrane disruption	Amphotericin B, sulfonamides
	Ion transport	Aminoglycosides, sulfonamides
	Phospholipase inhibition, leading to lysosomal dysfunction	Aminoglycosides
	Lipid peroxidation	Cephaloridine
	Oxidative enzyme inhibition	Tetracyclines
Interstitium	Mononuclear cell infiltration	Penicillins, cephalosporins, sulfonamides
Medulla	Prostaglandin inhibition, leading to ischemia and necrosis	Phenylbutazone, aspirin, phenacetin, acetaminophen

guarded as that for oliguric acute renal failure; however, the long-term prognosis is poor.[69]

Glomerulonephropathies often exhibit moderate to marked proteinuria, characterized by albuminuria, α_2-globulinuria, and immunoglobulinuria[75]; hypoalbuminemia; edema; and, often, hyperlipoidemia.[32,69,76] Proteinuria in humans is described as loss of more than 60 mg protein/kg/day,[77] although protein loss in glomerulonephropathies may be as high as 20 g protein/day.[69] The evidence for immune-mediated mechanisms includes the lack of correlation between the dosage and the severity of the lesions, as well as a lag between drug administration and the onset of glomerular lesions.[9] Patients with immune-mediated nephritides often have other clinical signs of immune-mediated disease, such as fever, rash, eosinophilia, hematuria, proteinuria, renal insufficiency, and, perhaps, polyarthritides.[61,62] Patchy fluorescence because of irregular immune complex deposition on the glomerular basement membranes is a characteristic finding in immunofluorescence evaluation of renal biopsy specimens.[9] When drugs associated with SLE-like syndromes have been given to the patient, serum antinuclear antibody titers and LE cell identification should be considered definitive tests.[69] The histologic changes of glomerulopathies consist of thickening and splitting of the glomerular basement membrane and loss of podocyte foot processes. Irregular thickening and scalloping of the glomerular basement membrane may be sufficiently prominent to be recognized by light microscopy with periodic acid–Schiff (PAS) staining methods. The cells of the glomerulus become swollen and laden with fat vacuoles, making the glomerulus appear hypercellular. Bowman's capsule may be distended, but only rarely is the glomerular space obliterated.[9]

Tubular damage can also result in proteinuria, although less extensive than that seen after glomerular damage. Proteins are liberated from the tubular epithelium, as are enzyme markers for the subcellular localization of the tubular injury, analogous to the use of serum alanine aminotransferase and alkaline phosphatase as enzyme markers for hepatocellular injury and biliary obstruction, respectively. In addition, tubular proteinuria can result from incomplete resorption of low-molecular-weight filtered proteins, such as lysozyme and β_2-microglobulin. Concentrations of several specific enzyme and serum protein markers of tubular damage are increased after aminoglycoside administration.[78–85] Although N-acetylglucosaminidase is frequently used as a clinical marker, evidence suggests that quantitation of the urinary excretion of N-acetylglucosaminidase does not distinguish between nonnephrotoxic and nephrotoxic patients being treated with aminoglycosides.[85] Of the other markers of renal tubular injury, γ-glutamyltransferase and β_2-microglobulin excretion are the most reliable. Excretion of these markers increases four to five days before any increase in the serum creatinine or the urea nitrogen concentrations occurs. Perhaps the best indicator of renal tubular damage is a dramatic increase in the fractional excretion of β_2-microglobulin.[86] With this method, quantitative urine collection is not needed; and many clinical laboratories are able to quantitate β_2-microglobulin. The fractional excretion of sodium also rises above 1% in patients with tubular necrosis or tubular obstruction.[69] When damage has progressed further, tubular necrosis occurs, and there is subsequent formation of urinary casts.[87]

Management

The first step in the treatment of drug-related nephropathies is to discontinue use of the drug. If the drug must be used, dosage adjustments should be made to prevent accumulation of drug in the patient.[88] Clinical reversal of signs attributable to glomerular changes may occur if the inciting cause of the immune complex formation is either withdrawn or filtered out through various forms of dialysis.

Therapy for polyuric renal failure includes intense fluid therapy, because significant fluid losses can occur during this time. For oliguric renal failure, urine production must be started immediately, by either osmotic or loop diuresis. If urine production has not started, dialysis, with maintenance of renal blood flow, is imperative.

Therapy for glomerulopathies is directed toward increasing protein production to counteract the marked proteinuria and hypoproteinemia. Diets high in caloric density and quality proteins slow endogenous protein catabolism.[75] Anabolic steroids, such as stanozolol, also promote protein anabolism.[75] For the edema that accompanies hypoproteinemia, diuretics can be given until the serum albumin concentration rises to within the normal range. Specific therapy for drug-related glomerulopathies includes corticosteroids, anticoagulants, and immunosuppressive drugs, such as cyclophosphamide, cyclosporine, and azathioprine.[48,89,90] Because the use of these drugs for immune-mediated nephropathies is controversial and because the drugs are occasionally nephrotoxic themselves, high-dose prednisolone (1.5 to 2.0 mg/kg) as alternate-day therapy is regarded as the treatment of choice for immune-mediated glomerulonephropathies.[69] Heparin may prevent the intraglomerular coagulation process associated with chronic renal failure[89,90] and may also replenish the negative charges lost from the visceral epithelial foot processes.[12] Antiinflammatory drugs may also alleviate some of the glomerular damage that results from immune complex-precipitated glomerular inflammation.[89] Hypertension, which often accompanies glomerulonephropathies, can be treated by restriction of salt intake and administration of diuretics, β-adrenergic blockers, and vasodilators.[69] Overloading the patient with antigen occasionally solubilizes the antigen–antibody complexes and decreases the deposition of immune complexes.[24]

Most tubular nephrotoxicities are reversible because the tubular epithelium can regenerate if the tubular basement membrane is still intact. Therefore, supportive therapy for acute tubular necrosis is very important. Fluid diuresis and administration of diuretics can be lifesaving.[91,92] Diuresis improves renal blood flow, rather than renal tubular function, and it promotes solute excretion by bulk flow as well.[69] Loop diuretics are less effective than mannitol for improvement of GFR and renal blood flow, and furosemide may even exacerbate aminoglycoside-induced nephrotoxicity.[93] Hydralazine also significantly improves renal blood flow. Because of the large number of vasodilatory dopamine receptors in the renal cortex, substantial temporary improvement of renal perfusion can be achieved by intravenous infusion of dopamine (2 to 5 µg/min/kg).[69,94] Several free oxygen radical scavengers may prove useful in the future, but their efficacy has not been demonstrated clinically.[95]

Hyperkalemia also accompanies acute oliguric renal failure, and hyperkalemic cardiotoxicity is responsible for the early mortality that is associated with acute renal failure. Intravenous infusion of calcium gluceptate (0.1 mEq/kg Ca^{++}) antagonizes the cardiotoxicity of severe hyperkalemia (> 8.0 mEq potassium/L). For moderate hyperkalemia (5.5 to 8.0 mEq potassium/L), intravenous 20% glucose can be administered with or without intravenous regular insulin, 0.12 to 0.25 U/kg, both of which promote movement of extracellular potassium into the cells.[69] Potassium intake should be restricted, even in the parenteral fluids. The amount of sodium in sodium bicarbonate may exacerbate the already hyperosmolar state associated with the accumulation of uremic compounds in the bloodstream, and sodium bicarbonate should thus be used cautiously. Other signs of uremia can be treated with histamine$_2$ antagonists, antiemetics, and phosphate binders.[69,91]

Conclusions

Given the structural and functional heterogeneity of mammalian nephrons, not all species, or even all breeds within a species, will have the same degree of nephrotoxic susceptibility to all therapeutic agents.[96] Furthermore, extrapolation of nephrotoxic potential across species lines is also dependent on the relative size and metabolic rates of each species. Therefore, allometric equations for improving interspecies and intraspecies comparisons[97] must be incorporated before the reports in one species can be used to direct therapeutic strategy with a potentially nephrotoxic compound.

Drug-related nephropathies may be encountered more frequently as additional therapeutic agents become available to the clinician. The underlying mechanisms of glomerular and tubular pathophysiology are related to disruptions of membrane functions and interactions, cellular metabolism, or induction of immune-mediated disease. Diagnosis of these problems is dependent on the causal association with treatment and documentation of renal disease by standard methods. Management of drug-related nephropathies is the same as that for any case of acute renal failure, glomerulonephritis, or interstitial nephritis.

REFERENCES

1. Brenner BM, Ichikawa I, Deen WM: Glomerular filtration, in Brenner BM, Rector FC (eds): *The Kidney*, ed 2. Philadelphia, WB Saunders Co, 1981, pp 289–327.
2. Burg MB: Renal handling of sodium, chloride, water, amino acids, and glucose, in Brenner BM, Rector FC (eds): *The Kidney*, ed 2. Philadelphia, WB Saunders Co, 1981, pp 328–370.
3. Schnermann J, Levine DZ: Tubular control of glomerular filtration rate in single nephrons. *Can J Physiol Pharmacol* 53:325–330, 1975.
4. Maher JF: Clinicopathologic spectrum of drug nephrotoxicity. *Adv Intern Med* 30:295–316, 1984.
5. Baylis C: The mechanism of the decline in glomerular filtration rate in gentamicin-induced acute renal failure in the rat. *J Antimicrob Chemother* 6:381–388, 1980.
6. Luft FC, Aronoff GR, Evan AP, et al: The effect of aminoglycosides on glomerular endothelium: A comparative study. *Res Commun Chem Pathol Pharmacol* 34:89–95, 1981.
7. Luft FC, Aronoff GR, Evan AP, et al: The renin–angiotensin system in aminoglycoside-induced acute renal failure. *J Pharmacol Exp Ther* 220:433–439, 1982.
8. Bulger RE, Eknoyan G, Purcell DJ, Dobyan DC: Endothelial characteristics of glomerular capillaries in normal, mercuric chloride-induced, and gentamicin-induced acute renal failure in the rat. *J Clin Invest* 72:128–141, 1983.
9. Gartner H-V: Drug-associated nephropathy. Part I: Glomerular lesions. *Curr Top Pathol* 69:143–181, 1980.
10. Batsford SR, Rohrbach R, Riede UN, et al: Effects of D-penicillamine administration to rats, induction of renal changes: Preliminary communication. *Clin Nephrol* 6:394–397, 1976.
11. Wehner H: Nierenveranderungen bei Behandlung mit Azathioprin. *Res Exp Med* 14:361–365, 1975.
12. Cheville NF: The kidney, in Cheville NF (ed): *Cell Pathology*, ed 2. Ames, IA, Iowa State University Press, 1983, pp 559–588.
13. Kanwar YS: Biology of disease. Biophysiology of glomerular filtration and proteinuria. *Lab Invest* 51:7–21, 1984.
14. Porter GA, Bennett WM: Toxic nephropathies, in Brenner BM, Rector FC (eds): *The Kidney*, ed 2. Philadelphia, WB Saunders Co, 1981, pp 2045–2108.
15. Caulfield JP, Farquhar MG: Loss of anionic sites from the glomerular basement membrane in aminonucleoside nephrosis. *Lab Invest* 39:505–512, 1978.
16. Couser WB, Salant DJ, Stilmant MM, et al: The effects of the aminonucleoside puromycin and nephrotoxic serum on subepithelial immune-deposit formation in passive Heymann nephritis. *J Lab Clin Med* 94:917–932, 1979.
17. Kronenberg KH, Scholl A, Schmulling RM, et al: Glomerulare Fruhveranderungen bei der Daunomycin-Nephrose. *Verh Dtsch Ges Pathol* 56:602–606, 1972.
18. Weening JJ, Fleuren GJ, Hoedemaeker PJ: Demonstration of antinuclear antibodies in mercuric chloride-induced glomerulopathy in the rat. *Lab Invest* 39:405–411, 1978.
19. Hertz PH, Yager H, Richardson JA: Probenecid-induced nephrotic syndrome. *Arch Pathol* 94:241–243, 1972.
20. Kelley VE, Cavallo T: Glomerular permeability. Transfer of native ferritin in glomeruli with decreased anionic sites. *Lab Invest* 39:547–553, 1978.
21. Kerjaschki D: Polycation-induced dislocation of slit diaphragms and formation of cell junctions in rat kidney glomeruli. *Lab Invest* 39:430–440, 1978.
22. Slauson DO, Lewis RM: Comparative pathology of glomerulonephritis in animals. *Vet Pathol* 16:135–164, 1979.
23. Rehan A, Johnson KJ, Wiggins RC, et al: Evidence for the role of oxygen radicals in acute nephrotoxic nephritis. *Lab Invest* 51:396–403, 1984.
24. Osborne CA, Jeraj K: Glomerulonephropathy and the nephrotic syndrome, in Kirk RW (ed): *Current Veterinary Therapy VIII*. Philadelphia, WB Saunders Co, 1980, pp 1053–1062.
25. Kovnat P, Labovitz E, Levison SP: Antibiotics and the kidney. *Med Clin North Am* 57:1045–1063, 1973.
26. Bacon PA, Tribe CR, MacKenzie JC, et al: Penicillamine nephropathy in rheumatoid arthritis. *Q J Med* 180:661–684, 1976.
27. Nagi AH, Alexander F, Barabas AZ: Gold nephropathy in rats—Light and electron microscopic studies. *Exp Mol Pathol* 15:354–362, 1971.
28. Silverberg DS, Kidd EG, Shnitka TK, et al: Gold nephropathy. A clinical and pathological study. *Arthritis Rheum* 13:812–825, 1971.
29. Owens CJ, Yarbrough DR, Brackett NC: Nephrotic syndrome following topically applied sulfadiazine silver therapy. *Arch Intern Med* 134:332–335, 1974.
30. Blomgren SE, Condemi JJ, Vaughan JH: Procainamide-induced lupus erythematosus. *Am J Med* 52:338–348, 1972.
31. Lima JJ: Procainamide, in Evans WE, Schentag JJ, Jusko WJ (eds):

Applied Pharmacokinetics. Spokane, WA, Applied Therapeutics, 1980, pp 404–435.

32. Matthes KJ: Drug-induced proteinuria. *Contrib Nephrol* 24:109–114, 1981.

33. Tisher CC: Anatomy of the kidney, in Brenner BM, Rector FC (eds): *The Kidney*, ed 2. Philadelphia, WB Saunders Co, 1981, pp 3–75.

34. Bonner FW, Bach PH, Dobrota M: The biochemistry of the kidney, in Bach PH, Bonner FW, Bridges JW, Lock EA (eds): *Nephrotoxicity: Assessment and Pathogenesis*. New York, John Wiley & Sons, 1982, pp 27–53.

35. Berndt WO: Renal tubular function, in Bach PH, Bonner FW, Bridges JW, Lock EA (eds): *Nephrotoxicity: Assessment and Pathogenesis*, New York, John Wiley & Sons, 1982, pp 54–65.

36. Levinsky NG: Pathophysiology of acute renal failure. *N Engl J Med* 296:1453–1457, 1977.

37. Oken DE: Local mechanisms in the pathogenesis of acute renal failure. *Kidney Int* 10:594–596, 1976.

38. Stein JH, Patak RV, Lifschitz MD: Acute renal failure: Clinical aspects and pathophysiology. *Contrib Nephrol* 14:118–141, 1978.

39. Carlton WW, Engelhardt JA: Chloroform nephrosis, male mouse, in Jones TC, Mohr U, Hunt RD (eds): *Urinary System. Monographs on Pathology of Laboratory Animals*. Berlin, Springer-Verlag, 1986, pp 225–228.

40. Ackerman DM, Hook JB: Biochemical interactions and nephrotoxicity. *Fundam Appl Toxicol* 4:300–314, 1984.

41. Anders MW: Metabolism of drugs in the kidney. *Kidney Int* 18:636–647, 1980.

42. Davis BB, Mattamal MB, Zeuser TV: Renal metabolism of drugs and xenobiotics. *Nephron* 27:187–196, 1981.

43. Omura T, Sato R: The carbon monoxide-binding pigment of liver microsomes. I. Evidence for its hemoprotein nature. *J Biol Chem* 239:2370–2378, 1964.

44. Fowler BA, Hook GER, Lucier GW: Tetrachlorodibenzo-*p*-dioxin induction of renal microsomal enzyme systems: Ultrastructural effects on pars recta (S₃) proximal tubule cells of the kidney. *J Pharmacol Exp Ther* 203:712–721, 1977.

45. Hook JB, McCormack KM, Kluwe WM: Biochemical mechanisms of nephrotoxicity. *Rev Biochem Toxicol* 3:53–78, 1979.

46. Williams PD, Holohan PD, Ross CR: Gentamicin nephrotoxicity. II. Possible membrane changes. *Toxicol Appl Pharmacol* 61:243–251, 1981.

47. Kaloyanides GJ: Aminoglycoside-induced functional and biochemical defects in the renal cortex. *Fundam Appl Toxicol* 4:930–948, 1984.

48. Chahwala SB, Harpur ES: An investigation of the effects of aminoglycoside antibiotics on Na⁺, K⁺-ATPase as a possible mechanism of toxicity. *Res Commun Chem Pathol Pharmacol* 35:63–78, 1982.

49. Bennett WM, Plamp CE, Parker RA, et al: Alterations in organic ion transport induced by gentamicin nephrotoxicity in the rat. *J Lab Clin Med* 95:32–39, 1980.

50. Klotman PE, Yarger WE: Reduction of renal blood flow and proximal bicarbonate reabsorption in rats by gentamicin. *Kidney Int* 24:634–638, 1983.

51. Kuo CH, Maitu K, Sleight SD, et al: Lipid peroxidation: A possible mechanism of cephaloridine-induced nephrotoxicity. *Toxicol Appl Pharmacol* 67:78–88, 1983.

52. Kuo CH, Hook JB: Depletion of renal glutathione content and nephrotoxicity of cephaloridine in rabbits, rats and mice. *Toxicol Appl Pharmacol* 63:292–302, 1982.

53. Zbinden G: Experimental renal toxicity, in Rouiller C, Muller AF (eds): *The Kidney: Morphology, Biochemistry, Physiology, vol II.* New York, Academic Press, 1969, pp 401–476.

54. Gillette JR: A perspective on the role of chemically reactive metabolites of foreign compounds in toxicity. I. Correlation of changes in covalent binding of reactive metabolites with changes in the incidence and severity of toxicity. *Biochem Pharmacol* 23:2785–2794, 1974.

55. McMurtry RJ, Snodgrass WR, Mitchell JR: Renal necrosis, glutathione depletion and covalent binding after acetaminophen. *Toxicol Appl Pharmacol* 46:87–100, 1978.

56. Tachibana M, Mizukoshi D, Kuriyama K: Inhibitory effects of kanamycin on glycolysis in the cochlea and kidney—Possible involvement in the formation of oto- and nephrotoxicities. *Biochem Pharmacol* 25:2297–2300, 1976.

57. Lipsky JJ, Leitman PS: Aminoglycoside inhibition of renal phosphatidylinositol phospholipase C. *J Pharmacol Exp Ther* 220:282–292, 1982.

58. Hostetler KY, Hall LB: Inhibition of kidney lysosomal phospholipases A and C by aminoglycoside antibiotics: Possible mechanism of aminoglycoside toxicity. *Proc Natl Acad Sci USA* 79:1663–1667, 1982.

59. Feldman S, Wang MY, Kaloyanides GJ: Aminoglycosides induce a phospholipidosis in the renal cortex of the rat: An early manifestation of nephrotoxicity. *J Pharmacol Exp Ther* 220:514–520, 1982.

60. Riviere JE, Hinsman EJ, Coppoc GL, et al: Single dose gentamicin nephrotoxicity in the dog: Early functional and ultrastructural changes. *Res Commun Chem Pathol Pharmacol* 33:403–418, 1981.

61. Baldwin DS, Levine BB, McCluskey RT, et al: Renal failure and interstitial nephritis due to penicillin and methicillin. *N Engl J Med* 279:1245–1252, 1968.

62. Silverstein RL, Eigenbrodt EH, McPhaul JJ: Interstitial nephritis caused by methicillin. Studies in a case complicating staphylococcal sepsis with acute glomerulonephritis. *Am J Clin Pathol* 76:316–321, 1981.

63. Sabatini S: Pathophysiology of drug-induced papillary necrosis. *Fundam Appl Toxicol* 4:909–921, 1984.

64. Reeves WB, Foley RJ, Weinman EJ: Nephrotoxicity from nonsteroidal anti-inflammatory drugs. *South Med J* 78:318–322, 1985.

65. Gunson DE: Renal papillary necrosis in horses. *JAVMA* 182:263–266, 1983.

66. Murray MJ: Phenylbutazone toxicity in a horse. *Compend Contin Educ Pract Vet* 7:S389–S394, 1985.

67. Read WK: Renal medullary crest necrosis associated with phenylbutazone therapy in horses. *Vet Pathol* 20:662–669, 1983.

68. Collins LG, Tyler DE: Experimentally induced phenylbutazone toxicosis in ponies: Description of the syndrome and its prevention with synthetic prostaglandin E₂. *Am J Vet Res* 46:1605–1615, 1985.

69. Cowgill LD: Diseases of the kidney, in Ettinger SJ (ed): *Textbook of Veterinary Internal Medicine*, ed 2. Philadelphia, WB Saunders Co, 1983, pp 1760–1860.

70. Finco DR, Coulter DB, Barsanti JA: Simple, accurate method for clinical estimation of glomerular filtration rate in the dog. *Am J Vet Res* 42:1874–1877, 1981.

71. Grauer GF: Clinicopathologic evaluation of early renal disease in dogs. *Compend Contin Educ Pract Vet* 7:32–38, 1985.

72. Fettman MJ, Allen TA, Wilke WL, et al: Single-injection method for evaluation of renal function with ¹⁴C-inulin and ³H-tetraethylammonium bromide in dogs and cats. *Am J Vet Res* 46:482–485, 1985.

73. Shea PH, Maher JF, Horak E: Prediction of glomerular filtration rate by serum creatinine and β₂-microglobulin. *Nephron* 29:30–35, 1981.

74. Watson ADJ, Church DB, Fairburn AJ: Postprandial changes in plasma urea and creatinine concentrations in dogs. *Am J Vet Res* 42:1878–1880, 1981.

75. August JR, Loar AS, Saunders GR, et al: Membranous glomerulonephropathy and nephrotic syndrome in a cat. *Compend Contin Educ Pract Vet* 7:363–368, 1985.

76. Osborne CA, Polzin DJ: Azotemia: A review of what's old and what's new. Part I. Definitions of terms and concepts. *Compend Contin Educ Pract Vet* 5:497–508, 1983.

77. Merrill JP: Glomerulonephritis (first of three parts). *N Engl J Med* 290:257–266, 1974.

78. Adelman RD, Halsted CC, Jordan GW, et al: Use of urinary activities in the early detection of aminoglycoside nephrotoxicity: A study in children and adults receiving gentamicin or netilmicin. *Proc West Pharmacol Soc* 24:261–264, 1981.

79. Beck PR, Thomson RB, Chaudhuri AKR: Aminoglycoside antibiotics and renal function: Changes in urinary γ-glutamyltransferase excretion. *J Clin Pathol* 30:432–437, 1977.

80. Crowell WA, Divers TJ, Byars TD, et al: Neomycin toxicosis in calves. *Am J Vet Res* 42:29–34, 1981.

81. Davey PG, Geddes AM, Cowley DM: Study of alanine aminopeptidase as a test of gentamicin nephrotoxicity. *J Antimicrob Chemother* 11:455–465, 1983.

82. Kaye WA, Griffiths WC, Camara PD, et al: The significance of β-2 microglobinuria associated with gentamicin therapy. *Ann Clin Lab Sci* 11:530–537, 1981.

83. Lechi A, Rizzotti P, Mengoli C, et al: Lactic dehydrogenase isoenzymes in urinary tract infections and aminoglycoside nephrotoxicity. *Infection* 11:64–65, 1983.

84. Schentag JJ, Suftin TA, Plaut ME, et al: Early detection of aminoglycoside nephrotoxicity with urinary β-2-microglobulin. *J Med* 9:201–209, 1978.

85. Reed MD, Vermeulen MW, Stern RC, et al: Are measurements of urinary enzymes useful during aminoglycoside therapy? *Pediatr Res* 15:1234–1239, 1981.

86. Roxe DM: Current status of renal clearances. *Ann Clin Lab Sci* 11:279–282, 1981.

87. Schentag JJ, Gengo FM, Plaut ME, et al: Urinary casts as an indicator of renal tubular damage in patients receiving aminoglycosides. *Antimicrob Agents Chemother* 16:468–474, 1979.

88. Riviere JE, Davis LE: Renal handling of drugs in renal failure, in Bovee KC (ed): *Canine Nephrology*. Media, PA, Harwal Publishing Co, 1984, pp 643–685.

89. Merrill JP: Glomerulonephritis (third of three parts). *N Engl J Med* 290:374–381, 1974.

90. Simon NM, Rosenberg MJ: Medical treatment of glomerular diseases. *Med Clin North Am* 62:1157–1181, 1978.

91. Brown SA, Barsanti JA, Crowell WA: Gentamicin-associated acute renal failure in the dog. *JAVMA* 186:686–690, 1985.

92. Riviere JE, Traver DS, Coppoc GL: Gentamicin toxic nephropathy in horses with disseminated bacterial infection. *JAVMA* 180:648–651, 1982.

93. Adelman RD, Spangler WL, Beason F, et al: Frusemide enhancement of netilmicin nephrotoxicity in dogs. *J Antimicrob Chemother* 7:431–440, 1981.

94. Seri I, Tulassay T, Kiszel J, et al: The use of dopamine for the prevention of the renal side effects of indomethacin in premature infants with patent ductus arteriosus. *Int J Pediatr Nephrol* 5:209–214, 1984.

95. Paller MS: Free radical scavengers in mercuric chloride-induced acute renal failure in the rat. *J Lab Clin Med* 105:459–463, 1985.

96. Valtin H: Structural and functional heterogeneity of mammalian nephrons. *Am J Physiol* 233:F491–F501, 1977.

97. Hackbarth H, Buttner D, Gartner K: Intraspecies allometry: Correlation between kidney weight and glomerular filtration rate vs. body weight. *Am J Physiol* 242:R303–R305, 1982.

KEY FACTS

- The nephrotoxic potential of aminoglycosides, penicillins, cephalosporins, and sulfonamides is dependent on dose, duration of treatment, and the particular drug formulation being used.
- Clinical signs of toxicity are referable to renal tubular necrosis, renal papillary necrosis, or immune-mediated interstitial nephritis.
- Basic treatment of adverse renal drug reactions includes administration of parenteral fluids, which may be specifically supplemented, and discontinuation of the eliciting drug.

Drug-Related Nephropathies
Part II. Commonly Used Drugs*

Jeffery A. Engelhardt, MS, DVM
Department of Microbiology, Pathology, and Public Health

Scott Anthony Brown, DVM, PhD†
Department of Veterinary Physiology and Pharmacology

School of Veterinary Medicine
Purdue University
West Lafayette, Indiana

Several therapeutic agents used in veterinary medicine cause or have a high potential to cause drug-induced renal disease. Part I of this two-part series described specific nephrotoxic mechanisms. This article discusses the mechanisms, diagnosis, management, and prevention of the renal toxicity associated with some of the commonly used drugs in veterinary medicine. The most frequently used of these agents as well as the clinical signs and treatment of the nephrotoxicity are outlined in Table I.

Numerous therapeutic agents are excreted from the body via the kidney, either as the parent drug or as metabolites. As a result, the kidney is exposed to high concentrations of many compounds, which form a continuum from nontoxic to highly toxic. The physiologic basis for the exposure of the kidney to high concentrations of foreign compounds was presented in Part I of this series.

Aminoglycosides
Incidence and Predisposing Factors

Aminoglycosides are used in patients with severe gram-negative infections. Gentamicin is the parenteral aminoglycoside used most frequently in companion animal medicine; streptomycin, amikacin, and tobramycin are also commonly used. All aminoglycosides are nephrotoxic and ototoxic, but each has an intrinsic capacity to damage renal proximal tubules, apparently as a function of the number of ionizable amino groups in the chemical structure. Neomycin, the most nephrotoxic aminoglycoside, should not be administered parenterally. The other nephrotoxic aminoglycoside antibiotics, in decreasing order of toxic potential, are as follows: gentamicin, tobramycin, amikacin, and streptomycin.

The incidence of gentamicin-induced nephrotoxicity in human medicine is 10% to 25% when serum concentrations of gentamicin are not monitored.

*Published as Purdue University Agricultural Experiment Station Journal Paper Number 10,722.

†Dr. Brown's present address is Department of Veterinary Physiology and Pharmacology, College of Veterinary Medicine, Texas A&M University, College Station, Texas.

TABLE I

Common Clinical Signs and Treatment Strategies for Specific Drug-Related Nephropathies

Drug	Clinical Signs	Treatment
Aminoglycosides	Acute renal failure, proteinuria, hematuria, hyperphosphatemia, hypoalbuminemia, elevated serum urea nitrogen (SUN)/creatinine levels	Discontinue drug; fluids, oral calcium, oral sodium, oral potassium
Amphotericin B	SUN >50 mg/dl, metabolic acidosis, hypokalemia, hematuria, cylindruria, proteinuria, pyuria	Discontinue drug; fluids, intravenous dopamine, oral sodium
Methoxyflurane	Acute renal failure	Fluids, electrolytes
Arsenicals	Proteinuria, cylindruria, vomiting, diarrhea	Dimercaprol (early), then penicillamine, fluids, intravenous dopamine
Cephalosporins (cephaloridine)	Acute renal failure	Discontinue drug; fluids, vitamin E
Penicillins	Acute renal failure, hematuria, systemic hypersensitivity reactions	Discontinue drug; value of corticosteroids or immunosuppressive agents uncertain
Tetracyclines	Acute renal failure, Fanconi-like syndrome (proteinuria, glycosuria)	Fluids
Sulfonamides	Acute renal failure, sulfonamide crystalluria	Urine alkalization, fluid diuresis
Nonsteroidal antiinflammatory drugs	None or acute renal failure, ulcers (oral, gastrointestinal), edema	Discontinue drug or reduce dose; fluids and/or plasma, intravenous dopamine

When the dose is adjusted to attain peak gentamicin serum concentrations of 8 to 10 μg/ml and trough concentrations (concentrations in the serum immediately before the next dose) of less than 2 μg/ml, the incidence of nephrotoxicity is less than 5%. Gentamicin-induced acute renal failure in clinical patients has been reported in veterinary medicine, but the reports have not specified the rate of occurrence of gentamicin-induced nephrotoxicity, indicating only that it remains a problem in severely ill patients.[1,2]

Mechanisms

Aminoglycosides are eliminated almost exclusively by glomerular filtration. Active uptake of aminoglycosides by the proximal tubules leads to accumulation of these drugs within the proximal tubular epithelium. The aminoglycosides then interfere with mitochondrial function and with normal lysosomal maturation and turnover. The result is accumulation of lysosomes within the cells as well as a decrease in cellular respiration, culminating in acute tubular necrosis. Part I of this series contains additional information on this mechanism.

Because aminoglycosides accumulate in the proximal tubules, protracted dosing increases the likelihood of nephrotoxicity. Factors that predispose a patient to aminoglycoside nephrotoxicity include prolonged therapy (more than five days), elevated trough serum concentrations (≥ 2 μg/ml for gentamicin and tobramycin, ≥ 5 μg/ml for amikacin), preexisting renal disease, and concurrent administration of cytotoxic or other nephrotoxic drugs. Dehydration,

even the subclinical dehydration caused by overzealous use of diuretics, can make animals more susceptible to the nephrotoxic potential of aminoglycosides.[3,4] Concurrent antiprostaglandin therapy exacerbates aminoglycoside nephrotoxicity, perhaps by inhibiting prostaglandin E_2, which may protect the kidney from toxic insults.[5,6] Interestingly, experimentally induced diabetes mellitus protects animals from renal accumulation of gentamicin and subsequent nephrotoxicity.[7-9]

Clinical Signs and Diagnosis

Clinical signs of aminoglycoside-induced nephrotoxicity are referable to acute tubular necrosis and subsequent acute renal failure. Diagnosis is based on a documented history of continued aminoglycoside therapy and the presence of the clinical signs of acute tubular necrosis. Initially, proteinuria resulting from release of intracellular proteins or decreased uptake of normally reabsorbed low-molecular-weight proteins (β_2-microglobulin) may be evident. Clinical laboratory values indicating increased urinary excretion of enzyme markers of renal proximal tubular damage, such as γ-glutamyltransferase, can reveal whether tubular damage has occurred. Later in the progression of the disease, urine-concentrating ability may be impaired and polyuria may be seen. Oliguria is a much poorer prognostic sign, but most cases of aminoglycoside-induced nephrotoxicity present clinically as nonoliguric acute renal failure. Sequential urinary cast counts may be quick, easy indicators of renal tubular damage; and increased numbers of urinary casts often appear earlier than the usual clinical indexes of renal failure, including altered serum urea nitrogen and creatinine concentrations.[10] Other laboratory changes that occur frequently include hematuria, hyperphosphatemia, hypoalbuminemia, and disorders in potassium balance.[1]

Therapy and Prevention

Aside from discontinuation of the aminoglycoside, treatment is generally supportive, as in any animal with acute tubular necrosis and renal failure. Aggressive fluid therapy is needed unless the patient is anuric or oliguric, in which case dialysis may be the only effective treatment. Because aminoglycosides compete with calcium in the mitochondria, oral calcium supplementation is effective in ameliorating aminoglycoside nephrotoxicity.[11,12] Prevention of electrolyte imbalances has been shown to benefit patients receiving aminoglycoside therapy, and oral sodium and potassium loading has been found to decrease experimental aminoglycoside nephrotoxicity.[13-15] For patients in which aminoglycosides have been administered at excessive dose rates, a novel approach involves treatment with carbenicillin or ticarcillin to complex and, thus, prevent renal uptake of the circulating aminoglycoside.[16] This therapy must be instituted early in the toxic process, because ticarcillin and carbenicillin will not affect aminoglycosides already taken up by the proximal renal tubules. If the patient can be supported through the crisis, the proximal tubules will regenerate to a certain extent, even in the face of continued exposure to aminoglycosides.[17,18]

The peak serum gentamicin concentration in humans has been positively correlated with successful treatment of persistent bacteremias.[19,20] In one study, the only significant difference between cure and failure in patients with gram-negative pneumonia was peak serum gentamicin concentration.[20] Furthermore, efficacy against pathogens and decreased nephrotoxicity were associated more closely with high intermittent peak concentrations than with continuous levels near or above the minimum inhibitory concentration (MIC).[21-24] Nephrotoxicity has been associated more closely with elevated trough concentrations, especially trough concentrations of greater than 2 μg/ml,[25,26] than with peak concentrations.[27] In humans, peak serum gentamicin concentrations should be at least 5 μg/ml, and preferably 8 to 12 μg/ml, for optimum therapy.[20]

Comprehensive reviews in human medicine have demonstrated that when nomograms were used to adjust a dose because of a patient's age, sex, hematocrit, fever, sepsis, weight, and creatinine clearance, the incidence of nephrotoxicity was 23% to 26%.[28,29] When dosages are individualized in humans, with therapeutic drug monitoring used to achieve peak concentrations of 6 to 8 μg/ml and trough concentrations of approximately 1 μg/ml, however, the incidence of gentamicin-induced nephrotoxicity decreases to below 4%, and frequently to below 1%.[30-34] Therapeutic monitoring of aminoglycosides may also benefit veterinary patients.[35] Peak concentrations of 6 to 10 μg/ml for gentamicin and tobramycin (25 to 30 μg/ml for amikacin) are correlated with effective treatment of the infection, whereas allowing the trough concentrations of gentamicin and tobramycin to drop below 2 μg/ml (below 5 μg/ml for amikacin) decreases the incidence of aminoglycoside-related nephrotoxicity dramatically. Individualized dosage adjustment in the face of renal dysfunction is mandatory for preventing accumulation of aminoglycosides in the kidney and further renal tubular damage.[36] Decreasing the total dose by increasing the dosage interval reduces the incidence of nephrotoxicity more than does decreasing the dose alone.[37] Alternatively, the dosage interval can be increased by a factor equal to the ratio of the patient's serum creatinine concentration to the normal serum creatinine concentration.

Amphotericin B
Incidence and Predisposing Factors

Amphotericin B is an effective agent for the treatment of several systemic fungal diseases. Alone or in combination with ketoconazole, amphotericin B is used for the treatment of blastomycosis, histoplasmosis, cryptococcosis, and coccidioidomycosis.[38,39] Reversible renal dysfunction develops in more than 80% of human patients receiving amphotericin B.[40] The same renal dysfunction occurs uniformly in veterinary patients as well.[38]

Mechanisms

In dogs, amphotericin B causes intense vasoconstriction that cannot be prevented by ganglionic or adrenergic blockade.[41] Renal blood flow decreases more than does glomerular filtration, indicating disproportionate afferent arteriolar vasoconstriction. Sodium loading decreases amphotericin B nephrotoxicity,[41,42] but the occurrence of renin-induced alterations in renal vascular resistance has not been confirmed.

In addition, amphotericin B alters the normal sterol–lipid interactions of the distal renal tubular epithelial membranes, thereby disrupting the normal permeability of the distal tubules. A theory unifying these two effects of treatment with amphotericin B may involve the tubuloglomerular feedback system of the macula densa and the distal tubules. Incorporation of amphotericin B into the distal tubular membrane may increase chloride permeability and, thus, activate the tubuloglomerular feedback system. Renal blood flow and the glomerular filtration rate would decrease as a result.[41]

Clinical Signs and Diagnosis

Clinical signs of amphotericin B nephrotoxicity consistently include serum urea nitrogen (SUN) concentrations of greater than 50 mg/dl. Treatment is often adjusted on the basis of the azotemic response of the patient. Other clinical signs include distal tubular acidosis with urinary loss of bicarbonate and potassium.[43] Subsequent acidemia and hypokalemia may be evident as a result of the distal tubular acidosis. Cylindruria, hematuria, pyuria, and proteinuria, which may be evident before the onset of azotemia, can be used as guides to amphotericin B dosing later in the treatment.

Treatment and Prevention

Because amphotericin B nephrotoxicity is reversible, discontinuation of the drug will result in the return of renal function to nearly normal levels, although complete recovery of previous renal functional capacity is uncommon. Supportive therapy and correction of any acidosis or electrolyte imbalance are necessary. Infusion of dopamine may relieve the renal vasoconstriction if complete renal shutdown has occurred.

Prevention of amphotericin B nephrotoxicosis depends on titration during therapy to minimize the risk of azotemia. Oral sodium loading may decrease the occurrence of azotemia by altering the tubuloglomerular feedback system.[42] Concurrent administration of mannitol, which has been used to decrease the rise in SUN concentration for a given dose of amphotericin B, is indicated in patients with preexisting renal disease that requires amphotericin B treatment.[38] Serum urea nitrogen concentrations can be used as a guide to therapy with amphotericin B and should be determined before each treatment. If the SUN concentration rises above 50 mg/dl, administration should be discontinued until it drops to less than 35 to 40 mg/dl, at which time treatment can be reinstituted.[39]

Methoxyflurane
Incidence and Predisposing Factors

Methoxyflurane nephrotoxicity, a dose-dependent occurrence in human anesthesiology, has not been fully documented in veterinary medicine. In humans, the incidence of nephrotoxicity increases with concurrent use of tetracyclines and aminoglycosides as well as with dehydration and obesity.[43] Concurrent administration of enzyme-inducing drugs, such as phenobarbital, may accelerate the production of toxic metabolites of methoxyflurane.[44] Because the nephrotoxicity is dose related, the risk of nephrotoxicity increases with the duration of anesthesia. Studies of dogs in which methoxyflurane anesthesia was maintained for three hours did not demonstrate any clinical signs of nephrotoxicity.[45] Increased serum inorganic fluoride concentrations, one of the causes of methoxyflurane-induced nephrotoxicity, however, were observed. Human studies show that subclinical toxicity occurs at 2.5 to 3.0 MAC-hr (minimum alveolar anesthetic concentration multiplied by the duration of anesthesia) and that clinical toxicity occurs only at ≥ 5.0 MAC-hr, at which serum inorganic fluoride concentrations are 90 to 120 μM.[44] Thus, dogs may be no less susceptible than humans to methoxyflurane-induced nephrotoxicity, but they are at reduced risk because of the shorter duration of anesthesia in canine surgery.

Mechanisms

Metabolism of methoxyflurane produces two compounds that exert their adverse effects in different manners.[44] Oxalic acid, one of the metabolites, can crystallize in the renal tubules and cause obstructive and, often, anuric renal failure. The main mechanism of methoxyflurane nephrotoxicity, however, is the production of inorganic fluoride, which causes tubular necrosis in a dose-dependent manner. Human nephrotoxicity resulting from methoxyflurane has been strongly correlated with serum concentration and urinary excretion of the inorganic fluoride ion.[44]

Clinical Signs and Diagnosis

The clinical signs of methoxyflurane nephrotoxicity are attributable to renal tubular necrosis and acute renal failure. In humans, polyuric renal failure may persist for weeks, while oliguric renal failure offers a much poorer prognosis.[43] In dogs in which methoxyflurane anesthesia was maintained for three hours, polyuria and polydipsia were the only effects observed. No laboratory parameters of renal function were altered after three hours of methoxyflurane anesthesia.[45] Inorganic fluoride concentrations of greater than 90 μM, however, are an indication that nephrotoxicity may develop. Diagnosis is based on clinical signs and documentation of recent or multiple surgeries in which methoxyflurane was the anesthetic.

Treatment and Prevention

Treatment is directed toward maintenance of proper fluid and electrolyte balance while the patient is in the polyuric state. If anuria or oliguria is present, dialysis may be the only alternative.

Thiacetarsamide and Other Trivalent Arsenicals
Incidence

Thiacetarsamide, a trivalent arsenical, is used as an adulticide against *Dirofilaria immitis*. It is used universally as the first part of a three-part treatment regimen for heartworm disease.

Mechanisms

Trivalent arsenicals have a high affinity for the sulfhydryl moieties of proteins and enzymes. Because renal cortical tissue is rich in sulfur-containing proteins, the kidney is a target for trivalent arsenicals.[46] Binding of arsenicals to the sulfhydryl groups denatures the proteins and consequently disrupts the enzymes and membrane transport processes that regulate the passage of electrolytes and sugars. In addition, the enzymes that protect the kidney from oxidant damage also are denatured, leaving the kidney much more susceptible to oxidant damage by normally innocuous substances. Furthermore, several enzymes crucial to normal glucose utilization, most notably the pyruvate dehydrogenase system, are inhibited.[46]

Clinical Signs and Diagnosis

The glomerulus is often the first part of the nephron to be affected adversely by trivalent arsenicals, with the development of proteinuria. Later, tubular necrosis and degeneration occur, leading to oliguria, proteinuria, and cylindruria.[47] Other nonrenal signs of arsenic intoxication include gastrointestinal discomfort, difficulty in swallowing, projectile vomiting, and profuse diarrhea.[46] Diagnosis is based on clinical signs, documented exposure to thiacetarsamide, and, perhaps, laboratory confirmation of blood concentration of arsenic above the normal range.

Treatment and Prevention

Treatment of thiacetarsamide-induced nephrotoxicosis, as for other types of acute renal failure, is supportive. If used early, dimercaprol (British anti-Lewisite or BAL) at a dosage of 2.2 mg/kg every six hours may chelate the arsenic and allow regeneration of the sulfhydryl-containing enzymes. Oral penicillamine (approximately 3.5 mg/kg every six hours) may be administered for one to two days after completion of dimercaprol therapy. An alternative is dimercaptosuccinic acid, which is less toxic than dimercaprol and can be given orally. No oral medication should be used if the animal is vomiting. Activated charcoal can adsorb any of the arsenical remaining in the gastrointestinal tract. Treatment of the arsenic-induced hypotension may be crucial for preventing both renal shutdown and circulatory shock. Dopamine infusion or fluid replacement therapy is indicated in these cases.[46] If the animal can be maintained through the acute crisis, the renal tubular epithelium will regenerate.[47]

Cephalosporins
Incidence and Predisposing Factors

Cephalosporins are a group of semisynthetic antimicrobial agents that are bactericidal to most species of gram-positive and several species of gram-negative bacteria. Although several cephalosporins are available for clinical use, only cephaloridine is approved by the U.S. Food and Drug Administration for use in dogs and cats.[48]

Cephaloridine is the most nephrotoxic of the currently available cephalosporins. Cephaloridine nephrotoxicity has been reported as a serious adverse drug reaction in humans but has not been widely reported in dogs or cats.[49]

Mechanisms

Cephaloridine inhibits renal cation transport; the impaired cation transport interferes with drug excretion and potentiates accumulation of drug within the renal cortex.[50] Accumulated cephaloridine depletes cortical glutathione,[51] which leads to membrane lipid peroxidation and necrosis of renal tubular cells.[52] Vitamin E and selenium partially inhibit the peroxidation by minimizing the effect of oxidizing radicals.[53,54]

Clinical Signs and Diagnosis

The administration of high doses of cephaloridine to laboratory animals of various species results in dose-related nephrotoxicity characterized by acute necrosis of the proximal renal tubules.[55] The clinical signs of cephaloridine-induced nephrotoxicity result from the proximal tubular damage and the resultant acute renal failure. Diagnosis is based on a documented history of high-dose cephaloridine therapy and clinicopathologic confirmation of acute renal failure.

Therapy and Prevention

Discontinuation of cephaloridine should be accompanied by supportive care. Fluid therapy and supplementation with vitamin E would be useful. Although documentation of cephaloridine-induced nephrotoxicity in dogs and cats is lacking, caution should be exercised when using this antimicrobial agent because of its high nephrotoxic potential.

Penicillins
Incidence and Predisposing Factors

The penicillins are a widely available group of natural and semisynthetic antimicrobial agents that are bactericidal to several gram-positive and some gram-negative species of bacteria.[56] Penicillins are not directly nephrotoxic; rather, the production of nephrotoxicity is dependent on an immune-mediated hypersensitivity reaction to the penicillin derivatives. All forms of penicillin have the potential to induce hypersensitivity reactions; and animals are predisposed by repeated, intermittent use of these agents. The interstitium is the portion of the kidney that is most often affected, although other components of the kidney can also be involved.

Mechanisms

The pathogenesis of the hypersensitivity reaction is unclear. Deposits of complement, immunoglobulin, and penicilloyl hapten have been detected along the tubular and glomerular basement membranes.[57] The initial step may be the binding of the penicillin hapten to structural proteins of the renal interstitium and tubular and glomerular membranes, with the subsequent formation of a stable hapten–protein conjugate. Cellular and humoral mechanisms are involved in the production of glomerulonephritis or tubulointerstitial nephritis.[58]

Clinical Signs and Diagnosis

The clinical signs of hypersensitivity nephritis are similar to those of acute renal failure; however, other signs of hypersensitivity, including fever and, possibly, skin rash, may be present. Hematuria is a consistent observation. Documented use of a penicillin, especially penicillin G, is necessary, although ampicillin, carbenicillin, oxacillin, nafcillin, and amoxicillin as well as the cephalosporins can provoke hypersensitivity nephritis.[58]

Therapy and Prevention

The optimum therapy for drug-induced allergic interstitial nephritis is still uncertain. Discontinuation of the offending agent is necessary. The use of corticosteroids or immunosuppressive agents remains controversial. Use of penicillins and cephalosporins should be avoided in patients with histories of antibiotic-induced allergic interstitial nephritis.

Tetracyclines
Incidence and Predisposing Factors

Tetracyclines, a group of natural or semisynthetic antimicrobial agents that are bacteriostatic for a wide variety of gram-positive and gram-negative bacteria, are used widely in veterinary medicine. The use of tetracyclines can lead to progressive azotemia through the antianabolic effects of these drugs. In addition, the use of outdated tetracyclines can cause a reversible Fanconi-like syndrome, a renal tubular defect characterized by proteinuria, glycosuria, aminoaciduria, hypercalciuria, hyperphosphaturia, and uricosuria.[58] There are few indications for the use of tetracyclines in animals that have any degree of renal insufficiency.[49,58] Despite widespread clinical use, reports of nephrotoxicity are uncommon.[59]

Mechanisms

Administration of tetracyclines to animals with preexisting renal disease can worsen the uremia. This action may not be the result of a direct toxic effect. Rather, increasing amounts of nitrogenous waste products accumulate, presumably because of the antianabolic effects of tetracyclines. These waste products can cause some of the clinical signs of uremia in a patient.

Clinical Signs and Diagnosis

The clinical signs of tetracycline-induced nephrotoxicity are referable to acute renal failure, and diagnosis is based on a documented history of tetracycline use. Proteinuria and glycosuria are the criteria for diagnosis of the Fanconi-like syndrome, which can be reversed.

Therapy and Prevention

Renal impairment can be slowly reversed once use of the drug has been discontinued. Management should proceed as for any animal in acute renal failure. As mentioned earlier, the tetracyclines should not be used in animals with preexisting renal disease.

Sulfonamides
Incidence and Predisposing Factors

The sulfonamides are a group of antimicrobial agents that are structural analogues of para-aminobenzoic acid, a constituent of folic acid. Sulfonamides are bacteriostatic for all gram-positive and several species of gram-negative bacteria. The sulfonamides are excreted via the kidney, and the insolubility of these drugs in the urine of some species has not been documented in the dog or cat. Sulfonamide-induced nephrotoxicity is related to decreased urine output and precipitation of the drug in the renal tubules, and thus these agents should be used with care in animals with impaired renal function.[60]

Mechanisms

Although the production of renal tubular damage by sulfonamides has not been described, crystallization and precipitation in the renal tubules can cause epithelial necrosis, leading to acute renal failure. Immune-mediated glomerulonephritis, vasculitis, interstitial nephritis, and tubular cell edema have been documented in humans and a few laboratory animal species.[61] Crystals become more numerous with increasing urine acidity. Renal tubular damage results from disruption of epithelial cell membranes by crystals and from tubular obstruction.[43]

Clinical Signs and Diagnosis

Clinical signs are referable to acute renal failure; and diagnosis is based on clinical signs, a history of drug use, and the presence of sulfonamide crystalluria.

Therapy and Prevention

Therapy consists of urine alkalization to solubilize formed crystals with concurrent fluid diuresis. Adequate hydration of the patient must be maintained during sulfonamide therapy to minimize the potential for crystal formation.

Nonsteroidal Antiinflammatory Agents
Incidence and Predisposing Factors

Analgesic nephropathy in humans has been associated with the use of several nonsteroidal antiinflammatory drugs (NSAIDs), especially aspirin, phenacetin, indomethacin, and phenylbutazone.[62] These agents, along with acetaminophen and other NSAIDs, are available for use in veterinary medicine. In most species, however, and most notably in the cat, acetaminophen causes a hepatotoxicity syndrome.[63] Phenylbutazone, on the other hand, has been incriminated as the cause of renal papillary necrosis, especially in horses. A similar syndrome is produced in cattle and sheep by phenothiazines.[64] Phenylbutazone is most widely used in equine medicine, but it is also used in canine and feline patients.[65]

Mechanisms

Nonsteroidal antiinflammatory drugs exert their action and cause toxicity by inhibiting cyclooxygenase, also known as prostaglandin synthetase. Cyclooxygenase converts arachidonic acid into cyclic endoperoxides, which are then converted into various prostaglandin derivatives.[66] Inhibition of renal synthesis of prostaglandins, especially PGE_2, causes reduction of renal blood flow to the cortex, medulla, and papillary regions. The action of renal PGE_2 is presumed to involve direct vasodilation and blunting of the renin–angiotensin II system. Inhibition of PGE_2 thus causes direct reduction in renal blood flow and enhances the effects of the renin–angiotensin II system.[67] The latter effect is further augmented by the increased vasoconstrictive action of thromboxane A_2.[66] The ischemia is most pronounced in the renal papilla.

Diagnosis

The most common morphologic alteration resulting from the use of NSAIDs is renal papillary necrosis; an infarction forms a well-demarcated focal zone of necrosis, with sequestration of tissue fragments and necrotic cellular debris in the renal papilla. Secondary renal cortical lesions, consisting of renal tubular dilation, filtrate retention, and interstitial edema, also develop.[68] These lesions are generally reversible.[69] Animals with renal papillary necrosis may or may not have the clinical signs of acute renal failure.[68–70] A documented history of the use of analgesic agents and supporting clinicopathologic data are therefore necessary. Renal papillary necrosis can be induced in horses at typical doses (8.8 mg/kg),[71] especially when the animals have been dehydrated and have been treated for more than four consecutive days. Animals may have concomitant protein-losing enteropathy, with resultant panhypoproteinemia.[71] Other clinical signs that may be seen include oral, gastric, duodenal, and colonic ulcers as well as edema.[69]

Treatment and Prevention

Initially, the drug should be discontinued or at least used at a reduced dose.[71] Another nonsteroidal antiinflammatory agent should not be substituted because the mechanisms of action for all of these agents are similar and the damage would thus continue.[66] Fluid and/or plasma therapy may be indicated, depending on the degree of fluid and protein loss. Maintenance of adequate hydration and reduction of the duration of analgesic use would minimize adverse drug reactions. Although still experimental, the use of intravenous dopamine infusion to preserve adequate renal blood flow may be beneficial.[72]

Conclusions

Several of the most commonly used therapeutic agents have the potential to cause drug-induced renal disease. Problems related to aminoglycoside therapy can be decreased by altering the dose schedule and the duration of therapy. Cephaloridine has not been proven to be nephrotoxic in dogs and cats, but the potential for renal damage exists. Renal damage resulting from the inhibition of prostaglandins may be a problem with the nonsteroidal antiinflammatory drugs and should be addressed on an individual basis in each case.

Even with the adverse side effects of the therapeutic agents discussed, their use is necessary under many circumstances. Prudent use and observation for adverse clinical signs should decrease the incidence of untoward responses during therapy.

REFERENCES

1. Brown SA, Barsanti JA, Crowell WA: Gentamicin-associated acute renal failure in the dog. *JAVMA* 186:686–690, 1985.
2. Riviere JE, Coppoc GL, Hinsman EJ, et al: Species-dependent gentamicin pharmacokinetics and nephrotoxicity in the young horse. *Fundam Appl Toxicol* 3:448–457, 1983.
3. Adelman RD, Spangler WL, Beasom F, et al: Furosemide enhancement of experimental gentamicin nephrotoxicity: Comparison of functional and morphological changes with activities of urinary enzymes. *J Infect Dis* 140:342–352, 1979.
4. Adelman RD, Spangler WL, Beasom F, et al: Furosemide enhancement of netilmicin nephrotoxicity in dogs. *J Antimicrob Chemother* 7:431–440, 1981.
5. Assael BM, Chiabrando C, Gagliardi L, et al: Prostaglandins and aminoglycoside nephrotoxicity. *Toxicol Appl Pharmacol* 78:386–394, 1985.
6. McNeil JS, Jackson B, Nelson L, et al: The role of prostaglandins in gentamicin-induced nephrotoxicity in the dog. *Nephron* 33:202–207, 1983.
7. Cronin RE, Splinter KL, Ferguson ER, et al: Gentamicin nephrotoxicity: Protective effect of diabetes on cell injury. *Miner Electrolyte Metab* 9:38–44, 1983.
8. Elliott WC, Houghton DC, Gilbert DN, et al: Experimental gentamicin nephrotoxicity: Effect of streptozotocin-induced diabetes. *J Pharmacol Exp Ther* 233:264–270, 1985.
9. Vaamonde CA, Bier RT, Gouvea W, et al: Effect of duration of diabetes on the protection observed in the diabetic rat against gentamicin-induced acute renal failure. *Miner Electrolyte Metab* 10:209–216, 1984.
10. Riviere JE, Coppoc GL: Selected aspects of aminoglycoside antibiotic nephrotoxicosis. *JAVMA* 187:508–509, 1981.
11. Bennett WM, Elliott WC, Houghton DC, et al: Reduction of experimental gentamicin nephrotoxicity in rats with dietary calcium loading. *Antimicrob Agents Chemother* 22:508–512, 1982.
12. Humes HD, Sastrasinh M, Weinberg JM: Calcium is a competitive inhibitor of gentamicin–renal membrane binding interactions and dietary calcium supplementation protects against gentamicin nephrotoxicity. *J Clin Invest* 73;134–147, 1984.
13. Bennett WM, Hartnett MN, Gilbert D, et al: Effect of sodium intake on gentamicin nephrotoxicity in the rat. *Proc Soc Exp Biol Med* 151:736–738, 1976.
14. Dobyan DC, Cronin RE, Bulger RE: Effect of potassium depletion on tubular morphology in gentamicin-induced acute renal failure in dogs. *Lab Invest* 47:586–594, 1982.
15. Heller J: Effect of some simple manoeuvres on the course of acute renal failure after gentamicin treatment in rats. *Int Urol Nephrol* 16:243–251, 1984.
16. English J, Gilbert DN, Kohlhepp S, et al: Attenuation of experimental tobramycin nephrotoxicity by ticarcillin. *Antimicrob Agents Chemother* 27:897–902, 1985.
17. Gilbert DN, Houghton DC, Bennett WM, et al: Reversibility of gentamicin nephrotoxicity in rats: Recovery during continuous drug administration. *Proc Soc Exp Biol Med* 160:99–103, 1979.
18. Laurent G, Toubeau G, Maldague P, et al: Tubular regeneration in rat kidney cortex during treatment with gentamicin at a low dose. *Arch Toxicol* 7(Suppl):459–463, 1984.
19. Jackson CG, Riff LJ: *Pseudomonas* bacteremia: Pharmacology and other bases for failure of treatment with gentamicin. *J Infect Dis* 124:S185–S191, 1971.
20. Noone P, Pattison JR, Davies DG: The effective use of gentamicin in life-threatening sepsis. *Postgrad Med* 50:S9–S16, 1974.
21. Gerber AU, Craig WA, Brugger HP, et al: Impact of dosing intervals on activity of gentamicin and ticarcillin against *Pseudomonas aeruginosa* in granulocytopenic mice. *J Infect Dis* 147:910–917, 1983.
22. Herscovici L, Lemeland JF, Dalion J, et al: Pyelonephrite aigue experimentale traitment par tobramycine influence du rhythme d'administration sur l'efficacite la tolerance renale. *Pathol Biol* 32:450–454, 1984.
23. Powell SH, Thompson WL, Luthe MA, et al: Once-daily vs. continuous aminoglycoside dosing: Efficacy and toxicity in animal and clinical studies of gentamicin, netilmicin, and tobramycin. *J Infect Dis* 147:918–932, 1983.
24. Reiner NE, Bloxham DD, Thompson WL: Nephrotoxicity of gentamicin and tobramycin given once daily or continuously in dogs. *J Antimicrob Chemother* 4:85–101, 1978.
25. Dahlgren JG, Anderson ET, Hewitt WL: Gentamicin blood levels: A guide to nephrotoxicity. *Antimicrob Agents Chemother* 8:58–62, 1975.
26. Takemoto RT, McGhan WF, Fushiki MR, et al: Gentamicin nephrotoxicity: Application of multivariate analysis. *Clin Pharm* 1:544–548, 1982.
27. Bennett WM, Plamp CE, Gilbert DN: The influence of dosage regimen on experimental nephrotoxicity: Dissociation of peak serum levels from renal failure. *J Infect Dis* 140:576–580, 1979.
28. Schentag JJ, Plaut ME, Cerra FB, et al: Aminoglycoside nephrotoxicity in critically ill surgical patients. *J Surg Res* 26:270–279, 1979.
29. Smith CR, Lipsky JJ, Laskin OL, et al: Double-blind comparison of the nephrotoxicity and auditory toxicity of gentamicin and tobramycin. *N Engl J Med* 302:1106–1109, 1980.
30. Burton ME, Vasko MR, Brater DG: Comparison of drug dosing methods. *Clin Pharmacokinet* 10:1–37, 1985.
31. Cipolle RJ, Seifert R, Zaske DE: Systematically individualized tobramycin dosage regimens. *J Clin Pharmacol* 20:570–580, 1980.
32. Heissler J, Pancorbo S: Comparison of gentamicin and tobramycin nephrotoxicity in patients receiving individualized pharmacokinetic dosing regimens. *Am Soc Hosp Pharm Midyear Clin Meet*:217, 1980.
33. Zaske DE, Cipolle RJ, Rotschafer JC, et al: Gentamicin pharmacokinetics in 1,640 patients: Method for control of serum concentrations. *Antimicrob Agents Chemother* 21:407–411, 1982.
34. Zaske DE, Cipolle RJ, Strate RG: Gentamicin dosage requirements: Wide interpatient variations in 242 surgery patients with normal renal function. *Surgery* 87:164–169, 1980.

35. Sojka JE, Brown SA: Pharmacokinetic adjustment of gentamicin dosing in horses with sepsis. *JAVMA* 189:784–789, 1986.
36. Riviere JE, Coppoc GL: Dosage of antimicrobial drugs in patients with renal insufficiency. *JAVMA* 178:70–72, 1981.
37. Riviere JE, Carver MP, Coppoc GL, et al: Pharmacokinetics and comparative nephrotoxicity of fixed-dose versus fixed-interval reduction of gentamicin dosage in subtotal nephrectomized dogs. *Toxicol Appl Pharmacol* 75:496–509, 1984.
38. Legendre AM, Selcer BA, Edwards DF, et al: Treatment of canine blastomycosis with amphotericin B and ketoconazole. *JAVMA* 184:1249–1254, 1984.
39. Pyle RL: Clinical pharmacology of amphotericin B. *JAVMA* 179:83–84, 1981.
40. Sande MA, Mandell GL: Antimicrobial agents. Antifungal and antiviral agents, in Gilman AG, Goodman LS, Rall TW, Murad F (eds): *The Pharmacological Basis of Therapeutics*, ed 7. New York, Macmillan Publishing Co, 1985, pp 1219–1239.
41. Porter GA, Bennett WM: Nephrotoxic acute renal failure due to common drugs. *Am J Physiol* 241:F1–F8, 1981.
42. Heidemann HT, Gerkens JF, Spickard WA, et al: Amphotericin B nephrotoxicity in humans decreased by salt repletion. *Am J Med* 75:476–481, 1983.
43. Thornhill JA: Toxic nephropathy, in Kirk RW (ed): *Current Veterinary Therapy VII. Small Animal Practice*. Philadelphia, WB Saunders Co, 1980, pp 1047–1052.
44. Mazze RI: Methoxyflurane nephropathy. *Environ Health Perspect* 15:111–119, 1976.
45. Pedersoli WM: Serum fluoride concentration, renal, and hepatic function test results in dogs with methoxyflurane anesthesia. *Am J Vet Res* 38:949–953, 1977.
46. Klaassen CD: Heavy metals and heavy-metal antagonists, in Gilman AG, Goodman LS, Rall TW, Murad F (eds): *The Pharmacological Basis of Therapeutics*, ed 7. New York, Macmillan Publishing Co, 1985, pp 1605–1627.
47. Tsukamoto H, Parker HR, Gribble DH, et al: Nephrotoxicity of sodium arsenate in dogs. *Am J Vet Res* 44:2324–2330, 1983.
48. Thomson RD, Quay JF, Webber JA: Cephalosporin group of antimicrobial drugs. *JAVMA* 185:1109–1114, 1984.
49. Appel GB, Neu HC: The nephrotoxicity of antimicrobial agents. *N Engl J Med* 296:663–670, 722–728, 784–787, 1977.
50. Wold JS, Turnipseed SH, Miller BL: The effect of renal cation transport inhibition in cephaloridine nephrotoxicity. *Toxicol Appl Pharmacol* 47:115–122, 1975.
51. Kuo CH, Hook JB: Depletion of renal glutathione content and nephrotoxicity of cephaloridine in rabbits, rats and mice. *Toxicol Appl Pharmacol* 63:292–302, 1982.
52. Kuo CH, Maita K, Sleight SD, et al: Lipid peroxidation: A possible mechanism of cephaloridine-induced nephrotoxicity. *Toxicol Appl Pharmacol* 67:78–88, 1983.
53. Cojocel C, Laeschke KH, Inselmann G, et al: Inhibition of cephaloridine-induced lipid peroxidation. *Toxicology* 35:295–305, 1985.
54. Cojocel C, Hannemann J, Baumann K: Cephaloridine-induced lipid peroxidation initiated by reactive oxygen species as a possible mechanism of cephaloridine nephrotoxicity. *Biochim Biophys Acta* 834:402–410, 1985.
55. Welles JS, Gibson WR, Harris PN, et al: Toxicity, distribution and excretion of cephaloridine in laboratory animals. *Antimicrob Agents Chemother* 19:863–869, 1966.
56. Wishart DF: Recent advances in antimicrobial drugs: The penicillins. *JAVMA* 185:1106–1108, 1984.
57. Wright NG, Nash AS: Experimental ampicillin glomerulopathy. *J Comp Pathol* 94:357–361, 1984.
58. Fillastre JP, Kleinknecht D, Godin M, et al: Antibiotic nephrotoxicity, in Bach PH, Bonner FW, Bridges JW, Lock EA (eds): *Nephrotoxicity: Assessment and Pathogenesis*. New York, John Wiley & Sons, 1982, pp 413–421.
59. Lairmore MD, Alexander AF, Powers BE, et al: Oxytetracycline-associated nephrotoxicosis in feedlot calves. *JAVMA* 185:793–795, 1984.
60. Bushby SRM: Sulfonamide and trimethoprim combinations. *JAVMA* 176:1049–1053, 1980.
61. Porter GA, Bennett WM: Toxic nephropathies, in Brenner BM, Rector FC (eds): *The Kidney*, ed 2. Philadelphia, WB Saunders Co, 1981, pp 2045–2108.
62. Johnson WJ: Nephrotoxicity of non-steroidal antiinflammatory drugs. *Mayo Clin Proc* 55:120–125, 1980.
63. Cullison RF: Acetaminophen toxicosis in small animals: Clinical signs, mode of action and treatment. *Compend Contin Educ Pract Vet* 6(4):315–321, 1984.
64. Salisbury RM: Mortality in lambs and cattle following the administration of phenothiazine. *NZ Vet J* 17:187–191, 1969.
65. Gabel AA, Tobin T, Ray RS, et al: Phenylbutazone in horses: A review. *J Equine Med Surg* 1:221–225, 1977.
66. Hornych A: Role of prostaglandins in drug nephrotoxicity. *Contrib Nephrol* 42:220–232, 1984.
67. Sabatini S: Pathophysiology of drug-induced papillary necrosis. *Fundam Appl Toxicol* 4:909–921, 1984.
68. Read WK: Renal medullary crest necrosis associated with phenylbutazone therapy in horses. *Vet Pathol* 20:662–669, 1983.
69. Murray MJ: Phenylbutazone toxicity in a horse. *Compend Contin Educ Pract Vet* 7(7):S389–S394, 1985.
70. Gunson DE: Renal papillary necrosis in horses. *JAVMA* 182:263–266, 1983.
71. Collins LG, Tyler DE: Phenylbutazone toxicosis in the horse: A clinical study. *JAVMA* 184:699–703, 1984.
72. Seri I, Tulassay T, Kiszel J, et al: The use of dopamine for the prevention of the renal side effects of indomethacin in premature infants with patent ductus arteriosus. *Int J Pediatr Nephrol* 5:209–214, 1984.

KEY FACTS

- Glomerulonephritis is associated with immune-complex deposition and results in glomerular injury.
- Four types of glomerulonephritis apparently exist in dogs and cats: proliferative, membranous, membranoproliferative, and chronic.
- Recent reports of membranoproliferative glomerulonephritis in a group of related Doberman pinschers and membranous glomerulonephritis in sibling cats imply that genetic factors play a role in the development of the disease.
- Glomerulonephritis is characterized by pathologic proteinuria in the absence of urinary tract inflammation.
- Rational treatment for this disorder includes restricted-protein diets and platelet-inhibitor drugs, such as aspirin.

Glomerulonephritis in Dogs and Cats

Albert E. Jergens, DVM
Department of Medicine and Surgery
College of Veterinary Medicine
University of Missouri
Columbia, Missouri

Glomerulonephritis is a disease characterized by morphologic and functional abnormalities primarily affecting the renal glomeruli. Secondary changes involving the renal tubules, interstitial tissue, and blood vessels can become evident with progressive glomerular disease.[1] Clinical glomerulonephropathies are now recognized with greater frequency in dogs[2,3] and cats.[1] Glomerulonephritis is a frequent cause of progressive renal failure in dogs.[1,4] Primary glomerulonephritis of unknown cause affects the kidneys only. Secondary glomerulonephritis results from inflammatory disease processes in other tissues, including canine pyometra,[5,6] systemic lupus erythematosus,[7] endocarditis,[8] feline leukemia virus infection,[9,10] infectious hepatitis,[11,12] malignancies,[13–15] chronic pancreatitis,[13,14] and infection with *Dirofilaria immitis*.[16,17]

There is no breed or sex predisposition for the development of canine or feline glomerulonephritis. Generally, the disease is encountered in dogs over five years of age.[18] Recent reports of membranoproliferative glomerulonephritis in a group of related Doberman pinschers[19] and membranous glomerulonephritis in sibling cats[20,21] imply that genetic factors play a role in the development of the disease. Immunologically mediated injury to the glomeruli is an important phenomenon in humans. Numerous, well-documented cases indicate that immunologic mechanisms also are involved in the development of glomerulonephritis in dogs and cats. In the vast majority of cases, the causative factors responsible for the development of glomerulonephritis in domestic animals are unknown.

Glomerular Anatomy and Physiology

The renal glomerulus consists of a network of highly branched capillaries enclosed by a capsule (Bowman's capsule) that is continuous with the epithelial lining of the proximal convoluted tubule. This capillary tuft is supplied by an afferent arteriole and drained by an efferent arteriole. The glomerulus comprises several components, including capillary endothelial cells, visceral and parietal epithelial cells, mesangial cells and the mesangial matrix, and the capillary basement membrane.[1] The parietal epithelial cells line the inner

Originally published in Volume 9, Number 9, September 1987

surface of Bowman's capsule, and the visceral epithelial cells line the outside of the glomerular basement membrane.[1] These cells contain podocytes (footlike processes) that project into the glomerular basement membrane. Slit pores spaced between podocytes are considered to be the sites of glomerular filtration.[22] The mesangial cells located between epithelial cells are believed to provide structural support to the glomerular basement membrane. In addition, these cells are part of the reticuloendothelial system and have phagocytic properties.

Glomerular filtrate passes through the capillary wall and the glomerular basement membrane and between podocytes to the glomerular lumen. Filtration occurs as a result of osmotic pressure gradients and hydrostatic pressure in the efferent arteriole.[23] Most substances with a molecular weight greater than 68,000 daltons,[24] as well as substances bound to transport proteins, do not normally pass through the glomerular capillary wall. Plasma proteins, such as albumin (molecular weight of 69,000 daltons), can be excluded from the glomerular filtrate because of their electrical charge and their size. Negatively charged sialoproteins along the glomerular capillary wall facilitate the passage of cationic protein molecules and hinder the movement of such anionic proteins as albumin.[24]

Functional Response to Injury

The nephron is a complex structure with limited regenerative capacity. Once damaged, new, functionally intact nephrons cannot be produced. Irreversible glomerular damage usually results in repair by replacement fibrosis and scarring.[1] This does not imply that all forms of glomerular disease are clinically irreversible, however. Glomeruli respond to injury in one of four basic mechanisms: (1) cellular proliferation of glomerular cells, (2) basement membrane thickening with resultant increase in plasma proteins, (3) leukocyte infiltration into injured glomerular tufts, and (4) hyalinization of glomeruli with secondary glomerular destruction.[18,22]

Cellular proliferation of endothelial, epithelial, and mesangial cells to replace damaged cells is a common response to glomerular injury. Endothelial and mesangial swelling and hyperplasia often occur in acute glomerular injury[1] and are potentially reversible conditions.[25] Mesangial cell hyperplasia is believed to reflect the increased phagocytic function of these cells.[26,27] Inflammatory states involving the glomeruli result in the exudation of leukocytes (polymorphonuclear neutrophil leukocytes) after complement activation. High numbers of these cells can cause significant damage to the glomerular capillaries by release of their lysosomal enzymes.

Damage to the glomerular capillary wall is associated with loss of inflammatory products into the urine; these can be detected by urinalysis. The visceral epithelial podocytes commonly fuse together in response to glomerular injury. This fusion results in increased glomerular permeability, which augments protein leakage into the glomerular filtrate. Additional studies have shown that proteinuria, as a consequence of alteration of the negative charges on the

glomerular capillary wall, occurs before podocyte fusion.[28,29] Thickening of the glomerular basement membrane also is common with glomerulonephritis. This is associated with the presence of abnormal structures—such as immune complexes, immunoglobulins, or fibrin—deposited along the basement membrane.

Morphologic Response to Injury

Morphologic and definitive diagnosis of glomerulonephritis can be made with the diagnostic tools of light, fluorescence, and electron microscopy. Specimens for examination are obtained by laparotomy, laparoscopy, necropsy, or percutaneous renal biopsy techniques.[30] Early attempts to classify canine glomerulonephritis into proliferative and membranous forms proved to be too restrictive.[4] Four types of glomerulonephritis apparently exist in dogs and cats: proliferative, membranous, membranoproliferative, and chronic.

Proliferative Glomerulonephritis

Proliferative glomerulonephritis is associated with hypercellularity of the glomerular tuft as a result of mesangial cell proliferation. The increased cellularity can be augmented by a proliferation of epithelial cells and the infiltration of polymorphonuclear neutrophil leukocytes.[31] Narrowing of glomerular capillary lumina as a result of the increased cellularity results in compromised renal blood flow and a reduction in glomerular filtration rate.

Membranous Glomerulonephritis

Membranous glomerulonephritis is characterized by pronounced, diffuse thickening of the glomerular basement membrane. Unlike proliferative glomerulonephritis, a reduction in glomerular cellularity occurs. This is the most common form of glomerulonephritis in cats. Glomerular basement membrane thickening results from the subepithelial deposition of immune complexes that stimulate glomerular basement membrane synthesis by epithelial cells.[26] Diagnosis of canine and feline membranous glomerulonephritis is based on the recognition of characteristic histopathologic criteria.[32] In cases of feline membranous glomerulonephritis, there is an apparent correlation with the degree of pathology and the severity of renal dysfunction.[32] The pattern of glomerular changes reportedly is similar in cats and dogs.[33]

Membranoproliferative Glomerulonephritis

Membranoproliferative glomerulonephritis involves a glomerular lesion characterized by cellular proliferation and glomerular basement membrane thickening. This is considered to be an intermediate glomerular lesion that can progress to generalized chronic glomerulonephritis and chronic renal failure.

Chronic Glomerulonephritis

Chronic glomerulonephritis is the most severe form and probably results from exacerbation of the previously described milder forms. The lesions are usually irreversible and are characterized by the presence of progressive glomerular scarring.

Immunologic Aspects

As stated, the cause of most cases of glomerulonephritis in dogs and cats is unknown. Clinical and experimental evidence suggests that immunologic mechanisms play a major role in the development of glomerulonephritis in domestic animals.[1,34-37] There evidently are two distinct immunologic mechanisms responsible for the majority of glomerular injuries: immune-complex glomerulonephritis, in which there is deposition of immune complexes in the glomeruli, and anti-basement-membrane glomerulonephritis, in which antibodies are produced against the glomerular basement membrane. Immune-complex deposition is the most common mechanism and accounts for 70% to 80% of cases of immunologically mediated glomerular disease in humans.[38,39]

Immune-Complex Glomerulonephritis

Circulating complexes of antigen and antibody are the primary factors initiating immune-complex glomerulonephritis. The complexes are deposited in the renal glomeruli as a result of the filtration function of these glomeruli. Any chronic disease state or persistent exposure to an antigen can stimulate immune-complex formation. Complement is a complex group of proteolytic enzymes identified as C1 through C9.[40] The activation of complement as a result of antigen-antibody interactions serves as a catalyst for the initial immunologic events, the secondary inflammatory response, and renal tissue damage. A major immunopathogenic effect of the complement is to attract neutrophils to sites of antibody deposition by the generation of chemotactic factors, principally C_3, C_5, and C_{576}.[14] Neutrophils destroy offending immune complexes by phagocytosis and extracellular release of lysosomal enzymes.[23] In addition to destroying immune complexes, these enzymes expose and digest glomerular basement membrane material, which leads to exposure of glomerular basement membrane collagen.

Glomerular membrane collagen serves as a potent platelet aggregator,[41] which promotes further platelet aggregation and release of such additional vasoactive substances as histamine and serotonin.[42] The increased capillary vascular permeability allows for further immune-complex deposition and neutrophilic chemotaxis.[43] Hageman factor (Factor XII), which also is activated by exposed glomerular membrane collagen, initiates the intrinsic coagulation pathway[35]; accumulation of fibrin polymers in the glomeruli results. Activated Hageman factor also activates the complement system, which increases capillary permeability and attracts additional neutrophils.[44] The result is a self-perpetuating cycle of inflammation-mediated tissue damage.

The formation and location of immune complexes in the glomeruli are influenced by many factors. Circulating immune complexes are normally cleared from the blood by the reticuloendothelial system. The macromolecules accumulate in the circulation from accelerated production or from impaired clearance.[45] Large, insoluble complexes formed in antibody excess are rapidly cleared and destroyed by cells of the reticuloendothelial system.[45] By contrast, intermediate-sized complexes formed in the presence of moderate antigen excess remain in solution and escape physiologic destruction. These complexes are deposited in various tissues, such as the glomeruli, and initiate inflammation.[1,46]

Hydrodynamic factors—such as turbulent blood flow, high filtration pressure, and trapping of solute particles by the slit pores—favor immune-complex deposition and resultant glomerular damage. The size of the immune complexes also can affect their ability to pass through capillary walls.[47,48] Recently, immune-complex receptors have been found on human glomerular epithelial and mesangial cells.[49-51] Although their role is disputed, they are believed to aid in the removal of circulating immune complexes. A phagocytic role for mesangial cells also has been postulated. Attempts to demonstrate the presence of these receptors on the glomeruli of domestic animals have failed.

Anti-Basement-Membrane Glomerulonephritis

Anti-basement-membrane glomerulonephritis is the second immunologic mechanism responsible for glomerulonephritis in dogs and cats. It is characterized by the localization of anti-glomerular basement membrane antibodies produced by the host and deposited in the glomerular capillary wall. This form of glomerulonephritis is of interest chiefly in the laboratory and has been experimentally induced in dogs.[52,53] Circulating antibodies, produced by immunization, react with glomerular basement membrane antigens and readily bind to them. After binding to the glomerular basement membrane, inflammation occurs that is identical to that with immune-complex disease. Elution of antibody from affected tissue, application to normal kidney, and staining with appropriate fluorescein-labeled antisera are required to confirm diagnosis of this disease.[54] Naturally occurring cases of anti-glomerular basement membrane disease have not been demonstrated in dogs and cats.[55-59]

Immunofluorescence Studies

The diagnosis of immune-mediated glomerular disease depends on evidence of immune-system participation in causing the functional and morphologic abnormalities. The demonstration of complement and immunoglobulins in renal tissues by immunofluorescence methods has been the primary tool affording rapid, reliable definition of immune-mediated renal disease. Because both immunologic mechanisms stimulate an inflammatory response with variable glomerular injury, they cannot be differentiated with certainty on the basis of clinical, laboratory, or light microscopy findings. Each has a characteristic immunofluorescence pattern, however.

Immune-complex disease generally manifests discontinuous, granular immune complexes on glomerular or tubular basement membranes. This fluorescence pattern has been termed *granular* and *lumpy-bumpy*.[1,26] Renal disease caused by the deposition of anti-glomerular basement membrane antibodies shows a smooth, diffuse, linear immunofluorescence pattern. This represents deposits of antibody and complement that coincide with the convolutions of the basement membrane.[1,26] Recently, immunoperoxidase techniques have been applied to the study of feline glomerulonephritis with encouraging results.[60] These techniques are used in the same manner as fluorescent-dye conjugates.[61] Renal tissue specimens incubated with an immunoenzyme reagent react with a substrate for the enzyme and produce a tissue-localized, colored precipitate. This reaction can be observed by conventional light microscopy methods.

The results of immunofluorescence and immune-complex studies can be misleading. Immunofluorescence findings can be negative in some cases of immune-mediated renal disease. In addition, fluorescent glomerular deposits are not pathognomonic for renal disease. Their presence can result from a normal physiologic process to remove pathogenic and nonpathogenic complexes from the body.[62]

Clinical Presentation

Patients can present with myriad clinical signs that might not suggest glomerulonephropathy. Clinical signs related to conditions that might have precipitated the glomerular injury (e.g., heartworms, feline leukemia virus, pyometra, and systemic lupus erythematosus) can be observed. The salient feature of glomerulonephritis is persistent proteinuria in the absence of urinary tract inflammation. An accurate assessment of renal proteinuria is critical in documenting substantial glomerular injury. Normal urine protein excretion values of less than 400 mg/day or less than 30 mg/kg/day[63-65] have been established for dogs. Urinary protein losses in excess of these values and consisting primarily of albumin are highly suggestive of pathologic glomerular proteinuria.

Recent studies patterned after those in humans[66] have determined that the urinary excretion of creatinine remains steady in the presence of a stable glomerular filtration rate.[67] Preliminary studies support the premise of stable protein clearance throughout the day in dogs.[68] The effectiveness of the protein-to-creatinine ratio in a single urine specimen as a predictor of the daily loss of urine protein has been demonstrated in dogs.[68] In a limited study, this assay was proven to be an extremely sensitive, specific screening tool for canine proteinuria. Twenty-four-hour collection of urine remains the most accurate method for quantitating urinary protein excretion.

Prolonged proteinuria can lead to the nephrotic syndrome, a condition characterized by proteinuria, hypoalbuminemia, hypercholesterolemia, and peripheral edema or ascites.[69,70] Because albumin is the principal protein responsible for the maintenance of plasma-colloidal osmotic pressure, excessive urinary losses lead to a significant reduction of oncotic pressure and to subsequent disturbances in fluid balance.[36] The result is an extravasation of fluid from the intravascular compartments into the extra-

vascular spaces. Hypercholesterolemia associated with hypoalbuminemia is related to the decrease in plasma oncotic pressure, which stimulates hepatic lipogenesis. Gross or microscopic hematuria is infrequently observed as a result of glomerular capillary injury.[18,70] The presence of granular or hyaline casts on urine sediment examination is highly suggestive of glomerular disease.[70] Other clinical signs that can be evident in progressive cases of glomerulonephropathies include uremia, polyuria, polydipsia, weight loss, and lethargy.[1,18,19,32,36,46,56]

Treatment

Treatment of glomerulonephritis remains a difficult and often unrewarding task. Because most cases of canine and feline glomerulonephritis are mediated by immunologic mechanisms, corticosteroids or immunosuppressive agents would appear to be of considerable benefit. The literature contains numerous reports of giving corticosteroids to human patients with immune-complex glomerulonephritis. The results of immunosuppressive therapy in these patients have been generally disappointing.[71-75] Use of these agents was originally based on the expectation that they would suppress antibody production or the inflammatory reactions initiated by immune complexes and complement. There has been no evidence to substantiate the hypothesis that naturally occurring glomerulonephritis is associated with hyperactivity or overstimulation of the immune system, however. At least one report attributed the successful management of glomerular disease and concurrent nephrotic syndrome to immunosuppressive therapy.[76] Another study reported spontaneous remission without treatment.[36]

The unpredictable variability and the lack of controlled clinical studies commend judicious use of corticosteroids and immunosuppressive agents in the treatment of glomerulonephritis.[36] Recent recommendations discouraging their use are based on the following assumptions: (1) these agents might inhibit beneficial tissue responses to injury; (2) renal failure might be aggravated by the catabolic effects of corticosteroids; and (3) these agents might favor the production of active immune complexes, causing further glomerular injury.

In humans, success in the treatment of glomerulonephritis has been obtained through the use of platelet-inhibitor drugs, such as aspirin and dipyridamole. The rationale for their use stems from the demonstrations of platelet activation in glomerulonephritis.[42,77,78] The mechanisms of action of these agents are believed to cause a reduction in platelet–vascular wall interaction and an inhibition of platelet and renal production of prostaglandins.[71] A recent controlled study of membranoproliferative glomerulonephritis in humans demonstrated that these agents can delay the progression to end-stage disease.[71]

Dietary modification can be an important, often overlooked tool in the treatment of glomerulonephritis and chronic renal failure. Recent studies indicate that the progression of chronic renal failure might be influenced by dietary protein intake.[79] Increased dietary protein increases renal blood flow in dogs and cats. Sustained hyperfiltration as a result of high dietary protein ingestion is believed to injure the glomerular microvasculature.[80] This damage results in increased glomerular permeability, which leads to pathologic proteinuria. Low-protein diets might protect against the progression of renal failure by minimizing these hemodynamic alterations and the development of glomerular sclerosis.[79]

The ideal level of protein restriction is unknown and can vary with the individual. A diet initiating therapy that provides 2.0 to 2.5 g of protein/kg daily has been recommended.[79] An optimal diet should strive to minimize protein intake and subsequent progressive glomerular pathology while maintaining adequate nutrition. Patients with the nephrotic syndrome might require additional sources of dietary protein to compensate for excessive urinary protein losses of albumin and antithrombin III. The increased permeability accompanying glomerulonephritis results in selective urinary loss of antithrombin III and a greater tendency toward thrombosis.[81] Similarly, hypoalbuminemia as a consequence of the nephrotic syndrome promotes platelet hypersensitivity and can aggravate the potential for thrombosis.[82] Although thromboembolism is a reported complication of glomerular disease in dogs, this disorder was observed infrequently in a recent retrospective study.[83]

Conclusion

The prognosis in most cases of canine and feline glomerulonephritis remains obscure because of the lack of information on the natural history of the disease. If the underlying causes of acute glomerulonephritis can be properly identified and removed, the morphologic and functional glomerular changes are theoretically reversible.[23] By contrast, changes such as fibrosis and glomerular tuft atrophy are irreversible.[36] Pharmacologic inhibition of platelet function and dietary protein restriction are promising forms of therapy that should be evaluated in future controlled studies. Substantial evidence now suggests that glucocorticoids are deleterious and inappropriate in the therapeutic management of glomerular disease. Guarded prognoses are warranted until more is known about the causes, clinical course, and therapeutic regimens of glomerulonephritis in dogs and cats.

REFERENCES

1. Osborne CA, Vernier RL: Glomerulonephritis in the dog and cat: A comparative review. *JAAHA* 9:101–127, 1973.
2. Muller-Peddinghaus R, Trautwein G: Spontaneous glomerulonephritis in dogs. II. Correlation of glomerulonephritis with age, chronic interstitial nephritis, and extrarenal lesions. *Vet Pathol* 14:121–127, 1977.
3. Muller-Peddinghaus R, Trautwein G: Spontaneous glomerulonephritis in dogs. I. Classification and immunopathology. *Vet Pathol* 14:1–13, 1977.
4. Murray M, Wright NG: A morphologic study of canine glomerulonephritis. *Lab Invest* 30:213–221, 1974.
5. Asheim A: Pathogenesis of renal damage and polydipsia in dogs with pyometra. *JAVMA* 147:736–745, 1965.
6. Obel A, Nicander L, Asheim A: Light and electron microscopical studies of the renal lesions in dogs with pyometra. *Acta Vet Scand* 5:146–178, 1964.
7. Lewis RM: Animal model: Canine systemic lupus erythematosus. *Am J Pathol* 69:537–540, 1972.
8. Highman B, Roshe J, Altland PO: Endocarditis and glomerulonephritis in dogs with aortic insufficiency. Production by single bacterial inoculation and effect of cortisone. *Arch Pathol* 65:388–394, 1958.
9. Mackey L: Feline leukemia virus and its clinical effects in cats. *Vet Rec* 96:5–11, 1975.
10. Anderson LJ, Jarrett WFH: Membranous glomerulonephritis associated with leukemia in cats. *Res Vet Sci* 12:179–180, 1971.
11. Morrison WI, Wright NG: Detection of immune complexes in the serum of dogs infected with canine adenovirus. *Res Vet Sci* 21:119–121, 1976.
12. Wright NG, Morrison WI, Thompson H, et al: Mesangial localization of immune complexes in experimental canine adenovirus glomerulonephritis. *Br J Exp Pathol* 55:458–465, 1974.
13. Lewis RJ: Canine glomerulonephritis: Results from a microscopic evaluation of fifty cases. *Can Vet J* 17:171–176, 1976.
14. Slauson DO, Lewis RM: Comparative pathology of glomerulonephritis in animals. *Vet Pathol* 16:135–164, 1979.
15. Hottendorf GJ, Nielson SW: Pathogenic report of twenty-nine necropsies on dogs with mastocytoma. *Pathol Vet* 5:102–121, 1968.
16. Aikawa M, Abramowsky C, Powers KG, et al: Dirofilariasis: Glomerulonephropathy induced by *Dirofilaria immitis* infection. *Am J Trop Med Hyg* 30:84–91, 1981.
17. Casey HW, Splitter GA: Membranous glomerulonephritis in dogs infected with *Dirofilaria immitis*. *Vet Pathol* 12:111–117, 1975.
18. Lewis RM, Center SA: Primary diseases affecting glomeruli, in Bovee KC (ed): *Canine Nephrology*. Media, PA, Harwal Publishing Co, 1984, pp 461–479.
19. Wilcock BP, Patterson JM: Familial glomerulonephritis in Doberman pinscher dogs. *Can Vet J* 20:244–249, 1979.
20. Nash AS, Wright NG: Membranous nephropathy in sibling cats. *Vet Rec* 113:180–182, 1983.
21. Crowell WA, Barsanti JA: Membranous glomerulonephropathy in two feline siblings. *JAVMA* 182:1244–1245, 1983.
22. Drazner FH: Glomerulonephritis in the dog and cat. *Compend Contin Educ Pract Vet* 1(8):604–612, 1979.
23. Krakowka S: Glomerulonephritis in dogs and cats. *Vet Clin North Am* 8:629–639, 1978.
24. Grauer GF: Clinicopathologic evaluation of early renal disease in dogs. *Compend Contin Educ Pract Vet* 7(1):32–39, 1985.
25. Mostofi FK, Antonovych TT, Limas E: Patterns of glomerular reaction to injury. *Hum Pathol* 2:233–252, 1971.
26. Robertson JL: Immunologic injury to the kidney and the renal response, in Bovee KC (ed): *Canine Nephrology*. Media, PA, Harwal Publishing Co, 1984, pp 439–460.
27. Vernier RL, Mauer SM, Fish AJ, et al: The mesangial cell in glomerulonephritis. *Adv Nephrol* 1:31–46, 1971.
28. Michael AF, Blau E, Vernier RL: Glomerular polyanion. Alteration in aminonucleoside nephrosis. *Lab Invest* 23:649–657, 1970.
29. Ryan GB, Karnovsky MJ: An ultrastructural study of the mechanisms of proteinuria in aminonucleoside nephrosis. *Kidney Int* 8:219–232, 1975.
30. Jeraj K, Osborne CA, Stevens JB: Evaluation of renal biopsy in 197 dogs and cats. *JAVMA* 181:367–369, 1982.
31. Clinical article: Glomerular disease in the dog. *Vet Rec* 95:61–62, 1974.
32. Nash AS, Wright NG, Spencer AJ, et al: Membranous nephropathy in the cat: A clinical and pathological study. *Vet Rec* 105:71–77, 1979.
33. Wright NG, Nash AS, Thompson H, et al: Membranous nephropathy in the cat and dog: A renal biopsy and follow-up study of sixteen cases. *Lab Invest* 45:269–277, 1981.
34. Jeraj KP, Vernier RL, Polzin D, et al: Idiopathic immune complex glomerulonephritis in dogs with multisystem involvement. *Am J Vet Res* 45:1699–1705, 1984.
35. Morrison WI, Wright NG: Immunopathological aspects of canine renal disease. *J Small Anim Pract* 17:139–148, 1976.
36. Osborne CA, Hammer RF, Resnick JS, et al: Natural remission of nephrotic syndrome in a dog with immune-complex glomerular disease. *JAVMA* 168:129–137, 1976.
37. Osborne CA, Hammer RF, Stevens JB, et al: Immunologic aspects of glomerular disease in the dog and cat. *Gaines Symp* 1976.

38. McCluskey RT: Immunologic mechanisms in renal disease, in Heptinstall RH (ed): *The Pathology of the Kidney*, ed 2. Boston, Little, Brown & Co, 1974, p 273.

39. Wilson CB, Dixon FJ: Diagnosis of immunopathologic renal disease. *Kidney Int* 5:389-401,1974.

40. Wells JF: Immune mechanisms in tissue damage, in Fudenberg HH (ed): *Basic and Clinical Immunology*. Los Altos, CA, Lange Medical Publications, 1976.

41. Cameron JS: Platelets and glomerulonephritis. *Nephron* 18:253-258, 1977.

42. Lindsay RM, Clark WF: Platelet destruction in renal disease. *Semin Thromb Hemost* 8:138-155, 1982.

43. Jones JV: Immunological mechanism in disease. *Practitioner* 214: 493, 1975.

44. McKay DG: Participation of components of the blood coagulation system in the inflammatory response. *Am J Pathol* 67:181-204, 1972.

45. McCluskey RT, Bhan AK: Immune complexes and renal disease. *Clin Immunol Allerg* 1:397-414, 1981.

46. Werner LL, Gorman NT: Immune-mediated disorders of cats. *Vet Clin North Am* 14:1039-1064, 1984.

47. Osborne CA, Hammer RF, Stevens JB, et al: The glomerulus in health and disease. A comparative review of domestic animals and man. *Adv Vet Sci Comp Med* 21:207-285, 1977.

48. Vogt A, Batsford S: Local immune complex formation and pathogenesis of glomerulonephritis. *Contrib Nephrol* 43:51-63, 1984.

49. Burkholder PM, Oberley TD, Barber TA, et al: Immune adherence in renal glomeruli. Complement receptor sites on glomerular capillary epithelial cells. *Am J Pathol* 86:635-651, 1977.

50. Shin ML, Gelfand MC, Nagle RB, et al: Localization of receptors for activated complement on renal visceral epithelial cells of human renal glomerulus. *J Immunol* 118:869-873, 1977.

51. Foidart JB, Salmon JP, Berthoux FJ, et al: Binding of soluble immune complexes to human glomerular complement receptors. *Kidney Int* 15:303-310, 1979.

52. McPhaul JJ, Grey GJ, Wagner DF, et al: Nephrotoxic canine glomerulonephritis. *Kidney Int* 6:123-127, 1974.

53. Wright NG, Thompson H, Cornwell HJC: Canine nephrotoxic glomerulonephritis. *Vet Pathol* 10:69-86, 1973.

54. Dibartola SP, Spaulding GL, Chew DJ: Urinary protein excretion and immunopathologic findings in dogs with glomerular disease. *JAVMA* 177:73-77, 1980.

55. Halliwell RE: Autoimmune diseases in domestic animals. *JAVMA* 181:1088-1096, 1982.

56. Wright NG, Fisher EW, Morrison WI, et al: Chronic renal failure in dogs: A comparative clinical and morphological study of chronic glomerulonephritis and chronic interstitial nephritis. *Vet Rec* 98:288-293, 1976.

57. Osborne CA, Jeraj K: Underlying cause of glomerulopathy remains a mystery. *DVM* 19:9, 1979.

58. Banks KL, Henson JB: Immunologically mediated glomerulitis of horses. *Lab Invest* 26:708-715, 1972.

59. Wilson CB, Dixon FJ: Anti-glomerular basement membrane antibody-induced glomerulonephritis. *Kidney Int* 3:74-89, 1973.

60. Arthur JE, Lucke VM, Newby TJ, et al: An immunohistological study of feline glomerulonephritis·using the peroxidase-antiperoxidase method. *Res Vet Sci* 37:12-17, 1984.

61. Taylor C: Immunoperoxidase techniques: Practical and theoretical aspects. *Arch Pathol Lab Med* 102:113-121, 1978.

62. Markman RV, Sutherland JC, Mardiney MR: The ubiquitous occurrence of immune complex localization in the renal glomeruli of normal mice. *Lab Invest* 29:111-120, 1973.

63. Barrett RE: Azotemia and proteinuria, in Ettinger SJ (ed): *Textbook of Veterinary Internal Medicine*, ed 2. Philadelphia, WB Saunders Co, 1983, pp 141-145.

64. Dibartola SP, Chew DJ, Jacobs G: Quantitative urinalysis including 24-hour protein excretion in the dog. *JAAHA* 16:537-545, 1980.

65. Barsanti JA, Finco DR: Protein concentration in urine of normal dogs. *Am J Vet Res* 40:1583-1588, 1979.

66. Ginsburg M, Chang BS, Matarese RA, et al: Use of single voided urine samples to estimate quantitative proteinuria. *N Engl J Med* 309:1543-1546, 1983.

67. Vestergaard P, Leverette R: Constancy of urinary excretion. *J Lab Clin Med* 51:211-218, 1958.

68. White JV, Olivier NB, Reimann K, et al: Use of protein-to-creatinine ratio in a single urine specimen for quantitative estimation of canine proteinuria. *JAVMA* 185:882-885, 1984.

69. Bovee KC: Clinical and laboratory evaluation of renal function, in Bovee KC (ed): *Canine Nephrology*. Media, PA, Harwal Publishing Co, 1984, pp 219-233.

70. Lewis RM, Spaulding G: Clinicopathologic interpretation of immune-mediated renal disease. *Cornell Vet* 68 (Suppl 7): 158-163, 1978.

71. Donadio JV, Anderson CF, Mitchell JC, et al: Membranoproliferative glomerulonephritis: A prospective clinical trial of platelet-inhibitor therapy. *N Engl J Med* 310:1421-1426, 1984.

72. Adams DA, Maxwell MH, Bernstein D: Corticosteroid therapy of glomerulonephritis and the nephrotic syndrome: A review. *Chron Dis* 15:29, 1962.

73. Black DAK, Rose G, Breger OB: Controlled trial of prednisone in adult patients with nephrotic syndrome. *Br Med J* 3:421, 1970.

74. Ehrenreich T, Porush JG, Churg J, et al: Treatment of idiopathic membranous nephropathy. *N Engl J Med* 295:741-746, 1976.

75. Grupe WE, Makker SP, Ingelfinger JR: Chlorambucil treatment of frequently-relapsing nephrotic syndrome. *N Engl J Med* 295:746-749, 1976.

76. De Schepper J, Hoorens J, Matteeuws D, et al: Glomerulonephritis and the nephrotic syndrome in a dog. *Vet Rec* 95:433-436, 1974.

77. Clark WF, Friesen M, Linton AL, et al: The platelet as a mediator of tissue damage in immune complex glomerulonephritis. *Clin Nephrol* 6:287-289, 1976.

78. George CRP, Clark WF, Cameron JS: The role of platelets in glomerulonephritis. *Adv Nephrol* 5:19-65, 1975.

79. Polzin DJ, Osborne CA, Leininger JR: The influence of diet on the progression of canine renal failure. *Compend Contin Educ Pract Vet* 6(12):1123-1129, 1984.

80. Brenner BM, Meyer TW, Hostetter TH: Dietary protein intake and the progressive nature of kidney disease: The role of hemodynamically mediated glomerular injury in the pathogenesis of progressive glomerular sclerosis in aging, renal ablation, and intrinsic renal disease. *N Engl J Med* 307:652-659, 1982.

81. Green RA: Clinical implications of antithrombin III deficiency in animal diseases. *Compend Contin Educ Pract Vet* 6(6):537-546, 1984.

82. Green RA, Russo EA, Greene RT, et al: Hypoalbuminemia-related platelet hypersensitivity in two dogs with nephrotic syndrome. *JAVMA* 186:485-488, 1985.

83. Center SA, Smith CA, Wilkinson E, et al: Clinicopathologic renal immunofluorescent and light microscopic features of glomerulonephritis in the dog: 41 cases (1975-1985). *JAVMA* 190:81-90, 1987.

UPDATE

Recent clinical investigations have shed new light on the pathogenesis, diagnosis, and therapy of glomerulonephritis in dogs and cats. It now appears that glomerular injury may result from a reaction to circulating immune complexes that accumulate in the glomerulus or form in situ. Progressive glomerular injury occurs as a consequence of inflammatory reaction (e.g., cellular infiltrate, complement activation, and cellular membrane damage) and the adaptive measure (e.g., glomerular hyperfiltration) that follows as the intact nephrons compensate for reduced nephron mass. Patients at high risk for glomerular proteinuria include those with infectious diseases, neoplasia, chronic inflammatory diseases, endocrine diseases (especially diabetes mellitus and hyperadrenocorticism), and those receiving glucocorticoid drugs.

Pathologic glomerular proteinuria remains the salient finding in glomerulonephritis. Routine urinalysis of affected patients reveals marked proteinuria (usually in excess of that which is appropriate for the patient's urine specific gravity) accompanied by few abnormalities in urine sediment. In both dogs and cats, the presence of pathologic proteinuria can be easily detected by calculating the urine protein:creatinine (UP/UC) ratio. Determination of the UP/UC ratio is a rapid, sensitive, and convenient method for the detection and estimation of daily urinary protein loss. Veterinary studies have shown that this ratio correlates well to 24-hour protein loss, and that it is not adversely influenced by prior feeding or collection method (e.g., cystocentesis or voided or catheterized urine specimens). The following criteria have been established:

- In dogs, UP/UC values < 0.5 are considered normal and UP/UC values > 1.0 are considered abnormal. If the UP/UC value is between 0.5 and 1.0, the author recommends repeating the ratio or performing a 24-hour collection for total urine protein determination.
- In cats, UP/UC values > 0.7 are considered abnormal.

Cornerstones of therapy for glomerulonephritis include dietary protein restriction and the use of platelet inhibitor drugs such as aspirin to reduce hypercoagulability. Although the exact degree of protein restriction remains controversial, considerable scientific evidence suggests that a reduction in dietary protein intake may be beneficial. High-protein diets have been implicated in hyperfiltration, glomerular capillary hypertension, and glomerulosclerosis of remaining functional nephrons in some species. Low-protein diets may also decrease the nausea that may accompany uremia, decrease the severity of renal azotemia, and lessen the magnitude of proteinuria in patients with glomerulonephritis. A variety of commercially prepared or home-made diets that are protein restricted, low in calcium, and low in phosphorus may be fed.

Low-dose aspirin therapy (0.5–2.5 mg/kg PO q 24 hr) is recommended to reduce inflammation, hypercoagulability, and thromboembolism associated with significant proteinuria. Aspirin therapy is convenient and may be administered on an outpatient basis. Systemic hypertension may occur in up to 80% of canine patients and may require dietary restriction of sodium. Judicious use of angiotensin-converting enzyme (ACE) inhibitors may ameliorate hypertension and may be beneficial in minimizing progressive glomerular injury. Consider an initial treatment with enalapril (0.25 to 0.5 mg/kg PO q 12–24 hr) or captopril (0.5 to 2.0 mg/kg PO q 8–24 hr); then titrate the dosage according to blood pressure. Further dosage reductions may be necessary in animals with reduced glomerular filtration (e.g., renal failure).

In summary, glomerulonephritis remains a diagnostic and therapeutic challenge to veterinarians. Biologic response to therapy may vary and is often unpredictable. Appropriate supportive therapy, as outlined in this article, may prolong survival and delay progression to chronic renal failure.

Renal Tubular Acidosis

KEY FACTS

- Renal tubular acidosis (RTA) is a group of disorders characterized by hyperchloremic metabolic acidosis.
- Proximal renal tubular acidosis, which is also known as type II renal tubular acidosis, results from a proximal tubular defect in bicarbonate reabsorption and is often associated with multiple defects in tubular resorption, which is known as Fanconi syndrome.
- Distal (type I) renal tubular acidosis is associated with a defect in secretion of hydrogen ions by distal tubules.
- Clinical consequences of renal tubular acidosis result from persistent metabolic acidosis, which may subsequently result in metabolic bone disease, severe electrolyte imbalances, and urolithiasis.

Texas A&M University
Debra L. Zoran, DVM

Iowa State University
Albert E. Jergens, DVM

RENAL tubular acidosis (RTA) is a group of disorders characterized by hyperchloremic metabolic acidosis occurring secondary to diminished renal tubular hydrogen ion secretion during renal sufficiency.[1-8] Kidneys play a critical role in the regulation of acid-base balance by reabsorbing filtered bicarbonate and by promoting the excretion of acids generated by metabolic processes. The reabsorption of filtered bicarbonate is one of the primary responsibilities of proximal tubules. In acid-base homeostasis, distal tubules are important in secreting hydrogen ions (H+). Abnormalities in proximal or distal tubular function can result in the development of renal tubular acidosis. Renal tubular acidosis is commonly divided into two groups based on the location of dysfunction within renal tubules. Proximal (type II) renal tubular acidosis involves a defect in bicarbonate reabsorption; distal (type I) renal tubular acidosis is associated with defective hydrogen ion secretion. A hyperkalemic form of distal renal tubular acidosis, which is only recognized in humans, is called type IV renal tubular acidosis. The objectives of this article are to describe renal acid-base homeostasis and the pathophysiology of proximal and distal renal tubular acidosis. The diagnosis and management of both syndromes are also discussed.

URINE ACIDIFICATION AND ACID-BASE HOMEOSTASIS

Acid-base homeostasis is regulated by several mechanisms, including neutralization of acids by body buffers, respiratory elimination of carbon dioxide, and renal regulation of bicarbonate reabsorption and hydrogen ion excretion.[1] Kidneys play a pivotal role in maintaining normal acid-base balance and restoring homeostasis during acidosis or alkalosis. Reabsorption of most filtered bicarbonate is necessary before the daily acid load can be excreted because bicarbonate loss in urine is equivalent to adding hydrogen ions to the body.[1] Proximal tubules normally reabsorb approximately 80% to 85% of filtered bicarbonate[1-5,9] while remaining bicarbonate is reabsorbed by the loops of Henle and distal nephrons. Bicarbonate reclamation from filtrate in the proximal tubular lumen involves a complex system of ion dissociations and exchanges (Figure 1). Proximal tubular epithelial cells generate hydrogen ions from carbon dioxide and water in a reaction that is catalyzed by carbonic anhydrase (CA). Carbon dioxide and water combine to form carbonic acid (H_2CO_3), which rapidly dissociates into hydrogen ions and bicarbonate ions. Bicarbonate is returned to peritubular capillaries, while the newly formed hydrogen ions are secreted into the tubular lumen in exchange for sodium.

The energy required for the exchange of hydrogen ions and sodium is provided by a sodium–potassium adenosinetriphosphatase pump.[3] Sodium ions in tubular fluid may also move into tubular epithelial cells because of differences in concentration gradient or as a result of a carrier protein that transports sodium into cells and hydrogen ions out of cells. A similar series of processes involving car-

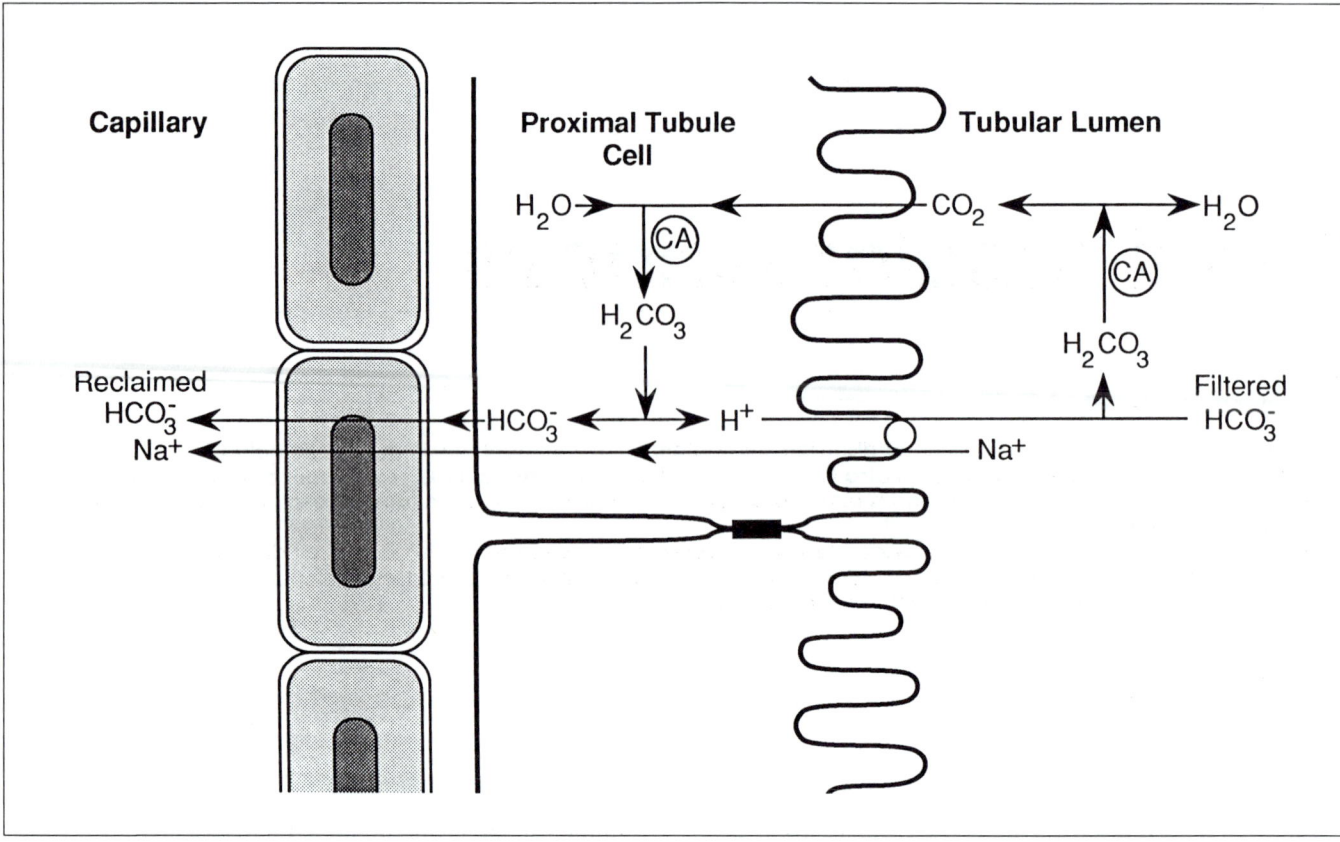

Figure 1—Schematic drawing of a proximal tubule segment. Shown are a cross section of the peritubular capillary, endothelium separating the tubular cell and capillary, and tubular lumen as well as the ion dissociations and exchanges that occur in the proximal tubules.

bonic anhydrase occurs within the tubular lumen. The net effect of these processes in the proximal tubule is that for each secreted hydrogen ion, one bicarbonate ion is added to plasma; normal plasma bicarbonate concentration is therefore maintained.

Distal tubules play an important role in acid-base homeostasis by secreting hydrogen ions (Figure 2). Distal tubules secrete hydrogen ions by means of a proton pump that actively transports hydrogen ions from cells into the tubular lumen without exchange or cotransport of ions.[10] This pump is regulated by pH and voltage gradients and requires energy derived from sodium–potassium adenosinetriphosphatase.[3] The pH of tubular fluid is partially regulated by buffers; the voltage gradient is influenced by the rate of sodium reabsorption. Sodium reabsorption by distal tubules is primarily controlled by the effects of aldosterone.

THE EXCRETION of hydrogen ions secreted by tubules involves combining hydrogen ions with ammonia or other buffers. Most hydrogen ions within tubular fluid are buf-

fered by phosphoric acid. This process is commonly called titratable acidity because the quantity of hydrogen ions that are buffered in this manner is measured by determining the amount of sodium hydroxide that must be added to urine to titrate the pH to 7.4.[1] The amount of hydrogen ions buffered by phosphoric acid increases as the tubular fluid pH decreases; however, the ability of titratable acids to enhance hydrogen ion excretion is limited because of the inability of the kidneys to increase phosphorous excretion markedly.

Another important buffer system within the distal nephron is production of ammonia by tubular cells.[9] Ammonia is generated by metabolism of amino acids, especially glutamine. The metabolism of glutamine to ammonia depends on pH and results in additional ammonia generation in cases of acidemia and decreased ammonia in cases of alkalemia. Ammonia formed within tubular cells diffuses into the lumen because of the concentration gradient of the lumen and low urine pH. In the tubular lumen, hydrogen ions bind to ammonia to form an ammonium ion (NH_4^+), which is a polar and water-soluble compound that cannot diffuse back into cell cytoplasm. This phenomenon is called ion trapping. Continued formation of ammonium

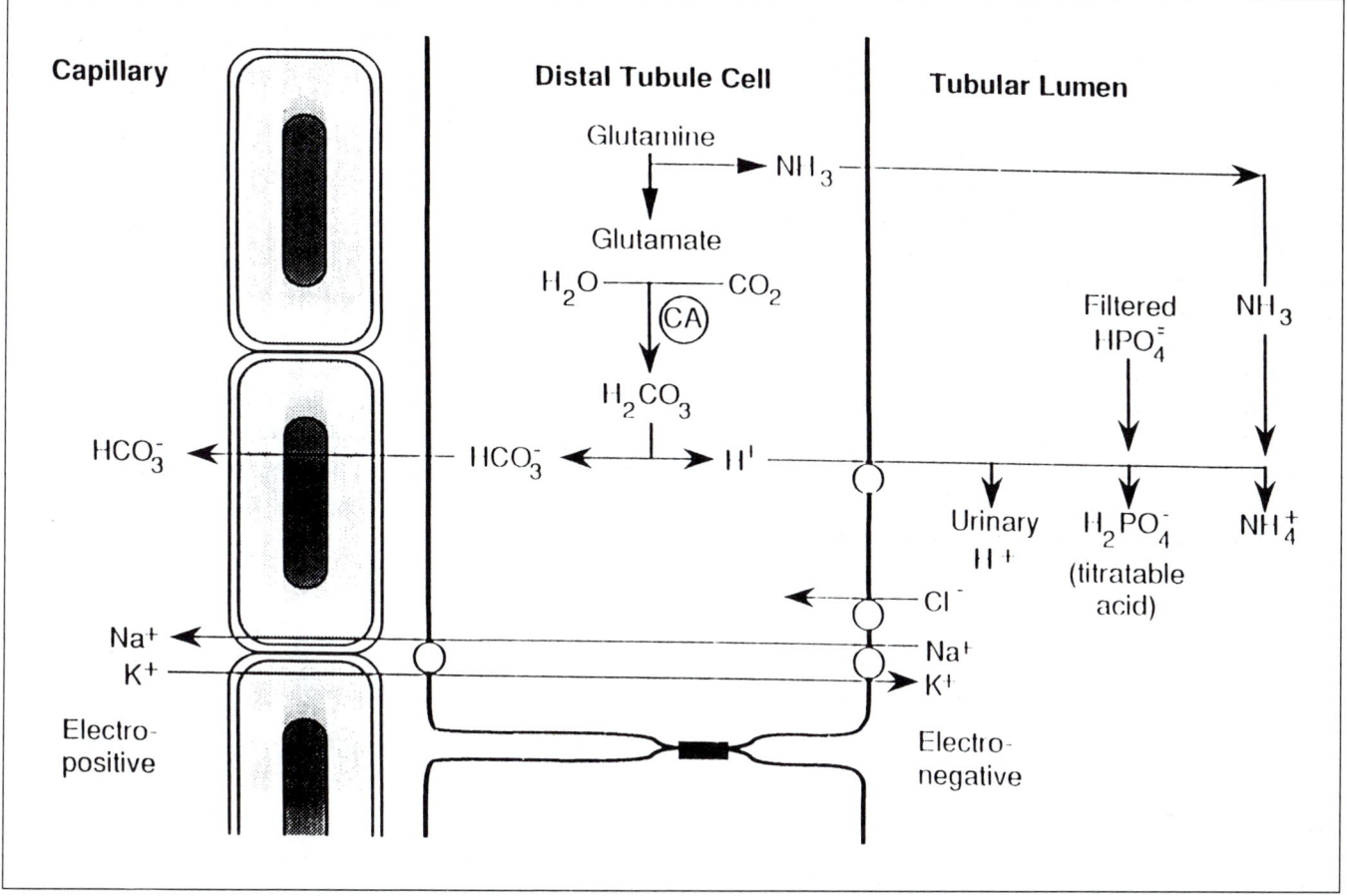

Figure 2—Schematic drawing of a cross section of a distal tubule. Depicted are the major structures (the peritubular capillary, renal tubular cell, and the tubular lumen); major ion exchange events associated with distal acidification are also represented.

ions in tubular fluid maintains urine ammonia concentration at low levels, thereby favoring continued ammonia diffusion into the lumen down its concentration gradient. The ability of the kidneys to augment ammonia production is a primary adaptive response to prolonged or severe acidemia.

DISTAL RENAL TUBULAR ACIDOSIS

The classic type of renal tubular acidosis (also called distal renal tubular acidosis) is the most common form in humans. This type is associated with a greater number of clinical abnormalities because of the associated chronic metabolic acidosis. Distal renal tubular acidosis occurs when defective hydrogen ion secretion causes metabolic acidosis resulting from the inability of the kidneys to excrete an acid load. In dogs and cats with distal renal tubular acidosis, urine pH is often greater than 7.0 despite severe acidemia.[3,4,6-8,11] The disorder is associated with hypokalemic and hyperchloremic metabolic acidosis and may result in nephrocalcinosis and osteomalacia if acidosis is left untreated.[5,6,11,18] Cases of distal renal tubular acidosis involving dogs and cats have infrequently been reported

in the veterinary literature. Previously reported cases include three cats[12,13,15] and one dog, which also had multiple defects of proximal tubular function.[14] In the two feline cases, pyelonephritis was reported to occur in addition to distal renal tubular acidosis[12,15]; the third case described a cat with hepatic lipidosis and distal renal tubular acidosis.[13]

Mechanisms responsible for defective hydrogen ion secretion in cases of distal renal tubular acidosis are poorly defined but include (1) back leak or gradient defects,[4,7,8,16] (2) secretory failure or proton pump defects,[4,7,17,18] and (3) voltage-dependent defects.[4,7,8,17] The distal tubules have tight epithelial junctions that allow formation of steep concentration and electric gradients.[6] These gradients are responsible for regulating hydrogen ion transport, which is primarily mediated by the proton pumps present in the plasma cell membrane. Medullary-collecting ducts have the largest number of cells containing proton pumps and thus are responsible for the highest rate of proton secretion.[6] Development of a distal acidification defect was first hypothesized to result from inability of the cells in the medullary-collecting ducts to generate or maintain a steep hydrogen ion gradient.[7] It is now recognized that several mechanisms, including secretory failure or voltage-dependent defects, may be responsible for defective hydrogen ion excretion or may contribute to the disorder.[7,8,16-18]

Evidence of abnormal proton pump activity in humans has been obtained by stimulating maximum urine acidification with infusions of sodium sulfate or by administering sodium bicarbonate and measuring urine carbon dioxide partial pressure (Pco_2) concentrations.[8,16,18] Sodium bicarbonate and sodium sulfate enhance distal renal tubular hydrogen ion secretion by increasing delivery of sodium to the distal nephron.[8,18] The reason for measuring urine carbon dioxide partial pressure after sodium bicarbonate loading is that hydrogen ion secretion must be intact for urine carbon dioxide partial pressure to increase. Bicarbonate in urine combines with secreted hydrogen ions to form carbonic acid, which then dissociates into water and carbon dioxide. This dissociation traps carbon dioxide in urine and thus allows urine concentration to be measured. Human patients with distal renal tubular acidosis resulting from defective hydrogen ion secretion therefore have alkaline urine and inappropriately low urine carbon dioxide partial pressure values after administration of bicarbonate. A similar response would be expected in dogs and cats with distal renal tubular acidosis after bicarbonate administration.

A THIRD possible mechanism for impaired distal tubular acidification of urine is the voltage-dependent form of renal tubular acidosis. This condition results from failure to generate and maintain negative luminal voltage differences in the distal nephron.[7] A decrease in luminal electronegativity occurs when sodium reabsorption by distal tubules is impaired. As sodium transport decreases, the ability of distal tubules to acidify urine also decreases.[7] Lithium therapy in humans has been implicated in causing distal renal tubular acidosis by this mechanism because lithium competes with sodium ions for exchange in the distal nephron, thereby resulting in decreased hydrogen ion secretion by reduced sodium ion transport.[7]

The clinical signs associated with distal renal tubular acidosis are often vague and nonlocalizing. Lethargy is the most frequently observed abnormality during physical examination. Muscle weakness, paralysis, polyuria and polydipsia, vomiting, and constipation have been reported in humans.[4,6] When systemic acidosis is left untreated, distal acidification defects are often associated with severe clinical complications, including osteomalacia, pathologic fractures, nephrocalcinosis, and nephrolithiasis.[3,5,6,7] Table I shows laboratory abnormalities and clinical complications of renal tubular acidosis in dogs and cats. The most consistent abnormality that occurs in routine biochemical profiles is hypokalemia. Hypokalemia is believed to result from enhanced kaliuresis and from the use of potassium as a substitute cation for hydrogen ions in exchange for sodium

TABLE I
Laboratory Abnormalities and Clinical Complications of Renal Tubular Acidosis[5,6]

Abnormalities	Proximal	Distal
Serum potassium	Normal to low	Severely decreased
Serum phosphate	Low	Normal
Serum bicarbonate	15–18 mEq/L	≤10–12 mEq/L
Urinalysis		
Glucose	Often present	Absent
Amino acids	Often present	Absent
Phosphate	Often present	Absent
Urine calcium	Normal	High
Urine bicarbonate	≥15%	≤5%
Urine pH		
If $HCO_3^- = 24$ mEq/L	>6.0	>6.0
If $HCO_3^- = 15$–18 mEq/L	5.5–8.0	>6.0
Clinical Complications		
Bone disease	Rare	Common
Nephrolithiasis and nephrocalcinosis	Rare	Common
Renal insufficiency	Rare	Often present

ions.[4] Blood-gas analysis for serum bicarbonate levels is also consistently abnormal and may be less than 10 mEq/L in severe cases of distal renal tubular acidosis.

Diagnosis

The first step in diagnosing distal renal tubular acidosis is detection of metabolic acidosis. Because renal tubular acidosis disorders result in hyperchloremic metabolic acidosis, determination of the anion gap may help characterize the cause of acidosis.[19] Potential causes of hyperchloremic metabolic acidosis (also called normal anion gap acidosis) include diarrhea, mild renal failure, and renal tubular acidosis.[1,19,20] Such drugs as carbonic anhydrase inhibitors and oral acidifying agents (e.g., methionine) also may cause hyperchloremic acidosis.[19] Because renal tubular acidosis is uncommon in companion animals, it is useful first to exclude more common causes of hyperchloremic metabolic acidosis. A thorough history, complete blood cell count, serum biochemical profile, and urinalysis are very often useful in excluding other causes.

U RINE pH must be carefully determined if distal renal tubular acidosis is suspected. A urine pH that is greater than 5.5 is associated with systemic acidemia and suggests renal tubular acidosis. Microscopic examination of urine sediment and urine culture should be performed to determine if urease-producing microbes are the cause of the alkaline urine pH. Excretion of electrolytes in urine collected for 24 hours may also be evaluated in suspected cases of distal renal tubular acidosis.[21,22] Humans with distal renal tubular acidosis excrete less than 5% of filtered bicarbonate but excrete excessive amounts of calcium and potassium in urine[4,5,6] (Table I). Mild to moderate hypokalemia may result from potassium loss in urine.[4,6,11] Although a similar electrolyte excretion profile would be expected in dogs and cats with distal renal tubular acidosis, to date it has been documented in only one cat and one dog.[13,15] Survey abdominal radiography is used to confirm metabolic bone disease, nephrocalcinosis, or calcium-containing uroliths. These radiographic abnormalities are more prevalent in patients with distal renal tubular acidosis than in those with proximal renal tubular acidosis and may be valuable in differentiating between the two disorders.

Use of specific tests to assess renal handling of bicarbonate or acid may be necessary to confirm diagnosis in some cases of distal renal tubular acidosis. A commonly used test is administration of sodium bicarbonate and subsequent measurement of urine carbon dioxide partial pressure concentrations.[2,4,7] The intravenous bicarbonate infusion dose should be sufficient to sustain an increase in serum bicarbonate concentration of 0.5 to 1.0 mEq/L/hr.[11] In patients with distal tubular acidification defects, there is no increase in urine carbon dioxide partial pressure concentration despite filtration of large amounts of bicarbonate. If patients with distal renal tubular acidosis have high urine pH values associated with systemic acidemia, the exogenous bicarbonate test is unnecessary.

A challenge test based on administration of ammonium chloride to evaluate the ability of the kidneys to excrete acid has also been described.[6] An oral dose of ammonium chloride (0.2 g/kg given in divided doses for one hour) is administered with subsequent measurement of urine pH for six hours.[11] Normal dogs have maximally acidified urine within a range of 5.4 to 5.9, whereas dogs with distal renal tubular acidosis have a urine pH above 6.0.[11] This test is often unnecessary because animals with renal tubular acidosis typically have metabolic acidemia that maximally stimulates excretion of acids by the kidneys. Because the challenge tests have been performed primarily in humans, the applicability and accuracy of the tests for use in companion animals are unknown.

Treatment

Treatment of distal renal tubular acidosis should focus on correcting any underlying disorders that cause renal tubular dysfunction. Examples of disorders that have been reported to cause renal tubular acidosis in humans include systemic lupus erythematosus, multiple myeloma, obstructive uropathies, and primary hyperparathyroidism[14] (Table II). Supportive treatment of distal renal tubular acidosis is usually required and focuses on correction of systemic aci-

demia with alkali therapy. In humans, the amount of bicarbonate required to correct acidemia varies but is generally less than 2 mEq/kg/day.[2,7,11,18] Bicarbonate may be orally administered as tablets, powder (baking soda), or a solution. Several nonbicarbonate preparations are also available as alkali substitutes and may contain one or more of the following ingredients: sodium citrate, citric acid, or potassium citrate.[2] Doses of the nonbicarbonate preparations have not been established for dogs or cats but could be extrapolated to the amount of bicarbonate necessary to correct acidemia. Some side effects of oral bicarbonate administration in humans include metabolic alkalosis, abdominal bloating, and production of excessive intestinal gas. The use of citrate-containing products is therefore sometimes preferred to pure bicarbonate in long-term therapy. Correction of metabolic acidemia results in reduced risk of metabolic bone disease and associated hypercalciuria, thereby potentially minimizing formation of calcium-containing uroliths.

POTASSIUM replacement in addition to alkali therapy may be necessary because profound potassium depletion may occur in animals with distal renal tubular acidosis.[11] Several potassium replacement elixirs are available for dogs and cats; the dose should be titrated to the individual needs of the patient. Vitamin D therapy is occasionally recommended for use in humans with metabolic bone disease[3]; however, use in dogs and cats with distal renal tubular acidosis has not been evaluated. Clients should be informed that lifelong therapy with frequent reevaluation of their pet's metabolic status is often necessary.

PROXIMAL RENAL TUBULAR ACIDOSIS

The most commonly observed form of renal tubular acidosis in dogs is proximal or type II renal tubular acidosis. Proximal renal tubular acidosis has only been reported in dogs and, in most cases, occurs in conjunction with other defects of proximal tubular function, which are collectively known as Fanconi syndrome.[24-29] Proximal renal tubular acidosis is associated with impaired ability of the proximal tubule to reabsorb filtered bicarbonate. Massive bicarbonate excretion results. The distal tubules have some ability to increase reabsorption of filtered bicarbonate. A reduction in serum bicarbonate concentration occurs in proximal renal tubular acidosis to a serum level that is generally between 15 and 18 mEq/L.[6] Serum bicarbonate levels stabilize in this range because the remaining filtered bicarbonate is reabsorbed by the distal nephron and, as a result, metabolic acidemia remains mild.

Because of the self-limiting nature of proximal renal tubular acidosis, the severity of the disorder is minimized and clinical complications are fewer than with distal renal tubular acidosis. Dogs with proximal renal tubular acidosis

TABLE II
Causes of Proximal and
Distal Renal Tubular Acidosis in Humans[1,4,6,7,18]

Distal	Proximal
Primary or idiopathic	Primary or idiopathic
Hereditary	Hereditary
Immunologic and hypergammaglobulinemic disorders	Secondary to heritable systemic disease
Sjögren's syndrome	Cystinosis
Systemic lupus erythematosus	Lowe's syndrome
Multiple myeloma	Wilson's disease
Idiopathic hypergammaglobulinemia	Fructose intolerance
Thyroiditis	Renal disorders
Cryoglobulinemia	Amyloidosis
Primary biliary cirrhosis	Multiple myeloma
Chronic active hepatitis	Renal transplant rejection
Interstitial nephropathies	Medullary cystic disease
Obstructive uropathy	Drugs and toxins
Analgesic nephropathy	Heavy metals
Renal transplant rejection	Acetazolamide
Medullary sponge kidney	Outdated tetracycline
Altered calcium metabolism	Mercaptopurine
Primary hyperparathyroidism	Streptozotocin
Vitamin D intoxication	Sulfonamides
Idiopathic hypercalciuria	Arginine and lysine
Drugs and toxins	Hyperparathyroidism
Amphotericin B	Hypervitaminosis D
Toluene	Vitamin D deficiency
Lithium	
Cyclamate	
Carbonic anhydrase B deficiency	

also retain adequate ability to acidify urine by distal tubular hydrogen ion secretion, thereby reducing the degree of metabolic acidemia if compared with distal renal tubular acidosis patients. The urine of affected animals may be acid or alkaline, depending on the time that the specimen is collected.[11] Urine is very alkaline and hydrogen ion excretion is minimal if massive bicarbonaturia is occurring. As soon as steady state levels of serum bicarbonate are attained and bicarbonate excretion ceases, hydrogen ion secretion returns to normal and the urine becomes appropriately acid (Table I).

The Fanconi syndrome is a generalized defect in proximal tubular transport; proximal renal tubular acidosis frequently occurs as part of this defect.[6,7,18,23] The Fanconi syndrome consists of congenital or acquired defects in proximal tubular reabsorption of bicarbonate, glucose, phosphate, potassium, uric acid, and amino acids[1,7,18] (Table I). Glucosuria occurs in patients with normal blood glucose concentrations, a phenomenon that also occurs with primary renal glucosuria. Determination of concentrations of serum and urine glucose assists in differentiating between impaired tubular reabsorption of glucose and hyperglycemic glucosuria.[1] Because patients with proximal renal tubular acidosis do not have hypercalciuria, nephrocalcinosis and nephrolithiasis are not observed. The development of metabolic bone disease is also unusual because the mild degree of metabolic acidemia results in less bone buffering of excess acid; however, kaliuresis and hypokalemia may be severe with proximal renal tubular acidosis and Fanconi syndrome. Hypokalemia in proximal renal tubular acidosis may also be aggravated by alkali therapy initiated to correct metabolic acidemia.

THE CAUSE and pathogenesis of Fanconi syndrome associated with proximal renal tubular acidosis are poorly defined. In humans, Fanconi syndrome has been reported to result from various factors, including inherited diseases, drugs, and toxins as well as disorders causing generalized metabolic dysfunction (Table II). The most likely explanation for the proximal tubular defect in humans is insufficient energy production for active reabsorption of glucose, amino acids, and electrolytes.[23] This theory is supported by animal studies in which maleic acid that was given to rats altered renal mitochondrial function causing excretory defects and tubular changes similar to those defects seen in patients with Fanconi syndrome.[23] Other proposed mechanisms in humans include altered permeability of the tight junctions between tubular cells permitting back flux of glucose, electrolytes, and amino acids; defective coupling of metabolism and transport in the proximal tubule; and defective luminal cell membrane permeability.[23] None of the proposed mechanisms has been proven in dogs.

Fanconi syndrome has been reported most frequently in basenjis but has also been reported in a Yorkshire terrier and a Pomeranian.[24–29] The tubular defect is hereditary in basenjis.[25–27] The progression of renal disease in this breed is quite variable and depends greatly on the severity of the underlying defects.

Diagnosis

The identification of a patient with proximal renal tubular acidosis may be an incidental finding because the disease is self-limiting and usually causes few clinical signs. The existence of common extrarenal causes of hyperchloremic metabolic acidosis should be excluded before considering a diagnosis of renal tubular acidosis. Urinalysis plays an integral role in initial diagnostic evaluation. Patients with proximal renal tubular acidosis may have appropriately acid urine because they retain the ability to secrete hydrogen ions in distal tubules. Detection of glucosuria in a normoglycemic patient may indicate primary renal glucosuria or proximal renal tubular acidosis with Fanconi syndrome. Additional tests may be helpful, including measurement of urine electrolyte and amino acid excretion by means of urine collection for a 24-hour period.[11] If the tests are inconclusive, bicarbonate challenge is the preferred provocative test.[11] The same protocol described in diagnosis of distal renal tubular acidosis is used for the sodium bicarbonate challenge. In humans with proximal renal tubular acidosis, urine bicarbonate levels after sodium bicarbonate challenge exceed 15% when serum bicarbonate levels approach normal.[1] Excessive urine excretion of electrolytes, glucose, and amino acids is observed if the patient has concurrent Fanconi syndrome.[1,11] The normal electrolyte excretion levels in dogs have been described.[22] In most cases, diagnosing Fanconi syndrome and proximal renal tubular acidosis is uncomplicated.

Treatment

Identifying and removing the underlying cause of the proximal tubular defect, such as acetazolamide administration, represent the cornerstone of therapy. When a specific cause is not identified, however, treatment of proximal renal tubular acidosis is directed at supportive therapy. As in cases of distal renal tubular acidosis, correction of metabolic acidemia by means of alkali therapy is the primary consideration. Bicarbonate supplementation for correction of acidemia is complicated, however, because bicarbonate administration contributes to a greater loss of bicarbonate in urine.[1] In humans with proximal renal tubular acidosis, the amount of bicarbonate required for therapy is usually between 5 and 10 mEq/kg/day.[3] Because the acidosis is self-limiting, bicarbonate therapy may not be required for all patients; in humans, bicarbonate therapy is not always initiated.[3,5] Potassium supplementation in proximal renal tubular acidosis is essential because bicarbonaturia increases urinary potassium loss and may deplete body potassium stores.[1] Oral potassium supplementation and frequent monitoring of serum potassium concentrations are recommended for patients with proximal renal tubular acidosis.[8] Low-salt diets and diuretics have been suggested as helpful adjunct therapy in human patients because bicarbonate reabsorption improves in conditions of mild volume depletion.[3,4,6] Human patients with hypophosphatemia may require phosphate and vitamin D supplementation to prevent development of metabolic bone disease.[3,4] Whether such therapy is required in dogs or cats is unknown.

SUMMARY

Renal tubular acidosis in dogs and cats describes two syndromes characterized by hyperchloremic metabolic acidosis in the presence of renal sufficiency. Distal renal tubular acidosis is defined as defective hydrogen ion secretion by distal tubules and has currently been reported more frequently in cats than in dogs. Distal renal tubular acido-

sis is associated with more clinical complications than is proximal renal tubular acidosis because of the severity and persistence of metabolic acidemia. Proximal renal tubular acidosis is more commonly recognized in dogs than in cats and occurs because of a defect in proximal tubular reabsorption of bicarbonate. Therapy of both syndromes is directed at correcting any identified underlying cause, but amelioration of metabolic acidemia and supportive therapy for associated complications remain the primary focus of treatment.

About the Authors

Dr. Zoran is affiliated with the Department of Animal Science at Texas A&M University and Dr. Jergens with the College of Veterinary Medicine, Iowa State University. Both are Diplomates of the American College of Veterinary Internal Medicine.

REFERENCES

1. Rose BD: *Clinical Physiology of Acid-Base and Electrolyte Disorders*, ed 2. New York, McGraw-Hill Book Co, 1984.
2. Chan JCM: Renal tubular acidosis. *J Pediat* 102(3):327–339, 1983.
3. Pohlman T, Hruska KA, Menon M: Renal tubular acidosis. *J Urol* 132(9):431–436, 1984.
4. Rocher LL, Tannen RL: The clinical spectrum of renal tubular acidosis. *Ann Rev Med* 37:319–331, 1986.
5. Davidman M, Schmitz P: Renal tubular acidosis: A pathophysiologic approach. *Hosp Pract* 23(1A):77–96, 1988.
6. Quintanilla AP: Renal tubular acidosis. *Postgrad Med* 67(4):60–73, 1980.
7. Batlle DC: Renal tubular acidosis. *Med Clin North Am* 67(4):859–878, 1983.
8. Batlle DC, Kurtzman MA: Distal renal tubular acidosis: Pathogenesis and classification. *Am J Kidney Dis* 1(6):328–344, 1982.
9. Gluck SL: Cellular and molecular aspects of renal hydrogen transport. *Hosp Pract* 24(5A):149–166, 1989.
10. Koeppen BM, Steinmetz PR: Basic mechanisms of urinary acidification. *Med Clin North Am* 67(4):753–768, 1983.
11. Polzin DJ, Osborne CA: Detection and management of canine renal tubular acidosis. *Proc 4th Annu ACVIM Vet Forum* 4:67–69, 1986.
12. Watson ADJ, Culvenor JA, Middleton DJ, et al: Distal renal tubular acidosis in a cat with pyelonephritis. *Vet Rec* 119(7):65–68, 1986.
13. Brown SA, Spyridakis LK, Crowell WA: Distal renal tubular acidosis and hepatic lipidosis in a cat. *JAVMA* 189(10):1350–1352, 1986.
14. DiBartola SP, Leonard PO: Renal tubular acidosis in a dog. *JAVMA* 180(1):70–73, 1982.
15. Drazner FH: Distal renal tubular acidosis associated with chronic pyelonephritis in a cat. *Calif Vet* 6:15–19, 1980.
16. Batlle DC, Sehy JT, Roseman MK, et al: Clinical and pathophysiologic spectrum of acquired distal renal tubular acidosis. *Kidney Int* 20:389–396, 1981.
17. Halperin ML, Goldstein MB, Richardson RMA, et al: Distal renal tubular acidosis syndromes: A pathophysiologic approach. *Am J Nephrol* 5:1–8, 1985.
18. Batlle DC, Arruda JAL: Renal tubular acidosis syndromes. *Min Elect Metab* 5:83–99, 1981.
19. Polzin DJ, Osborne CA: Clinical significance of anion gap. *Proc 4th Annu ACVIM Vet Forum* 5:4.71–4.76, 1986.
20. Orsini JA: Pathophysiology, diagnosis, and treatment of clinical acid-base disorders. *Compend Contin Educ Pract Vet* 11(5):593–604, 1989.
21. Vaden SL, Babineau C, Ford RB: Comparison of methods to evaluate urine electrolyte concentrations in normal dogs. *Proc 7th Annu ACVIM Vet Forum* 7:1050, 1989.
22. DiBartola SP, Chew DJ, Jacobs G: Quantitative urinalysis including 24-hour protein excretion in the dog. *JAAHA* 16:537–546, 1980.
23. Chesney RW: Etiology and pathogenesis of the Fanconi syndrome. *Min Elect Metab* 4:303–316, 1980.

24. McEwan MA, Macartney L: Fanconi syndrome in a Yorkshire terrier. *J Small Anim Pract* 28:737–742, 1987.
25. Breitschwerdt EB, Ochoa R, Waltman C: Multiple endocrine abnormalities in basenji dogs with renal tubular dysfunction. *JAVMA* 182(12):1348–1353, 1983.
26. Easley JR, Breitschwerdt EB: Glucosuria associated with renal tubular dysfunction in three basenji dogs. *JAVMA* 168(10):938–943, 1976.
27. Bovee KC, Joyce T, Blazer-Yost B, et al: Characterization of renal defects in dogs with a syndrome similar to the Fanconi syndrome in man. *JAVMA* 174(10):1094–1100, 1979.
28. Bovee KC: Renal dysplasia and renal Fanconi syndrome in the dog. *Proc 4th Annu ACVIM Vet Forum* 4:13.41–13.42, 1986.
29. Brown SA, Rakich PM, Barsanti J, et al: Fanconi syndrome and acute renal failure associated with gentamicin therapy in a dog. *JAAHA* 22(5):635–640, 1986.

UPDATE

Since 1991, new bits of information about renal tubular acidosis (RTA) and Fanconi syndrome have surfaced intermittently. Most of the recent investigations of RTA involve research animals. However, some findings may be relevant to companion animals, and those have been added to this article for the sake of completeness. Readers seeking a review of the clinical aspects of RTA in humans should peruse the 5th edition of Maxwell and Kleeman's *Clinical Disorders of Fluid and Electrolyte Metabolism,* which is an excellent source of recent information.[1]

The research of Dafnis and coworkers, who examined the effects of proton pump inhibitors on renal tubular function, has the most potential significance to veterinary clinicians.[2] Their recent studies revealed that H^+-K^+-ATPase inhibitors induced distal RTA in rats.[2] The rats were given the drug for 10 days, which suggests that these effects occur rapidly. The agent evaluated in this study was vanadate, but omeprazole or other proton pump inhibitors could also be expected to cause a similar response. Although the effects of proton pump inhibitor therapy on distal renal tubular acidification have not yet been evaluated in dogs or cats, reduced H^+ ion secretion by the renal tubules may be a potential adverse effect of these agents. The clinical significance of this possibility awaits further clarification through studies examining the effects of these drugs in companion animals.

The occurrence of proximal RTA or the more generalized disorder of tubular function, Fanconi syndrome, is sporadic and clinical manifestations usually are mild. Proximal RTA and Fanconi syndrome tend to occur secondary to drug therapy or metabolic (particularly immunologically mediated) diseases. The recent literature cites a case in which Fanconi syndrome and interstitial nephritis were reported in conjunction with ranitidine therapy in a human.[3] In addition, myeloma-associated Fanconi syndrome was recently examined by Aucouturier and coworkers.[4]

New potential causes of proximal or distal RTA continue to be reported in the literature, but diagnostic tests and methods of treatment remain essentially the same. Once RTA is diagnosed, the clinician's primary goal is to identify the underlying cause and, if possible, correct it. The clinician's secondary goal is to control any overt metabolic acidosis that may further complicate the patient's condition; this is likely to occur only in distal RTA.

REFERENCES

1. Halperin ML, Carlisle EJF, Donnelly S, et al: Renal tubular acidosis, in Narins RG (ed): *Clinical Disorders of Fluid and Electrolyte Metabolism,* ed 5. New York, McGraw-Hill, 1994, pp 875–910.
2. Dafnis E, Spohn M, Lonis B, et al: Vanadate causes hypokalemic distal renal tubular acidosis. *J Physiol* 265:F449–F453, 1992.
3. Neilakantappa K, Gallo GR, Lowenstein J: Ranitidine associated interstitial nephritis and Fanconi syndrome. *Am J Kid Dis* 22(2):333–336, 1993.
4. Aucouturier P, Bauwens M, Khamlichi A: Monoclonal Ig L chain and L chain V domain fragment crystallization in myeloma-associated Fanconi's syndrome. *J Immunol* 150(8:1):3561–3568, 1993.

KEY FACTS

- Polycystic kidney disease is associated with progressive displacement of functional renal tissue with multiple, enlarging cysts.
- Multiple genetic and acquired factors can influence clinical manifestations of the disease.
- Cysts develop from abnormal tubules, the cells of which apparently secrete fluid into the cyst cavity.
- Pending further studies, treatment of feline polycystic kidney disease is limited to management of progressive renal failure.

Feline Idiopathic Polycystic Kidney Disease

Jody P. Lulich, DVM
Carl A. Osborne, DVM, PhD
Patricia A. Walter, DVM, MS
Department of Small Animal
  Clinical Sciences

Timothy D. O'Brien, DVM, PhD
Department of Veterinary Pathobiology

College of Veterinary Medicine
University of Minnesota
St. Paul, Minnesota

Polycystic kidney disease (PCKD) is a disorder characterized by displacement of significant portions of normally differentiated renal parenchyma by multiple cysts.[1] In humans, polycystic kidney disease is inherited as an autosomal dominant or recessive trait.[2] Lack of genealogic information precludes a precise diagnosis of inherited polycystic kidney disease in most adult cats. The fact that 8 of 10 cats with bilateral polycystic kidneys evaluated at the University of Minnesota Veterinary Teaching Hospital and elsewhere have been long-haired suggests a familial tendency in this species.[3,4] A report of possible polycystic kidneys in several generations of long-haired cats in South Carolina supports this hypothesis.[5]

Etiopathogenesis

Until recently, the consensus was that polycystic kidney disease in mice was an inherited phenomenon. Recent research, however, indicates that renal cyst formation in a particular strain of mice requires exposure to as yet undefined environmental factors. For example, a strain of mouse (Carworth Farm White-Werder) that commonly develops polycystic kidneys when housed in conventional laboratory environments does not develop the disease in germfree environments.[6] Various agents (drugs, endotoxins, and hormones), singly and in combination, have been associated with the development of renal cysts in animals.[7-10]

The role of acquired factors in the development of this disease in humans also is noteworthy. Human patients without familial histories of polycystic kidneys commonly develop renal parenchymal cysts after years of peritoneal dialysis or hemodialysis.[11] These observations allude to the crucial role that environmental factors play in the development and progression of polycystic kidney disease in some patients with or without a hereditary predisposition to the disorder.

Light-microscopic and macropuncture studies of humans with polycystic kidney disease indicate that cysts are dilated segments of nephrons.[12] The results of biochemical analysis of cyst fluid from one cat are indicative of cystic dilation of nephron segments (see the Case Study). The reduced concentrations of glucose in cyst fluid is compatible with tubular reabsorption of glucose; the marked elevations of creatinine in cyst fluid compared with that in serum is compatible with tubular modification of glomerular filtrate. De-

TABLE I
Benzodiazepines Used to Stimulate Appetite in Anorectic Cats

Agent	Dose	Route	Frequency	Dose Form
Diazepam (Valium®—Roche Products)	0.2–0.3 mg/kg	Oral	Every 12 to 24 hours	2-mg tablets
Oxazepam (Serax®—Wyeth Laboratories)	0.2–0.4 mg/kg	Oral	Every 24 hours	10-mg capsules
Flurazepam hydrochloride (Dalmane®—Roche Products)	0.2–0.4 mg/kg	Oral	Every four to seven days	15-mg capsules

creases in total carbon dioxide concentration in cysts might reflect tubular activity to decrease systemic acid excess.

The range of solute concentrations among cysts might suggest that cysts develop from various locations within the nephron. The degree of change between the solute concentration in serum and that in the cyst should reflect the activity of the nephron segment that becomes cystic. Cysts derived from proximal nephron segments can have solute concentrations similar to those of serum. Cystic segments of functioning distal nephrons are expected to have lower concentrations of sodium, chloride, and total carbon dioxide and higher concentrations of potassium and creatinine.

Precise causative mechanisms responsible for the development of multiple cysts in both kidneys of cats are unknown. In humans, it has been popular to incriminate hypertrophy and hyperplasia of renal tubular epithelium as an early event.[2,13] According to this line of reasoning, the proliferating epithelium eventually causes outflow obstruction, which leads to progressive dilation of tubular lumens.

An alternative hypothesis is that there is an intrinsic defect in tubular basement membranes. Defects in the supporting framework are considered to contribute to cyst formation by allowing dilation and ballooning of tubular walls, similar to that which occurs during the formation of an aneurysm. Concomitant cysts in other organs, especially the liver, support the possibility of a generalized basement membrane defect.

Clinical Manifestations

Irrespective of its cause, polycystic kidney disease is typically characterized by progressive cyst enlargement and compression of adjacent parenchyma, which leads to progressive, irreversible renal failure. It is probable that early stages of the disease are associated with mild clinical signs and normal kidney size. Cats with polycystic kidney disease eventually develop nonspecific signs of anorexia, weight loss, depression, and dehydration.

Enlarged, bosselated[a] kidneys were detected by abdominal palpation in 9 of 10 cats with polycystic kidney disease

---

[a]The root word *boss* is derived from the French *boce*, meaning hump or swelling. In common usage, the root is applied to a raised part or protruding ornament on a flat surface (as in *embossed*). In medical lingo, *bosselated* refers to a structure covered by numerous rounded protuberances.

confirmed at the University of Minnesota Veterinary Teaching Hospital. The cat without palpably enlarged renal cysts was not azotemic; small cysts were confirmed by renal ultrasonography. Antemortem diagnosis of polycystic kidneys often necessitates the use of ultrasonography, contrast radiography, aspiration of fluid from cysts, or exploratory celiotomy.

Therapy

No specific treatment for polycystic kidney disease is currently available. Therapy therefore should be directed at delaying the progression and consequences of renal failure.[14] Therapy to minimize deficits and excesses in fluid, nutritional, acid-base, and electrolyte balance can include the following steps: (1) correct dehydration with enteral or with parenteral fluid, (2) offer protein- and phosphorus-restricted diets formulated for cats with primary renal failure, (3) give alkalinizing agents (e.g., sodium bicarbonate) to maintain adequate acid-base balance, (4) consider oral phosphorus-binding agents (aluminum carbonate, aluminum oxide, or calcium citrate) to control hyperphosphatemia, and (5) provide water-soluble vitamins (B and C) to replace deficits resulting from decreased consumption and urinary loss. Serial patient evaluation is essential to monitoring therapeutic response. Such invasive procedures as urinary catheterization and renal biopsy, however, should be used with extreme caution.

Chronic renal failure is commonly associated with nonregenerative anemia resulting from erythropoietic failure.[15] In humans with polycystic kidneys and renal failure, chronic regenerative anemia and polycythemia have been documented.[16] It has been hypothesized that compression of renal parenchyma (by enlarging cysts) causes local tissue hypoxia and stimulates erythropoietin production.[17] The regenerative anemia in some cats with polycystic kidney disease might be caused by a similar mechanism (see the Case Study). If this is true, the use of erythropoietic stimulating agents (e.g., anabolic steroids) to increase red blood cell mass might be unnecessary.

Anorexia, a frustrating problem in cats with renal failure, can be minimized by giving benzodiazepine tranquilizing agents (Table I). In our experience, oxazepam at a dosage of 0.4 mg/kg daily has been effective in improving the appetite of anorectic cats with renal failure. Fluraze-

TABLE II
Hematologic Values

Parameter	Day 1	7	13	28	40	72	88	Normal Values [a]
Hematocrit (%)	20.6	19.5	21.9	19.7	23.0	19.7	17.1	30–45
Protein (g/dl)[b]	9.1	8.7	8.2	8.2	8.6	8.4	8.7	6.0–7.5
Red blood cell count ($10^6/\mu l$)	3.92	3.87	4.26	4.40	5.13	4.35	3.94	5.0–10.0
Reticulocyte count (%)								
Total	5.9	36.3	64.7	32.0	23.4	60.0	38.3	1.4–10.8[c]
Aggregate	0.6	0.9	0.3	0	0	0.1	0.3	0–0.4
Punctate	5.3	35.4	64.4	32.0	23.4	59.9	38.0	1.4–10.8
White blood cell count ($10^3/\mu l$)	11.8	8.7	5.6	9.0	9.2	8.5	8.8	5.5–19.5
Neutrophils	10.56	7.83	4.51	6.84	6.99	7.69	8.18	2.5–12.5
Bands	0	0	0	0	0	0	0	0–0.3
Lymphocytes	0.71	0.39	0.87	1.71	1.01	0.72	0.4	1.5–7.0
Monocytes	0.21	0.44	0.06	0	0.28	0.09	0.13	0–0.85
Eosinophils	0.41	0	0.17	0.45	0.92	0	0.09	0–0.75
Basophils	0	0.4	0	0	0	0	0	Rare

[a] Normal values taken from Duncan JR, Prasse KW: *Veterinary Laboratory Medicine*, ed 2. Ames, IA, Iowa State University Press, 1986, p 229.
[b] Plasma protein determined by refractometry.
[c] Reticulocyte count normal values taken from Cramer DV, Lewis RM: Reticulocyte response in the cat. *JAVMA* 160:61–67, 1972.

pam hydrochloride has been equally effective and has longer duration. These drugs should be employed cautiously because the type and frequency of adverse effects associated with their use in cats with renal failure have not been evaluated.

Treatment of infected cysts might require special consideration. The acidic nature of cyst fluid and its containment by an epithelial barrier might inhibit the establishment of bactericidal concentrations of commonly used acidic antibiotics (e.g., cephalosporins and penicillins) within cysts. Alkaline, lipid-soluble antibiotics (e.g., trimethoprim-sulfonamide combinations, chloramphenicol, tetracycline, and clindamycin), which penetrate the epithelial barrier and become ionized and trapped within cysts, have been recommended for humans with polycystic kidney disease and can be considered for cats with the disease.[11]

Prognosis

Based on our experience of 10 cats with polycystic kidney disease, survival times are primarily related to the degree of renal failure at the time of diagnosis and its rate of progression rather than on detection of polycystic kidneys per se. Affected young cats typically died within weeks after diagnosis of the disease or were euthanatized because of severe renal dysfunction. If not evaluated by necropsy, polycystic kidney disease in young cats can be included as an unrecognized cause of perinatal deaths.[18]

Older adult cats (8 to 11 years of age) with polycystic kidneys apparently have more tolerance of their azotemic status; this favors improved short-term survival. Long-term survival of adult cats depends on the rate of progression of renal failure after appropriate therapy. In our series, the longest period of survival after diagnosis and therapy was more than 16 months (the patient is still alive). Of seven adult cats with polycystic kidney disease available for follow-up evaluation at the University of Minnesota Veterinary Teaching Hospital, the mean survival time was at least 5.5 months.

Case Study

The following study illustrates findings typical of naturally occurring polycystic kidney disease in adult domestic cats.

Data Base

A 10-year-old, spayed female, Persian cat was referred to the University of Minnesota Veterinary Teaching Hospital with a history of bilateral renomegaly, anorexia, weight loss, and azotemia of six months duration. Because the referring veterinarian considered neoplasia likely, aspiration biopsies from both kidneys were obtained. Evaluation of the aspirates revealed fluid containing many red blood cells and white blood cells.

Pertinent findings obtained by physical examination at the time of admission to the University of Minnesota Veterinary Teaching Hospital included depression and mild dehydration (5% loss of body weight). Both kidneys were palpably enlarged, nonpainful, and extensively bosselated.

Preliminary diagnostic procedures included complete blood cell count, serum chemistry profile, urinalysis, quantitative urine culture, and survey abdominal radiographs. Nonregenerative anemia (a hematocrit of 20.6% without elevated reticulocyte numbers or polychromasia) was detected (Table II). Serum chemistry values confirmed azotemia (creatinine was 9.3 mg/dl and urea nitrogen was 108 mg/dl). Additional serum chemistry abnormalities in-

TABLE III
Serum Chemistries and Renal Cyst Chemistries

Parameter	Day 1 Serum	Day 7[a] Serum	Day 7[a] Cyst	Day 13[a] Serum	Day 13[a] Cyst	Day 28[a] Serum	Day 28[a] Cyst	Day 40[a] Serum	Day 40[a] Cyst	Day 72[a] Serum	Day 72[a] Cyst	Day 88 Serum
Creatinine (mg/dl)	9.3	8.0	12	6.5	12.2	5.7	8.5	5.9	7.8	5.3	6.1	8.3
Urea nitrogen (mg/dl)	108	86	108	89	113	141	168	133	156	117	132	163
Sodium (mEq/L)	153	156	147	156	147	159	149	159	166	156	155	152
Chloride (mEq/L)	120	114	116	122	116	120	115	118	129	123	127	118
Potassium (mEq/L)	3.0	3.5	2.2	3.6	2.6	3.8	3.3	4.0	3.8	4.3	3.8	4.1
Phosphorus (mg/dl)	16.1	12.0	6.6	9.4	11.2	15.1	12.2	12.2	10.7	13.5	12.9	16.2
Magnesium (mg/dl)	3.1	2.9	3.0	1.6	2.0	2.1	2.1	2.1	1.9	2.1	2.3	3.2
Glucose (mg/dl)	136	102	3	83	2	88	0	96	7	102	5	113
Total carbon dioxide (mEq/L)	9.7	16.0	10.1	16.0	9.4	14.2	6.9	16.6	11.8	11.9	7.3	10.6

[a]Renal cyst fluid and blood for serum chemistries were obtained concurrently.

cluded elevations of phosphorus and magnesium concentrations and reduction in total carbon dioxide concentration (Table III).

Considering the dehydration, the patient's urine specific gravity (1.009) was inappropriately low (Table IV). *Escherichia coli* bacteria in excess of 100,000/ml were cultured from urine removed by cystocentesis. Bilateral renomegaly was identified by survey radiography (Figure 1). The length of each kidney was five times the length of the second lumbar vertebra.

Although a diagnosis of primary renal failure was established, the underlying cause was not yet known. Renal ultrasonography was performed to evaluate parenchymal consistency and structural integrity. Multilocular anechoic areas characterized by distal enhancement were detected within the cortex and medulla of both kidneys.[19] Normal renal pelvic architecture and position were maintained (Figure 2). These findings are consistent with cyst formation within renal parenchyma.[20]

Aerobic bacterial cultures from aspirates of 12 cysts

TABLE IV
Urinalysis and Urine Culture Results from Samples Collected by Cystocentesis

Parameter	Day 1	Day 7	Day 13	Day 28	Day 40	Day 72	Day 88
Specific gravity	1.009	1.011	1.011	1.010	1.010	1.008	1.010
pH	6.0	6.0	6.0	5.25	6.0	6.0	5.5
Color	Light yellow	Light yellow	Colorless	Light yellow	Light yellow	Light yellow	Light yellow
Protein[a]	1+	1+	1+	1+	1+	0	1+
Bilirubin[a]	0	0	0	0	0	0	0
Occult blood[a]	2+	3+	3+	3+	3+	3+	3+
Red blood cells per high-power field (×450)	5–10	4	10–17	2	0	6	20
White blood cells per high-power field (×450)	Too numerous to count	30	2	2	1	1	0
Sediment	Many bacteria	Few epithelial cells	Negative	Few epithelial cells	Few epithelial cells, few fat droplets	Negative	Few epithelial cells, few fat droplets
Urine culture	*Escherichia coli* ($>10^5$/ml)	Negative	Negative	Negative	Negative	Negative	Negative

[a]Values represent semiquantitative evaluations based on a scale of 0 to 4, without consideration of urine volume.

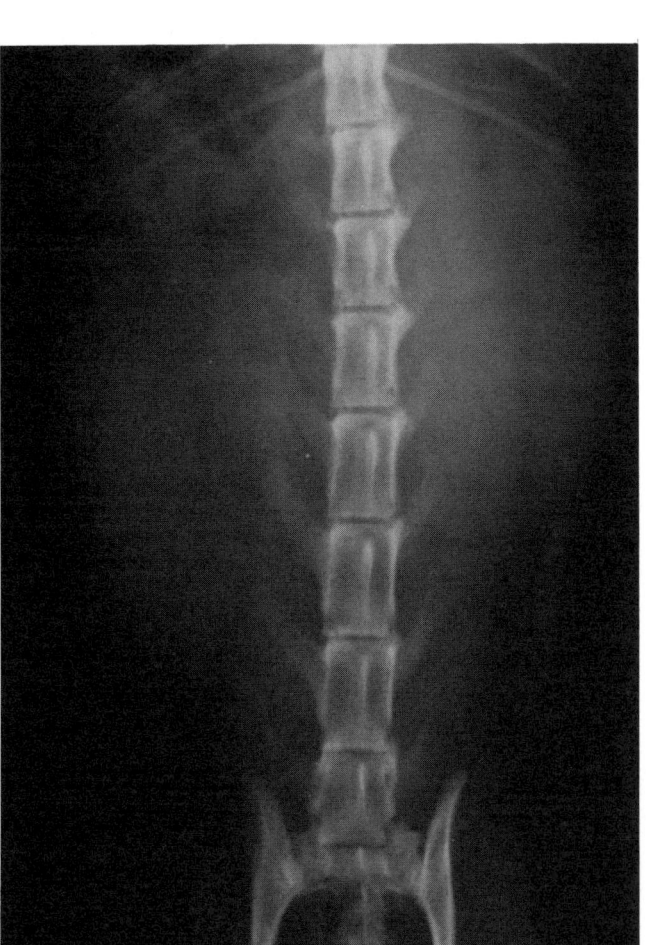

Figure 1—Ventrodorsal survey abdominal radiograph of a 10-year-old, female, Persian cat with polycystic kidneys. The large, diffuse images of both kidneys are apparent.

from both kidneys were negative. Cyst fluid concentrations of creatinine and urea nitrogen were elevated compared with those of serum; phosphorus, glucose, and total carbon dioxide concentrations were decreased (Table III). Non-regenerative anemia was detected initially. Subsequent hemograms indicated red blood cell regeneration, however, as evidenced by marked reticulocytosis (Table II). This regenerative response might have minimized the rate of progression of anemia assumed to be associated with renal failure.

Diagnostic Conclusions

The patient's data were consistent with a diagnosis of polycystic kidneys with concomitant azotemic primary renal failure. Related abnormalities included hyperphosphatemia, hypermagnesemia, metabolic acidosis, regenerative anemia, and *E. coli* urinary tract infection apparently limited to the excretory pathway.

Therapeutic Approach

Specific therapy for urinary tract infection consisted of amoxicillin trihydrate/clavulanate potassium (Clavamox®—Beecham Laboratories) at a dosage of 7.2 mg/kg twice daily. Because no specific treatment for polycystic kidneys is currently available, initial supportive therapy was directed toward minimizing deficits and excesses in fluid, electrolyte, nutritional, and acid-base balance. The patient received replacement and maintenance polyionic fluids (lactated Ringer's solution) intravenously during the first 24 hours of hospitalization. Sodium bicarbonate, 37 mg/kg twice daily, also was given orally.

The patient was discharged with instructions for the owners to encourage water consumption, continue oral

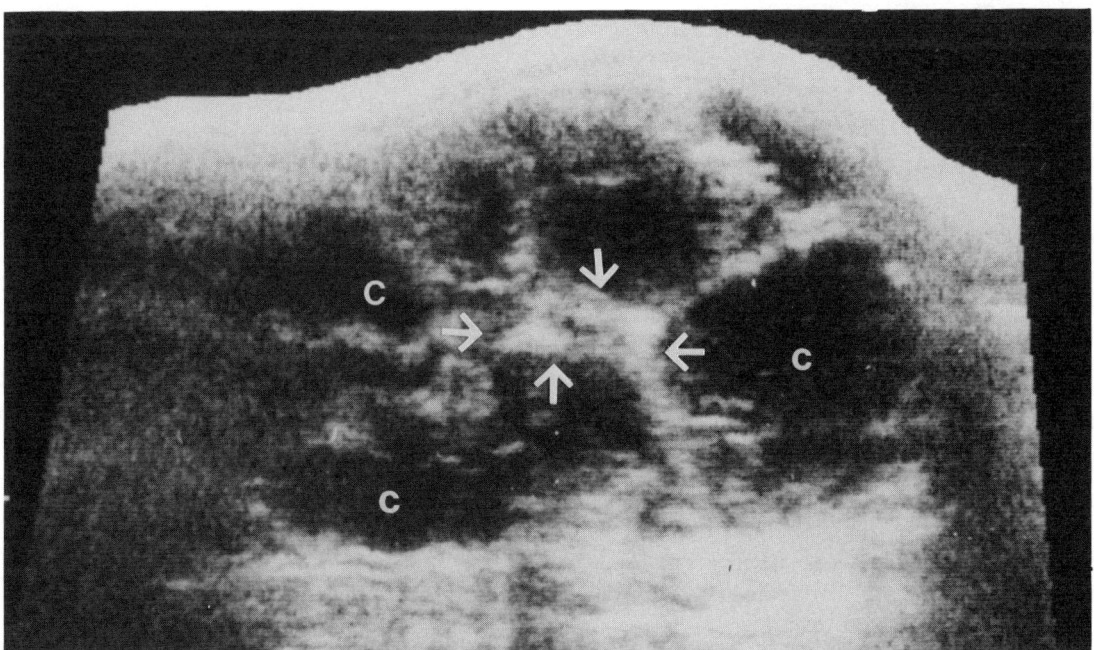

Figure 2—Sagittal static-B sonogram of the right polycystic kidney of the patient in Figure 1. The renal sinus echo, demonstrating the renal pelvis and peripelvic fat, is maintained (*arrows*). The multiple anechoic areas represent cysts (*c*).

TABLE V
Renal Cyst Chemistries[a]

Parameter	Mean	± Standard Deviation	Range	Serum Concentration[b]
Creatinine (mg/dl)	9.1	1.5	7.5–12.1	7.6
Urea nitrogen (mg/dl)	159.4	13.9	139–185	109
Sodium (mEq/L)	151.0	4.8	139–160	151
Chloride (mEq/L)	122.8	11.1	104–157	120
Potassium (mEq/L)	2.79	0.19	2.4–3.2	3.0
Glucose (mg/dl)	11.1	19.9	0–77	98
Total carbon dioxide (mEq/L)	6.0	2.1	2.9–11.1	10.6

[a]Values represent concentrations from 19 cysts aspirated during celiotomy.
[b]Renal cyst fluid and blood for serum chemistries were obtained concurrently.

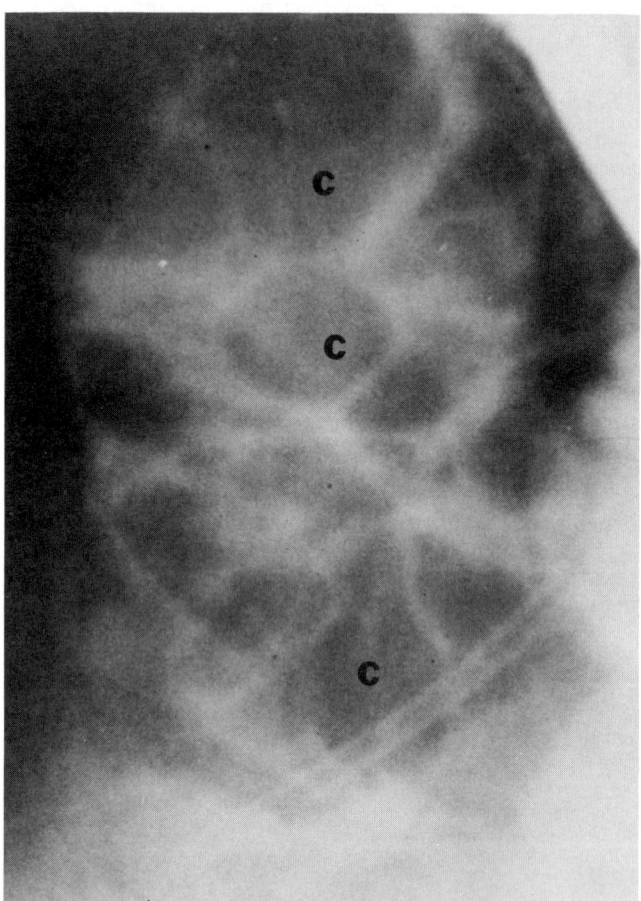

Figure 3—Semiselective renal angiogram of the patient in Figure 1 during celiotomy. This radiograph was exposed seven seconds after the injection of radiographic contrast medium. Opacified septa of vascularized or filtering portions of the right kidney outline the nonopacifying cysts (c).

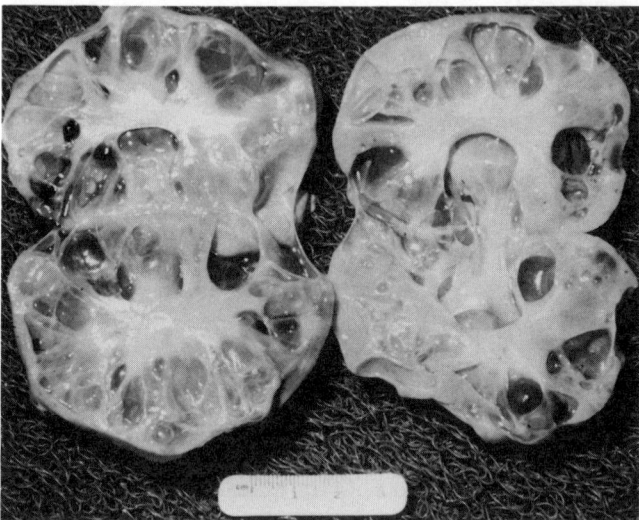

Figure 4—Photograph of sagittally sectioned, polycystic kidneys from the patient in Figure 1.

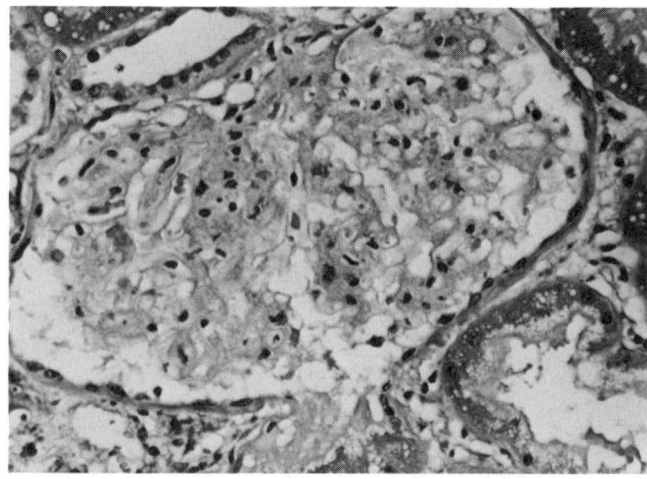

Figure 5—Photomicrograph of a glomerulus from the right kidney of the patient in Figure 1. Note the increase in the mesangium and the segmental increase in thickness of the glomerular capillary walls. (6-μm section, periodic acid–Schiff stain, original magnification ×450)

medications, and offer a diet formulated for cats with renal failure (Prescription Diet Feline k/d®—Hill's Pet Products). In the event of anorexia, the owners were advised to encourage eating by feeding small quantities of food frequently and by placing food in the cat's mouth.

The patient returned to the hospital one week later for a follow-up examination. The owners had noticed a slight improvement in the cat's activity, but partial anorexia continued. The owners were instructed to continue previous therapy with the addition of flurazepam hydrochloride at a dosage of ⅛ to 1/16 of a 15-mg capsule once weekly to stimulate the patient's appetite. The appetite improved immediately and increased progressively for the next two months.

Blood, urine, and cyst fluid were serially sampled and analyzed at approximately two-week intervals. Results were used to evaluate the progression of disease and to modify treatment. Creatinine concentrations gradually declined at each visit, but they did not return to normal (Table III). Because serum phosphorus concentrations remained elevated, the contents of aluminum hydroxide capsules (Amphojel®—Wyeth Laboratories) at a dosage of 70

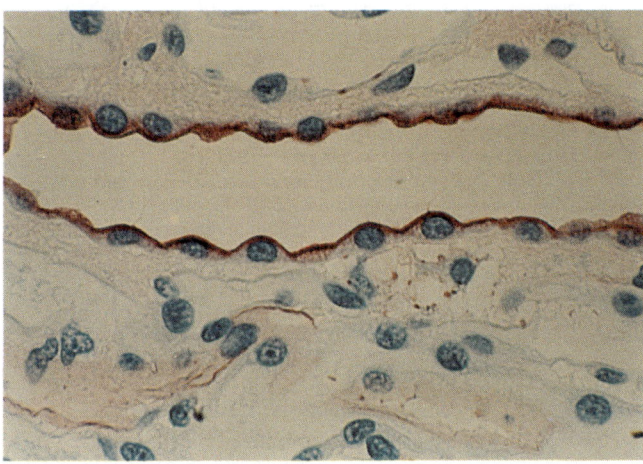

Figure 6—Photomicrograph of a section of collecting duct obtained from the kidney of a normal, adult, Domestic Shorthair cat. The collecting duct epithelial cells are brown as a result of binding with peanut lectin and subsequent staining by the avidin-biotin-peroxidase method. (4-μm section, original magnification ×205)

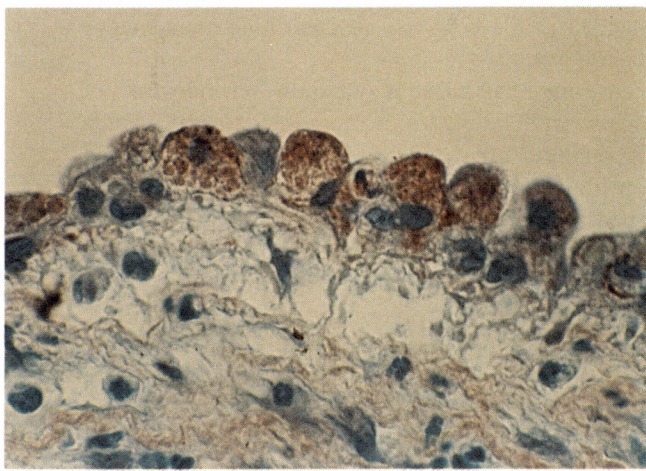

Figure 7—Photomicrograph of a section of the right kidney obtained from the patient in Figure 1. Some of the epithelial cells lining one of the renal cysts are brown as a result of binding with peanut lectin and of subsequent staining by the avidin-biotin-peroxidase method (compare with Figure 6). (4-μm section, original magnification ×128)

mg/kg/day were added to the food. To maintain positive fluid balance, the patient also received 180 ml of polyionic fluids (lactated Ringer's solution) subcutaneously.

The patient progressively improved during the next three months but subsequently became anorectic and depressed. The owners became discouraged and requested that the cat be euthanatized. This outcome was unfortunate because the abrupt elevations in serum creatinine and urea nitrogen concentrations with clinical dehydration suggested that the problems were reversible (Table III).

Before euthanasia, the cat was anesthetized to permit further in vivo evaluation of the origin of the renal cysts. Evaluation of cyst fluid concentrations of creatinine and urea nitrogen were elevated compared with those of the serum; concentrations of phosphorus, glucose, and total carbon dioxide were decreased (Table V). These findings are consistent with tubular modification of glomerular filtrate. A catheter was placed in the abdominal aorta for semiselective renal angiography. The angiogram revealed numerous radiolucent renal cysts separated by thin, interconnecting septa of renal parenchyma (Figure 3).

Necropsy Findings

The renal parenchyma of both kidneys was markedly displaced by hundreds of irregular cysts; the largest measured approximately 2 cm in diameter (Figure 4). Cyst contents varied from clear, serous fluid to reddish brown, opaque fluid. Bile-duct and hepatic parenchyma contained smaller cysts measuring 1 to 5 mm in diameter. Findings consistent with secondary renal hyperparathyroidism consisted of bilateral parathyroid hyperplasia and mineralization of the aorta, the gastric mucosa, and the renal tubular basement membranes.

Light-microscopic examination of the kidneys demonstrated loss of cortical and medullary renal tubules as well as focal areas of interstitial fibrosis containing accumulations of plasma cells. Most of the glomeruli were sclerotic. Viable glomeruli were characterized by varying degrees of glomerular capillary-wall thickening and increases in the mesangial matrix (Figure 5). The proximal convoluted tubules were hypertrophic with moderately dilated lumens. The remainder of the urinary tract was normal.

Special Studies

In an effort to identify the origin of renal cysts, sections of polycystic kidney and normal cat kidney were evaluated for the binding of four lectins. Formalin-fixed, paraffin-embedded kidney sections 4 μm thick and mounted on chrome-alum coated slides were stained. Biotinylated lectin binding to renal tubules were evaluated using the avidin-biotin-peroxidase staining procedure.[21] In the normal cat kidney, peanut (*Arachis hypogaea*) lectin, soybean (*Glycine maximum*) lectin, and *Dolichos biflorus* lectin all stained the distal tubules and the collecting ducts (Figure 6). The three lectins also stained some areas of the cysts (Figure 7).

In contrast, in normal cats, wheat germ (*Triticum vulgaris*) lectin stained all epithelial components of the nephron from the visceral epithelial cells of the glomerulus to the distal collecting ducts and also stained many cyst epithelial cells. Some cyst epithelial cells did not stain with any of these lectins, however. In noncystic portions of polycystic kidneys, epithelial cells lining moderately dilated and atrophying tubules often failed to stain with any of the lectins. Because none of these lectins specifically stained only the proximal tubules, we could not confirm or exclude the possibility of cysts forming from the proximal tubules and the loops of Henle. The results indicate that some portions of the cysts were derived from distal tubules and collecting ducts, however (Figures 6 and 7).

REFERENCES

1. Earl DP, Kark RM, Lange K, et al (eds): *Handbook of Kidney Nomenclature and Nosology.* Boston, Little, Brown & Co, 1975, p 139.
2. Welling LW, Grantham JJ: Cystic and developmental diseases of the kidney, in Brenner BM, Rector FC (eds): *The Kidney.* Philadelphia, WB Saunders Co, 1986, pp 1341–1376.
3. Northington JW, Juliana MM: Polycystic kidney disease in a cat. *J Small Anim Pract* 18:663–666, 1977.
4. Battershell D, Garcia JP: Polycystic kidney in a cat. *JAVMA* 154:555–565, 1969.
5. Cowgill WA, Hubbell JJ, Riley JC: Polycystic renal disease in related cats. *JAVMA* 175:286–288, 1979.
6. Werder AA, Amos MA, Neilsen AH, et al: Comparative effects on the development of cystic kidney disease in CFWwf mice. *J Lab Clin Med* 103:399–407, 1984.
7. Carone FA: Diphenylthiazole-induced renal cystic disease, rat, in Jones TC, Mohr U, Hunt RD (eds): *Urinary System.* New York, Springer-Verlag, 1986, pp 262–267.
8. Gardner KD, Reed WP, Evan AP, et al: Endotoxin provocation of experimental renal cystic disease. *Kidney Int* 32:329–334, 1987.
9. Dobyan DC, Hill C, Lewis T, et al: Cyst formation in rat kidney induced by cis-platinum administration. *Lab Invest* 45:260–268, 1981.
10. Carone FA, Rowland RG, Petlman SG, et al: The pathogenesis of drug-induced renal cystic disease. *Kidney Int* 5:411–421, 1974.
11. Grantham JJ: Polycystic kidney disease: Hereditary and acquired. *Kidney* 17:19–23, 1984.
12. Huseman R, Grady A, Welling D, et al: Macropuncture study of polycystic disease in adult kidneys. *Kidney Int* 18:375–385, 1980.
13. Evan AP, Gardner KD, Bernstein J: Polypoid and papillary epithelial hyperplasia: A potential cause of ductal obstruction in adult polycystic disease. *Kidney Int* 16:743–750, 1979.
14. Osborne CA, Polzin DJ: Conservative medical management of feline chronic polyuric renal failure, in Kirk RW (ed): *Current Veterinary Therapy VIII. Small Animal Practice.* Philadelphia, WB Saunders Co, 1983, pp 1008–1018.
15. Fisher JW: Mechanism of the anemia of chronic renal failure. *Nephron* 25:106, 1980.
16. Rosse WF, Waldmann TA, Cohen P: Renal cysts, erythropoietin and polycythemia. *Am J Med* 34:76–81, 1963.
17. Golde D, Hocking WG, Koeffler HP, et al: Polycythemia: Mechanisms and management. *Ann Intern Med* 95:71–87, 1981.
18. Lulich JP, Osborne CA, Lawler DF, et al: Urologic disorders of immature cats. *Vet Clin North Am [Small Anim Pract]* 17:663–696, 1987.
19. Walter PA, Johnston GR, Feeney DA, et al: Renal ultrasonography in healthy cats. *Am J Vet Res* 48:600–607, 1987.
20. Ralls PW, Halls J: Hydronephrosis, renal cystic disease and renal parenchymal disease. *Semin Ultrasound* 2:49–60, 1981.
21. Hsu SM, Raine L, Fanger H: Use of avidin-biotin-peroxidase complex (ABC) in immunoperoxidase techniques: A comparison between ABC and unlabeled antibody (PA) procedures. *J Histochem Cytochem* 29:577–580,1981.

UPDATE

Acute Renal Failure. Part II. *(continued from page 30)*

- Correct persistent dehydration (see original text)
- Provide for insensible losses (13 to 20 ml/kg/day)
- Replace urinary and gastrointestinal losses.

Some clinicians factor in a 3% to 5% estimate for subclinical dehydration in renal failure patients, regardless of physical examination findings. Urine volume is quantitated in 6 to 8 hour intervals and replaced during an equivalent period, in addition to other calculated amounts. Overhydration of oliguric patients and further dehydration of polyuric patients should be avoided.

Fluid composition during long-term maintenance therapy should be tailored to the individual patient. After the initial rehydration with normal saline, other polyionic fluids designed to provide buffering capacity and electrolyte replacement (e.g., lactated Ringer's solution, Normosol-R, Plasma-Lyte) are often used in the first few days of treatment, particularly when ongoing gastrointestinal losses are great. For longer term therapy, lower-sodium solutions designed to meet maintenance fluid needs (e.g., half-strength lactated Ringer's solution or 0.45% saline in 2.5% dextrose, Normosol-M, or Plasma-Lyte 56 and 5% dextrose injection) may be more appropriate, particularly when ongoing losses consist primarily of free water losses in polyuria.[1] Alternating administration of 5% dextrose solutions with high-sodium replacement solutions may also be effective in preventing hypernatremia in patients requiring long-term fluid therapy. Other acute renal failure patients continue to require balanced isotonic solutions. Potassium supplementation is usually required in excess of amounts supplied in commercial fluids (see Table I, original text), and serial monitoring of serum electrolytes is recommended as the best way to determine maintenance fluid composition.

Recovering renal tissue may require several weeks of fluid support. The best indicators of recovery include reduced blood urea nitrogen, serum creatinine, and serum phosphorous concentrations accompanied by lessened clinical signs of uremia. Biochemical parameters often do not return to normal, but may stabilize at an acceptable level of azotemia. As these positive indicators are observed and oral intake of food and fluid increases, tapering of fluid therapy can begin. Fluid volumes usually can be reduced by 25% to 50% daily for several days. During this process, monitor the patient carefully. If progressive dehydration or azotemia occurs, attempt to taper the fluid volume more slowly.

ADDITIONAL REFERENCE

1. Chew DJ: Fluid therapy during intrinsic renal failure, in DiBartola SF (ed): *Fluid Therapy in Small Animal Practice.* Philadelphia, WB Saunders, 1992, pp 554–572.

Clinical Experience with Peritoneal Dialysis in Small Animals

KEY FACTS

- Peritoneal dialysis is a means of maintaining metabolic balance in small animals with reversible renal failure.
- Peritonitis is a common problem in small animals undergoing peritoneal dialysis.
- Omentectomy and placement of a column-disk catheter provide reliable access for peritoneal dialysis.
- Alleviating uremia by means of aggressive dialysis is a significant factor in improving the patient's nutritional status.

Colorado State University
Leslie J. Carter, MS   Wayne E. Wingfield, MS, DVM

Mark Morris Associates
Topeka, Kansas
Timothy A. Allen, DVM

A SIGNIFICANT NUMBER of animals with reversible renal failure succumb to metabolic imbalance before kidney regeneration can occur. Dialysis is a way of maintaining metabolic balance until renal function returns. Peritoneal dialysis is an established treatment for renal failure in humans; the use of peritoneal dialysis in animals is increasing as dialysis procedures are refined. Peritoneal dialysis is more adaptable for use in animals than is hemodialysis; hemodialysis requires expensive equipment, highly trained technicians, and surgical vascular intervention.

The purpose of this article is to discuss some of the special problems and complications of peritoneal dialysis in small animals. Although successful peritoneal dialysis in animals has been demonstrated,[1] potential problems include the dialysate bag volume, hydration assessment, peritoneal catheters, peritonitis, pleural effusion, and nutritional support. If the clinician is aware of these potential complications, the use of peritoneal dialysis to treat reversible renal failure can be successful.

DEFINITION

Dialysis is the movement of solutes and water from one solution to another across a semipermeable membrane. Peritoneal dialysis is a process in which dialysate (a dialysis solution) is cycled through the peritoneal cavity by an implanted catheter. Dialysate contains physiologic concentrations of electrolytes and varying concentrations of dextrose. The dialysate within the peritoneal cavity is surrounded by the highly vascular peritoneal membrane, which serves as a semipermeable dialyzing membrane between the blood and the dialysate. Because of concentration gradients between these two solutions, the molecules of low molecular weight, toxins, and fluid move across the membrane. With each dialysis exchange cycle, toxins and excess water are removed from the body, other ions equilibrate at physiologic concentrations, and metabolic imbalances are minimized.

Continuous ambulatory peritoneal dialysis (CAPD), the dialysis method most commonly utilized in animals, uses a system in which dialysate in a collapsible bag is infused into the peritoneal cavity through tubing connected to a surgically placed peritoneal catheter. After remaining in the abdomen for a prescribed period (dwell time), the dialysate is drained back into the bag. The used bag is aseptically replaced with a new bag of dialysate. This procedure is repeated as often as necessary to control uremia.[2] Basic peritoneal dialysis procedures in dogs and cats have been described in the literature.[2]

Originally published in Volume 11, Number 11, November 1989

DIALYSATE VOLUME

Peritoneal dialysate is available in 250- and 500-ml as well as one-, two-, and three-liter plastic containers. For small animals, the recommended dialysate infusion volume is 30 ml/kg. Because the infusion volume for an average adult human is approximately two liters, bags smaller than two liters of dialysate can be difficult to obtain. With continuous ambulatory peritoneal dialysis, the dialysate bag remains connected to the tubing after infusion. The same bag is used to drain the effluent dialysate. For a small animal, such as a cat, only a small portion of a two-liter bag is infused; after the effluent is drained, the majority of dialysate is discarded. Attempts to minimize dialysate waste by transferring small quantities to other containers may lead to peritonitis.

RECENTLY, a dialysis method for infants has been described. In this method, a single large bag of dialysate is used for multiple, small-volume exchanges.[3] To achieve accurate volumes of dialysate for each infusion, the dialysate bag is weighed on a bedside scale. This method also is well suited for use in small animals. First, a two-liter bag of dialysate is connected to the transfer tubing and is placed on a balance scale (Figure 1). The scale is positioned at a level adjacent to and slightly above the patient. The weight of the full bag is recorded, and the weight of the infusion volume is calculated (30 ml × body weight [(kg)]/1000 ml) and then subtracted from the weight of the two-liter bag. The scale is then set to this weight. Next, the roller clamp on the transfer tubing is opened to start dialysate infusion. When the scale balances, delivery of the dialysate is completed and infusion is stopped by closing the roller clamp. After an appropriate dwell time, the peritoneal effluent is drained back into the same bag and mixed with the dialysate. The process is repeated without changing the dialysate bag. Effective dialysis can occur when used dialysate is mixed with fresh dialysate until the concentration of uremic toxins in the dialysate balances with that of the blood.

The frequency of reuse for a single bag varies with infusion volume, bag size, and dwell time. Using 250-ml infusion volumes at one exchange per hour, we have dialyzed an 8-kg dog for four hours with a single two-liter bag of dialysate. Ultrafiltrate, which is excess body water osmotically pulled into the dialysate, is measured as the extra fluid volume in the bag when it is disconnected. This technique significantly reduces the number of bag exchanges and amount of wasted dialysate. The risk of peritonitis also is greatly reduced because the dialysis system is opened less frequently. Other advantages of this single-bag technique include increased ultrafiltrate removal and less loss of protein in dialysate effluent.[3]

HYDRATION ASSESSMENT

Because anuric or oliguric animals cannot regulate fluid balance, it is important to manage hydration. Although

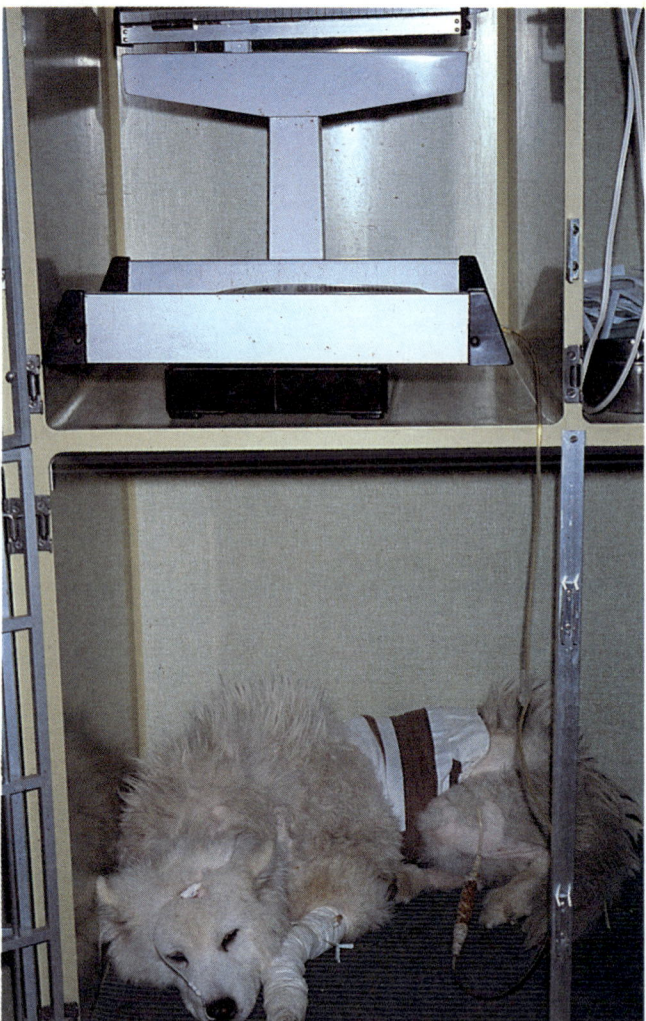

Figure 1—A method for delivering accurate dialysate volumes using a single, large bag of dialysate.

overhydration may lead to pulmonary edema or heart failure, underhydration could compromise perfusion to regenerating kidneys. Central venous pressure and changes in body weight are the most objective parameters for monitoring hydration of patients receiving peritoneal dialysis. Because central venous pressures within the normal range of 3 to 5 cm H_2O indicate optimal hydration, fluids should be adjusted according to deviations from these values. Long-term maintenance of central venous catheters is often difficult because of the risk of thrombosis and phlebitis, catheter rotation requirements, and accidental removal.

In the absence of a central catheter, important factors of hydration assessment include skin turgor, mucous membrane moisture, chemosis, and enophthalmos. These parameters, however, may be altered for reasons unrelated to hydration. Skin turgor can be altered with loss of subcutaneous fat, mucous membranes may be dry because of panting, chemosis may occur secondary to allergens, and patients with muscle atrophy may appear enophthalmic.

Packed cell volume and total serum protein concentration also are frequently used to assess hydration in a normal patient. Packed cell volume may not be a reliable indicator of hydration in patients with renal failure because anemia often develops subsequent to uremia. Total serum protein concentration may be low because of cachexia and protein loss in the urine and/or the dialysate. Frequent and careful monitoring of changes in body weight therefore appears to be the best method for assessing fluid balance in veterinary dialysis patients.

IN ADDITION TO altering oral and/or intravenous fluid administration, hydration can be adjusted by varying the concentration of dextrose in the dialysate. Dialysate is available in dextrose concentrations of 1.5%, 2.5%, and 4.25%. The most hypertonic dialysate (4.25% dextrose, 485 mOsm/L) is used for severely overhydrated patients to remove excess fluid from the body; 2.5% dextrose dialysate (396 mOsm/L) is used for mildly overhydrated patients. The mildly hypertonic 1.5% dextrose dialysate (346 mOsm/L) is used with supplemental intravenous fluids, if required, for normoeuvolemic patients. Frequent monitoring and adjustments are necessary to balance the animal's rapidly changing hydration status.

PERITONEAL CATHETERS

Peritoneal catheters are available in straight, curled, and column-disk types. The fenestrated straight and curled catheters float free in the abdominal cavity and are prone to occlusion with omentum, intestine,[1] or fibrin plugs. Occlusion also may be aggravated in dogs and cats because of their natural posture. Outflow obstruction, which precludes effective dialysis, can result in accumulation of uremic toxins. Therefore, catheter replacement is required if the obstruction cannot be relieved by sterile flushing. Prophylactic heparinization of dialysate (250 to 1000 IU/L) is recommended for the first few days of dialysis to prevent occlusion caused by fibrin clot formation secondary to catheter insertion trauma.

The column-disk catheter is surgically secured against the ventral peritoneal wall and is designed to alleviate outflow occlusion. This catheter appears to be the best for veterinary patients,[1] although omental wrapping frequently occurs unless omentectomy is performed (Figure 2). Omentectomy at the time of surgical catheter placement has been performed to reduce the incidence of catheter obstruction.[4] We routinely perform omentectomy at the time of peritoneal catheter placement. This procedure is accomplished by pulling as much omentum as possible through the incision made for the peritoneal catheter and then ligating the omentum and excising it (Figure 3). The omental stub is allowed to retract into the peritoneal cavity, and the peritoneal catheter is then placed. This procedure is performed to eliminate catheter occlusion caused by omental wrapping.

Dialysate leakage from the peritoneal cavity at the catheter insertion site or through herniations in the abdominal wall is another complication associated with catheters. This leakage is evidenced by swelling of subcutaneous tissue or prepuce or by pericatheter drainage (Figure 4). Ideally, the surgical site should be permitted to heal for several days before use, allowing time for the growth of fibrin into the catheter's Dacron™ cuffs and for subsequent formation of a seal at the incision site and subcutaneous tunnel. Immediate initiation of dialysis, however, is usually necessary to alleviate a uremic crisis. Decreasing the exchange volume and rate may help to reduce leakage. If subcutaneous fluid accumulation and dialysate leakage are severe, effective dialysis cannot be accomplished. If leakage is not alleviated by adjusting the dialysate regimen, surgical correction is needed.

PERITONITIS

Peritonitis is a major complication of peritoneal dialysis. In humans maintained on continuous ambulatory peritoneal dialysis, reports of peritonitis range from 0.4 to 5.2 episodes per patient year of dialysis.[5,6] Peritonitis is the most frequent reason human patients withdraw from continuous ambulatory peritoneal dialysis and transfer to other forms of dialysis.[5]

Peritonitis is diagnosed by any two of the following criteria: (1) cloudy or bloody dialysate effluent with inflammatory cells (more than 200 cells/μl, primarily neutrophils), (2) detection of organisms in a Gram-stained or cultured effluent, and (3) clinical signs of peritonitis.[7] In patients with peritonitis, an increased number of white blood cells causes the dialysate to appear cloudy. Dialysate effluent may also appear turbid and/or bloody in the absence of peritonitis because of cellular debris and fibrin secondary to trauma associated with catheter placement. This sign usually disappears within the first few days of dialysis.

In humans, gram-positive organisms originating from the skin or upper airway flora account for approximately 70% of peritoneal infections.[5] Another 25% of infections is caused by gram-negative skin or bowel contaminants[5]; fungal infections are responsible for approximately another 5%.[5] Clinical signs of peritonitis in humans and animals include anorexia, depression, fever, diarrhea, vomiting, and abdominal tenderness. Cloudy dialysate with a negative bacterial culture and a negative cytologic evaluation suggests a sterile peritonitis caused by chemical or mechanical irritation of the peritoneum. Eosinophilia in the dialysate effluent may also accompany noninfectious peritonitis.[8]

THE PRIMARY CAUSE of peritonitis in patients undergoing peritoneal dialysis is contamination of the tubing spike during bag exchanges.[5] Peritonitis is occasionally caused by bowel perforation or infection of the subcutaneous tunnel in which the catheter tubing is inserted.[5] Although peritonitis can be life threatening, this condition is usually responsive to antimicrobial therapy. Peritonitis secondary to bowel perforation or to subcutaneous tunnel or fungal infection carries a more guarded prognosis.[5] At

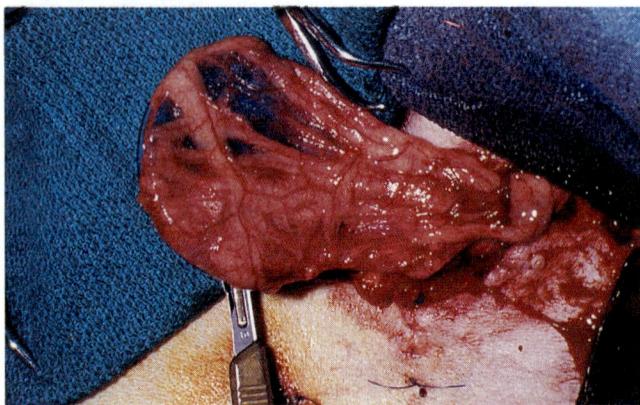

Figure 2—A column-disk catheter encapsulated within the omentum of a dog.

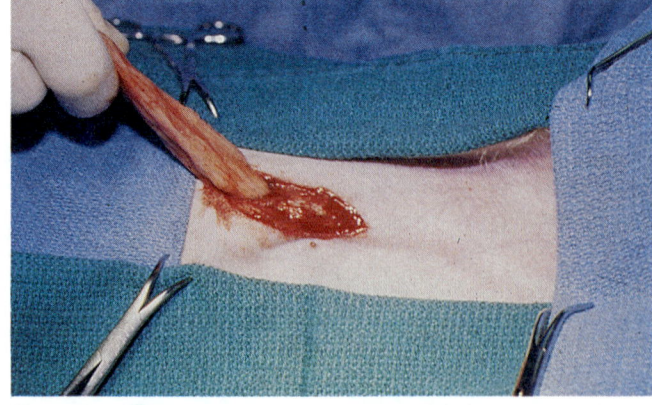

Figure 3—Canine omentum being pulled through a catheter incision for excision.

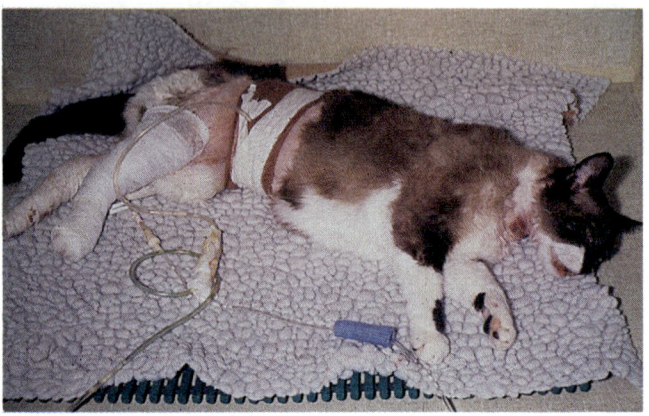

Figure 4—Subcutaneous accumulation of dialysate in a cat with pericatheter leakage.

the first sign of cloudy dialysate effluent, a microbial culture should be obtained and a cytologic evaluation performed. If the white blood cell count in the effluent is greater than 200 cells/μl, a broad-spectrum antibiotic, such as a cephalosporin, should be administered systemically or added to the dialysate (i.e., cephalothin at 250 mg per two-liter bag) until the infective organism is identified.[7] Antimicrobial therapy should be adjusted according to the antimicrobic susceptibility results. To minimize fibrin formation and adhesions, heparin should be added to dialysate (250 to 1000 IU/L) during episodes of peritonitis.[7]

If appropriate systemic antibiotics are used, intraperitoneal antibiotics are not necessary.[9] Antibiotic doses are easier to regulate through systemic administration, especially when using the single-bag, multiple-exchange technique. One study showed that cephalosporins were not bactericidal in peritoneal dialysis solutions.[6] Although aminoglycosides have been recommended for treatment of peritonitis caused by gram-negative organisms,[7] the nephrotoxicity of these antibiotics demonstrates that they should be used with caution. Suggested antimicrobial agents and doses recommended for addition to dialysate are given in Table I.[7]

A prophylactic saline wash followed by saline–iodine wash of the peritoneal cavity has been recommended for preventing peritonitis after contamination of the dialysis system.[7] Isotonic saline is instilled after a dialysate exchange of the same volume is made, and then the solution is immediately drained from the peritoneal cavity. This saline rinse removes any dialysate residue before the iodine solution is instilled. This procedure is necessary because dextrose in the dialysate converts iodine to iodide, thus making the solution inactive. Next, isotonic saline with 0.2 ml of 2% iodine per liter is infused and allowed to remain for four minutes. This solution is then drained, and regular dialysis exchanges are resumed. This procedure is performed once a day for five days. If peritonitis develops, the concentration of iodine may be doubled and the flush frequency increased to twice a day. If the peritonitis is not controlled within 24 hours, the dialysate is cultured and treatment with cephalothin and heparin is initiated.[7]

Some researchers have reported increased morbidity and mortality in dogs with experimentally induced peritonitis lavaged with povidone-iodine–saline solution compared with dogs lavaged with saline alone.[10] The quantity of iodine used in that study, however, was much greater than the 0.2 ml of 2% iodine recommended in the saline–iodine flush.

PREVENTION IS the best treatment for peritonitis. Strict aseptic technique, including the wearing of a surgical mask and gloves, should be used during bag exchanges. Exchanges also should be performed in a low-traffic area. All connections in the system should be wrapped with povidone-iodine–soaked gauze and then a sterile gauze wrap. Medicine ports on the dialysate bag should be prepared before use, and an aseptic injection technique should be followed. If disconnection occurs, all tubing ends that are contaminated should be soaked in 10% povidone-iodine solution for five minutes and reconnected using sterile technique. A saline flush followed by saline–iodine flush, prophylactic antibiotic therapy with a cephalosporin, or both should be instituted. The patient and the surrounding environment should be kept as clean as possible.

TABLE I
Antimicrobial Agents for Use in Dialysate

Antibiotic	Dose (per liter of dialysate)
Cephalothin	125 mg
Ampicillin	50 mg
Sulfadiazine and trimethoprim	25 mg and 5 mg
Clindamycin	50 mg
Tobramycin[a]	5 mg
Ticarcillin	100 mg
Vancomycin hydrochloride[a]	30 mg
Cloxacillin sodium	100 mg
Amikacin sulfate	50 mg
Gentamicin[a]	5 mg
Amphotericin B (for fungal peritonitis)	5 mg
Penicillin G[a]	50,000 IU/L

[a]Not to be mixed with heparin.

PLEURAL EFFUSION

An unexpected complication occurred when a dog became severely dyspneic and had a diminishing return of dialysate two days after beginning peritoneal dialysis. Chest radiographs demonstrated severe bilateral pleural effusion without an apparent diaphragmatic defect (Figure 5). Two liters of a straw-colored fluid was removed by thoracentesis. To determine whether the effusion originated from the peritoneal cavity, methylene blue was infused with the peritoneal dialysate and allowed to dwell. No dye was observed in the fluid obtained by thoracentesis one hour later. Radiographic contrast material was introduced into the peritoneal cavity in an attempt to demonstrate a pleuroperitoneal communication. The contrast material did not appear in the thorax. Dextrose concentration of the pleural fluid was 350 mg/dl; the serum dextrose concentration was 112 mg/dl. Although there was no demonstrable communication between the pleural and peritoneal cavities, it is believed that the pleural fluid contained dialysate because of a high dextrose content and because there was a temporal relationship between the initiation of dialysis, the decreased dialysate return, and the development of pleural effusion.

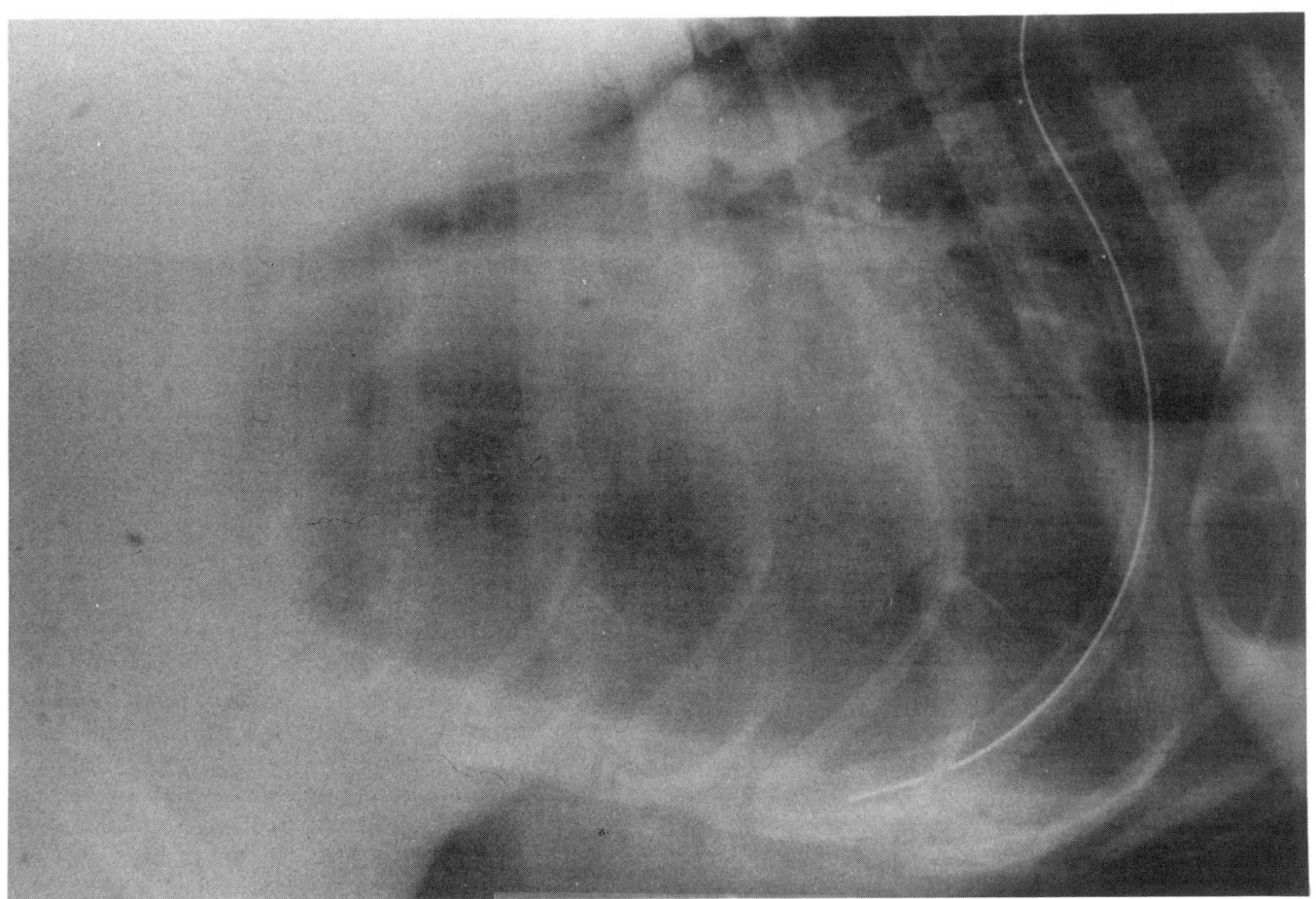

Figure 5—A radiograph of pleural effusion in a young adult, mixed-breed, neutered male dog undergoing peritoneal dialysis. The chest drain is visible.

SEVERAL REPORTS describe acute, massive, right-sided hydrothorax as a rare complication of continuous ambulatory peritoneal dialysis in humans.[11-17] The condition was characterized by dyspnea, chest pain, and a decreasing dialysate return within 4 to 48 hours after initiation of peritoneal dialysis. When peritoneal dialysis was discontinued, the hydrothorax resolved. Attempts to demonstrate a pleuroperitoneal connection by infusing methylene blue, radiopaque medium, or aggregated isotopes with dialysate and subsequently inspecting the pleural fluid for these agents were not always successful. Occasionally, gross anatomic defects in the diaphragm were observed during surgery or at autopsy.[12] The diaphragm may rupture when abdominal pressure is created by repeated distention of the peritoneal cavity with large volumes of dialysate and ultrafiltrate.[11,12,16] Pleuroperitoneal connections may also exist around major vessels and the esophagus.[13] Increased intraabdominal pressure and negative intrathoracic pressure may produce a large pressure gradient, thus driving fluid into the pleural cavity.[13] Increased intraabdominal pressure may also contribute to pleural effusion by intensifying pulmonary artery pressure.[11]

If no anatomic defects are apparent, transfer of fluid from the peritoneal to the pleural cavity most likely occurs through subdiaphragmatic lymphatics.[11,14] Hydrothorax that is secondary to continuous ambulatory peritoneal dialysis in humans is almost exclusively right sided; the supply of lymphatics is richer in the right side of the diaphragm than in the left side.[11,14] Because the canine mediastinum is less complete than that of humans, it may account for the bilateral effusion in dogs. Hypoventilation caused by an increase in abdominal fluid also may decrease the lymphatic removal of pleural fluid.[11]

Thoracentesis has been indicated to relieve hydrothorax and may be performed intermittently or continuously with an indwelling chest tube.[13,15] Pleurodesis with talc insufflation has been successfully used to seal the pleural cavity in humans with hydrothorax caused by peritoneal dialysis.[17] Pleural dialysis has been successfully performed as an alternative to peritoneal dialysis in dogs.[18]

In humans, massive hydrothorax has been resolved by decreasing dialysate volume and dwell time and/or by performing dialysis with the patient in a semisitting, upright position.[15,16] Posture compliance is difficult to achieve in animals. Adjustments can be made in dialysate volume and dwell time, but dialysis efficiency may be compromised.

NUTRITION

One of the most discouraging problems associated with peritoneal dialysis in animals is the inability to provide adequate nutritional support. Adequate protein intake is necessary for body maintenance, metabolism, and repair, especially for the regenerating renal tubular epithelium. Although practitioners can successfully dialyze dogs with renal failure, many patients die of malnutrition.[1,19] Because the uremic patient is usually plagued with refractory anorexia, nausea, and vomiting, malnutrition can become critical if renal failure is prolonged. As caloric deficit increases with inadequate nutrition, catabolism of endogenous proteins accelerates, thus aggravating uremia and further increasing nausea. Accumulation of gastrin normally eliminated by the kidney can lead to gastrointestinal ulcers. Uremic gastritis also contributes to anorexia, nausea, and vomiting. Necrotic lesions of the tongue can occur, thus making prehension and mastication of food painful. Hypertonic dialysis fluid reduces appetite.[20] The continual pressure and mechanical irritation of dialysate infusion and drainage also can aggravate an anorectic condition.

ANOTHER PROBLEM is the continual loss of protein through the dialysate. Loss of protein in children receiving peritoneal dialysis has been estimated to be between 0.19 and 0.28 g/kg/day.[21] During episodes of peritonitis, protein loss is increased.

Dextrose in dialysate may be a source of energy. In one study, glucose uptake in children was demonstrated to range from 1.9 to 2.2 g/kg/day (3.75 kcal/g).[22] Another study demonstrated that 800 to 3000 kcal/day also may be supplied this way.[23] Amino acids, rather than dextrose, have been proposed as osmotic agents in dialysate.[24] This method could be a way of providing amino acids as well as minimizing protein loss. The human peritoneum has been successfully used as a route for total parenteral nutrition.[25]

Intravenous hyperalimentation, which is used widely in humans, has many drawbacks in veterinary medicine, such as maintenance of central catheters, expense, and limited availability. As more insight is gained into the problems of animals, this procedure should become an important method of nutritional maintenance. Currently, such intravenous supplements as amino acid and lipid infusions, which are reported to be beneficial in humans, may also be used in animals.[25,26] Enteral nutrition by orogastric or nasogastric tube feeding, pharyngostomy, or gastrostomy is an option but is contraindicated if the animal is continuously vomiting. Jejunostomy at the time of peritoneal catheter placement requires a large abdominal incision and can increase the potential for dehiscence and dialysate leakage.

PHARMACOLOGIC AGENTS used to control vomiting include cimetidine (Tagamet®—Smith, Kline & French) to reduce uremic gastroenteritis[27] and phenothiazine derivatives. In our experience, however, these agents are rarely effective in controlling vomiting in severely uremic patients. We use cimetidine and phenothiazine derivatives when effective and nasogastric or intermittent orogastric tube feeding when tolerated. In general, we have found that alleviating uremia with aggressive dialysis seems to be the key factor in decreasing vomiting and thus improving the appetite and general nutritional status of the patient.

About the Authors

Ms. Carter and Dr. Wingfield, who is a Diplomate of the American College of Veterinary Emergency and Critical Care, are affiliated with the Department of Clinical Sciences, College of Veterinary Medicine and Biomedical Sciences, Colorado State University, Fort Collins, Colorado. Dr. Allen, who is a Diplomate of the American College of Veterinary Internal Medicine, is affiliated with Mark Morris Associates, Topeka, Kansas.

REFERENCES

1. Thornhill JA, Hartman J, Boon GD, et al: Support of an anephric dog for 54 days with ambulatory peritoneal dialysis and a newly designed peritoneal catheter. *Am J Vet Res* 45(6):1156–1161, 1984.
2. Thornhill JA: Peritoneal dialysis in the dog and cat: An update. *Compend Contin Educ Pract Vet* 3(1):20–34, 1981.
3. Warady BA, Stall C, Paulsen J, et al: A unique approach to peritoneal dialysis in infants. *Am J Kidney Dis* 7:235–240, 1986.
4. Salusky IB, Kopple JD, Fine RN: Continuous ambulatory peritoneal dialysis in pediatric patients: A 20-month experience. *Kidney Int* 24:101–105, 1983.
5. Levey AS, Harrington JT: Continuous peritoneal dialysis for chronic renal failure. *Medicine* 61(5):330–339, 1982.
6. Appleby DH, John J: Effect of peritoneal dialysis solution on the antimicrobial activity of cephalosporins. *Nephron* 30:341–344, 1982.
7. Thornhill JA, Riviere JE: Peritonitis associated with peritoneal dialysis: Diagnosis and treatment. *JAVMA* 182:721–724, 1983.
8. Humayun HM, Ing TS, Daugirdas JT, et al: Peritoneal fluid eosinophilia in patients undergoing maintenance peritoneal dialysis. *Arch Intern Med* 141:1172–1173, 1981.
9. Root ER, Kanarek KS: Management of renal failure: Emphasis on peritoneal dialysis in the neonate. *J Fla Med Assoc* 70:814–820, 1983.
10. Lores ME, Ortiz JR, Rosello PJ: Peritoneal lavage with povidone-iodine solution in experimentally induced peritonitis. *Surg Gynecol Obstet* 153:33–38, 1981.
11. Rudnick MR, Coyle JF, Beck LH, McCurdy DK: Acute massive hydrothorax complicating peritoneal dialysis, report of 2 cases and a review of the literature. *Clin Nephrol* 12(1):38–44, 1979.
12. Grefberg N, Danielson BG, Benson L, Pitkanen P: Right-sided hydrothorax complicating peritoneal dialysis. *Nephron* 34:130–134, 1983.
13. Seebaran AR, Patel PL: Acute massive hydrothorax—A rare complication of peritoneal dialysis. *S Afr Med J* 60:827–828, 1981.
14. Singh S, Vaidya P, Dale A, Morgan B: Massive hydrothorax complicating continuous ambulatory peritoneal dialysis. *Nephron* 34:168–172, 1983.
15. Milutinovic J, Wu W, Lindholm DD, Lapp NL: Acute massive unilateral hydrothorax: A rare complication of chronic peritoneal dialysis. *South Med J* 73:827–828, 1980.
16. Townsend R, Fragola JA: Hydrothorax in a patient receiving continuous ambulatory peritoneal dialysis. *Arch Intern Med* 142:1571–1572, 1982.
17. Scheldewaert R, Bogaerts Y, Panwels R, et al: Management of a massive hydrothorax in a CAPD patient: A case report and a review of the literature. *Peritoneal Dial Bull* 2:69–72, 1982.
18. Shahar R, Holmberg DL: Pleural dialysis in the management of acute renal failure in two dogs. *JAVMA* 187:952–954, 1985.
19. Rubin J, Jones Q, Quillen E, Bower JD: A model of long-term peritoneal dialysis in the dog. *Nephron* 35:259–263, 1983.
20. Young GA, Hobson SM, Young SM, et al: Adverse effects of hypertonic dialysis fluid during CAPD. *Lancet* 2:1421, 1983.
21. Broyer M, Niaudet P, Champion G, et al: Nutritional and metabolic studies in children on continuous ambulatory peritoneal dialysis. *Kidney Int* 24:106–110, 1983.
22. Salusky IB, Fine RN, Nelson P, et al: Nutritional status of children undergoing continuous ambulatory peritoneal dialysis. *Am J Clin Nutr* 38:599–611, 1983.
23. DeSanto NG, Capodicasa G, Senatore R, et al: Glucose utilization from dialysate in patients on continuous ambulatory peritoneal dialysis (CAPD). *Int J Artif Organs* 2(3):119–124, 1979.
24. Oreopoulos DG, Katirtzoglou A: Continuous ambulatory peritoneal dialysis (CAPD): A life sustaining treatment without artificial organs. *Int J Artif Organs* 2(6):268–269, 1979.
25. Giordano C, Capodicasa G, DeSanto NG: Artificial gut for total parenteral nutrition through the peritoneal cavity. *Int J Artif Organs* 3(6):326–330, 1980.
26. Abel RM, Beck CH, Abbott WM, et al: Improved survival from acute renal failure after treatment with intravenous essential L-amino acids and glucose. *N Engl J Med* 288:695–699, 1973.
27. Thornhill JA: Control of vomiting in the uremic patient, in Kirk RW (ed): *Current Veterinary Therapy. VIII.* Philadelphia, WB Saunders Co, 1983, pp 1022–1024.

UPDATE

Since publication of our original article, we have gained experience using a modified dialysate delivery system and exchange procedure sequence. In the standard CAPD connection system, a single length of transfer tubing connects to the surgically implanted dialysis catheter tubing at one end and is spiked to the dialysate bag at the other end. The system remains connected and closed except for a brief time during bag exchanges and the patient 'wears' the collapsed or partially collapsed bag and tubing between exchanges. Alternatively, the Y-set disconnect system uses a Y-shaped transfer tubing connecting to the dialysis catheter at one end and to the dialysate bag and a drainage bag on either end segment of the Y. The Y-set may be disconnected from the patient after each exchange, and depending on manufacturer and protocol, the transfer tubing infused with disinfectant and disconnected ends capped with disinfectant filled caps.

During an exchange, the Y-set is connected to the catheter tubing and a *flush/drain/fill* procedure performed utilizing roller clamps on each segment. A small volume of dialysate is *flushed* from the dialysate bag to the drainage bag. Next the dwell volume is *drained* from the peritoneal cavity into the drainage bag. Then fresh dialysate is *filled* into the peritoneal cavity.[1] This sequence allows any contaminants potentially introduced during connection to be flushed into the drainage bag before dialysate is introduced to the peritoneal cavity. Even with routine disconnection, this system, along with a modified exchange procedure sequence, has significantly reduced the rate of peritonitis in humans maintained on peritoneal dialysis.[2–10] Additionally, since small volumes of fresh dialysate are easily delivered and the patient is freed from 'wearing' the dialysate bag and system between exchanges, complications of dialysate waste and cumbersomeness associated with bag size become inconsequential.

We dialyzed an 11 kilogram, 10-year-old, spayed female, mixed breed dog in acute renal failure secondary to complications of transitional cell carcinoma and related surgery for approximately five months using this system (Delmed Freedom Set, Delmed Inc., Concord, CA 94520). Two days after ureteral transposition and bladder tumor resection, the dog became anuric and BUN and serum creatinine rose to 112 and 7.5 mg/dl, respectively. A column-disk dialysis catheter was surgically placed and peritoneal dialysis begun using 250 ml infusion volumes and one to two hour dwell times. Accurate delivery of dialysate was accomplished by using a cage-side scale to deliver the calculated weight of the infusion volume. A standard, straight connection system was utilized. The day after dialysis was initiated, BUN dropped to 86 mg/dl and serum creatinine to 6.7 mg/dl. Seven days after initiation of dialysis the dog was switched to a Y-set disconnect system and infusion volume was increased to 500 ml. The owner was trained to perform the dialysis exchanges and the dog was sent home to receive eight exchanges per day (three hour dwell times). Within six days the exchanges were further decreased to four per day (six hour dwell times). BUN at that time was 42 mg/dl and serum creatinine 3.5 mg/dl. The dog produced only scant amounts of urine for several weeks postoperatively. The dog underwent chemotherapy for transitional cell carcinoma and was maintained on 3 to 4 dialysis exchanges per day. One episode of antibiotic sensitive subclinical peritonitis occurred when the dog chewed through its transfer tubing. Approximately four and one half months from dialysis initiation, the dog's renal function stabilized and she was weaned off dialysis. The dialysis catheter was infused with a heparin solution and left in place. The dog did well for approximately another 5 months when its tumor recurred. The tumor was refractory to chemotherapy and the patient was euthanatized.

In the past, the dialysis regimen in humans has been adjusted empirically, based on the patient's life style, compliance, and clinical symptoms. Many patients are thought to be underdialyzed utilizing standard dialysis prescriptions which fail to account for patient size, residual kidney function, or nutritional status.[11–13] Quantitative assessment of dialysis adequacy based on urea and creatinine kinetics is being used to individualize dialysis prescription parameters. Weekly urea and/or creatinine clearances (peritoneal and residual renal) and Kt/V index are analyzed for acceptable values (K = total urea clearance in ml/minute; t = time on dialysis in minutes; V = the volume of distribution of urea as total body water corrected for body surface area).[14–16] These analyses would appear to have greater application in chronically dialyzed (greater than one week) veterinary patients versus those acutely dialyzed, but more experience is needed to determine their usefulness.

Lastly, amino acids are now commonly being used intermittently with glucose as an osmotic agent in dialysate to ameliorate protein calorie malnutrition associated with peritoneal dialysis due to appetite suppression and increased protein loss in dialysate. Amino acids have approximately twice the osmotic effectiveness of glucose and therefore a solution of 1% amino acids is used in one out of four daily exchanges. Benefits other than improvement of nitrogen balance include decreased hyperglycemia and plasma triglyceride and cholesterol levels as glucose load is decreased.[17–19]

REFERENCES

1. Lane IF, Carter LJ, Lappin MR: Peritoneal dialysis: An update on methods and usefulness, in Kirk RW (ed): *Current Veterinary Therapy XI.* Philadelphia, WB Saunders Co, 1992, pp 865–870.
2. Holley JL, Bernardini J, Piraino B: Infecting organisms in continuous ambulatory dialysis patients on the Y-set. *Am J Kidney Dis* 23(4):569–573, 1994,
3. Viglino G, Colombo A, Cantu P, et al: In vitro and in vivo efficacy of a new connector device for continuous ambulatory peritoneal dialysis. *Perit Dial Inc* 13 Suppl 2:S148–S151, 1993.
4. Port FK, Held PJ, Nolph KD, et al: Risk of peritonitis and technique failure by CAPD connection technique: A national study. *Kidney Int* 42(4):967–974, 1992.
5. Stramignoni E, Maffei S, Bonello F, et al: Peritoneal complications of continuous ambulatory peritoneal dialysis. *Minerva Urol Nefrol* 44(1):57–61, 1992.
6. Burkart JM, Jordan JR, Durnell TA, Case LD: Comparison of exit-site infections in disconnect versus nondisconnect systems for peritoneal dialysis. *Perit Dial Int* 12(3):317–320, 1992.
7. Dryden MS, McCann M, Wing AJ, Phillips I: Controlled trial of a Y-set dialysis delivery system to prevent peritonitis in patients receiving continuous ambulatory peritoneal dialysis. *J Hosp Infect* 20(3):185–192, 1992.
8. Scalamogna A, De-Vecchi A, Castelnovo C, et al: Long-term incidence of peritonitis in CAPD patients treated by the Y-set technique: Experience in a single center. *Nephron* 55(1):24–27, 1990.
9. Piraino B, Bernardini J, Sorkin MT: The effect of the Y-set on catheter infection rates in continuous ambulatory peritoneal dialysis patients. *Am J Kidney Dis* 16(1):46–50, 1990.
10. Fetter MA, Blackley MC: Further experience with the Delmed Freedom Set and the *Flush Drain/Fill* sequencing. *Adv Perit Dial* 6:141–143, 1990.
11. Mooraki A, Kliger AS, Gorhan-Brennan NL, et al: Weekly KT-V urea and selected outcome criteria in 56 randomly selected CAPD patients. *Adv Perit Dial* 9:92–96, 1993.
12. Gotch F, Gentile DE, Schoenfeld PY: CAPD prescription in current clinical practice. *Adv Perit Dial* 9:69–72, 1993.
13. Keshaviah P: Adequacy of CAPD: A quantitative approach. *Kidney Int* Suppl 38:S160–S164, Oct 1992.
14. Arkouche W, Delawari E, My H, et al: Quantification of adequacy of peritoneal dialysis. *Perit Dial Int* 13 Suppl 2:S215–S218, 1993.
15. Selgas A, Baja MA, Fernandez-Reyes MJ, Bosque E, et al: An analysis of adequacy of dialysis in a selected population on CAPD for over 3 years: The influence on urea and creatinine kinetics. *Nephrol Dial Transplant* 8(11):1244–1253, 1993.
16. Acchiardo SR, Kraus AP Jr, Kaufman PA, et al: Evaluation of CAPD prescription. *Adv Perit Dial* 7:47–50, 1991.
17. Bruno M, Bagnis C, Marangella M, et al: CAPD with an amino acid dialysis solution: A long-term, cross-over study. *Kidney Int* 35:1189–1194, 1989.
18. Hanning RM, Balfe JW, Zlotkin SH: Effectiveness and nutritional consequences of amino acid-based vs glucose-based dialysis solutions in infants and children receiving CAPD. *Am J Clin Nut* 46:22–30, 1987.
19. Khanna R, Wu G, Rodella H, Oreopoulos D: Use of amino acid containing solution in CAPD patients. *Perit Dial Bull* 4(3) Jul-Sep Suppl:S121–S124, 1984.

Canine Urolithiasis: Diagnosis, Treatment, and Prevention

University of Minnesota

Carl A. Osborne, DVM, PhD

Jody P. Lulich, DVM, PhD

Joseph W. Bartges, DVM, PhD

Rosama Thumchai, DVM

Lawrence J. Felice, PhD

Lisa K. Unger, CVT

Lori A. Koehler, CVT

Kathleen A. Bird, CVT

Laurie Swanson, CVT

Urolithiasis may affect 1.5% to 3.0% of all dogs admitted for medical care. Recurrence of urolithiasis following the removal or dissolution of a urinary calculus is common. Uroliths always result from one or more underlying inherited, congenital, and/or acquired disorders. Therefore, the detection of uroliths is not the endpoint, but rather is the beginning, of the diagnostic investigation.

This article consists primarily of clinical recommendations for the diagnosis, management, and prevention of canine urolithiasis presented as tables and algorithms. After reading the introductory comments, consult the index of tables for specific information. A reference list has been provided to direct the reader to further information.

BIRTH AND GROWTH OF UROLITHS

Urolith formation may be divided into two complementary but separate phases: initiation and growth. Initiating events are not the same for all types of uroliths. In addition, factors that cause a urolith may be different from those that foster its growth. The initial step in the development of a urolith is the formation of crystal nidus (embryo). This phase of initiation of urolith formation, called *nucleation*, depends on supersaturation of urine with calculogenic crystalloids. The degree of supersaturation may be influenced by the magnitude of renal excretion of the crystalloids, urine pH, crystallization inhibitors, and/or crystallization promoters in urine. Further growth of the crystal nidus depends on its ability to remain in the urinary system, the degree and duration of supersaturation of urine with crystalloids identical to or different from that of the nidus, and the physical characteristics of the crystal nidus.

OVERVIEW OF PATIENT EVALUATION AND DIAGNOSIS

The importance of an appropriate physical examination and history to the evaluation of urolithiasis is emphasized. Information to be gathered from the client should include answers to the following questions:

- What is the dog's diet history?
- Has there been any change in the dog's water consumption or eating habits?
- Have there been prior medical problems?
- Has there been a change in micturition in terms of character, frequency, quantity, pollakiuria, polyuria or polydipsia, oliguria or anuria, or incontinence?
- Has there been any change in the color or odor of the dog's urine?
- Have there been any systemic signs?
- Has any therapy (including diet) been given?
- If so: what, how much, for how long, and what was the response?

The physical examination should include temperature, pulse, respiratory rate, body weight, skin pliability, and/or thorough evaluation of all body systems, with particular attention to the urinary system. Rectal palpation of the urethra should be performed on all dogs, even females.

A complete urinalysis should be performed; a urine sample may be submitted or saved for urine culture. Laboratory analysis (e.g., complete blood cell counts and serum chemistry analyses) should be performed, or samples should be saved for possible future analysis prior to the initiation of therapy. Survey radiographs of the entire urinary tract should be obtained. Intravenous urography should be considered for patients with renal or ureteral uroliths; intravenous urography or contrast and double-contrast urethrocystography should be considered for patients with cystic and/or urethral calculi. Ultrasonography of the entire urinary system can be performed. Uroliths retrieved during voiding—with the aid of a urinary catheter or by voiding urohydropropulsion—should be submitted only to a laboratory that uses quantitative techniques of analysis (see Table 8).

OVERVIEW OF MEDICAL MANAGEMENT OF CANINE UROLITHS

1. Institute appropriate medical therapy (see index of tables). Consider surgical correction if uroliths are obstructing urine outflow and/or if correctable abnormalities predisposing to urolith recurrence are identified (see Table 22). Consider voiding urohydropropulsion for urocystoliths small enough to pass through the urethra (see Table 20).
2. Eradicate or control urinary tract infections.
3. Initiate therapy with a calculolytic diet. Ideally, no other supplements or food should be fed. Combine with appropriate drug therapy, if necessary (see index of tables).
4. Devise a protocol to monitor efficacy of therapy.
   a. Try to avoid diagnostic follow-up studies that require urinary catheterization. If they are required, give appropriate pericatheterization antimicrobial agents to prevent iatrogenic urinary tract infections.
   b. Evaluate serial urinalyses (including urine pH, specific gravity, and microscopic examination of sediment) for crystals and bacteria. Remember that crystals may form in urine that is stored at room temperature or refrigerated, and these may be in vitro artifacts.
   c. Perform serial radiography to detect the location(s), number, size, density, and shape of recurrent uroliths.
5. If uroliths increase in size or do not begin to decrease in size after approximately 4 weeks of appropriate medical management, alternative methods should be considered. Difficulty in inducing complete dissolution of uroliths by creating urine that is undersaturated with the suspected or known calculogenic crystalloids should prompt consideration that the wrong mineral was identified, the urolith is composed of different minerals, or the owner or the patient is not complying with medical recommendations.
6. Once uroliths are dissolved or surgically removed, it is important to devise a long-term management plan.

Index of Tables and Figures

TABLE 1

Mineral Composition of 30,642 Canine Uroliths Evaluated at the Minnesota Urolith Center by Quantitative Methods (1981 to 1994)

Predominant Mineral Type	Proportion of Predominant Mineral (%)	Number of Uroliths	%
Magnesium Ammonium Phosphate 6H$_2$O		16,542	54.0
	100	(9654)	(31.5)
	70–99[a]	(6888)	(22.5)
Magnesium Hydrogen Phosphate 3H$_2$O		2	<0.1
	100	(1)	(<0.1)
	70–99[a]	(1)	(<0.1)
Calcium Oxalates		8557	27.9
Calcium Oxalate Monohydrate	100	(2706)	(8.8)
	70–99[a]	(2560)	(8.4)
Calcium Oxalate Dihydrate	100	(1009)	(3.3)
	70–99[a]	(1194)	(3.9)
Calcium Oxylate Monohydrate & Dihydrate	100	(767)	(2.5)
	70–99[a]	(321)	(1.1)
Calcium Phosphates		237	0.8
Calcium Phosphate	100	(58)	(0.2)
	70–99[a]	(85)	(0.3)
Calcium Hydrogen Phosphate 2H$_2$O	100	(48)	(0.2)
	70–99	(45)	(0.2)
Tricalcium Phosphate	70–99	(1)	(<0.1)
Purines		2130	7.0
Ammonium Acid Urate	100	(1546)	(5.1)
	70–99[a]	(359)	(1.2)
Sodium Acid Urate	100	(112)	(0.4)
	70–99[a]	(20)	(≤0.1)
Sodium Calcium Urate	100	(33)	(0.1)
	70–99[a]	(11)	(<0.1)
Ammonium Calcium Urate	70–99[a]	(1)	(<0.1)
Uric Acid	100	(11)	(<0.1)
	70–99[a]	(7)	(<0.1)
Xanthine	100	(23)	(<0.1)
	70–99[a]	(7)	(<0.1)
Cystine		405	1.3
	100	(389)	(1.3)
	70–99[a]	(16)	(<0.1)
Silica		356	1.2
	100	(232)	(0.8)
	70–99[a]	(124)	(0.4)
Dolomite	100	1	<0.1
Mixed[b]		623	2.0
Compound[c]		1755	5.7
Matrix		32	0.1
Drug Metabolite		2	<0.1
Total		30,642	100%

[a]Urolith composed of 70–99% of mineral type listed; no nucleus and shell detected.
[b]Uroliths did not contain at least 70% of mineral type listed; no nucleus or shell detected.
[c]Uroliths contained an identifiable nucleus and one or more surrounding layers of a different mineral type.

TABLE 2
Mineral Composition of 366 Canine Nephroliths Evaluated by Quantitative Methods

Predominant Mineral Type	*Proportion of Predominant Mineral (%)*	*Number of Uroliths*	*%*
Calcium oxalate		140	38.3
Calcium oxalate • 1H$_2$O	70–100	(116)	(31.7)
Calcium oxalate • 2H$_2$O	70–100	(18)	(4.9)
Calcium oxalate • 1H$_2$O & 2H$_2$O	70–100	(6)	(1.6)
Calcium phosphate		12	3.3
Calcium apatite	70–100	(11)	3.0
Calcium hydrogen phosphate 2H$_2$O	70–100	(1)	0.3
Magnesium ammonium phosphate	70–100	124	33.9
Purines		38	10.4
Ammonium acid urate	70–100	(33)	(9.0)
Sodium acid urate	70–100	(2)	(0.5)
Calcium sodium urate	70–100	(2)	(0.5)
Xanthine	70–100	(1)	(0.3)
Silica	70–100	1	0.3
Mixed		22	6.0
Compound		22	6.0
Matrix		5	1.4
TOTAL		366	100

TABLE 3
Problem-Specific and Therapeutic-Specific Database for Diagnosis and Management of Urolithiasis

1. Obtain appropriate history and perform physical examination, including rectal examination of urethra.
2. Perform complete urinalysis; save aliquot for possible determination of mineral concentration.[a]
3. Obtain quantitative urine culture and determine urine urease activity; test for antimicrobial susceptibility if bacterial pathogens are identified. Consider attempts to isolate ureaplasmas if urease-positive urine is bacteriologically sterile.
4. Perform complete blood cell count.
5. Freeze aliquot of serum collected at time of venipuncture to obtain complete blood cell count for possible determination of urea nitrogen, creatinine, calcium and/or uric acid concentrations.
6. Obtain radiographs.
   a. Take survey radiographs of entire urinary system.
   b. Consider IV urography for patients with renal or ureteral uroliths.
   c. Consider IV urography or contrast cystography for patients with bladder uroliths.
   d. Consider contrast urethrography for patients with urethral uroliths.
   e. Ultrasonography is recommended, if the equipment is available.
7. Determine mineral composition of uroliths.
   a. Quantitatively analyze uroliths passed during micturition or retrieved during diagnostic procedures.
   b. Use results obtained from history, physical examination, laboratory examination, and radiography to determine probable mineral composition of uroliths.
8. Initiate therapy to eradicate UTI, if present.
9. Initiate therapy for urolithiasis.
   a. Initiate therapy to promote dissolution of uroliths that are amenable to medical therapy.
      i. Formulate follow-up protocol to monitor dissolution of uroliths.
      ii. Formulate alternative treatment options if uroliths do not dissolve or if problems such as recurrent outflow obstruction occur.
   b. Remove uroliths by voiding urohydropropulsion.
   c. Use nephrotomy or cystotomy to remove uroliths.
      i. During surgical procedure, remove bladder or kidney biopsy specimens for microscopic examination.
      ii. Correct any anatomic defects that are present.
      iii. Compare the number of uroliths removed during surgery with the number identified by radiography.
      iv. Postsurgical radiographs should be obtained to evaluate the completeness of urolith removal.
      v. Submit uroliths for quantitative analysis.
10. Once uroliths are surgically removed or medically dissolved, initiate therapy to prevent their recurrence.
11. Formulate follow-up protocol with clients.

[a]The patient's diet should be the same as it was when the uroliths formed. Alternatively, one may use a standard diet designed to promote reproducible excretion of minerals in the urine of normal animals.

TABLE 4
Urine pH Values Commonly Associated with Formation of Uroliths in Dogs

Urolith Type	pH
Sterile struvite	>6.5
Infection-induced struvite	>7.0
Calcium phosphate	>7.0
Calcium oxalate	<7.0
Ammonium acid urate	<7.0
Cystine	<7.0
Silica	<7.0

TABLE 5
Common Characteristics of Some Urine Crystals

Type of Crystal	Appearance	pH Range in Which Crystal is Commonly Found [a]		
		Acidic	Neutral	Alkaline
Ammonium urate	Yellow-brown spherulites; thorn apples	+	+	±
Amorphous urates	Amorphous or spheroid yellow-brown structures	+	±	−
Bilirubin	Reddish-brown needles or granules	+	−	−
Calcium carbonate	Large yellow-brown spheroids with radial striations, or small crystals with spheric, ovoid, or dumbbell shapes	−	±	+
Calcium oxalate dihydrate	Small colorless envelopes (octahedral form)	+	+	±
Calcium oxalate monohydrate	Small spindles, "hemp seed," or monohydrate dumbbells	+	+	±
Calcium phosphate	Amorphous, or long, thin prisms	±	+	+
Cholesterol	Flat, colorless plates with corner notch	+	+	−
Cystine	Flat, colorless hexagonal plates	+	+	±
Hippuric acid	Four- to six-sided, colorless, elongated plates or prisms with rounded corners	+	+	±
Leucine	Yellow-brown spheroids with radial and concentric laminations	+	−	−
Ammoniomagnesium phosphate	Three- to six-sided, colorless prisms	±	+	+
Sodium urate	Colorless or yellow-brown needles or slender prisms, sometimes in clusters or sheaves	+	±	−
Sulfa metabolites	Sheaves of needles with central or eccentric binding; occasionally fan-shaped clusters	+	±	−
Tyrosine	Fine colorless or yellow needles arranged in sheaves or rosettes	+	−	−
Uric acid	Diamond or rhombic rosettes, or oval plates, structures with pointed ends; occasionally six-sided plates	+	−	−
Xanthine	Amorphous, spheroid, or ovoid yellow-brown structures	+	±	−

[a]The symbol (+) means the crystals commonly occur at this pH; the symbol (±) means that crystals may occur at this pH, but are more common at another pH; the symbol (−) means that crystals are uncommon at this pH.

TABLE 6
Typical Radiographic Characteristics of Uroliths Commonly Encountered in Dogs

Mineral Type	Degree of Radiopacity	Shape
Cystine	+ to ++	Smooth, usually small, round to oval
Calcium oxalate dihydrate	++++	Often rough, round to oval (occasionally jackstone)
Calcium oxalate monohydrate	+++	Often smooth, round (occasionally jackstone)
Magnesium ammonium phosphate (struvite)	+ to ++++	Smooth, round or faceted, occasionally assuming the shape of renal pelvis, ureter, bladder, or urethra; sometimes laminated
Calcium phosphate	++++	Smooth, round or faceted
Ammonium urate and uric acid	0 to ++	Smooth, but occasionally irregular; round or oval
Silica	++ to ++++	Typically jackstone
Mixed and compound	+ to ++++	Varies with composition. May have detectable nucleus and shell
Maxtrix	0 to +	Usually round, but may be influenced by location

TABLE 7
Radiodense Structures That May Resemble Nephroliths

Mineralized renal parenchyma

Radiodense intestinal ingesta

Radiodense medications in the intestinal tract

Large abdominal thela

Calcified lymph nodes

Osseous metaplasia of transitional epithelium

Cholecystoliths

TABLE 8
Checklist of Factors that Suggest the Probable Mineral Composition of Canine Uroliths

1. Urine pH
   a. Struvite and calcium apatite uroliths - usually alkaline (Tables 4 and 5). Sterile struvite uroliths may be observed with urine pH 6.5 or higher.
   b. Ammonium urate uroliths - acid to neutral.
   c. Cystine uroliths - acid.[a]
   d. Calcium oxalate - often acid to neutral.[a]
   e. Silica - acid to neutral.[a]
2. Identification of crystals in uncontaminated fresh urine sediment, preferably at body temperature.
3. Type of bacteria, if any, isolated from urine.
   a. Urease-producing bacteria, especially staphylococci and less frequently *Proteus* spp., are typically associated with canine struvite uroliths. Ureaplasmas may cause struvite uroliths in dogs.
   b. Urinary tract infections often are absent in patients with calcium oxalate, cystine, ammonium urate, and silica uroliths.
   c. Calcium oxalate, cystine, ammonium urate, and silica uroliths may predispose patients to urinary tract infections; if infections are caused by urease-producing bacteria, struvite may precipitate around metabolic uroliths.
4. Radiographic density and physical characteristics of uroliths (Table 6).
5. Serum chemistry evaluation
   a. Hypercalcemia may be associated with calcium-containing uroliths.
   b. Hyperuricemia may be associated with uric acid or urate uroliths.
   c. Hyperchloremia, hypokalemia, and acidemia may be associated with distal renal tubular acidosis and calcium phosphate or struvite uroliths.
6. Urine chemistry evaluation
   a. Patient should be consuming either a standardized diagnostic diet or the same diet that was consumed when the uroliths formed.
   b. Excessive quantities of one or more minerals contained in the urolith are expected. The concentration of crystallization inhibitors may be decreased.
7. Breed of dog and history of occurrence of uroliths in patient's ancestors or littermates.
8. Quantitative analysis of uroliths fortuitously passed during micturition, collected via catheter technique, or obtained by voiding urohydropropulsion (Table 20).

[a]Concomitant infection with urease-producing microbes may result in the production of alkaline urine.

TABLE 9
Summary of Recommendations for Medical Dissolution and Prevention of Canine Ammonium Urate, Sodium Urate, and Uric Acid Uroliths

1. Perform appropriate diagnostic studies, including complete urinalyses, quantitative urine culture, and diagnostic radiography. Determine precise location, size, and number of uroliths. The size and number of uroliths are not a reliable index of the probable efficacy of therapy.
2. If available, determine mineral composition of uroliths. If unavailable, estimate their composition by evaluating appropriate clinical data (Table 8).
3. Consider surgical correction if uroliths are obstructing urine outflow.
4. Determine baseline pretreatment serum uric acid concentrations and (if possible) fractional excretion of urine uric acid.
5. Initiate therapy with a low-purine calculolytic diet (e.g., Prescription Diet Canine u/d). No other food supplements should be fed to the patient. Compliance with dietary recommendation is suggested by reduction in serum urea nitrogen concentration (usually <10 mg/dl).
6. Initiate therapy with allopurinol at 30 mg/kg per day divided into two equal subdoses (a smaller dose is required in azotemic patients). Xanthine uroliths may form if a diet containing excessive purines is fed or if excessive allopurinol is given.
7. If necessary, administer sodium bicarbonate or potassium citrate orally to eliminate aciduria. Strive for a urine pH of approximately 7.
8. If necessary, eradicate or control urinary tract infections with appropriate antimicrobial agents. Maintain antimicrobial therapy during, and for an appropriate period following, urate urolith dissolution.
9. Devise a protocol to monitor efficacy of therapy:
   a. Try to avoid diagnostic follow-up studies that require urinary catheterization. If they are required, give appropriate pericatheterization antimicrobial agents to prevent iatrogenic urinary tract infection.
   b. Evaluate serial urinalyses. Urine pH, specific gravity, and microscopic examination of sediment for urate crystals are especially important. Remember, crystals formed in urine stored at room or refrigeration temperatures may represent in vitro artifacts.
   c. Serially evaluate the serum uric acid concentrations and (if possible) fractional excretion of urine uric acid.
   d. Evaluate urolith(s) location(s), number, size, density, and shape, at approximately monthly intervals. Intravenous urography may be used for radiolucent uroliths located in the kidneys, ureters, or urinary bladder. Retrograde contrast urethrocystography may be required for radiolucent uroliths located in the bladder and urethra.
   e. If necessary, perform quantitative urine cultures. They are especially important in patients that were infected prior to therapy and in patients that are catheterized during therapy.
10. Continue calculolytic diet, allopurinol, and alkalinizing therapy for approximately 1 month following disappearance of uroliths, as detected by radiography.
11. Prevention: Urate uroliths are highly recurrent. Preventative therapy should be directed at keeping urine concentrations of ammonia and uric acid to a minimum. This may be achieved by feeding a diet low in protein that also promotes an alkaline urine in dogs. The effectiveness of dietary management for the prevention of ammonium urate uroliths in dogs with portosystemic shunts is unknown. The long-term use of allopurinol is discouraged because of the potential for the development of xanthine uroliths.

TABLE 10
Expected Changes Associated with Medical Therapy of Ammonium Urate Uroliths

Factor	Pre-Therapy	During Therapy	Prevention Therapy
Polyuria	±	1+ to 3+	1+ to 3+
Pollakiuria	0 to 4+	↑ then ↓	0
Hematuria	0 to 4+	↓	0
Urine specific gravity	variable	1.004 to 1.015	1.004 to 1.015
Urine pH	<7.0	>7.0	>7.0
Urine inflammation	0 to 4+	↓	0
Urate crystals	0 to 4+	0	variable
Bacteriuria	0 to 4+	0	0
Bacterial culture of urine	0 to 4+	0	0
BUN (mg/dl)	variable	≤15	≤15
Urolith size and number	small to large	↓	0

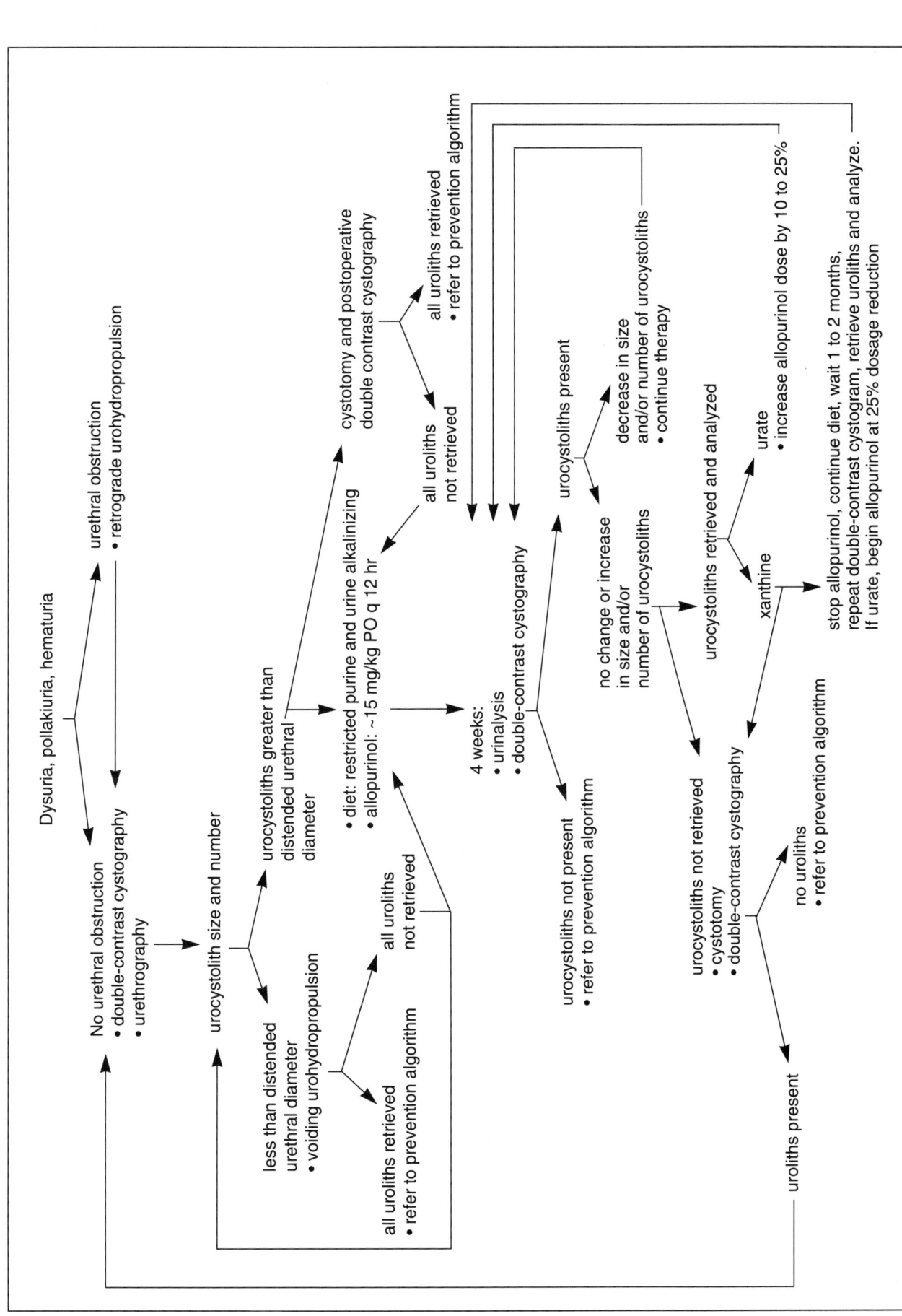

Figure 1—Algorithm for the medical management of canine ammonium urate urocystoliths.

TABLE 11
Risk Factors for Calcium Oxalate Urolithiasis and Recommendations to Minimize Them

Risk Factor	Pathologic Disorder	Therapeutic Management	
		Goal	*Method*
Hypercalciuria	*Intestinal Hyperabsorption:* Idiopathic	Dietary calcium reduction	Provide diet with reduced calcium (e.g., Prescription Diet u/d)
	Hypophosphatemia	Normalize vitamin D production by sustaining a normal serum phosphorous concentration	Provide phosphorous supplementation (e.g., Neutra-Phos-K®, Willen)
	Vitamin D excess	Limit excessive intestinal calcium absorption	Avoid oral vitamin D supplementation
	Renal Leak: Idiopathic	Promote renal calcium reabsorption	Consider thiazide diuretic?
	Renal tubular acidosis	Increase renal tubular reabsorption of bicarbonate to enhance calcium reabsorption	Provide oral alkali therapy (e.g., potassium citrate)
	Dietary protein excess	Increase renal tubular reabsorption of bicarbonate to enhance calcium reabsorption and promote adequate citrate excretion	Provide diet with reduced protein (e.g., Prescription Diet u/d)
	Dietary sodium excess	Minimize renal sodium and calcium excretion	Provide diet with reduced sodium (e.g., Prescription Diet u/d)
	Glucocorticoid excess	Decrease glucocorticoid-enhanced bone resorption and urine calcium excretion	Control hyperadrenocorticism and avoid glucocorticoid supplementation
	Excessive Skeletal Resorption: Primary hyperparathyroidism	Normalize skeletal calcium resorption, serum calcium concentration, and renal calcium filtration	Parathyroidectomy
	Pseudohyperparathyroidism	Control paraneoplastic parathyroid hormone-like activity	Neoplasm erradication or remission
	Osteolytic lesions	Minimize release of excessive skeletal calcium	Correct underlying bone disorder
Hyperoxaluria	Dietary oxalate excess	Avoid foods with high oxalate content	Provide diets low in oxalate (e.g., Prescription Diet u/d)
	Fat malabsorption	Decrease intestinal fat	Provide diet with reduced fat
	Vitamin C excess	Minimize precurser of oxalate	Avoid vitamin C supplementation
	Vitamin B_6 deficiency	Permit convention of glyoxylate (an oxalate precurser) to glycine	Provide adequate vitamin B_6
	Primary hyperoxaluria	Minimize oxalate synthesis	Provide excess vitamin B_6?
Hypocitraturia	Idiopathic	Promote citrate excretion	Provide oral potassium citrate (e.g., Urocit-K, Mission Pharmacal)
	Acidosis	Minimize acidosis	Provide oral alkali therapy (potassium citrate)
Defective macromolecular inhibitors	Inherited disorder?	Restore urinary concentration of effective inhibitors	Unknown

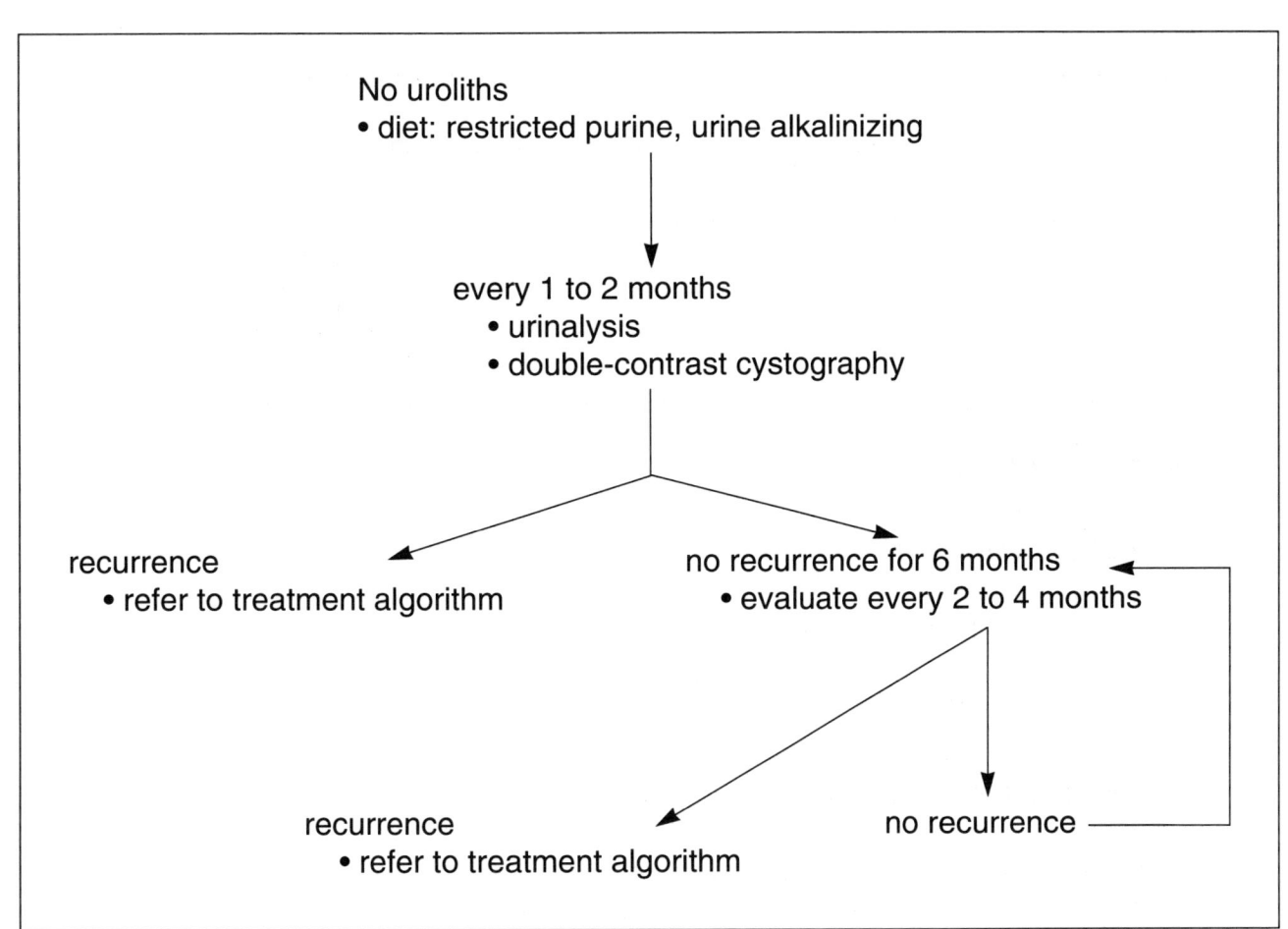

Figure 2—Algorithm for the prevention of canine ammonium urate uroliths.

TABLE 12
Summary of Distinguishing Clinical Manifestations of Different Types of Hypercalciuria

Feature	AH	RH	PHPT
Serum calcium	N	N	↑
Serum PTH	↓/N	↑	↑
Serum phosphorus	N/↑	N	↓/↑**
Urine calcium			
Fasting	N	↑	↑
Dx diet*	↑	↑	↑
Urine oxalate	N	N	N
Urine uric acid	N	N	N
Bone density	N	↓	↓
Calcium balance (total body)	Positive	Negative	Negative

AH = Absorptive hypercalciuria, RH = Renal-leak hypercalciuria, PHPT = Primary hyperparathyroidism, PTH = Parathormone.
 *Dx diet = Diagnostic diet used in the evaluation of normal and calcium oxalate urolith dogs.
**As glomerular filtration rate declines, phosphorus is retained in serum.

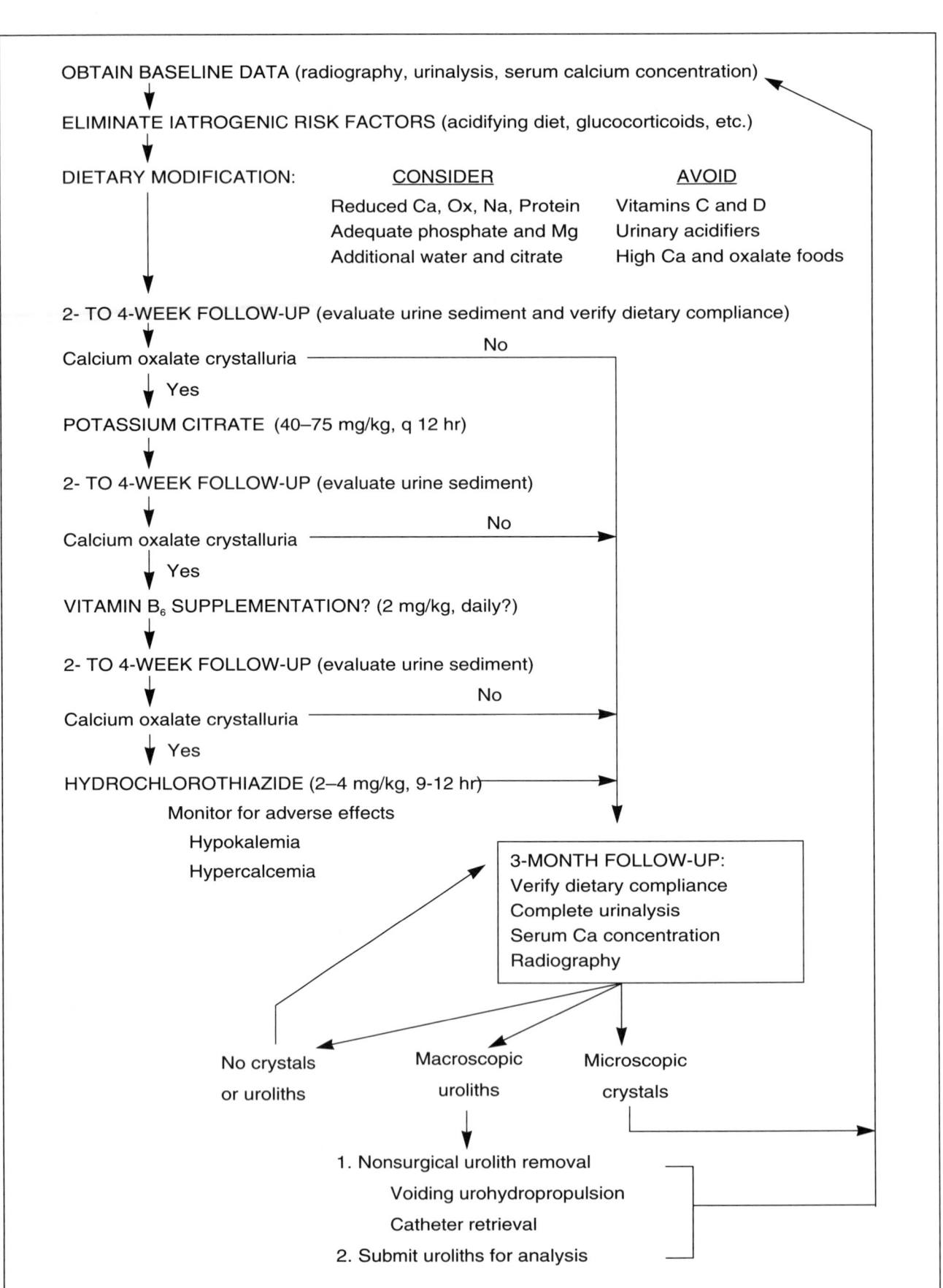

Figure 3—Algorithm for medical management of calcium oxalate uroliths.

TABLE 13

**Expected Changes Associated with Medical Therapy to
Minimize Recurrence of Calcium Oxalate Uroliths**

Factor	Pretherapy	Preventative Therapy
Polyuria	±	variable
Pollakiuria	0 to 4+	0
Hematuria	0 to 4+	0
Urine specific gravity	variable	1.004 to 1.015
Urine pH	<7.0	>7.0
Urine inflammation	0 to 4+	0
CaOx crystals	0 to 4+	0
Bacteriuria	0 to 4+	0
Bacterial culture of urine	0 to 4+	0
BUN (mg/dl)	>15	<15
Urolith size and number	small to large	0

TABLE 14

Summary of Recommendations for Management of Calcium Phosphate Uroliths

1. Surgery remains the most reliable way to remove active calcium phosphate uroliths from the urinary tract. However, we emphasize that surgery may be unnecessary for clinically inactive calcium phosphate uroliths. Small urocystoliths may be nonsurgically removed by voiding urohydropropulsion or by aspiration through a urinary catheter (Table 20). Medical therapy of patients with recurrent calcium phosphate uroliths should then be directed at removing or minimizing risk factors that contribute to supersaturation of urine with calcium phosphate.

2. Patients with hypercalcemia and primary hyperparathyroidism usually require surgery. Parathyroidectomy may result in dissolution of uroliths; it generally prevents their recurrence.

3. Several different medical protocols have been reported to be of value in humans with normocalcemic hypercalciuria. Ideally, the choice of therapy should be based on the cause of idiopathic hypercalciuria (see Tables 11 and 12).

   a. There has been little clinical experience in the use of drugs in dogs with calcium phosphate uroliths. However, medications that can enhance calcium excretion (such as glucocorticoids and furosemide) and those containing large quantities of sodium should be avoided, if possible.

   b. Diets designed to avoid excessive protein, sodium, calcium and vitamin D may be of benefit. Excessive restriction or supplementation of dietary phosphorus probably should be avoided. Enhancement of urine volume by feeding a canned diet (and/or a protein-restricted diet to reduce renal medullary urea), and encouraging water consumption may be of benefit. Although understandably difficult in some patients, fluid intake should be encouraged throughout the day to promote a constantly high urine volume. In humans, high-fiber diets have been shown to reduce intestinal absorption and urinary excretion of calcium.

   c. with the exception of Brushite, calcium phosphates tend to be less soluble in alkaline urine. The benefit to such patients of the use of appropriate dosages of acidifiers is unknown. Acidification tends to enhance urine calcium excretion and is a risk factor for calcium oxalate urolith formation. Pending further studies, we are unable to recommend the routine use of urine acidifiers for patients with calcium phosphate urolithiasis.

4. To our knowledge, medical dissolution of calcium phosphate uroliths has not been attempted in dogs with distal renal tubular acidosis (RTA). Diets designed to dissolve struvite uroliths are generally not expected to promote the dissolution of calcium phosphate uroliths, in part because they tend to promote acidemia and aciduria, thus potentially enhancing hypercalciuria and hypocitraturia. However, correction of hypercalciuria, hyperphosphaturia, and hypocitraturia by alkalinization therapy with potassium citrate might promote dissolution of these uroliths in patients with complete or incomplete distal RTA. Chronic alkalinization therapy apparently is beneficial in preventing calcium phosphate urolith formation in humans with distal RTA. Such therapy has been advocated for patients with complete or incomplete forms of distal RTA because it decreases urolith formation and nephrocalcinosis and increases urine citrate concentration. Oral administration of sodium chloride, long recommended for all forms of urolithiasis, may promote hypercalciuria and calcium phosphate urolith formation. Therefore, oral salt therapy is not recommended to promote diuresis in dogs with uroliths containing calcium salts.

TABLE 15
Summary of Recommendations for Medical Dissolution and Prevention of Canine Cystine Uroliths

1. Perform appropriate diagnostic studies, including complete urinalyses, quantitative urine culture, and diagnostic radiography. Determine precise location, size, and number of uroliths. The size and number of uroliths are not a reliable index of the probable efficacy of therapy.

2. If available, determine mineral composition of uroliths. If unavailable, determine their composition by evaluation of appropriate clinical data (Table 8).

3. Consider surgical correction if uroliths are obstructing urine outflow, and/or if correctable abnormalities predisposing to the recurrence of urinary tract infections are identified by radiography or other means. Small urocystoliths may be removed by voiding urohydropropulsion (Table 20).

4. Initiate therapy with calculolytic diet (e.g., Prescription Diet Canine u/d). No other food or mineral supplements should be fed to the patient. Compliance with dietary recommendation is suggested by reduction of serum SUN concentration (usually <10 mg/dl).

5. Initiate therapy with N-(2-mercaptoropionyl)-glycine (MPG) at a daily dosage of approximately 30 mg/kg body weight (divided into two equal subdoses).

6. If necessary, administer potassium citrate orally to eliminate aciduria. Strive for pH of approximately 7.5.

7. If necessary, eradicate or control urinary tract infections with appropriate antimicrobial agents.

8. Devise protocol for follow-up therapy.
   a. Try to avoid diagnostic follow-up studies that require urinary catheterization. If they are required, give appropriate pericatheterization antimicrobial agents to prevent iatrogenic urinary tract infection.
   b. Evaluate serial urinalyses. Urine pH, specific gravity, and microscopic examination of sediment for crystals are especially important. Remember that crystals formed in urine stored at room or refrigeration temperatures may represent in vitro artifacts.
   c. Perform serial radiography at monthly intervals to evaluate stone location(s), number, size, density, and shape. Intravenous urography may be used for radiolucent uroliths located in the kidneys, ureters, or urinary bladder. Antegrade contrast cystourethrography may be required for radiolucent uroliths located in the bladder and urethra.

9. Continue calculolytic diet, MPG, and alkalinizing therapy for approximately one month following disappearance of uroliths as detected by radiography.

10. Prevention: Use of a low protein diet which promotes an alkaline urine has been effective in preventing cystine urolith recurrence. If necessary, low doses of MPG may also be used.

TABLE 16
Expected Changes Associated with Medical Therapy of Cystine Uroliths

Factor	Pretherapy	During Therapy	Preventative Therapy
Polyuria	±	1+ to 3+	1+ to 3+
Pollakiuria	0 to 4+	↑ then ↓	0
Hematuria	0 to 4+	↓	0
Urine specific gravity	variable	1.004 to 1.014	1.004 to 1.014
Urine pH	<7.0	>7.0	>7.0
Urine inflammation	0 to 4+	↓	0
Urate crystals	0 to 4+	0	variable
Bacteriuria	0 to 4+	0	0
Bacterial culture of urine	0 to 4+	0	0
BUN (mg/dl)	variable	<15	≤15
Urolith size and number	small to large	↓	0

TABLE 17
Summary of Recommendations for Medical Dissolution of Canine Struvite Uroliths

A. Adult dogs with urinary tract infection:
1. Perform appropriate diagnostic studies, including complete urinalyses, quantitative urine culture, and diagnostic radiography. Determine precise location, size, and number of uroliths. The size and number of uroliths are not a reliable index of probable efficacy of therapy.
2. If feasible, determine mineral composition of uroliths. If not feasible, estimate their composition by evaluation of appropriate clinical data (Table 8).
3. Consider surgical correction if uroliths are obstructing urine outflow, and/or if correctable abnormalities predisposing to recurrent urinary tract infection are identified by radiography or other means. Small urocystoliths may be removed by voiding urohydropropulsion (Table 20).
4. Eradicate or control urinary tract infections with appropriate antimicrobial agents. Maintain antimicrobial therapy during, and for 3 to 4 weeks following, urolith dissolution.
5. Initiate therapy with calculolytic diets. No other food or mineral supplements should be fed to the patient. Compliance with dietary recommendations is suggested by reduction in SUN concentration (usually <10 mg/dl).
6. Devise a protocol to monitor efficacy of therapy.
   a. Try to avoid diagnostic follow-up studies that require urinary catheterization. If they are required, give appropriate pericatheterization antimicrobial agents to prevent iatrogenic urinary tract infection.
   b. Evaluate serial urinalyses. Urine pH, specific gravity, and microscopic examination of sediment for crystals are especially important. Remember: crystals formed in urine stored at room or refrigeration temperatures may represent in vitro artifacts.
   c. Perform serial radiography at monthly intervals to evaluate stone location(s), number, size, density, and shape.
   d. If necessary, perform quantitative urine cultures. They are especially important in patients that were infected prior to therapy, and in patients that were catheterized during therapy.
   e. Feed patients calculolytic diet for 1 month following the disappearance of uroliths on survey radiography.
   f. If uroliths increase in size during dietary management or do not begin to decrease in size after approximately 4 to 8 weeks of appropriate medical management alternative methods should be considered. Difficulty in inducing complete dissolution of uroliths by creating urine that is undersaturated with the suspected calculogenic crystalloid should prompt consideration that the wrong mineral component was identified, the nucleus of the uroliths is of different mineral composition than other portions of the urolith, and the owner of the patient is not complying with medical recommendations.
7. Consider administration of acetohydroxamic acid (25 mg/kg/day divided into two equal doses) to patients with persistent uroliths and persistent urease-producing microburia, despite the use of antimicrobial agents and calculolytic diet.

B. Adult dogs with persistently sterile urine:
1. Follow the protocol described above, but do not administer antimicrobial agents or acetohydroxamic acid.
2. Periodically culture urine specimens obtained by cystocentesis to detect secondary urinary tract infections. If UTI develops, initiate antimicrobial therapy.

C. Immature dogs
1. Use caution in consideration of use of protein-restricted diets in growing pups.
2. Short-term therapy with a calculolytic diet has been effective in dissolving struvite urocystoliths. If initiated, monitor the patient for evidence of nutritional deficiencies (especially protein malnutrition).
3. Acetohydroxamic acid has not been evaluated in growing pups.
4. Small urocystoliths may be removed by voiding urohydropropulsion (Table 20). Surgery remains the safest means of removing large uroliths from immature dogs.

TABLE 18
Expected Changes Associated with Medical Therapy of Cystine Uroliths

Factor	Pretherapy	During Therapy	Preventative Therapy
Polyuria	±	1+ to 3+	0
Pollakiuria	1+ to 4+	↑ then ↓	0
Hematuria	1+ to 4+	↓	0
Urine specific gravity	variable	1.004 to 1.014	normal
Urine pH	>7.0	≤6.5	variable
Urine inflammation	1+ to 4+	↓	0
Urate crystals	0 to 4+	0	variable
Bacteriuria	0 to 4+	↓ to 0	0
Bacterial culture of urine	0 to 4+	↓ to 0	0
BUN (mg/dl)	>15	≤10	variable
Urolith size and number	small to large	↓	0

TABLE 19
Summary of Recommendations for Prevention of Canine Silica Uroliths

1. Perform appropriate diagnostic studies, including complete urinalyses, quantitative urine culture, and diagnostic radiography. Determine precise location, size, and number of uroliths.
2. If available, determine mineral composition of uroliths. If unavailable, determine their composition by evaluation of appropriate clinical data (Table 8).
3. Small urocystoliths may be removed by voiding urohydropropulsion (Table 20). Consider surgical removal of larger uroliths that are causing clinical disease.
4. To prevent further growth of existing silica uroliths, or to prevent recurrence of surgically removed silica uroliths:
   a. Avoid use of diets containing substantial plant proteins, and especially avoid those containing soybean hulls or corn gluten feed.
   b. Enhance diuresis by adding moisture to the diet and/or stimulating thirst with supplemental sodium chloride.
   c. Avoid efforts to deliberately acidify urine.
5. If necessary, eradicate or control urinary tract infections with appropriate antimicrobial agents.

TABLE 20
Voiding Urohydropropulsion: A Nonsurgical Technique for Removing Small Urocystoliths

1. Perform appropriate diagnostic studies, including complete urinalysis, quantitative urine culture, and diagnostic radiography. Determine location, size, surface contour, and number of urocystoliths.
2. Anesthetize the patient, if needed.
3. If the urinary bladder is not distended with urine, moderately distend the urinary bladder with a physiologic solution (saline, Ringer's lactate, etc.) injected through a transurethral catheter. To prevent overdistension, palpate the bladder through the abdomen during infusion. Remove the catheter.
4. Position the patient so that the vertebral spine is approximately vertical.
5. Gently agitate the urinary bladder, with the objective of promoting gravitational movement of urocystoliths into the bladder neck.
6. Induce voiding by manually expressing the urinary bladder. Use steady digital pressure rather than an intermittent squeezing motion.
7. Collect urine and uroliths in a cup. Compare urolith number and size to those detected by radiography, and submit them for quantitative analysis.
8. If needed, repeat steps 3 through 7 until the number of uroliths detected by radiography is removed, or until uroliths are no longer voided.
9. Perform double-contrast cystography to insure that no uroliths remain in the urinary bladder. Repeat voiding urohydropropulsion if small urocystoliths remain.
10. Administer prophylactic antimicrobials for 3 to 5 days, or longer if needed.
11. Monitor for adverse complications such as hematuria, dysuria, bacterial urinary tract infection, and urethral obstruction with uroliths.
12. On the basis of quantitative mineral analysis of voided urocystoliths, formulate appropriate recommendations to minimize urolith recurrence or to manage uroliths remaining in the urinary tract.

TABLE 21
General Principles and Considerations for Surgical Management of Uroliths

PREOPERATIVE CONSIDERATIONS

1. Obtain all blood and urine samples before administering diagnostic (e.g., radiopaque contrast media) or therapeutic (e.g., antibiotics, fluids, etc.) agents. Quantitatively evaluate renal function.
2. Always radiograph the entire urinary tract to determine the location and number of uroliths. Contrast radiography and/or ultrasonography should be considered to evaluate the patency of the excretory pathway. Thoroughly evaluate the entire urinary tract for correctable anatomic abnormalities that may have initiated urinary infection and subsequent struvite urolithiasis.

OPERATIVE CONSIDERATIONS

1. Preserve renal organ function. Avoid the use of mattress sutures to repair nephrotomy incisions, because they cause additional irreversible loss of renal function due to infarction.
2. Remove renoliths before removing cystoliths in patients with multiple uroliths. If ureteroliths are present, or if small or fractured renoliths subsequently pass into the ureters, they may be flushed into the bladder from the renal pelvis.
3. Obtain urine samples for routine analysis and microbial culture if they could not be obtained before surgery. Obtain biopsy samples of the urinary tract at the time of nephrotomy, pyelotomy, cystotomy, and/or urethrotomy. Evaluation of biopsy samples may be of diagnostic and prognostic significance.
4. Make every effort to remove all uroliths. Thoroughly flush the affected lumen of the urinary tract with a sterile isotonic solution to remove small uroliths. Bacteria harbored inside struvite uroliths allow urinary tract infections to persist and predispose to the recurrence of struvite uroliths.

5. If possible, prevent suture material from penetrating the lumen of the urinary tract. Suture material may serve as a nidus for urolith formation by lowering the formation product. Nonabsorbable and multifilament sutures are more calculogenic than absorbable and monofilament sutures.
6. Save all uroliths for mineral analysis, possible culture, and possible microscopic examination. Culture of uroliths may help detect bacteria in patients receiving antimicrobial therapy before diagnostic urine culture and antimicrobial susceptibility tests are performed.

POSTOPERATIVE CONSIDERATIONS

1. Avoid the use of indwelling catheters, which are a common cause of iatrogenic urinary tract infections. If an indwelling catheter must be used, a closed system should be used when possible, for it minimizes retrograde migration of pathogens through the catheter lumen.
2. If multiple uroliths are present, evaluate the urinary tract radiographically following surgery. Immediate detection of uroliths that were inadvertently allowed to remain in the urinary tract is of prognostic significance. It may be erroneously assumed that the patient is highly predisposed to recurrent urolithiasis if residual uroliths are first detected on radiographs taken several weeks following surgery. Appropriate medical and/or surgical therapy should be formulated to manage residual uroliths.
3. Therapy should be designed to promote postoperative diuresis in patients undergoing nephrolithotomy. Increased urine flow minimizes the formation of blood clots in the renal pelves that have the potential to obstruct urine outflow and/or mineralize.

TABLE 22
Difficulties, Do's, and Don'ts of Urolith Management

1. Difficulties in the diagnosis of uroliths.
   a. Wrong "guesstimate" of mineral type (Table 8)
   b. Improper analysis (retrieval, submission, qualitative rather than quantitative technique)
   c. Uroliths composed of multiple minerals
   d. Uroliths not composed of minerals (matrix, drugs, foreign material)
2. Difficulties in the treatment of uroliths.
   a. Owner or patient noncompliance
   b. Inability to correct or control underlying disease process(es)
   c. Improper therapy
   d. Changed composition of uroliths during therapy
   e. Undesired influence of drug therapy
   f. Inadequate surgical retrieval
3. Difficulties in the prevention of uroliths.
   a. Owner or patient noncompliance
   b. Inability to correct or control underlying disease process

   c. No short-term or long-term plan formulated to prevent urolith recurrence
   d. Improper therapy
4. Urolith management DO's and DON'Ts
   a. DO
      1) Analyze uroliths by quantitative methods
      2) Obtain baseline data prior to therapy
      3) Serially monitor patient response to therapy
      4) Monitor compliance of owners and patients
      5) Retrieve and analyze recurrent uroliths
      6) Take radiographs of the urinary tract following surgery to remove uroliths.
   b. DON'T
      1) Rely on incomplete data
      2) Treat without obtaining baseline data
      3) Treat without serially monitoring the patient
      4) Assume the owner or patient is compliant

BIBLIOGRAPHY

Bartges JW, Osborne CA, Felice LJ: Acquired xanthine uroliths: Risk factor management, in Bonagura JD, Kirk RW (eds): *Current Veterinary Therapy, vol II.* Philadelphia, WB Saunders Co, 1992, pp 900–905.

Lulich JP, Osborne CA, Bartges JW, et al: Canine urolithiasis, in Ettinger SJ, Feldman EC (eds): *Internal Medical Disorders of the Dog and Cat.* Philadelphia, WB Saunders Co, in press.

Lulich JP, Osborne CA, Carlson M, et al: Nonsurgical removal of urocystoliths in dogs and cats by voiding urohydropropulsion. *JAVMA* 203:660–663, 1993.

Lulich JP, Osborne CA, Smith CL: Canine calcium oxalate urolithiasis: Risk factor management, in Bonagura JD, Kirk RW (eds): *Current Veterinary Therapy,* vol II. Philadelphia, WB Saunders Co, 1992, pp 892–899.

Osborne CA (ed): Symposium on canine urolithiasis: Part I—Etiopathogenesis and detection. *Vet Clin North Am* 16:1–206, 1986.

Osborne CA (ed): Symposium on canine urolithiasis: Part II—Treatment and prevention. *Vet Clin North Am* 16:1–206, 1986.

Osborne CA, Davis LS, Sanna JJ, et al: Identification and interpretation of crystalluria in domestic animals: A light and scanning electron microscopic study. *Veterinary Medicine* 85:18–37, 1990.

Osborne CA, Finco DR (eds): Canine and Feline Nephrology and Urology. Malvern, PA, Lea & Febiger, in press.

Osborne CA, Hoppe A, O'Brien TD: Medical dissolution and prevention of cystine urolithiasis, in Kirk RW (ed): *Current Veterinary Therapy, vol. 10.* Philadelphia, WB Saunders Co, 1989, pp 1189–1193.

Osborne CA, Lulich JP, Unger LK: Nonsurgical retrieval of uroliths for mineral analysis, in Bonagura JD, Kirk RW (eds): *Current Veterinary Therapy. vol. 11.* Philadelphia, WB Saunders Co, 1992, pp 886–889.

Osborne CA, Lulich JP, Unger LK, et al: Canine and feline urolithiasis: Relationship of etiopathogenesis to treatment and prevention, in Bojrab MJ (ed): *Disease Mechanisms in Small Animal Surgery.* Malvern, Lea & Febiger, 1993, pp 426–463.

Osborne CA, Polzin DJ: Nonsurgical management of obstructive urolithopathy. *Vet Clin North Am* 16:333–347, 1986.

Feline Urologic Signs: A Unifying Hypothesis of Causes

University of Minnesota

Carl A. Osborne, DVM, PhD

John P. Kruger, DVM, PhD

Jody P. Lulich, DVM, PhD

Rosama Thumchai, DVM

Joseph W. Bartges, DVM

David J. Polzin, DVM, PhD

K. D. Beauclair, MS

T. Molitor, PhD

Lisa K. Unger, CVT

Lori A. Koehler, CVT

Kathleen A. Bird, CVT

Laurie Swanson, CVT

Feline urologic syndrome (FUS) has traditionally been viewed as a distinct pathophysiologic entity initiated and perpetuated by multiple (often undefined) factors. However, available clinical and experimental data suggest that the term "FUS" represents a constellation of clinical signs associated with lower urinary tract disease in male and female cats. As with all species, feline lower urinary tract disease may result from fundamentally different causes that may be single, multiple and interacting, and/or unrelated (Table I).[1] Because the clinical signs of hematuria, dysuria, pollakiuria, and/or urethral obstruction are the common denominator of feline lower urinary tract disease, the acronym FUS should represent feline urologic signs rather than feline urologic syndrome.

FELINE UROLITHS

In a prospective diagnostic study of feline lower urinary tract disease performed at the University of Minnesota,[a] uroliths were detected in approximately 22% (32 of 143) of the cats.[1] Magnesium ammonium phosphate has been the most frequently encountered mineral in uroliths submitted to the Minnesota Urolith Center; however, approximately 46% of the uroliths are primarily composed of other minerals (Table II).[2] Similar findings have been reported by other investigators.[3,4]

STERILE STRUVITE UROLITHS

As reviewed elsewhere,[1] probable risk factors for formation of sterile struvite uroliths include: 1) mineral composition of diets, 2) energy content of diets, 3) moisture content of diets, 4) urine alkalinizing metabolites in diets, 5) quantity of diet consumed, 6) caloric density, 7) ad libitum versus meal

[a]Minnesota Urolith Center, Department of Small Animal Clinical Sciences, College of Veterinary Medicine, St. Paul, Minnesota 55108 (phone 612-625-4221)

TABLE I
Examples of Confirmed Causes of Lower Urinary Tract Disease in Cats

Metabolic (including nutritional)
Uroliths
  Struvite
  Calcium phosphates
    (calcium apatite; calcium hydrogen phosphate)
  Calcium oxalate
    (monohydrate and dihydrate)
  Ammonium urate
  Uric acid
  Cystine
  Xanthine
  Matrix
Urethral plugs
  Struvite crystals only
  Matrix only
    Inflammatory products
    Sloughed tissue
    Blood clots
  Matrix and struvite crystals
  Matrix and other crystals
    (e.g., calcium oxalate ammonium urate)
Inflammatory
  Infectious agents
  Viral (experimental)
  Bacterial
  Mycotic
  Parasitic
Noninfectious idiopathic

Anatomic abnormalities
  Congenital
    Urachal anomalies
    Persistent uterus masculinus
    Urethrorectal fistula
    Phimosis
  Acquired urethral strictures
Neoplastic
  Benign
    Papilloma (bladder)
    Cystadenoma (bladder)
    Leiomyoma (bladder)
  Malignant
    Transitional cell carcinoma (bladder and urethra)
    Squamous cell carcinoma (bladder)
    Adenocarcinoma (bladder)
    Unclassified carcinoma (bladder)
    Lymphosarcoma (bladder)
    Myxosarcoma (bladder)
    Prostatic adenocarcinoma (urethra)
    Endometrial adenocarcinoma (extraurinary)
Neurogenic
  Reflex dyssynergia
  Urethral spasm
  Hypotonic or atonic bladder (primary or secondary)
Iatrogenic
Traumatic

feeding schedules, 8) formation of concentrated urine, and 9) retention of urine. Elimination or control of these risk factors may result in dissolution of sterile struvite uroliths (Prescription Diet Feline s/d), and prevention of their recurrence.[5]

INFECTION-INDUCED STRUVITE UROLITHS

Probable risk factors for infection-induced struvite urolithiasis include: 1) infections with urease producing microbial pathogens, 2) abnormalities in local host defenses of the urinary tract that allow bacterial infections (including perineal urethrostomies), and 3) the quantity of urea (the substrate of urease) excreted in urine. Eradication of urinary tract infections with antimicrobial agents combined with consumption of magnesium-restricted acidifying diets (Prescription Diet Feline s/d) may result in dissolution of infection-induced struvite uroliths.[1,5]

CALCIUM OXALATE UROLITHS

The underlying causes of feline calcium oxalate uroliths have not been clearly established. Detectable hypercalcemia (11.1 to 13.5 mg/dl) may occur in some patients. Risk factors for calcium oxalate urolithiasis in nonhypercalcemic patients may include:

1) factors that promote hypercalciuria, 2) decreased crystallization inhibitors, 3) vitamin B-6 deficiency, 4) formation of concentrated urine, and 5) retention of urine. Factors that promote hypercalciuria include: 1) acidemia, 2) high dietary protein content, 3) high dietary sodium content, 4) excessive vitamin D, and 5) excessive vitamin C.[6]

Medical protocols that promote dissolution of calcium oxalate uroliths in cats are unavailable. Urocystoliths small enough to pass through the urethra may be removed by voiding urohydropropulsion.[7] Surgery remains as the only alternate for removal of larger active calcium oxalate uroliths. To minimize recurrence, consumption of nonacidifying, protein-restricted, and sodium-restricted diets should be considered.

AMMONIUM URATE UROLITHS

As reviewed elsewhere, there have been isolated case reports of uric acid and ammonium urate uroliths in cats during the past 20 years.[1] Although a renal tubular reabsorptive defect and portovascular anomalies have been incriminated as causes in a few cases, the cause of formation of most feline purine uroliths has not been established.[6] Probable risk factors for ammonium urate urolithiasis include: 1) in-

TABLE II

Mineral Composition of 6335 Feline Uroliths Evaluated by Quantitative Methods[a]

Predominant Mineral Type		Number of Uroliths	%
Magnesium Ammonium Phosphate $6H_2O$		3413	53.9
	100%	(2904)	(45.8)
	70–99%[b]	(509)	(8.0)
Magnesium Hydrogen Phosphate $3H_2O$		16	0.3
	70–99%[b]	(16)	(0.3)
Calcium Oxalates		2037	37.2
Calcium Oxalate Monohydrate			
	100%	(738)	(11.6)
	70–99%[b]	(704)	(11.1)
Calcium Oxalate Dihydrate			
	100%	(69)	(1.2)
	70–99%[b]	(234)	(3.7)
Calcium Oxalate Monohydrate & Dihydrate			
	100%	(269)	(4.2)
	70–99%[b]	(23)	(0.4)
Calcium Phosphates		68	1.1
Calcium Phosphate			
	100%	(23)	(0.3)
	70–99%[b]	(29)	(0.5)
Calcium Hydrogen Phosphate $6H_2O$			
	100%	(5)	(0.1)
	70–99%[b]	(9)	(0.2)
Tricalcium Phosphate			
	100%	(1)	(<0.1)
	70–99%[b]	(1)	(<0.1)
Uric Acid and Urates		432	6.8
Ammonium Acid Urate			
	100%	(327)	(5.2)
	70–99%[b]	(97)	(1.5)
Sodium Urate			
	70–99%[b]	(1)	(<0.1)
Uric Acid			
	100%	(4)	(0.1)
	70–99%[b]	(3)	(<0.1)
Cystine		22	0.3
Xanthine		9	0.1
Silica		0	0
Mixed[c]		118	1.9
Compound[d]		115	1.8
Matrix		106	2.0
Total		6335	100%

[a]Uroliths analyzed by polarized light microscopy and x-ray diffraction methods.
[b]Uroliths composed of 70–99% of mineral type listed; no nucleus and shell detected.
[c]Uroliths did not contain at least 70% of mineral type listed; no nucleus or shell detected.
[d]Uroliths contained an identifiable nucleus and one or more surrounding layers of a different mineral type.

creased urine uric acid concentration associated with consumption of purine precursors in the diet, 2) increased urine ammonia concentration, 3) formation of concentrated urine, and 4) retention of urine.

Medical protocols that consistently promote dissolution of ammonium urate uroliths in cats have not yet been developed. Urocystoliths small enough to pass through the urethra may be removed by voiding urohydropropulsion.[7] Surgery is the most reliable method to remove larger uroliths from the urinary tract. Prevention of recurrence should encompass consumption of diets low in purine precursors (e.g., low in liver), that promote formation of less acid urine (pH ± 7) that is not highly concentrated.

CALCIUM PHOSPHATE UROLITHS

Calcium phosphate uroliths may occur in association with primary hyperparathyroidism in humans and dogs, and this association has been made in cats.[1] Probable risk factors for calcium phosphate urolithiasis include: 1) factors that promote hypercalciuria, 2) alkaline urine pH (except for Brushite), 3) increased matrix (including blood clots), 4) decreased crystallization inhibitors, 5) formation of concentrated urine, and 6) retention of urine.

Protocols designed to dissolve or prevent calcium phosphate uroliths in cats have not been studied. Urocystoliths small enough to pass through the urethra may be removed by voiding urohydropropulsion.[7] Surgery remains the most reliable way to remove larger uroliths from the urinary tract. We emphasize that surgery may be unnecessary for clinically inactive calcium phosphate uroliths. Based on studies in other species, avoiding excessive dietary protein and sodium may prevent hypercalciuria.

CYSTINE UROLITHS

Cystine has been observed in several feline uroliths evaluated at our center. Feline cystine uroliths have also been encountered by other clinicians.[8] The major risk factor appears to be decreased renal tubular reabsorption of cystine following glomerular filtration. Formation of concentrated acid urine and retention of urine are also likely to be risk factors for cystine urolithiasis.

URINARY TRACT INFECTIONS
Viral Urinary Tract Infections

As reviewed elsewhere, there is considerable evidence that cell associated herpesvirus (bovine herpesvirus-4) can induce long-term viral urinary tract infections in cats in a laboratory setting.[9] However, reproducible evidence that cell-associated herpesvirus causes naturally occurring symptomatic feline lower urinary tract disease is lacking. Recent discovery of virus-like particles with morphologic characteristics similar to those of caliciviruses in crystalline matrix urethral plugs obtained from male cats with naturally occurring urethral obstruction is noteworthy[1] (Figure 1).

In a prospective clinical study performed at the University of Minnesota designed to detect the causes of lower urinary tract disease in 141 male and female cats with naturally occurring disease, a specific etiology could not be determined in 77 (53%) cats.[1] A cause-and-effect relationship among clinical signs and uroliths, bacterial urinary tract infections, anatomic abnormalities, neoplasms, and neurogenic diseases was not identified. However, the subsequent course of clinical signs in these cats was consistent with a viral etiology. Clinical signs of gross hematuria, dysuria, and pollakiuria resolved spontaneously without treatment.

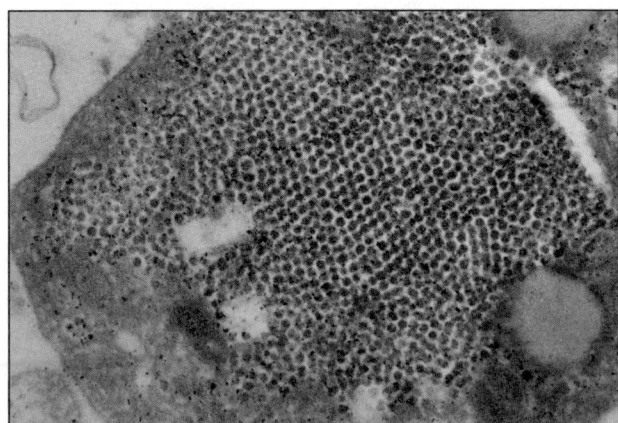

Figure 1—Transmission electron micrograph of a section of urethral plug obtained from a 3-year-old male domestic longhaired cat. Note virus particles contained within an unidentified cell. 80,000 × = original magnification (From Osborne CA: Feline matrix crystalline urethral plugs. A unifying hypothesis of causes. *J Small Animal Pract* 33:172–177, 1992. Reproduced with permission.)

BACTERIAL URINARY TRACT INFECTIONS

Bacterial urinary tract infections are associated with signs of lower urinary tract disease in 1 to 3% of cats that have not been treated with indwelling transurethral catheters or urethrostomy.[1,10] The infrequent occurrence of bacterial infections of the urinary tract of cats has been linked with their innate ability to produce highly concentrated, acidic urine that contains large quantities of urea.[11] The large quantity of Tamm-Horsfall mucoprotein present in feline urine may also minimize bacterial urinary tract infections. Following use of indwelling catheters, the prevalence of urinary tract infections may rise to 50%; following perineal urethrostomy, the prevalence may exceed 20%.[1,12,13]

Bacteria resembling cocci occasionally have been detected in crystalline-matrix urethral plugs obtained from male cats with naturally occurring urethral obstruction.[14] Detection of bacteria in the cytoplasm of leucocytes trapped in the plugs indicates that they were present at the time the urethral plugs formed.

FUNGAL URINARY TRACT INFECTIONS

Although uncommon, infections of the urinary tract of cats with fungal pathogens has been observed.[15] They most commonly occur in patients with impaired systemic or local host defenses. Fungal pathogens that produce urease may foster production of magnesium ammonium phosphate uroliths.

Experience with treatment of fungal urinary tract infections in cats is limited. In patients with asymptomatic fungal urinary tract infections, correction of

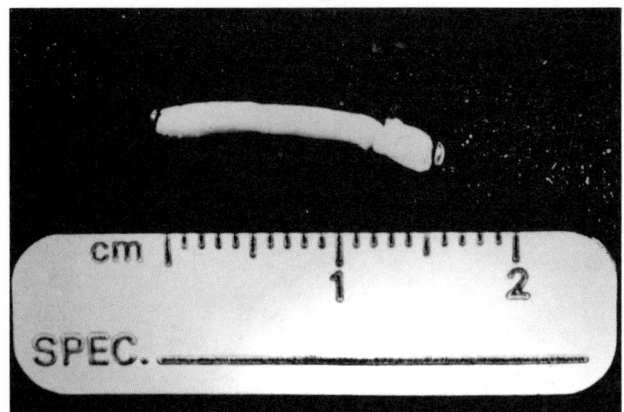

Figure 2—Matrix-crystalline urethral plug removed from an adult male domestic shorthaired cat. The mineral component of the plug was composed of magnesium ammonium phosphate.

identifiable predisposing factors and alkalinizing urine to a pH greater than 7.5 may be sufficient. We have not been successful in eradicating fungal urinary tract infections with alkalinization of urine alone. Patients that have concurrent clinical signs of lower urinary tract disease or other debilitating or complicating disorders may require additional specific antifungal therapy to eliminate these pathogens. Flucytosine, amphotericin B, ketaconazole, itraconazole, and fluconazole have been used to treat *Candida* spp urinary tract infections in humans. However, to date, there are no studies confirming the safety or efficacy of these drugs in the treatment of fungal urinary tract infection in cats.

MATRIX-CRYSTALLINE URETHRAL PLUGS
Etiopathogenesis

There are physical and probable etiopathogenic differences between feline uroliths and urethral plugs.[1,16] Therefore, these terms should not be used as synonyms.

The most commonly encountered form of naturally occurring feline urethral plugs contains relatively large quantities of matrix in addition to minerals (Figure 2). Minerals identified in matrix-crystalline plugs vary in composition (Table III). We presume that risk factors associated with formation of magnesium ammonium phosphate, calcium oxalate, calcium phosphate, ammonium urate, cystine and xanthine crystals contained in urethral plugs are similar to risk factors associated with formation of classical uroliths. Therefore, prevention or control of these risk factors should minimize recurrence of the crystalline components of urethral plugs.

The question about the specific composition of urethral plug matrix has not yet been answered. The observation that the urine concentration of Tamm-

Horsfall mucoprotein is increased in cats with lower urinary tract disease[17] prompts the hypothesis that this type of mucoprotein is a major component of plug matrix. Tamm-Horsfall mucoprotein has been identified in human and ovine uroliths.[18,19] It has also been identified as a local host defense mechanism against viral and bacterial urinary tract infections in other species.[20]

Light and transmission electron microscopic evaluation of naturally occurring feline urethral plugs have revealed that noncrystalline components of plugs also include red blood cells, white cells, epithelial cells, spermatozoa, virus-like particles, and bacteria (Figure 3).[14] It is likely that urethral plugs contain other inflammatory reactants as well.

HYPOTHESIS

We hypothesize that various combinations of two different etiologic events may lead to three different, but common, clinical manifestations of naturally occurring feline lower urinary tract disease (Figure 4).[14]

I. Urinary tract infections with viruses, and occasionally bacterial or fungal pathogens, lead to production of mucoprotein and inflammatory reactants, and the clinical signs of hematuria and dysuria (Figure 4). Urethral obstruction is a very uncommon clinical feature of this form of lower urinary tract disease as a noncrystalline gel of mucoprotein and inflammatory reactants can be passed through the urethra of female and male cats.

II. The presence of factors that promote crystal formation in urine, in absence of concomitant urinary tract infections that cause production of large quantities of mucoprotein and inflammatory reactants, leads to formation of classical uroliths (Figure 4; Table II). Urolithiasis affecting the lower urinary tract is typically characterized by hematuria and dysuria. Urethral obstruction may occur if small uroliths become lodged in the urethra.

III. The concomitant occurrence of urinary tract infection (I) and crystalluria (II) may lead to formation of matrix-crystalline plugs (III) that obstruct the urethra, especially of male cats (Figure 4). The same type of phenomenon is known to occur during formation of casts in renal tubular lumens.[21,22] Tamm-Horsfall mucoprotein may form a gel in tubular lumens that traps intact cells (cellular casts), disintegrating cells (granular casts), or lipid droplets (fatty casts). The process could also be compared to preparation of fruit jello; the matrix (comparable to gelatin) traps various types of crystals (comparable to fruit). The matrix may

TABLE III
Mineral Composition of 820 Feline Urethral Plugs Analyzed by Quantitative Methods[a]

Predominant Mineral Type		Number of Uroliths	%
Magnesium Ammonium Phosphate $6H_2O$		636	77.6
	100%	(540)	(65.9)
	70–99%[b]	(96)	(11.7)
Newberyite		3	0.4
	100%	(1)	(0.1)
	77–99%	(2)	(0.3)
Calcium Oxalate		14	1.7
Calcium Oxalate Monohydrate			
	100%	(4)	(0.5)
	70–99%[b]	(5)	(0.6)
Calcium Oxalate Dihydrate			
	100%	(2)	(0.2)
	70–99%[b]	(2)	(0.2)
Calcium Oxalate Monohydrate & Dihydrate		(1)	(0.1)
Calcium Phosphate		21	2.6
Calcium Phosphate			
	100%	(11)	(1.3)
	70–99%[b]	(7)	(0.9)
Calcium Hydrogen Phosphate $6H_2O$			
	100%	(2)	(0.3)
	70–99%[b]	(1)	(0.1)
Ammonium Acid Urate		6	0.7
	100%	(6)	(0.7)
Xanthine		1	0.1
Sulfadiazine		1	0.1
Mixed[c]		27	3.3
Matrix		113	13.4
Total		820	100%

[a]Urethral plugs examined by polarizing light microscopy and x-ray diffraction methods.
[b]Urolith composed of 70–99% of mineral type listed; no nucleus and shell detected.
[c]Uroliths did not contain at least 70% of mineral type listed; no nucleus or shell detected.

also trap red cells, white cells, epithelial cells, bacteria, and cells containing viruses. This hypothesis provides a plausible explanation of the observed association of virus particles in matrix-crystalline plugs containing crystals of different mineral composition (Table III).

TREATMENT OF URETHRAL PLUGS

Medical Treatment - Irrespective of the cause(s) of urethral obstruction, predictable clinical and biochemical abnormalities subsequently develop. They are characterized by systemic deficits and/or excesses in fluid (dehydration), electrolyte (hypercalcemia, hyperphosphatemia, etc.), and acid-base (metabolic acidosis) balance, and retention of metabolic wastes (creatinine, urea, other protein catabolites). The magnitude of these systemic abnormalities varies with the degree and duration of obstruction.

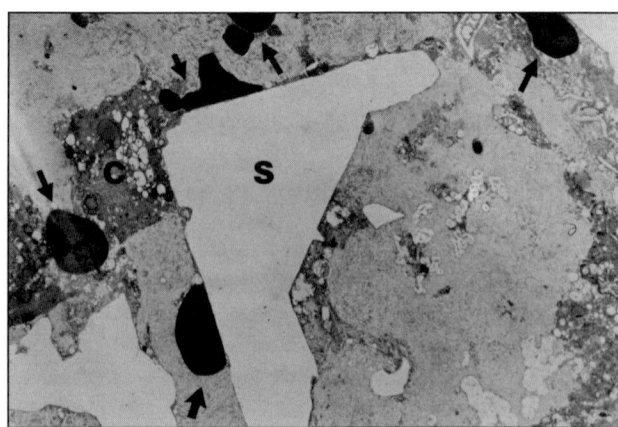

Figure 3—Electron micrograph of a section of a urethral plug removed from an 11-month-old male Siamese cat. Note the struvite crystal(s) red cells (arrows), unidentified cell(c), and cell fragments trapped in proteinaceous matrix.

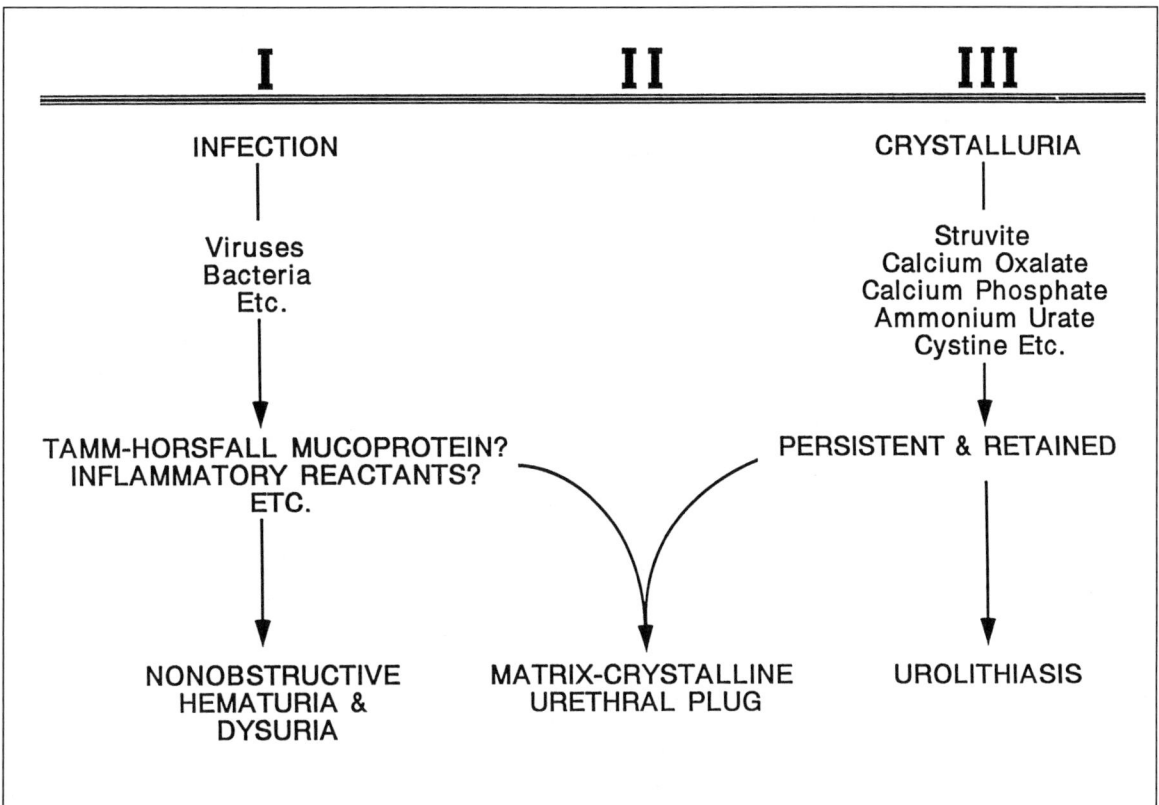

Figure 4—Schematic illustration of different manifestations of feline lower urinary tract disease associated with single or interacting underlying causes.

Obstructive uropathy that persists longer than about 24 hours usually results in postrenal uremia. This occurs because increased back pressure induced by obstruction to outflow impairs glomerular filtration, renal blood flow, and tubular function. Following obstruction of the urethra of normal cats, death will occur in 3 to 6 days. Damage to the mucosal surface of the urinary bladder may shorten survival time. Despite the potentially catastrophic outcome of urethral obstruction, the biochemical consequences of this disorder are potentially reversible provided appropriate supportive and symptomatic parenteral therapy is given. In severe cases, initiation of supportive therapy to correct hyperkalemia, metabolic acidosis, and volume depletion should be initiated immediately after decompression of the excretory pathway by cystocentesis (see the following section on reestablishing urethral patency for details).

The immediate need to remove urethral plugs within hours of their discovery precludes attempts to cause their dissolution over a period of days or weeks. However, it is often possible to repulse urethral plugs into the bladder lumen. Thus the question arises, can such plugs be dissolved by medical therapy? As previously described, urethral plugs contain a substantially greater quantity of matrix than do classical uroliths.

Although it is probable that medical protocols effective in inducing sterile struvite urolith dissolution would also be effective in dissolving the struvite crystalline component of urethral plugs located in the bladder lumen, such therapy may not result in dissolution of plug matrix. It should be emphasized that calcium oxalate and ammonium urate crystals have been identified in a few naturally occurring feline urethral plugs (Table III). These factors may account for lack of expected response to therapy in some patients.

Attempts to dissolve struvite crystals with urine acidifiers or diets designed to promote acid urine should not be initiated in cats with postrenal azotemia. The metabolic sequela of urethral obstruction, particularly severe metabolic acidosis, must be corrected before diets designed to acidify urine are utilized.

Reestablishment of Urethral Patency - Obstructive urethropathy may be caused by one or more intraluminal, mural, or extramural abnormalities located at one or more sites. It follows that reverse flushing solutions may be very effective in dissolving urethral plugs, but would have no effect on obstructive lesions located in the urethral wall or periurethral tissue. Inability to restore the patency by flushing the urethral lumen with a solution should arouse one's suspicion of a mural or periurethral lesion in addition to, or instead of, a firmly lodged urethral plug or ure-throlith.

Physical restraint alone, or in combination with topical anesthesia, may be sufficient for obstructed patients that are particularly docile or severely depressed. Wrapping the cat in a bath towel may help to protect the patient and the assistant. If local anesthetics are used to anesthetize the urethral mucosa, they should be administered only in a quantity sufficient to accomplish this goal. We do not recommend use of local anesthetic agents as primary reverse flushing solutions because they may induce systemic toxicity if absorbed in sufficient quantity. Their absorption may be enhanced by damage to the urothelium, and their toxic potential may be enhanced by postrenal uremia.

Because of an increased risk of adverse drug reactions associated with obstructive uropathy, pharmacologic restraint should be avoided when feasible. However, the risk of adverse drug reactions must be weighed against the possibility of iatrogenic trauma to the urethra in an uncooperative patient. If the disposition of the patient is such that attempts to dislodge the urethral obstruction are likely to be associated with additional damage to the urethra, or if there is a high risk of iatrogenic urinary tract infection, some form of pharmacologic restraint should be considered. Short-acting barbiturates (thiamyal) that are metabolized by the liver, propofol, and/or inhalant anesthetics may be considered if general anesthesia is required. Anesthetics must be given cautiously as dosages less than those recommended for patients with normal renal function are required in patients with postrenal azotemia. If ketamine hydrochloride is used, similar caution must be used since it is excreted in active form by the kidneys. Low doses (1 to 2 mg/kg/given intravenously) have been successfully used by many clinicians. However, if difficulty is encountered in relieving outflow obstruction, it is generally inadvisable to administer additional quantities of ketamine.

We recommend a step-by-step priority of procedures when attempting to restore urethral patency of an obstructed male cat. In order of priority they are: 1) massage the distal urethra; 2) attempt to induce voiding by gentle voiding of the urinary bladder; 3) cystocentesis; 4) retrograde urethral flushing; 5) combinations of 1 to 4; 5) diagnostic radiology to determine if cause of urethral obstruction is intraluminal, mural, and/or extramural; 6) surgical procedures.

Immediate Aftercare - After urine flow has been reestablished by nonsurgical techniques, most of the urine should be removed from the bladder lumen. It is unnecessary and inadvisable to remove all the urine from the bladder lumen because trauma associated with such efforts may aggravate the severity of blad-

der lesions. Manual compression may be used provided it does not require substantial pressure to induce voiding. Manual compression of the bladder is not necessarily the procedure of choice if an overdistended bladder has been recently decompressed by cystocentesis, since it may result in extravasation of urine into the bladder wall or peritoneal cavity. Alternative methods include use of a catheter and syringe, or cystocentesis. Each of these procedures has advantages or disadvantages that must be considered in light of the status of the urinary bladder and urethra of each patient. If the gross appearance of voided or aspirated urine suggests that reobstruction due to intraluminal debris is likely, removal of this material with saline or lactated Ringer's solution flushes of the bladder lumen may be of value in minimizing reobstruction. Particulate material located in the dependent portion of the bladder may be dispersed throughout the bladder lumen by digitally moving the bladder up and down, which may in turn facilitate aspiration of crystals, inflammatory reactants, and blood clots into the catheter and syringe. Local instillation of antimicrobial agents into the bladder lumen in attempt to prevent or treat urinary tract infection is of unproved value. Unless the bladder wall is hypotonic or atonic, the antimicrobial agent is likely to be voided soon after instillation. If circumstances dictate the need for antimicrobial agents, they should be given orally or parenterally to maximize their effectiveness.

The urinary bladder should be periodically evaluated following restoration of adequate urethral patency to ensure that urethral obstruction has not recurred and/or that the detrusor muscle is not hypotonic. Micturition induced by gentle digital compression of the bladder may facilitate evaluation of urethral patency.

Caution must be used when selecting various drugs for azotemic cats. Although glucocorticoid therapy has been advocated to minimize inflammatory swelling of the urethra, glucocorticoids may aggravate the severity of potentially life-threatening anemia by inducing protein catabolism (via gluconeogenesis). Likewise, administration of acidifying agents to azotemic cats may aggravate the severity of existing metabolic acidosis. Indiscriminate use of any drug in patients with renal dysfunction must be avoided because of potential adverse drug reactions associated with the uremic state.

Following relief of urethral obstruction, a transitory obligatory postobstructive diuresis may develop. Even though polyuric cats may consume some water, it is often insufficient to maintain proper fluid balance. Therefore, it may be necessary to supplement water intake by parenteral administration of rehydrating or maintenance fluids.

Indwelling Transurethral Catheters - We do not recommend routine use of indwelling urinary catheters in cats following relief of urethral obstruction because they may induce further damage to the urinary tract. Disruption of the glycosaminoglycan (GAG) coating of the urothelium as a result of indwelling urethral catheters may promote adherence of microbes and urinary tract infection. Disruption of the GAG coating may also facilitate adherence of crystals to the urothelium, facilitating their growth and/or aggregation.

Indwelling urinary catheters may be indicated following relief of urethral obstruction to: 1) facilitate measurement of urine formation rate during intensive care of critically ill cats, 2) promote recovery of detrusor atony by maintaining an empty bladder, and 3) prevent recurrence of urethral obstruction caused by urine precipitates or mural abnormalities in high risk patients. The likelihood of whether or not a cat will voluntarily resume micturition may be assessed by evaluation of: 1) the caliber of the urine stream during the voiding phase of micturition, 2) the abundance of material in urine with the potential to occlude the urethral lumen, and 3) the adequacy of detrusor tone immediately following relief of urethral obstruction.

When use of indwelling urinary catheters is deemed to be beneficial, several precautions will minimize catheter-induced complications. Sterilized catheters composed of soft, pliable material are preferred because they are less likely to cause trauma to the urinary tract. Catheters constructed of relatively inert material will minimize toxicity to adjacent tissues. To minimize injury to proximal portions of the urethra and especially the urinary bladder, insertion of an excessive length of catheter should be avoided. If the wall of the urinary bladder is not hypotonic, use of an open-ended catheter that extends only a short distance into the bladder lumen is recommended. To minimize ascending urinary tract infection, the urethral catheter should be connected to a closed sterilized drainage system when possible. Likewise, administration of a broad-spectrum antimicrobial agent such as ampicillin may be considered. However, since urinary tract infection by resistant microbes will develop in some patients during antimicrobial therapy, follow-up urine culture and susceptibility tests are essential to determine the need for, and the type of, additional antimicrobial therapy. An alternative is to consider administration of antibiotics during indwelling transurethral catheterization only if evidence of infection is detected. This will minimize the likelihood of infection caused by bacteria which are resistant to antimicrobial agents. If catheter-induced bacterial infection develops and remains asymptomatic, it may be treated with antibiotics following removal of the catheter. Urethral catheters should be removed within as short a time span as possible (12 to 36 hours) to minimize catheter-induced iatrogenic disease. The cat should then be observed for signs of a reobstruction during a 12- to 24-hour period before being discharged from the hospital.

In one study of cats with induced cystitis and indwelling transurethral catheters attached to a closed collection system, glucocorticoids increased the susceptibility of the cats to bacterial urinary tract infection without decreasing urinary tract infection.[23] Intravesicular injection of DMSO did not decrease the incidence of bacterial urinary tract infection or the severity of inflammation.[23]

Acknowledgment

The authors gratefully acknowledge the technical assistance of Annette DesLauriers, Chris Hall, Debbie Molls, Lori Schultz, and Marcia Johnson.

REFERENCES

1. Osborne CA, Kruger JM, Johnston GR, Polzin DJ: Feline lower urinary tract disorders, in Ettinger SJ (ed): *Textbook Of Veterinary Internal Medicine*, ed 2, vol 2. Philadelphia, PA, WB Saunders Co, 1989, pp 2057-2082.
2. Osborne CA, Sanna JJ, Unger LK, Clinton CW, Davenport MP: Analyzing the mineral composition of uroliths from dogs, cats, horses, cattle, sheep, goats, and pigs. *Vet Med* 84:750-764, 1989.
3. Ling GV, Franti CE, Ruby AL, Johnson DL: Epizootiologic evaluation and quantitative analysis of urinary calculi from 150 cats. *JAVMA* 196:1459-1462, 1990.
4. Sanders G, Hesse A, Leusmann DB: Experimental investigation of the genesis of struvite stones in cats. *Scanning Electron Microscopy* IV:1713-1719, 1986.
5. Osborne CA, Lulich JP, Kruger JM, Polzin DJ, Johnston GR, Kroll RA: Medical dissolution of feline struvite urocystoliths. *JAVMA* 196:1053-1063, 1990.
6. Osborne CA, Lulich JP, Bartges JW, Polzin DJ: Feline metabolic uroliths: Risk factor management, in Bonagura JD, Kirk RW (ed): *Current Veterinary Therapy*, XI. Philadelphia, WB Saunders Co, 1992.
7. Lulich JP, Osborne CA, Carlson M, et al: Nonsurgical removal of urocystoliths in dogs and cats by voiding urohydropropulsion. *JAVMA* 203:660-663, 1993.
8. DiBartola SP, Chew DJ, Horton ML: Cystinuria in a cat. *JAVMA* 198:102-104, 1981.
9. Kruger JM, Osborne CA: The role of viruses in feline lower urinary tract disease. *J Vet Int Med* 4:71-78, 1990.
10. Barsanti JA, Finco DR, Shotts EB, Blue J, Ross L: Feline urologic syndrome: Further investigation into etiology. *JAAHA* 18:391-395, 1982.
11. Lees GE, Osborne CA, Stevens JB: Antibacterial properties of urine: Studies of feline urine specific gravity, osmolality, and pH. *JAAHA* 15:135-141, 1979.
12. Gregory CR, Vasseur PB: Long-term examination of cats with perianal urethrostomy. *Vet Surg* 12:210-212, 1983.
13. Osborne CA, Caywood DD, Johnston GR, Polzin DJ, Lulich JP, Kruger JM: Comparison of perineal urethrostomy

(continues on page 223)

Bacterial Urinary Tract Infections: Invasion, Host Defenses, and New Approaches to Prevention

David F. Senior, BVSc
Department of Medical Sciences
College of Veterinary Medicine
University of Florida
Gainesville, Florida

The urinary tract, including the proximal urethra, is bacteriologically sterile in healthy individuals, even though the distal urethra and vulva or prepuce support a normal flora of bacteria. Normal individuals are resistant to bacterial urinary tract infection (UTI). Bacterial inoculation of the bladder in experimental animals usually fails to establish UTI beyond two to three days unless the uroepithelium is first damaged by a chemical or mechanical insult. Despite this normal high resistance to establishment of UTI in normal animals, some individuals are predisposed to recurrent UTI. Small animal practitioners are frequently confronted by patients with persistent or recurrent bacterial UTI that exists despite any demonstrable anatomic defects. Host defenses are remarkably efficient in healthy individuals, but in patients with recurrent UTI, disruption of protective mechanisms allows bacterial colonization. This article reviews facts and conjecture regarding bacterial invasion and host-defense mechanisms that have led to new approaches to the management of patients with recurrent UTI.

Bacterial Invasion

Most bacterial UTI is caused by microorganisms that ascend to the bladder via the urethra. Bacterial invasion depends on the special properties of uropathogens that allow them to colonize the uroepithelium. The process of infection involves initial colonization of the genitalia, passage or transport along the urethra, and finally adherence to the uroepithelial surface.

In humans, the original source of the infecting bacteria is almost always the fecal flora; however, the frequency with which a particular strain of bacteria causes UTI is not simply based on its occurrence in feces.[1] The fecal flora of humans is mostly composed of nonsporulating anaerobes such as *Bacterioides, Fusobacterium, Veillonella,* and *Bifidobacterium,* while the most common urinary pathogen is *Escherichia coli,* which represents less than 1% of the total flora.[1] Of the more than 150 known serotypes of *E. coli,* only five account for most UTI in humans.[1] In the dog, in which the fecal flora has not been well characterized, the same situation may exist. *Escherichia coli* has been reported to

TABLE I
Bacterial Isolates in Canine UTI

Bacterial Isolates	Percent of Total		
	Ref. 2 (n = 1400)	Ref. 3 (n = 187)	Ref. 4 (n = 40)
Escherichia coli	37.8	36.4	67
Staphylococcus aureus	14.5	18.7	6
Proteus mirabilis	12.4	31.0	3
α-hemolytic streptococci	10.7	8.6	—
Klebsiella pneumoniae	8.1	4.8	—
Pseudomonas	3.4	2.7	—
Enterobacter	2.6	5.9	3
Other Proteus spp.	2.4	—	—
β-hemolytic streptococci	1.9	—	6
Miscellaneous	6.1	—	—
Other staphylococci and micrococci	—	2.0	15

be the most commonly isolated uropathogen in dogs,[2-4] but serotyping apparently has not been performed (Table I). These data suggest that uropathogens possess unique properties enabling them to colonize the uroepithelium.[1]

Genital Colonization

The vulval flora is not the same as the fecal flora and does not include urinary pathogens in healthy women. Studies in women with recurrent bacterial UTI revealed that uropathogen colonization of the vulva preceded

TABLE II
Bacteria Isolated from the Prepuce and Vagina of Normal Dogs

Isolates	Frequency of Isolation (%)			
	Prepuce Ref. 7 (n = 20)	Prepuce Ref. 8 (n = 51)	Vagina Ref. 7 (n = 20) (intact)	Vagina Ref. 7 (n = 20) (spayed)
Staphylococcus aureus	60	20	70	55
Mycoplasma spp.	35	0	30	5
Corynebacterium	15	0	35	15
Staphylococcus epidermidis	15	31	5	10
Streptococcus canis	15	0	35	45
Escherichia coli	10	10	25	25
Moraxella spp.	10	0	10	0
Streptococcus viridans	10	8	20	15
Hemophilis spp.	5	0	0	0
Acinetobacter spp.	5	0	0	0
Flavobacterium spp.	5	0	5	0
Klebsiella pneumoniae	5	0	5	5
Proteus mirabilis	5	4	5	25
Streptococcus equisimilis	5	0	0	0
Enterobacter spp.	0	0	5	0
Pasteurella spp.	0	0	5	15
Pseudomonas aeruginosa	0	0	5	10
Streptococcus faecalis	0	0	5	10
No growth	10	14	0	0

bacterial cystitis.[5,6] When the vulval flora returned to normal, recurrent bacterial UTI ceased to occur.

Similar studies have not been performed in dogs, but the normal preputial and vaginal flora have been surveyed in a number of instances (Table II).[7-9] The most frequently found organisms in the canine vulva were *Staphylococcus aureus*, *Streptococcus canis*, *Corynebacterium* spp., *Mycoplasma* spp., and *E. coli. Proteus mirabilis* appeared to be more frequently isolated in spayed than in intact dogs. The isolates from the male prepuce were similar. By contrast, the most frequently recovered uropathogen is *E. coli*. Thus, the situation in the dog is somewhat analogous to that in humans, but it is not known if the enterobacteria in the normal flora are different serotypes than those that become uropathogens.

Passage Along the Urethra

Bacterial uropathogens must travel along the urethra to the bladder following genital colonization. It has been hypothesized that organisms can swim against the flow of urine or progressively grow along the urethral wall.[1] Turbulent urine flow caused by anatomic defects can assist ascent of bacteria into the bladder.[1] Anatomic urethral deformity that occurs during intercourse is a major factor in bacterial ascent along the urethra in women.[1] This phenomenon has not been studied in dogs.

Bacterial Adherence to Mucosal Surfaces

Recent evidence strongly supports a major role of bacterial adherence in colonization of vaginal[10,11] and urethral surfaces[12] and uroepithelial cells.[13] Bacterial adherence to epithelial surfaces is achieved by molecular binding between fimbriae or fibrillae and specific receptor sites on the uroepithelial surface (Figure 1).

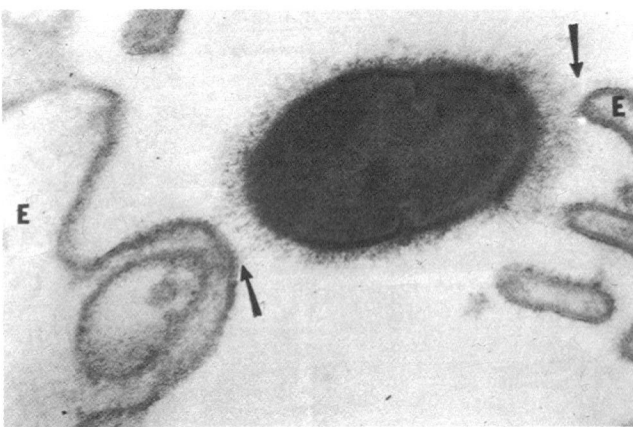

Figure 1—Electron micrograph of an ultrathin section of group A streptococcal cells (*center*) adherent to the villi of pharyngeal epithelial cell (*E*). The surface fibrillar network composed of protein-lipotechoic acid complexes appears to mediate the attachment of organisms to the epithelial cell membrane. (From Beachey EH, Ofek I: Epithelial cell binding of group A streptococci by lipotechoic acid on fimbriae denuded of M protein. *J Exp Med* 143:759-771, 1976. Reprinted with permission.)

Fimbriae and fibrillae are long, filamentous projections from gram-negative and gram-positive bacterial cell walls, respectively.

When bacteria approach the uroepithelial surface, they encounter a number of attractive and repulsive forces. Attractive forces due to fluctuating dipoles of similar frequency on both bacterial and epithelial surfaces are active over a relatively long distance. Also, long hydrophobic molecules extending from bacterial surfaces are attracted to the phospholipid epithelial cell membranes. Both of these forces tend to bring bacteria into close apposition with the uroepithelium; however, extremely close apposition is prevented by strong repulsive forces, because both the bacterial cell wall and the uroepithelium are negatively charged. The repulsive forces are only active over a short range. Thus, the opposing forces of attraction and repulsion allow bacteria to come very close to the uroepithelial surface, but repulsive forces prevent actual contact.

Bacterial adherence to uroepithelium is achieved by the fimbriae or fibrillae (Figure 2). Specific molecular structures on fimbriae and fibrillae, called *adhesins*, bind with complementary receptor sites on epithelial cell surfaces. Once a sufficient number of adhesin-receptor interactions occur, bacteria are permanently "docked" or attached. In this way, fimbriae and fibrillae bridge the gap between bacterial and epithelial surfaces.

The molecular structure of a number of adhesins and receptors has been established. Lipotechoic acid appears to be the adhesin on the fibrillae of group A streptococci.[14] The complementary epithelial receptor site remains unknown, but evidence suggests that it may be an albuminlike membrane protein or lipoprotein.[15] Certain strains of *E. coli* bind to mannose residues in the host cell membrane, while others bind to more complex carbohydrates, including hexosylceramide.[16,17] Although at least nine different adhesin-receptor systems have been found, probably many other systems remain to be identified. In addition, virus infection may induce new membrane receptors that recognize adhesins not previously recognized by uninfected cells.[18-20]

Although only one adhesin-receptor system has been identified for each of most bacteria, some may manifest more than one adhesin at the same time or may alter the adhesin type being expressed. The adhesins in some bacteria are controlled by genes in extrachromosomal DNA (plasmids).[21] The expression of adhesins may change rapidly, depending on growth phases. This phenomenon may be important in different phases of tissue invasion because adhesins render bacteria more susceptible to phagocytosis. Bacteria that undergo rapid phenotypic variation so that adhesins are not expressed once tissue invasion begins are less susceptible to phagocytosis (Figure 3).[15] The on-off switch for formation of bacterial adhesins is probably located in chromosomal DNA.[22]

Bacterial adherence is essential to subsequent tissue invasion. It also allows enhanced action by bacterial

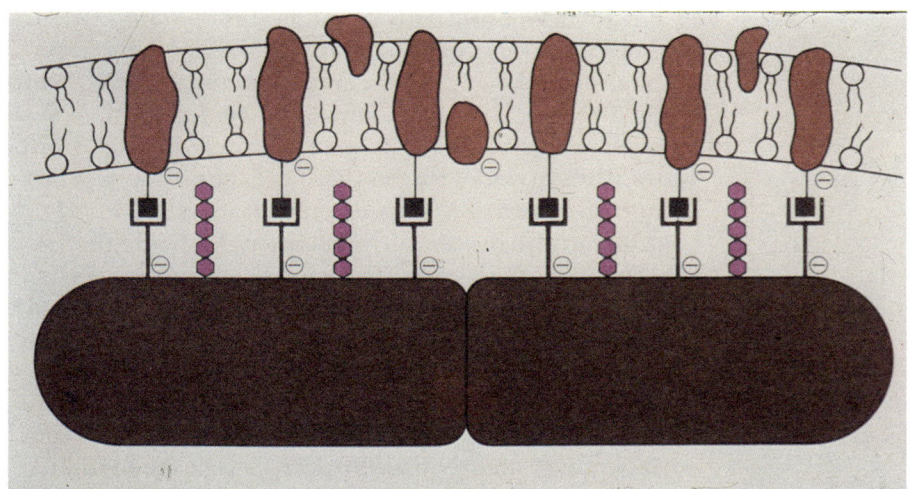

Figure 2—Attachment of a bacterial cell (*bottom*) via a specific adhesin to complementary receptors on the host cell membrane (*top*). To overcome the net negative charge on both the bacterial and host cell surfaces, hydrophobic molecules on the surface of bacteria are attracted toward the hydrophobic phospholipid molecules in the lipid bilayer membrane. (From Beachey EH [ed]: *Bacterial Adherence*. London, Chapman and Hall, 1980, pp 1-29. Reprinted with permission.)

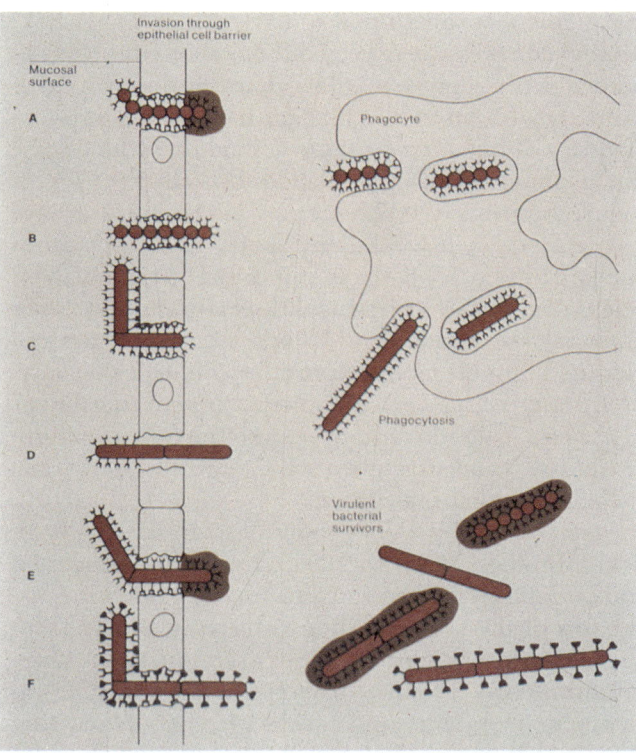

Figure 3—Diagrammatic representation of the adaptability of virulent bacteria to the pressures of their microenvironment. Adhesins that cause bacteria to adhere to the mucosal epithelial cells and that are also recognizable by phagocytic cells (*top right*) must be either masked with capsular material (*A and E*) or shed (*D and E*). Cells that do not shed or mask their adhesins tend to be ingested and killed by phagocytes (*top right*). (From Beachey EH, Eisenstein BI, Ofek I: *Bacterial Adherence in Infectious Diseases*. Kalamazoo, MI, The Upjohn Co, 1982, p 34. Reprinted with permission.)

nonpathogenic flora may exclude colonization by uropathogens and protect against UTI by a number of mechanisms. As the normal flora is bound to epithelial receptor sites, it may limit the accessibility of the epithelial surface to pathogenic bacteria.[24,25] Further, bacteriocins produced by the normal flora may disrupt the metabolism of uropathogens and prevent vaginal or preputial colonization. Bacteriocins are substances produced by one strain of bacteria that can interfere with the normal metabolism of other strains of bacteria.[26] Also, the normal flora may have a high affinity but a relatively low requirement for essential nutrients needed by uropathogens.[27,28] Thus, by occupying epithelial binding sites, producing bacteriocins and preferentially consuming essential nutrients, the normal vulval and preputial flora can play a protective role in preventing uropathogen colonization. Other factors may also be involved.

There is considerable evidence that secretory immunoglobulins in cervicovaginal mucus and in urine assist in preventing UTI in humans. When cervicovaginal mucus from women with recurrent UTI and from normal controls was incubated with the predominant fecal *E. coli* from the same individual, only 25% of women with recurrent UTI demonstrated antibody coating of the bacteria, compared with 77% of the normal controls.[6] In another study, the concentration of secretory IgA in 24-hour urine samples tended to be lower in women prone to recurrent UTI compared with that of normal controls (Figure 4).[29] Because antibody coating prevents bacterial adherence, specific antibody production may be an important protective mechanism. The reason for reduced antibody production has not been established.

The surface of the urethral epithelium has been studied by scanning electron microscopy in female dogs.[30] The surface of the proximal urethral epithelium has folds called *microplicae* when the lumen is contracted; the folds flatten when the lumen is expanded during voiding. This structure is similar to that observed in the bladder. The distal urethral epithelium has fingerlike projections called *microvilli* similar to those in the

toxins that can more readily interact with toxin receptor sites on the uroepithelial cell surface rather than being inactivated by urine and mucus-inactivating components.

Host Defenses

The vulval bacterial flora in normal human females does not include uropathogens.[23] Colonization of the normal vulval and preputial luminal membranes with

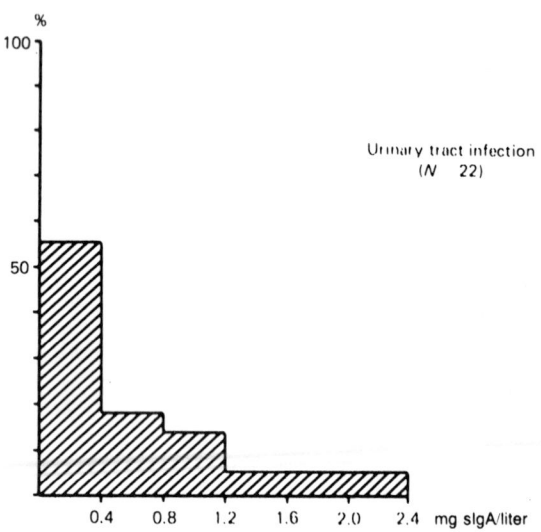

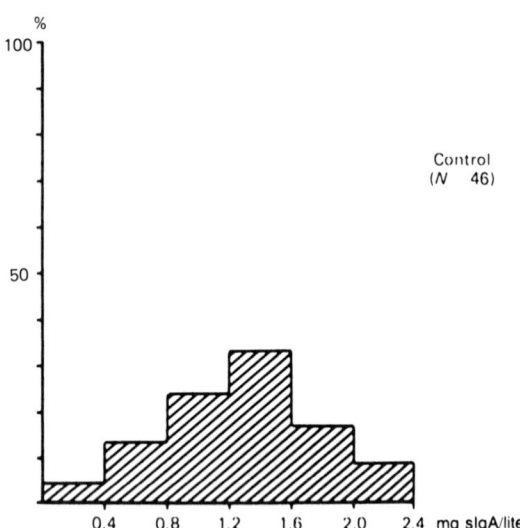

Figure 4—Frequency distribution of urinary secretory IgA concentration in 24-hour urine samples of women with recurrent urinary tract infection (*top*) and healthy control women (*below*). The distribution is approximately gaussian in control women; it is markedly skewed in women with a history of UTI. (From Riedasch G, Heck P, Rauterberg E, Ritz E: Does low urinary sIgA predispose to urinary tract infection? *Kidney Int* 23:759-763, 1983. Reprinted with permission.)

vagina. This structural difference is consistent with the presence or absence of a normal bacterial flora. The uroepithelium of the distal urethra and vagina supports a normal bacterial flora, while that of the bladder and proximal urethra does not. It has been suggested that these structural differences may be associated with resistance to bacterial colonization.[30]

The composition of urine appears to affect bacterial growth. Extremes of urine osmolality and pH tend to inhibit growth of many bacteria in rabbit, dog, and human urine.[31] In very concentrated urine, growth inhibition may not be due to hyperosmolality per se, but rather to high concentrations of urea, which is the most concentrated solute in urine.[31] Other unknown substances concentrated in urine can also inhibit bacterial growth. In dilute urine, growth inhibition may be due to lack of nutrients. Some strains of *Staph. aureus* and *Proteus* spp. exhibit relative resistance to high concentrations of urea, which may explain their frequent involvement in UTI. Compared with dogs with lower urinary tract disease, bacteria are rarely isolated from the urine of cats. This may be due to the physiologically normal hyperosmolality of cat urine.

Because urine can support bacterial growth, the one-way flow of constant urine entry from the ureters and repeated voiding is an important defense mechanism. Urine formation tends to dilute bladder urine bacterial counts, and frequent voiding eliminates bacteria from the bladder. The efficiency of this system is dependent on the rate of urine flow from the ureters, the frequency of voiding, and residual bladder volume after voiding. Decreased urine flow rate, prolonged periods between voiding, and a large residual bladder volume after voiding predispose the animal to bacteriuria (Table III).[1] Prolonged periods between voiding can occur in house-trained pets not given regular opportunities to urinate. Animals with an atonic bladder have a high residual bladder volume after urination. Bladder stone disease can also increase residual bladder volume.

Direct antibacterial properties of the mucosa have been proposed; however, in rabbits, this mechanism appears to play a relatively minor part in the bladder defense against UTI.[32] Mucosal secretion of a surface mucopolysaccharide layer composed of glycosaminoglycans is much more important to bladder defense. This protective barrier was shown to prevent attachment of bacteria, calcium, and protein to the uroepithelium of rabbits[32-34] and attachment of calcium oxalate crystals to the uroepithelium of rats.[35]

Destruction of the glycosaminoglycan layer by acid, neuraminidase,[34] or povidone-iodine[35] allows bacterial and calcium oxalate crystal attachment. Following disruption of the glycosaminoglycan layer, replacement with a synthetic sulfonated glycosaminoglycan given intraluminally prevents bacterial and crystalline attachment in rabbits and rats.[33,35] It is proposed that heavily sulfonated glycosaminoglycans coat the uroepithelium and attract dipolar water molecules that become tightly bound to the negatively charged sulfate groups. This layer of glycosaminoglycans plus "fixed" water molecules could provide a water barrier and thus mask highly charged regions on the cell surfaces.[33]

The production and secretion of the normal protective glycosaminoglycan layer appears to be under hormonal control by estrogen and progesterone in rabbits.[36] Peaks of the incidence of UTI prior to puberty and after menopause in celibate women have been suggested as evidence of a similar process in humans.[36,37] An increased incidence of UTI in spayed bitches may be further indirect evidence of the importance of a similar effect in the dog[36]; however, these effects may be multifactorial and not simply related to mucopolysaccharide production by bladder uroepithelium.

Secretion of mucosal mucopolysaccharide can be

TABLE III

Effect of Normal Voiding, Infrequent Voiding, and High Residual Bladder Volume on Urinary Bacterial Counts

Parameter Measured	Time (Minutes)	No. Bacteria[a]	Volume[b,c]	Bacteria/ml[d]
Normal voiding	0	100	1	100
(every 240	240	6400	241	27
minutes)	480	1699	241	7
	720	451	241	2
Prolonged urine	0	100[d]	1	100
retention (480 vs.	480	4.1×10^5	481	851
240 minutes)	960	3.5×10^6	481	7251
	1440	3.0×10^7	481	0.62×10^5
	1920	2.5×10^8	481	5.3×10^5
High residual	0	4000[d]	40	100
bladder volume	240	2.6×10^5	280	914
(40 vs. 1 ml)	480	2.3×10^6	280	8.4×10^3
	720	2.1×10^7	280	7.6×10^4
	960	2.0×10^8	280	7.0×10^5

[a]The number of bacteria doubles in 40 minutes.
[b]1 ml residual bladder volume
[c]1 ml/minute urine production rate
[d]100 bacteria/ml seeded into the initial urine

altered by oral administration of the licorice derivative carbenoxolone. This effect has been observed in rabbits and humans.[37] When carbenoxolone was given to rabbits following acid treatment and *E. coli* infection of the bladder, it enhanced the rate of clearance of infection compared with untreated control animals.[37]

In summary, a number of physiologic abnormalities have been identified in human patients prone to recurrent bacterial UTI, including reduced levels of secretory immunoglobulin in cervicovaginal mucus and urine, altered vaginal flora, abnormal bladder function, and an abnormal glycosaminoglycan layer in the bladder. More than one factor may be important in an individual patient, and other factors probably remain to be discovered.

New Approaches to Prevention of Infection

A number of approaches to infection prevention in susceptible patients have been suggested in view of recent knowledge about the pathogenesis of bacterial UTI.

Bacterial adherence is mediated by specific molecules, so that analogues that block the molecular site of attachment on bacterial or mucosal cell walls may prevent bacterial attachment. Mannose and similar molecules block the receptor sites for some strains of *E. coli*.[38] When a mannose residue was infused into the bladders of mice, mucosal colonization by simultaneously infused *E. coli* was greatly reduced.[38] The infused mannose residue probably combined with bacterial adhesin sites and prevented docking with mannoselike uroepithelial receptor sites. The choice of the mannose residue used is critical, because some types become incorporated into human epithelial cells and actually enhance bacterial attachment.[39,40]

The surface mucopolysaccharide layer composed of glycosaminoglycans that coats uroepithelial surfaces is a major natural barrier to bacterial colonization. In an experimental model of bacterial UTI, bladder infusion of heparin, a synthetic glycosaminoglycan, reduced bacterial attachment in rabbits after the natural glycosaminoglycan layer had been damaged by povidone-

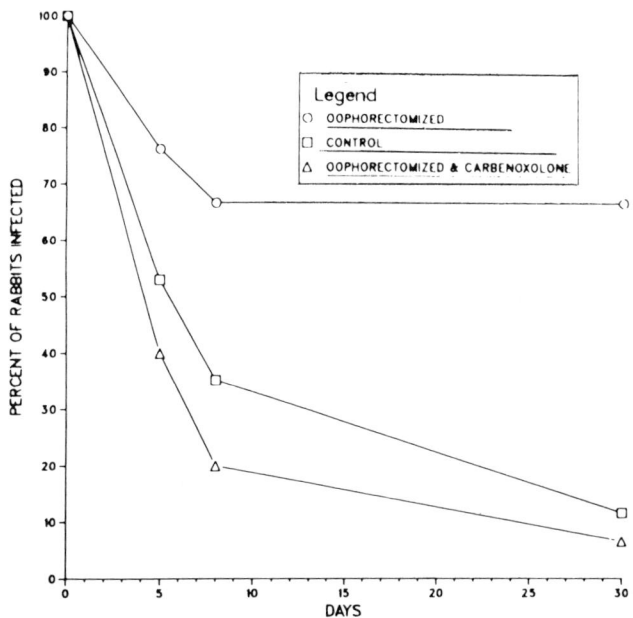

Figure 5—The ability of animals in three experimental groups of rabbits to clear induced *E. coli* urinary tract infections. Carbenoxolone appeared to correct delayed clearance observed in oophorectomized animals. (From Mooreville M, Fritz RW, Mulholland SG: Enhancement of the bladder defense mechanism by an exogenous agent. *J Urol* 130:607-609, 1983. Reprinted with permission.)

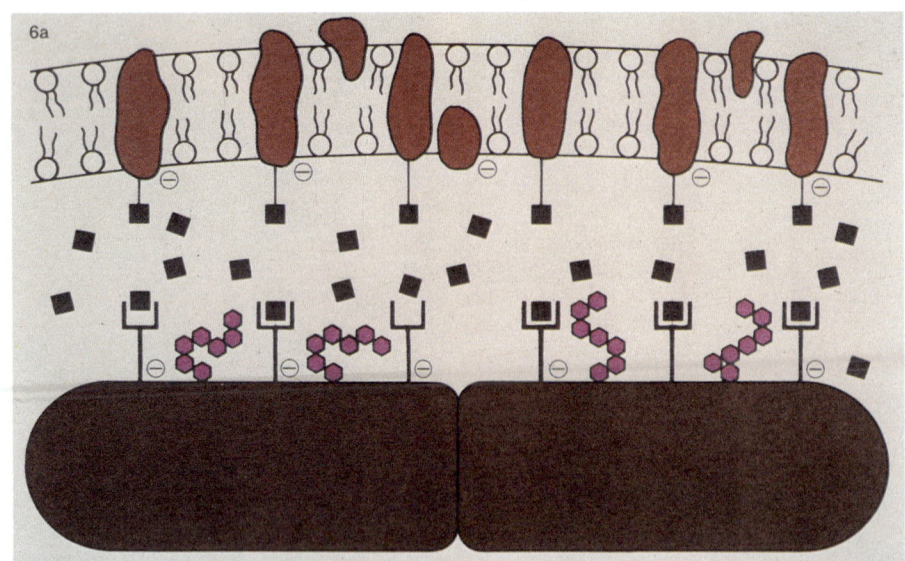

Figure 6—Specific blockade of bacterial adherence by an excess of isolated receptor analogue material. (From Beachey EH [ed]: *Bacterial Adherence*. London, Chapman and Hall, 1980, pp 1-29. Reprinted with permission.)

iodine treatment.[35] Carbenoxolone increased mucopolysaccharide production by epithelial surfaces. Oral administration of carbenoxolone corrected the reduced ability to clear experimental infection observed in oophorectomized rabbits (Figure 5).[37] Because heparin must be instilled into the bladder directly, its use in the clinical situation is limited. On the other hand, carbenoxolone was effective in experimental rabbits when given orally and may be a possible preventive measure.[37]

The synthetic glycosaminoglycan pentosanpolysulfate prevented bacterial adherence following acid damage of the endogenous mucopolysaccharide layer in rabbits.[41] There is some evidence that pentosanpolysulfate is excreted in the urine after oral administration, so this drug may be another nonspecific protective measure for chronically reinfected patients.[42]

Substances that interfere with bacterial expression of fimbrial adhesins would also be expected to prevent attachment and colonization. In vitro, subminimum inhibitory concentration urine concentrations of penicillin G suppressed fimbrial expression by resting group A streptococci and caused them to lose their adherence capacity.[43] Similarly, subminimum inhibitory concentration urine concentrations of penicillin, ampicillin, and amoxicillin prevented fimbriae formation and adherence of *E. coli* in the growth phase to human epithelial cells.[44-47] Subminimum inhibitory concentration levels of streptomycin caused production of large aberrant fimbriae by *E. coli*, and adherence to epithelial cells was impaired.[48] In humans and dogs, single daily administration of antibiotics at one half to one eighth the normal daily dose is well recognized as a preventive strategy for chronic recurrent bacterial UTI.[49,50] The success of this regimen may be partially due to interference with fimbrial formation by bacteria.

Production of fimbriae by *Salmonella typhimurium* appears to be under the control of cyclic AMP. Metabolic suppression of cyclic AMP by various sugars disrupted fimbriae formation in vitro,[51] so the use of other substances to disrupt bacterial metabolism and prevent normal fimbrial formation is a future possibility.

Substances that interfere with bacterial attachment and fimbrial formation or that coat the uroepithelial surface are likely to have a short-term effect confined to their period of administration. With an immunologic approach, long-term protection may be possible. A vaccine composed of fimbriae could cause production of an antifimbrial antibody. If the antibody were present in secretions, it could combine with the fimbriae, cover the adhesin-combining site, and prevent bacterial adherence (Figure 6). Fimbrial vaccines derived from certain pathogenic strains of *E. coli* have been given to pregnant cows and sows. Subsequent offspring that suckled colostrum rich in antibodies directed against *E. coli* fimbriae were protected against experimental *E. coli* enterocolitis.[52-54] Such vaccines are commercially available in some countries.[14] This principle has also been applied to the urinary tract, where a fimbrial vaccine directed against type 1 fimbriae prevented experimental pyelonephritis due to *E. coli* expressing type 1 fimbriae in rats.[55] More recently, a fimbrial vaccine prevented experimental pyelonephritis due to P-fimbriated *E. coli* in monkeys.[56]

At present, the immunologic approach to prevention of UTI is only a laboratory phenomenon. Many different adhesin receptor systems have been identified, and current work does not suggest that a broad-spectrum vaccine will soon be developed. Other, more practical, possibilities may become apparent, though, as the nature of bacterial adherence is further elucidated.

REFERENCES

1. O'Grady F: Urinary tract infection: Initiation and ascent, in Chisholm GD, Williams DI (eds): *Scientific Foundations of Urology*, ed 2. Chicago, Yearbook Medical Publishers Inc, 1982, pp 199-204.
2. Ling GV, Biberstein EC, Hirsch DC: Bacterial pathogens associated with urinary tract infections. *Vet Clin North Am [Small Anim Pract]* 9:617-630, 1979.
3. Finco DR: Urinary tract infections, in Kirk RW (ed): *Current Veterinary Therapy VII*. Philadelphia, WB Saunders Co, 1980, pp 1158-1161.
4. Kiristo A-K, Vasenius H, Sandholm M: Canine bacteriuria. *J Small Anim Pract* 18:707-712, 1977.
5. Stamey TA, Timothy M, Millar M, Mihara G: Recurrent urinary infections in adult women. The role of introital enterobacteria. *Calif Med* 115:1-19, 1971.
6. Stamey TA, Wehner N, Mihara G, Condy M: The immunologic basis of recurrent bacteriuria: Role of cervicovaginal antibody in enterobacterial colonization of the introital mucosa. *Medicine* 57:47-56, 1978.
7. Ling GV, Ruby AL: Aeorbic bacterial flora of the prepuce, urethra, and vagina of normal adult dogs. *Am J Vet Res* 39:695-698, 1978.
8. Allen WE, Dagnall GJR: Some observations on the aerobic bacterial flora of the genital tract of the dog and bitch. *J Small Anim Pract* 23:325-335, 1982.
9. Hinman F: Metal recolonization in bitches. *Trans Am Assoc Genitourinary Surg* 68:73-77, 1977.
10. Fowler JE, Stamey TA: Studies of introital colonization in women with recurrent urinary infections. VII. The role of bacterial adherence. *J Urol* 117:472-476, 1977.
11. Fowler JE, Stamey TA: Studies of introital colonization in women with recurrent urinary infections. X. Adhesive properties of *Escherichia coli* and *Proteus mirabilis*: Lack of correlation with urinary pathogenicity. *J Urol* 120:315-318, 1978.
12. Kallenius G, Winberg J: Bacterial adherence to periurethral epithelial cells in girls prone to urinary-tract infections. *Lancet* 2:540-543, 1978.
13. Svanborg-Eden C, Jodal V: Attachment of *Escherichia coli* to urinary sediment epithelial cells from urinary tract infection-prone and healthy children. *Infect Immunol* 26:837-840, 1979.
14. Beachey EH, Ofek I: Epithelial cell binding of group A streptococci by lipotechoic acid on fimbriae denuded of M protein. *J Exp Med* 143:759-771, 1976.
15. Beachey EH, Eisenstein BI, Ofek I: *Bacterial Adherence in Infectious Diseases. Current Concepts*. Kalamazoo, MI, The Upjohn Co, 1982.
16. Leffler H, Svanborg-Eden C: Glycolipid receptors for uropathogenic *Escherichia coli* on human erythrocytes and uroepithelial cells. *Infect Immunol* 34:920-929, 1981.
17. Kallenius G, Mollby R, Svensen SV, et al: The pk antigen as receptor for the hemagglutination of pyelonephritic *Escherichia coli*. *SEMS Microbiol Lett* 7:297-302, 1980.
18. Sanford BA, Shelokov A, Ramsay MA: Bacterial adherence to virus-infected cells: A cell culture model of bacterial superinfection. *J Infect Dis* 137:176-181, 1978.
19. Sanford BA, Smith N, Shelokov A, Ramsay MA: Adherence of group B streptococci and human erythrocytes to influenza A virus-infected MDCK cells (40424). *Proc Soc Exp Biol Med* 160:226-232, 1979.
20. Sanford BA, Smith N, Shelokov A, Ramsay MA: Adherence of influenza A viruses to group B streptococci. *J Infect Dis* 141:496-506, 1980.
21. Duguid JP, Old DC: Adhesive properties of enterobacteriacae, in Beachey EH (ed): *Bacterial Adherence. Receptors and Recognition Series B*, vol 6. London, Chapman and Hall, 1980, pp 184-217.
22. Eisenstein B: Genetic regulation of type 1 fimbriae in *Escherichia coli*. Transcriptional control and phase variation analyzed by a pil-lac operon fusion. *Science* 214:337-339, 1981.
23. Stamey TA: The role of introital enterobacteria in recurrent urinary tract infections. *J Urol* 109:467-472, 1973.
24. Sprunt K, Redman W: Evidence suggesting importance of role of interbacterial inhibition in maintaining balance of normal flora. *Ann Intern Med* 68:579-590, 1968.
25. Sprunt K, Leidy GA, Redman W: Prevention of bacterial overgrowth. *J Infect Dis* 123:1-10, 1971.
26. Nomura M: Colicins and related bacteriocins. *Ann Rev Microbiol* 21:257-284, 1967.
27. Brock TD: Principles of microbial ecology. Englewood Cliffs, NJ, Prentice Hall Inc, 1966, pp 114-139.
28. Savage DC, McAllister JS: Microbial interactions at body surfaces and resistance to infectious diseases, in Dunlop RH, Moon HW (eds): *Resistance to Infectious Disease*. Saskatoon, Canada, Modern Press, 1970, pp 113-127.
29. Reidasch G, Heck P, Rauterberg E, Ritz E: Does low urinary sIgA predispose to urinary tract infection? *Kidney Int* 23:759-763, 1983.
30. Mooney JK, Hinman F: Surface differences in cells of proximal and distal canine urethra. *J Urol* 111:495-501, 1974.
31. Lees GE, Osborne CA: Antibacterial properties of urine: A comparative review. *JAAHA* 15:125-132, 1979.
32. Parsons CL, Greenspan C, Mulholland SG: The primary antibacterial defense mechanism of the bladder. *Invest Urol* 13:72-76, 1975.
33. Parsons CL, Stauffer C, Schmidt JD: Bladder-surface glycosaminoglycans: An efficient mechanism of environmental adaptation. *Science* 208:605-607, 1980.
34. Shrom SH, Parsons CL, Mulholland SG: Vesical defence: Further evidence for a charge-related mucosal anti-adherence mechanism. *Surg Forum* 29:632-633, 1978.
35. Chang S-Y, Gill WB, Vermeulen CW: Povidone-iodine bladder injury in rats and protection with heparin. *J Urol* 130:382-385, 1983.
36. Mulholland SG, Qureshi SM, Fritz RW, Silverman H: Effect of hormonal deprivation on the bladder defense mechanism. *J Urol* 127:1010-1013, 1982.
37. Mooreville M, Fritz RW, Mulholland SG: Enhancement of the bladder defense mechanism by an exogenous agent. *J Urol* 130:607-609, 1983.
38. Aronson M, Medalia O, Schori L, et al: Prevention of colonization of the urinary tract of mice with *Escherichia coli* by blocking of bacterial adherence with methyl alpha-D-mannopyranoside. *J Infect Dis* 139:329-332, 1979.
39. Leffler H, Svanborg-Eden C: Glycolipid receptors for uropathogenic *Escherichia coli* on human erythrocytes and uroepithelial cells. *Infect Immun* 34:920-929, 1981.
40. Kallenius G, Mollby R, Hultberg H, et al: Structure of carbohydrate part of receptor on human uroepithelial cells for pyelonephritogenic *Escherichia coli*. *Lancet* 2:604-606, 1981.
41. Parsons CL, Pollen JJ, Anwar H, et al: Antibacterial activity of bladder surface mucin duplicated in the rabbit by exogenous glycosaminoglycan (sodium pentosanpolysulfate). *Infect Immun* 27:876-881, 1980.
42. Parsons CL, Schmidt JD, Pollen JJ: Successful treatment of interstitial cystitis with sodium pentosanpolysulfate. *J Urol* 130:51-53, 1983.
43. Alkan ML, Beachey EH: Excretion of lipotechoic acid by group A streptococci: Influence of penicillin on excretion and loss of ability to adhere to human oral epithelial cells. *J Clin Invest* 61:671-677, 1978.
44. Ofek I, Beachey EH, Eisenstein BI, et al: Suppression of bacterial adherence by sublethal concentrations of β-lactam aminoglycoside antibiotics. *Rev Infect Dis* 1:832-837, 1979.
45. Eisenstein BI, Ofek I, Beachey EH: Interference with mannose binding and epithelial cell adherence of *Escherichia coli* by sublethal concentrations of streptomycin. *J Clin Invest* 63:1219-1228, 1979.
46. Eisenstein BI, Beachey EH, Ofek I: Influence of sublethal concentrations of antibiotics on the expression of mannose-specific ligand of *Escherichia coli*. *Infect Immun* 28:154-159, 1980.
47. Svanborg-Eden C, Sandberg T, Stenquist K, Ahlstedt S: Decrease in adhesion of *Escherichia coli* to human urinary tract epithelial cells in vitro by subinhibitory concentrations of ampicillin: A preliminary study. *Infection* 6:S121-S123, 1978.
48. Eisenstein BI, Ofek I, Beachey EH: Loss of lectin-like activity in aberrant type 1 fimbriae of *Escherichia coli*. *Infect Immun* 31:792-797, 1981.
49. Stamey TA: Urinary tract infections in women, in Harrison JH, Gittes RF, Perlmutter AD, et al (eds): *Campbell's Urology*, ed 4. Philadelphia, WB Saunders Co, 1978, pp 451-479.
50. Ling GV: Treatment of urinary tract infections. *Vet Clin North Am* 9(4):795-804, 1979.
51. Saier MH Jr, Schmidt MR, Leibowitz M: Cyclic AMP-dependent synthesis of fimbriae in *Salmonella typhimurium*: Effects of cya and pts mutations. *J Bacteriol* 134:356-358, 1978.

52. Rutter JM, Jones GW: Protection against enteric disease caused by *Escherichia coli*: A model for vaccination with a virulence determinant. *Nature* 242:531-532, 1973.

53. Acres SD, Isaacson RE, Babiuk LA, Kapitany RA: Immunization of calves against enterotoxigenic colibacillosis by vaccinating dams with purified K99 antigen and whole cell bacterins. *Infect Immun* 25:121-126, 1979.

54. Isaacson RE, Dean EA, Morgan RL, Moon HW: Immunization of suckling pigs against enterotoxigenic *Escherichia coli*-induced diarrheal disease by vaccinating dams with purified K99 or 987 P pili: Antibody production in response to vaccination. *Infect Immun* 29:824-826, 1980.

55. Silverblatt FJ, Cohen LS: Antipili antibody affords protection against experimental ascending pyelonephritis. *J Clin Invest* 64:333-336, 1979.

56. Roberts JA, Hardaway K, Kaack B, et al: Prevention of pyelonephritis by immunization with P-fimbriae. *J Urol* 131:602-607, 1984.

UPDATE

Recently, ultra-low-dose calcitriol (Rocaltrol®, Roche Laboratories) 1 to 3 ng/kg orally once daily has been shown to directly suppress parathyroid hormone production in dogs and cats with chronic renal failure. Although this dose appears to suppress parathyroid hormone levels very effectively, intestinal calcium absorption may not be appreciably increased because serum calcium levels do not rise. Even so, low-dose calcitriol is not recommended if hyperphosphatemia (>6 mg/dl) is present. Anecdotal reports suggest that patients feel and act better when calcitriol is administered; however, these findings are subjective. At the moment, there is no evidence that direct suppression of hyperparathyroidism with calcitriol reduces the rate of progression and increases survival in dogs and cats with chronic renal failure. The available human capsules must be reformulated to provide the needed low dose. A specialty pharmacy, Island Pharmacy Services (1-800-328-7060), can provide reformulated capsules or liquid for oral dosing.

The anemia of chronic renal failure responds dramatically to treatment with erythropoietin (Epogen®, Amgen; Procrit®, Ortho Biotech) given at 50 to 100 u/kg weekly. The lower doses can maintain a raised hematocrit level once the initial target packed cell volume has been achieved. About 60% of treated dogs develop antibodies to erythropoietin, but only 20% develop sufficiently high levels to block the effect of the drug. The drug is very expensive and is probably best reserved for patients with profound anemia, in whom the effect will be dramatic. Owners report an almost immediate (with 2 days of onset of treatment) improvement in the patient's feeling of well being.

Enalapril (Enacard®, Merck) may provide useful antihypertensive effects in dogs with chronic renal failure. Enalapril may cause fewer gastrointestinal upsets than captopril.

Urinary Tract Neoplasms in Dogs and Cats

Steven E. Crow, DVM
Department of Small Animal
Clinical Sciences
College of Veterinary Medicine
Michigan State University
East Lansing, Michigan

Neoplasms of the urinary bladder occur in dogs with greater frequency than tumors of other urinary tract organs, presumably because of the storage function of the bladder. Increased contact time of carcinogens, especially chemicals, with urothelial cells is apparently responsible for this predilection. In cats, renal tumors are more common, presumably because lymphosarcoma may occur more often in this species.

Neoplasms of the canine or feline urinary tract are diagnostic and therapeutic challenges for veterinarians. Diagnosis is often delayed because of a lack of overt clinical signs or a partial response to empirical treatment. Because delay can result in considerable progression of the neoplasm, a majority of urinary tract tumors are extensive at the time of definitive diagnosis.

Most urinary tract neoplasms are malignant, and thus careful evaluation of affected animals is indicated. The diagnostic workup should be directed at identifying (1) the organ(s) primarily involved; (2) the exact size and location of the neoplasm; (3) metastatic foci, if present; and (4) serious intercurrent diseases. Without such information, appropriate decisions regarding treatment and prognosis cannot be made.

A histogenetic basis for classification of primary urinary tract neoplasms is given in Table I.

Renal Neoplasms

Renal tumors constitute from 1.6% to 2.5% and from 0.6% to 1.7% of all reported neoplasms in cats and dogs, respectively.[1-4] In humans, the incidence of renal cancer has been increasing in the past decade; males are affected approximately twice as often as females.[5] In humans, factors that increase the risk of renal cancer include smoking, urban living, a family history of renal cancer, and exposure to radiographic contrast material.

Nitrosamines and anthraquinones also have been identified as carcinogens in experiments; epithelial cells in the renal tubules concentrate these chemicals, thereby potentiating malignant transformation.[5] None of these factors, however, has been correlated with naturally occurring renal neoplasms in dogs or cats.[1] Male dogs do have an increased predilection,[4] which might suggest that sex hormones may influence the development and/or maintenance of tumor cells in the kidneys. Regression of renal tumors in some humans treated with progestins further supports the concept of sex hormone regulation of renal neoplasms.[1,5]

Most primary renal tumors are malignant. Adenocarcinomas (also

Originally published in Volume 7, Number 8, August 1985

TABLE I
Histogenetic Classification of Urinary Tract Neoplasms

Origin	Cell Type	Benign	Malignant
Tubular epithelium	Renal	Adenoma	Adenocarcinoma
Epithelium of conducting apparatus	Transitional	Papilloma	Transitional cell carcinoma
Embryonal rests of metanephros	Undifferentiated	Nephroblastoma (Wilms' tumor)	Renal carcinoma
Supporting tissue	Fibroblasts	Fibroma	Fibrosarcoma
	Muscle fibers	Leiomyoma	Leiomyosarcoma
		Rhabdomyoma	Rhabdomyosarcoma
	Neurons	Neurofibroma	Neurofibrosarcoma
	Endothelium	Angioma	Angiosarcoma
	Adipocytes	Lipoma	Liposarcoma

known as *hypernephromas, Grawitz's tumors,* or *renal cell carcinomas*) account for a majority of renal cancers in dogs. These tumors originate from tubular cells and have unpredictable growth patterns. Some adenocarcinomas remain localized for months, while others metastasize early in their course. Metastasis occurs hematogenously and may affect the lungs, liver, brain, skin, spleen, eyes, or bone.[6–8] Histology of a metastatic deposit can be so characteristic that it may foretell the presence of a primary renal adenocarcinoma before any clinical signs of the kidney; mass are evident. Renal adenocarcinomas occur in older dogs (an average age of eight years) and are usually unilateral, affecting one pole of the kidney; occasionally, bilateral involvement is observed. Gross characteristics vary from a soft multinodular mass to a hard fibrous tumor (Figure 1). Adenocarcinomas are sometime cystic in nature and may invade the renal pelvis, ureters, and adjacent blood vessels.[1,4,6,7]

Neoplasms of the renal pelvis are rare. When they occur, they usually arise from transitional epithelial cells. Clinical findings are similar to those seen with adenocarcinomas.

Embryonal nephroma (also called *nephroblastoma* or *Wilms' tumor*) arises from the primordial metanephros (i.e., from pluripotential vestigial cells that have retained their embryonal characteristics). These tumors may differentiate into epithelium as well as mesen-

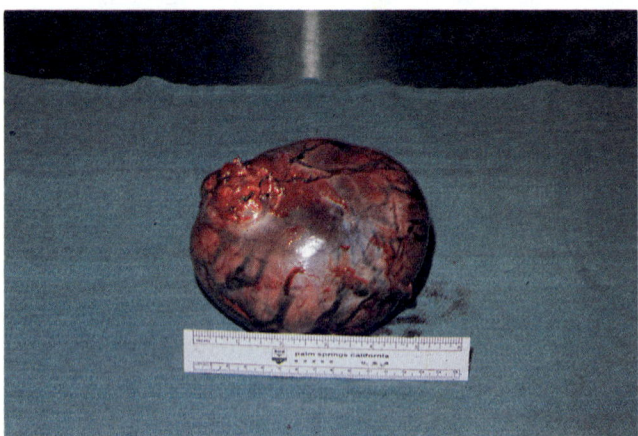

Figure 1A

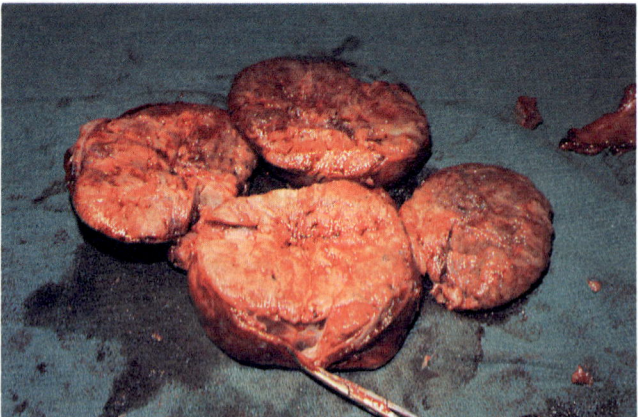

Figure 1B

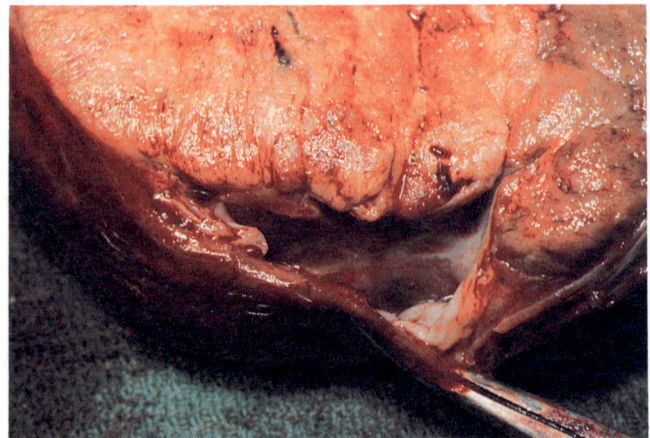

Figure 1C

Figure 1—(**A, B,** and **C**) Kidney removed from a dog with unilateral renal adenocarcinoma. This dog was presented for weight loss and anorexia of one-month duration. During surgery, a solitary hepatic metastatic nodule and retroperitoneal extension of the primary lesion were identified.

chymal tissues, such as muscle, cartilage, bone, or fat. In humans, embryonal nephroma accounts for 20% of childhood tumors and is usually diagnosed at three to four years of age.[9] Although this neoplasm is rare in dogs and cats, when it occurs it is seen in animals younger than two years of age.[3,4] While nephroblastomas in humans are usually malignant, many embryonal nephromas in dogs follow a benign course[1,9]; they are single, large masses that grow by expansion. Occasionally, invasion into perirenal tissue may be observed, and metastasis to the peritoneum and viscera has been recorded.[9]

Benign renal adenomas are rarely reported in animals.[1,2] The diagnosis of renal adenoma is controversial because it is not possible to determine biologic behavior by histologic criteria alone. Renal leiomyoma also has been reported in a dog.[10]

Metastatic or secondary renal tumors usually are not evident as clinical problems until they are in an advanced stage. In dogs, a variety of metastatic renal neoplasms have been reported, including hemangiosarcoma, malignant melanoma, and mammary adenocarcinoma.[1,11] The most common renal neoplasm in cats is lymphosarcoma; renal involvement is associated most often with the alimentary or multicentric forms of lymphosarcoma (Figure 2). Interestingly, only one fourth to one third of cats with renal lymphosarcoma shows a concurrent patent feline leukemia virus infection.[12] Renal lymphosarcoma also occurs in dogs.[1-3]

Paraneoplastic syndromes are commonly associated with renal neoplasms in humans and have been reported in dogs with kidney tumors as well. Erythrocytosis (polycythemia) associated with excessive secretion of erythropoietin or possibly resulting from local renal anoxia has been reported in a dog with hypernephroma.[13] A large left-flank mass may be mistaken for an enlarged spleen resulting from polycythemia vera. Careful palpation and anamnesis usually can guide the clinician to determining a correct diagnosis. Hypercalcemia occasionally is recognized; it may be caused by ectopic secretion of prostaglandin or parathormone or may be secondary to extensive bony metastasis. Lymphosarcoma and adenocarcinoma are tumors associated most frequently with these causes of hypercalcemia. Hypertrophic osteopathy has been reported in a cat with renal papillary adenoma.[14] In humans, other reported effects of renal neoplasms include fever, hepatomegaly, hypertension (resulting from increased renin activity), and amyloidosis.[5]

Anemia, hematuria, and fever are common clinical findings. . . .

The practitioner usually can diagnose renal tumors by evaluating clinical signs, a routine blood count and urinalysis, and radiographic studies. Anemia, hematuria, and fever are common clinical findings; however, these signs rarely are present concurrently. A mass and/or low-grade pain in the flank may be evident on abdominal palpation. Weight loss, muscle weakness (associated with hypercalcemia), polyuria, polydipsia, and hindlimb edema have also been observed.[1,3,7]

Although proteinuria and hematuria may be evident, the urinalysis can be normal in many cases. Nonregenerative anemia or erythrocytosis may be present. In humans with renal tumors, increased α_1 and α_2 globulins have been noted.[6] Advanced cases may exhibit renal failure, especially when both kidneys are involved.

Survey abdominal radiographs frequently can demonstrate a retroperitoneal mass (Figure 3). Excretory urography occasionally can be helpful in delineating a neoplasm from normal kidney tissue. Renal angiography or computer-assisted tomography (although rarely performed) can clarify the extent of renal masses.

Percutaneous or punch biopsies are easy to perform and may yield a diagnosis after cytologic and/or histologic evaluation. Cytologic evaluation of a fine-needle aspirate often can yield a definitive diagnosis when the enlarged kidney results from diffuse infiltration of the parenchyma with lymphosarcoma cells. Occasionally, exploratory laparotomy may be required to establish a diagnosis.

Survey thoracic radiographs should be taken before considering invasive diagnostic techniques. Multiple, round interstitial nodules are characteristic of pulmonary metastasis from adenocarcinomas (Figure 4). Other radiographic patterns are seen with metastatic foci caused by other types of renal neoplasms.

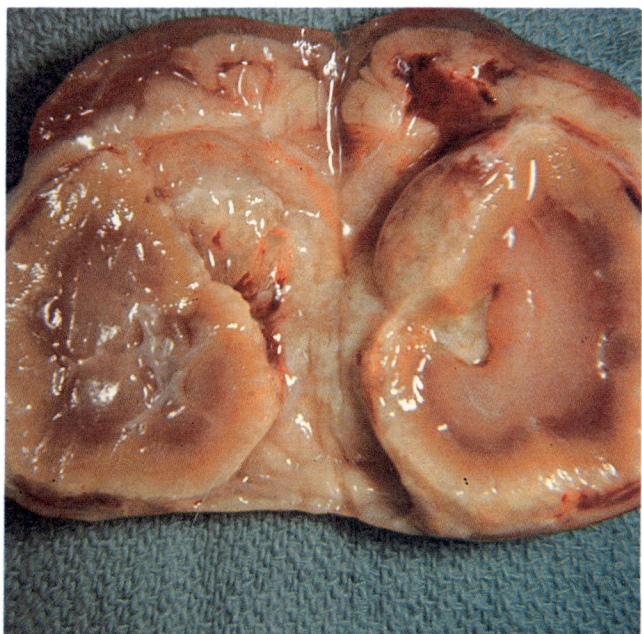

Figure 2—Kidney removed from a cat with renal lymphosarcoma. Both kidneys were severely infiltrated by abnormal lymphoid cells; the cat was azotemic.

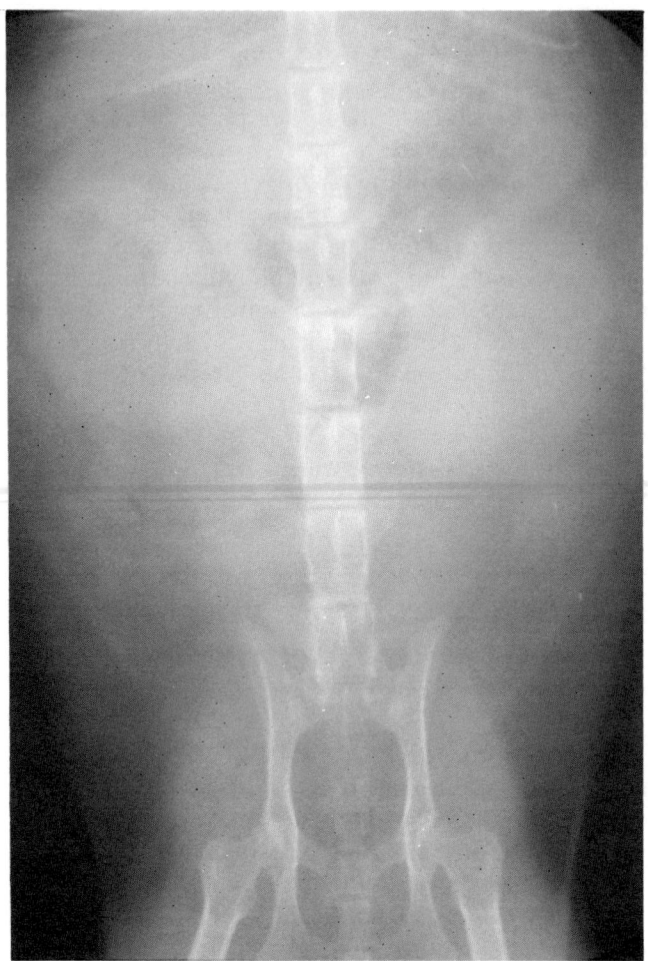

Figure 3—A survey abdominal radiograph of the cat mentioned in Figure 2. Two large, irregularly shaped kidneys can be visualized easily.

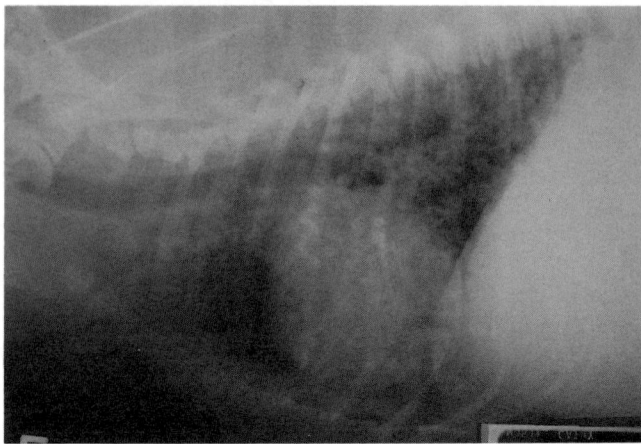

Figure 4—The multiple well-defined interstitial nodules in the lung fields represent pulmonary metastasis from a renal adenocarcinoma.

Renal neoplasms are usually treated by unilateral nephrectomy and ureterectomy[1]; obviously, neither mode of therapy can be applicable when renal involvement is bilateral. Most renal neoplasms are contained within the organ capsule at the time of diagnosis, permitting resection of the mass. When the caudal vena cava, lumbar musculature, or adrenal glands are invaded by a tumor, removal of the tumor rarely is possible. Highly aggressive or invasive renal carcinomas should receive adjuvant cytotoxic chemotherapy after a 10- to 14-day recovery period. Combinations of 5-fluorouracil (Fluorouracil—Roche Laboratories), doxorubicin hydrochloride (Adriamycin™—Adria Laboratories), and cyclophosphamide (Cytoxan®—Mead Johnson Pharmaceutical) have been used on occasion in dogs (Table II), but evidence for objective response has been lacking in most cases. As mentioned previously, renal carcinomas may be affected by androgens. In humans, treatment with medroxyprogesterone sometimes causes partial regression or arrests the growth of primary renal neoplasms.[15]

The efficacy of radiation or immunotherapy has not been reported for dogs or cats with renal adenocarcinomas.

Renal lymphosarcoma can be treated with combination chemotherapy, usually consisting of cyclophosphamide, vincristine, prednisone, and (more recently) L-asparaginase.[12] Dramatic reduction in organ size observed with other forms of this neoplastic disorder rarely is documented in cases of renal lymphosarcoma. More frequently, a partial remission can be achieved, with temporary reduction in the severity of clinical signs being the result. Long-term remission and survival are difficult to achieve in cats and dogs with this form of lymphosarcoma.[1,12]

TABLE II
Anticancer Drugs for Treating Carcinomas of the Urinary Tract in Dogs

Agent	Dose[a] and Route	Frequency
Systemic		
Cyclophosphamide	50–75 mg/m^2 orally	4 times weekly
	200–300 mg/m^2 intravenously	Every 7 days
Doxorubicin hydrochloride	30 mg/m^2 intravenously	Every 21 days
5-fluorouracil	200 mg/m^2 intravenously	Every 7 days
Intravesicular		
5-fluorouracil	300 mg/m^2 via catheter	Every 7 days
Triethylenethiophosphoramide	15–30 mg via catheter	Every 7–14 days

[a]m^2 = square meters of body surface.

Ureteral Tumors

Primary tumors of the ureters are very unusual in dogs and cats. Reported neoplasms include transitional cell carcinoma, papillary carcinoma, leiomyoma, and leiomyosarcoma.[1,16,17] The few ureteral neoplasms described have been unilateral and difficult to diagnose until they achieved considerable size or obstructed the ureter. Clinical signs are hematuria and lower back pain. Stiffness and acute lumbar pain may be observed when ureteral obstruction is present.[5]

Diagnosis can be confirmed by contrast urography in some cases. Very large masses are occasionally palpable ventral to the lumbar muscles. Most confirmed cases have been established by exploratory laparotomy. Computer-assisted tomography is helpful in identifying retroperitoneal masses in humans and would likely be beneficial in identifying mass lesions in dogs as well.

Treatment of ureteral neoplasms consists of unilateral nephroureterectomy. Because of the possibility of a ureteral tumor representing an extension or metastatic focus from a renal neoplasm and because hydroureter and hydronephrosis often are present, attempts at less radical tumor resection are not advised. No experience with radiation or chemical treatment of these lesions has been reported.

Urinary Bladder Neoplasms

In dogs, neoplasms of the urinary bladder far exceed those of other urinary tract organs; however, they are relatively rare in cats. The reason(s) for a decreased incidence of urinary bladder cancer in cats is unknown. Cats may alter chemical carcinogens differently than other species do, and thus these potentially toxic substances may not be presented to the bladder in adequate concentration or form to induce malignant transformation.[18-20]

... veterinarians should note and report multiple incidences of bladder neoplasia to public health officers.

In humans, bladder cancer is more common in males than in females; in dogs, however, females are affected more frequently. Risk factors identified in humans include pelvic irradiation, smoking, and exposure to aromatic amines among workers in aniline dye, paint, leather, and rubber factories. Aniline dye workers have a 30-fold greater likelihood of developing bladder cancer than the general public.[5,21] While no studies have confirmed a cause-and-effect relationship between such chemicals and natural-occurring bladder tumors in dogs, animal experiments and clinical studies in humans have implicated such drugs as phenacetin, saccharin

sodium, and cyclamate sodium as causes of bladder malignancies.[5,22,23] Cyclophosphamide unequivocally increases the risk of bladder neoplasia in humans[24]; a recent report implicated this drug as a probable cause of transitional cell carcinoma of the urinary bladder in a dog.[25] Abnormal metabolism of tryptophan is found in 50% of humans with bladder cancer, and tryptophan metabolites are known to be carcinogenic in animals.[5] Because of these associations, veterinarians should note and report multiple incidences of bladder neoplasia to public health officers.

Most neoplasms of the canine urinary bladder are malignant. Transitional cell carcinoma is the most prevalent.[18-20,26] Other malignant tumors include squamous cell carcinoma,[1] botryoid rhabdomyosarcoma,[27] chemodectoma,[28] leiomyosarcoma,[6,29-31] leiomyoma,[32] fibroma,[33] fibrosarcoma, and undifferentiated sarcoma.[1,2] Most bladder neoplasms are slow-growing masses that metastasize late in their natural history. Clinical signs include hematuria, strangury, and pollakiuria; dribbling of urine and nocturia are sometimes observed. Most dogs appear healthy and have a good appetite. Constitutional signs of severe systemic illness are noted only in very advanced cases where ureteral and/or urethral obstruction is present. Signs of uremia occur in these cases, and rapid progression to death is expected if total occlusion of urinary output occurs.[19]

Diagnosis is usually documented by urinalysis and cystography. Urinalysis may reveal evidence of hematuria and/or urinary tract infection (pyuria, bacteriuria, and/or proteinuria). Specific gravity of the urine can vary considerably because some dogs with bladder neoplasms voluntarily drink a large amount of water. This polydipsia is apparently psychogenic because concentration of urine is usually obtained during a water deprivation test.[19] Hematologic and biochemical parameters are usually within normal limits; however, serum creatinine and blood urea nitrogen concentrations are elevated in dogs with partial obstruction of the lower urinary tract. Examination of urinary sediment sometimes reveals from a few to many anaplastic epithelial cells (Figure 5); however, the author recommends caution in making a definitive diagnosis on the basis of a few clusters of epithelial cells, because atypical transitional cells can be found in dogs with cystitis.[1,19,21]

Hypertrophic osteopathy, which involves firm and often painful periosteal bone proliferation on long bones of the extremities, is a paraneoplastic syndrome occasionally associated with bladder neoplasms in dogs (Figure 6). This debilitating complication has been identified in dogs with transitional cell carcinoma,[34] botryoid rhabdomyosarcoma,[35] and neurofibrosarcoma.[36] The mechanism for the bony proliferation is unknown but presumably is related to the afferent innervation of the bladder by branches of the vagus nerves.

Survey abdominal radiographs are rarely diagnostic when bladder neoplasia is present but may be helpful in

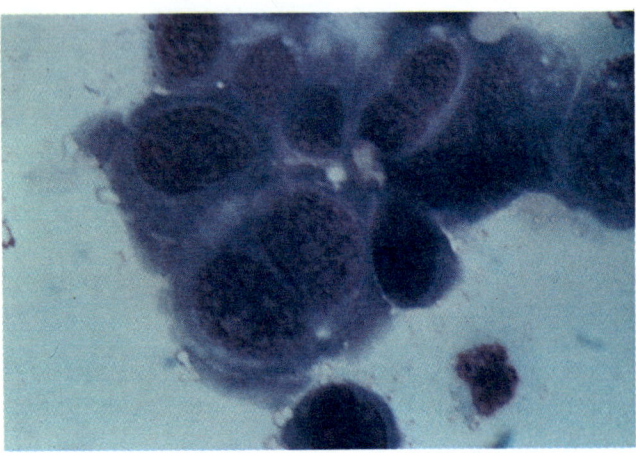

Figure 5—Cytologic results of a bladder wash obtained from a dog with transitional cell carcinoma. (Wright's stain, ×430) Note the binucleation, pleomorphism, anisokaryosis, and hyperchromatism suggestive of malignancy. (Courtesy of D. Weiss, Michigan State University)

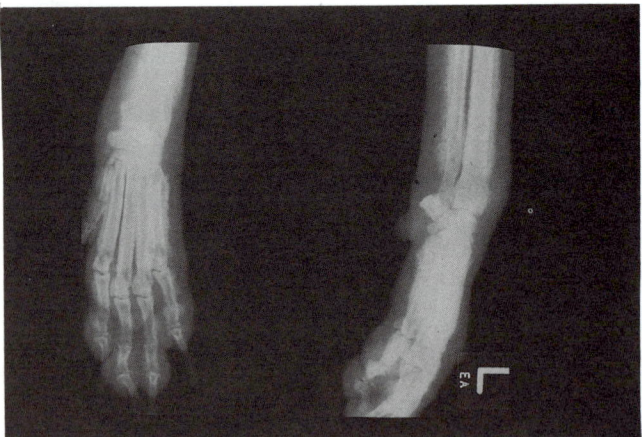

Figure 6—Radiographs of long bones in a dog with hypertrophic osteopathy associated with transitional cell carcinoma of the urinary bladder.

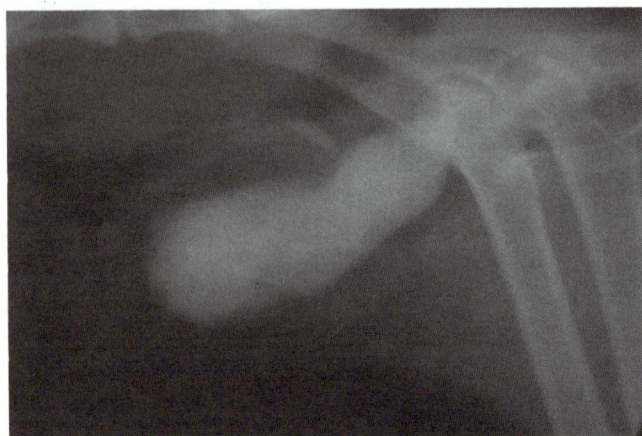

Figure 7—A double-contrast cystogram of a dog with a large filling defect in the trigonal area caused by transitional cell carcinoma. Also note the presence of bilateral hydroureter.

ruling out other disorders, such as prostatic disease and urolithiasis. Occasionally, sublumbar lymphadenopathy or osteolysis of lumbar vertebral bodies may be seen when a metastasizing bladder neoplasm is present. Contrast urography is usually needed to demonstrate the existence of a bladder neoplasm. Double-contrast cystography is most effective in delineating masses in the bladder wall and lumen (Figure 7). Radiographic abnormalities may include diffuse thickening of the bladder wall, ulceration, and space-occupying lesions, especially in the trigone. To evaluate the size and location of the renal pelves and ureters, an excretory urogram should be done before instilling negative contrast.[19,37] If frank hemorrhage is observed, care should be taken in performing negative-contrast cystography. The use of carbon dioxide is preferred to the use of air because of the risk of a fatal air embolism developing when using the latter.

Cystoscopy is the cornerstone for obtaining a diagnosis of bladder neoplasms in humans.[5] Unfortunately, this technique is rarely applicable in small animal practice. Most cystoscopes are either too large in diameter or too short to reach the bladder of a male dog; in a large female dog, however, a pediatric fiber-optic bronchoscope occasionally can be used to visualize the urinary bladder mucosa. Biopsies of suspicious areas can be obtained in such cases, thereby avoiding exploratory surgery. Percutaneous cystocentesis or fine-needle aspiration of the bladder wall can sometimes yield strong cytologic evidence of bladder neoplasia; however, exploratory surgery may be required to obtain a definitive diagnosis.[37] Before electing surgery for diagnostic measures, other therapeutic possibilities should be considered.

The prognosis for and treatment of bladder neoplasms depend on the exact location and extent of the primary mass as well as the presence or absence of regional and distant metastases. Clinical staging (Table III) should

be completed before treatment is initiated. Preinvasive carcinomas (rarely identified in animals) and small neoplasms are treated by partial cystectomy and occasionally with intravesical chemotherapy.

Unfortunately, bladder neoplasms are usually very advanced or in the trigonal area, making subtotal resection with retention of function impossible (Figure 8). Consequently, other methods of therapy need to be considered to treat most dogs and cats with bladder neoplasms.

Despite the difficulty encountered in resecting the primary mass, evidence of regional lymph node or distant organ metastasis usually is not apparent at first presentation. When metastasis is observed (usually several months after diagnosis), the sublumbar and iliac lymph nodes and lungs are affected most often.[18,20]

The goals for treating bladder tumors are the same as those for all antineoplastic therapy: control of the primary mass and prevention of development of metastatic foci. Specific objectives of regional control include relief of urinary discomfort, maintenance of urinary continence, and prevention of hydroureter and hydro-

TABLE III
Clinical Stages of Bladder Tumors in Dogs[a]

Category	Letter and Numeric Designation[b]	Description	Diagnostic Measures[c]
Primary tumor	T0	No evidence of primary tumor	Clinical examination, cystoscopy, urography or cystography, laparotomy
	T1S	Carcinoma in situ	
	T1	Superficial papillary tumor	
	T2	Tumor invading bladder wall, with duration	
	T3	Tumor invading neighboring organs (prostate, uterus, vagina, anal canal)	
Regional lymph nodes[d]	N0	No involvement of regional lymph nodes	Surgical examination (laparotomy, laparoscopy)
	N1	Regional lymph nodes involved	
	N2	Regional lymph nodes and juxta regional lymph nodes involved	
Distant metastasis	M0	No evidence of metastasis	Clinical examination, radiography of the thorax, laparotomy
	M1	Distant metastasis present (specify site or sites)	

[a]No stage grouping is recommended at present.
[b]Approved by the World Health Organization in 1979.
[c]If the appropriate numeric designation within a category cannot be determined after completing the diagnostic procedures indicated, the symbols Tx, Nx, or Mx should be used accordingly.
[d]The regional lymph nodes are the internal and external iliac lymph nodes. The juxta regional lymph nodes are the lumbar lymph nodes.

nephrosis. Segmental resection is associated with a high risk of recurrence; this method should be considered only if the tumor is solitary, is localized in the apical portion of the bladder, and can be removed with a 2-cm margin of healthy tissue. Many surgical procedures have been tried on humans with transitional cell carcinomas; most of the procedures involve radical or total cystectomy with urinary diversion. Total cystectomy is the complete removal of the bladder, prostate (in males), and urethra, while radical cystectomy involves both pelvic lymph node dissection and total cystectomy.

Several methods of urinary diversion, including ureteral and trigonal colostomy, ureteroileostomy, and gastrocystoplasty, have been attempted on dogs following cystectomy. None of these techniques, however, has been notably successful to date. Azotemia and diarrhea have been consistent postsurgical complications, although fecal continence is usually preserved; other complications include pyelonephritis and hyperchloremic acidosis. Gastrocystoplasty, which involves the formation of a substitute bladder from the gastric fundus, is technically difficult and requires frequent emptying of the collection pouch by the animal's owner; postoperative complications are common. At present, cystectomy apparently is an unacceptable solution for treating dogs and cats with bladder neoplasms.[a] Hopefully, the

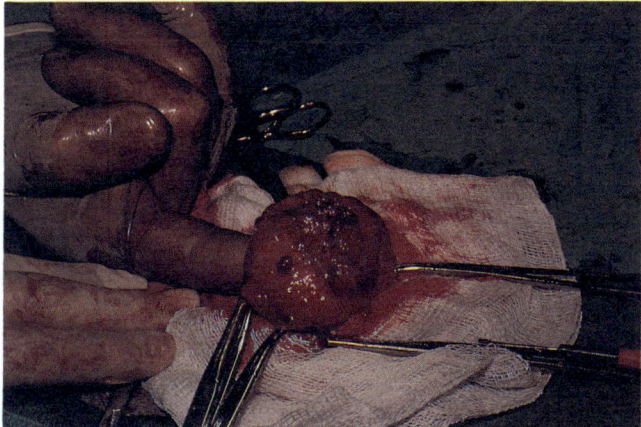

Figure 8—Diffuse infiltration of bladder mucosa and muscularis by transitional cell carcinoma. Note the markedly distended ureter just cranial to its entry into the urinary bladder.

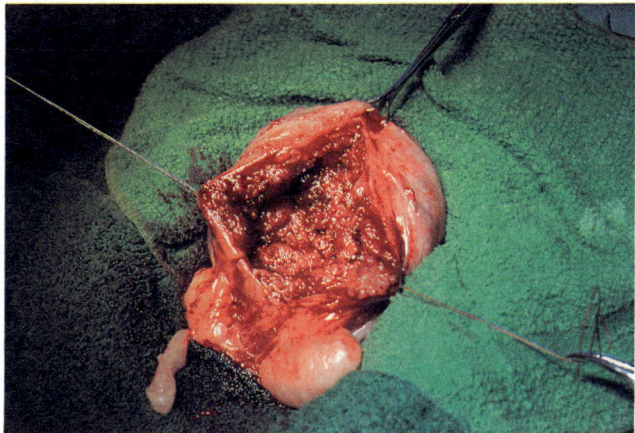

Figure 9—Application of single-fraction radiation intraoperatively. The bladder should be exposed and the remainder of the abdomen shielded with lead sheeting wrapped in sterile towels.

development of a synthetic bladder prosthesis will change that outlook in the next decade.

Although curative surgical treatment presently is not available for most animals with bladder neoplasms, other methods of treatment sometimes offer significant relief of clinical signs. Treating a coexisting urinary tract infection with antibacterial drugs or dissolving or removing urinary calculi may relieve the discomfort of straining for weeks to months.[a] Bacterial culture and susceptibility testing of urine should be done for all patients with suspected urinary tract infections superimposed on bladder neoplasms. Treatment with appropriate drugs should be continued until the infection is controlled or eliminated.

Chemical cauterization of the bladder should be considered when marked hematuria is noted. Moderate bleeding can be treated by giving the animal methenamine mandelate (10 mg/kg orally every six hours) to effect. Severe bleeding may require intravesicular instillation of ice-cold fluids or 1% formalin solution.[8] Diluted formalin should be used cautiously, with strict adherence to reported technique.[38]

Strangury and hematuria are the predominant clinical signs observed in dogs with urethral tumors.

Chemotherapy has not been used extensively in humans or animals with bladder cancer because of the locally invasive behavior of the tumors. In humans, responses have been short-lived, and improvement in survival time has not been shown with single-agent or combination chemotherapy. Agents with some demonstrated efficacy in treating bladder neoplasia include mycophenolic acid,[39] cyclophosphamide, doxorubicin hydrochloride, cisplatin, 5-fluorouracil, and triethylenethiophosphoramide (Thiotepa®—Lederle Laboratories).[40-43] Objective reduction of the tumor mass has not been reported in dogs with transitional cell carcinomas, but subjective responses have been noted in several cases. Apparent arrest of tumor growth and partial relief of clinical signs have been observed in dogs treated with 5-fluorouracil, doxorubicin hydrochloride, and cyclophosphamide systemically and with 5-fluorouracil and triethylenethiophosphoramide intravesically.[a]

Radiation therapy may be palliative in some animals with bladder neoplasms. External beam irradiation generally is not indicated because of the excessive scat-

ter-radiation effects on surrounding viscera,[44] but intraoperative radiation now is being evaluated at several veterinary schools. Doses of 15 to 20 Gray (1500 to 2000 rad) have been applied directly to an exposed tumor while the rest of the abdomen is shielded (Figure 9). Preliminary results indicate that this mode of treatment results in temporary arrest of many tumors and partial relief of clinical signs in some animals.[37,45]

Urethral Neoplasms

Recent reports indicate that urethral neoplasms are quite rare in dogs,[46,47] and tumors of the feline urethra were not observed in one multiinstitutional study.[2] The most commonly identified neoplasms of the canine urethra apparently are transitional cell carcinoma, squamous cell carcinoma, and adenocarcinoma. In a few instances, some of these neoplasms may represent extension of bladder or prostatic neoplasms rather than being primary urethral masses. Various other neoplasms have been reported to occur in the canine urethra.[1,46,47] As is the case with humans, female dogs have two times greater relative risk of developing urethral cancer than males do. It has been suggested that male dogs are spared because of the presence of prostatic secretions in their urethra, which may effectively dilute carcinogens that are present in urine in the urethral lumen.[46,47] Causes of urethral neoplasms in dogs are not known; but urethral cancer has been associated with gonorrheal urethritis, strictures, and transitional cell carcinoma of the bladder in humans.[5]

Strangury and hematuria are the predominant clinical signs observed in dogs with urethral tumors. These signs may exist for a few weeks to many months before the animal is presented by the owner; occasionally, complete obstruction of the lower urinary tract is present before the animal is examined by a veterinarian. In these advanced cases, such constitutional signs as vomiting and depression can be expected.

Diagnosis of a urethral mass can often be made by careful examination, including digital rectal and vaginal palpation. While some urethral tumors are diffuse, many are located in the distal urethra. Hematologic and serum chemistry determinations are usually within normal limits, except when obstruction is present. Elevations of serum urea nitrogen, creatinine, and phosphorus concentrations can be expected. Inability to pass a urethral catheter into the bladder should raise suspicion that a mass or stone is obstructing the lumen of the urethra.

Survey and contrast urethrography sometimes is helpful in delineating the extent of urethral masses. If inguinal and pelvic lymph nodes are enlarged, they should be aspirated to determine whether metastatic neoplastic cells are present. Cytologic evaluation of urine occasionally can confirm malignant epithelial cells.

Malignant urethral tumors frequently metastasize to distant sites. Consequently, thoracic and abdominal

---

[a]Walshaw R, Crow SE: Unpublished clinical observations of cases presented from 1977 to 1984. East Lansing, MI, Michigan State University.

radiographs should be evaluated before considering treatment. Careful perusal of the sublumbar region for evidence of lymphadenopathy as well as examination of the lumbosacral vertebral bodies and pelvic bone for bony extension and/or metastasis constitute important criteria for staging urethral neoplasms.

... splitting of the pelvis is often required to identify the extent of the tumor.

Diagnosis is usually made by surgical exploration of the pelvic urethra. A perineal or vaginal approach is difficult and often affords insufficient exposure of the lesion to permit resection. Consequently, splitting of the pelvis is often required to identify the extent of the tumor. Because these neoplasms tend to be diffuse in nature, complete resection cannot be accomplished in many cases. Extension into the bladder precludes urethrectomy and prepubic urethrostomy. Advanced cases may require radical surgery (e.g., urethrocystectomy with ureteral or trigonal intestinal implantation) to remove the visible neoplastic disease. When regional lymph nodes are grossly enlarged, block dissection should be attempted to remove the primary mass, affected lymph nodes, and intervening lymphatic vessels.

There are no reports of adjuvant chemotherapy after surgery has been performed on dogs with urethral tumors, but a case presented recently[a] had recurrent and metastatic transitional cell carcinoma after urethral resection; external beam irradiation resulted in complete regression of all visible lesions for several months.[a]

REFERENCES

1. Theilen GH, Madewell BR: Tumors of the urogenital tract, in Ettinger SJ (ed): *Textbook of Veterinary Internal Medicine—Diseases of the Dog and Cat.* Philadelphia, WB Saunders Co, 1974.
2. Priester WA, McKay FW: *National Cancer Institute Monograph 54. The Occurrence of Tumors in Domestic Animals.* Washington DC, U.S. Government Printing Office, 1980.
3. Baskin GB, De Paoli A: Primary renal neoplasms of the dog. *Vet Pathol* 14:591-605, 1977.
4. Hayes HM, Fraumeni JF: Epidemiological features of canine renal neoplasms. *Cancer Res* 37:2553-2556, 1977.
5. Casciato DA, Lowitz BB: *Manual of Bedside Oncology.* Boston, Little, Brown & Co, 1983.
6. Smith CW, Macy DW: Renal carcinoma with pulmonary metastasis. *Canine Practice*:34-41, 1976.
7. Burger GT, et al: Renal carcinoma in a dog. *JAVMA* 171:282-283, 1977.
8. Whitley RD, et al: Renal adenocarcinoma with ocular metastasis in a dog. *JAAHA* 16:949-953, 1980.
9. Sagartz JW, et al: Malignant embryonal nephroma in an aged dog. *JAVMA* 161:1658-1660, 1972.
10. Mills JHL, Orr JP: Canine renal leiomyoma—An unusual tumour. *Can Vet J* 18:76-78, 1977.
11. Crow SE, Bell TG, Wortman JA: Hematuria associated with renal hemangiosarcoma in a dog. *JAVMA* 176:531-533, 1980.
12. Weller RE, Stann SE: Renal lymphosarcoma in the cat. *JAAHA* 19:363-367, 1983.
13. Peterson ME, Zanjani ED: Inappropriate erythropoietin production from a renal carcinoma in a dog with polycythemia. *JAVMA* 179:995-996, 1981.
14. Nafe LA, Herron AJ, Burk RL: Hypertrophic osteopathy in a cat associated with renal papillary adenoma. *JAAHA* 17:659-662, 1981.
15. Samuels ML, Sullivan P, Howe CR: Medroxyprogesterone acetate in the treatment of renal cell carcinoma (hypernephroma). *Cancer* 22:525-529, 1968.
16. Liska WD Patnaik AK: Leiomyoma of the ureter of a dog. *JAAHA* 13:83-84, 1977.
17. Berzon JL: Primary leiomyosarcoma of the ureter in a dog. *JAVMA* 175:374-376, 1979.
18. Osborne CA, et al: Neoplasms of the canine and feline urinary bladder: Incidence, etiologic factors, occurrence, and pathologic features. *Am J Vet Res* 29:2041-2045, 1968.
19. Osborne CA, et al: Neoplasms of the canine and feline urinary bladder: Clinical findings, diagnosis and treatment. *JAVMA* 152:247-251, 1968.
20. Strafuss AC, Dean MJ: Neoplasms of the urinary bladder. *JAVMA* 166:1161-1163, 1975.
21. Whitmore WF: Bladder cancer. *CA [Cancer J Clin]* 28:170-177, 1978.
22. Conzelman GM Jr, Moulton JE: Dose-response relationships of the bladder tumorigen 2-naphthalamine: A study in beagle dogs. *J Natl Cancer Inst* 49:193-196, 1972.
23. Morrison AS, Buring JE: Artificial sweeteners and cancer in the lower urinary tract. *N Engl J Med* 302:537-541, 1980.
24. Wall RL, Clausen KP: Carcinoma of the urinary bladder in patients receiving cyclophosphamide. *N Engl J Med* 293:271-273, 1975.
25. Weller RE, Wolf AM, Oyejide A: Transitional cell carcinoma of the bladder associated with cyclophosphamide therapy in a dog. *JAAHA* 15:733-736, 1979.
26. Dill GS, McElyea U, Stookey JL: Transitional cell carcinoma of the urinary bladder in a cat. *JAVMA* 160:743-745, 1972.
27. Kelly DF: Rhabdomyosarcoma of the urinary bladder in dogs. *Vet Pathol* 10:375-384, 1973.
28. Patnaik AK, Lord PF, Liu S-K: Chemodectoma of the urinary bladder in a dog. *JAVMA* 164:797-800, 1974.
29. Burk RL, Meierhenry EF, Schaubhut CW: Leiomyosarcoma of the urinary bladder in a cat. *JAVMA* 167:749-751, 1975.
30. Seely JC, Cosenza SF, Montgomery CA: Leiomyosarcoma of the canine urinary bladder, with metastases. *JAVMA* 172:1427-1429, 1978.
31. Johnson TC: A report of two cases of neoplasm of the urinary bladder in dogs. *JAAHA* 15:357-359, 1979.
32. Patnaik AK, Greene RW: Intravenous leiomyoma of the bladder in a cat. *JAVMA* 175:381-383, 1979.
33. Birchard SJ, et al: Fibroma of the urinary bladder of a dog. *JAAHA* 18:63-66, 1982.
34. Brodey RS, Riser WH, Allen H: Hypertrophic pulmonary osteoarthropathy in a dog with carcinoma of the urinary bladder. *JAVMA* 162:474-478, 1973.
35. Halliwell WH, Ackerman N: Botryoid rhabdomyosarcoma of the urinary bladder and hypertrophic osteoarthropathy in a young dog. *JAVMA* 165:911-913, 1974.
36. Mandel M: Hypertrophic osteoarthropathy secondary to neurofibrosarcoma of the urinary bladder in a cocker spaniel. *VM SAC*:1307-1308, 1975.
37. Crow SE, Klausner JS: Management of transitional cell carcinomas of the urinary bladder, in Kirk RW (ed): *Current Veterinary Therapy VIII.* Philadelphia, WB Saunders Co, 1983.
38. Weller RE: Intravesical installation of dilute formalin for treatment of cyclophosphamide-induced hemorrhagic cystitis in two dogs. *JAVMA* 172:1206-1209, 1978.
39. Connolly JG, Halsall GM: Use of mycophenolic acid in superficial bladder cancer. *Urology* 5:131-132, 1975.
40. Carter SK, Wasserman TH: The chemotherapy of urologic cancer. *Cancer* 36:729-747, 1975.

41. Bush H, Thatcher N, Barnard R: Chemotherapy in the management of invasive bladder cancer. *Cancer Chemother Pharmacol* 3:87-96, 1979.
42. Murphy WM, Soloway MS: The effect of the thio-TEPA on developing and established mammalian bladder tumors. *Cancer* 45:870-875, 1980.
43. Jakse G, Hofstadter F, Marberger H: Intracavitary doxorubicin hydrochloride therapy for carcinoma in situ of the bladder. *J Urol* 125:185-190, 1981.
44. Matsumoto K, et al: Clinical evaluation of intraoperative radio-therapy for carcinoma of the urinary bladder. *Cancer* 47:509-513, 1981.
45. Turrell J: Intra-operative radiation therapy. *The Second Purdue Veterinary Cancer Society Workshop*. West Lafayette, IN, Purdue University, 1982.
46. Tarvin G, Patnaik AM, Greene R: Primary urethral tumors in dogs. *JAVMA* 172:931-933, 1978.
47. Wilson GP, Hayes HM, Casey HW: Canine urethral cancer. *JAAHA* 15:741-744, 1979.

Urinary Incontinence in Geriatric Dogs

Donald R. Krawiec, DVM, MS, PhD
Assistant Professor
Department of Veterinary Clinical Medicine
College of Veterinary Medicine
University of Illinois
Urbana, Illinois

Stanley I. Rubin, DVM, MS
Assistant Professor
Western College of Veterinary Medicine
University of Saskatchewan
Saskatoon, Saskatchewan, Canada

Urinary incontinence, as defined by the International Continence Society, is a condition where "involuntary loss of urine is a social or hygienic problem, and is objectively demonstrable."[1] Urinary incontinence is not a disease, nor is it caused by a single condition; however, it is a sign that can be linked to numerous causes. Common terms used in describing various types of incontinence (i.e., urge, stress, overflow, paradoxical, and reflex) mostly describe signs and do not define the problem in specific pathophysiologic or anatomic terms (Table I). Simply stated, there are two ways for incontinence to occur: either the pressure in the bladder is greater than the ability of the normal urethral sphincter to prevent emptying, or the urethral sphincter is too weak to inhibit voiding[2]; the pathophysiologic bases for either are varied.

Urinary incontinence occurs in two age groups: the very young as a result of congenital malformation or the adult as an acquired disorder.[3] In this article, the causes of urinary incontinence will be reviewed as they relate to the geriatric animal.

In three recent studies of adult dogs, the mean age of onset ranged from 5.3 to 8.3 years.[3-5] This finding indicates that urinary incontinence is most commonly a disorder of middle-aged to geriatric animals. While there is no specific predisposition based on age, the likelihood of occurrence increases with age. Acquired adult urinary incontinence can be a frustrating problem for both the owner and the pet. The owner is concerned for sanitary and aesthetic reasons; the pets react because they are reprimanded for something they cannot control. In an extreme case, the pet may be euthanatized.

Anatomy and Physiology of the Lower Urinary Tract

The lower urinary tract is composed of the bladder, which is lined with smooth muscle called the *detrusor muscle*, and the urethra, which consists of an internal smooth muscle sphincter continuing from the detrusor muscle and an external skeletal muscle sphincter.[6-8]

Sympathetic innervation of the bladder and urethra occurs via the hypogastric nerve, which emerges from the lumbar spinal cord (L1 to L2). Stimulation of β receptors of the bladder causes the detrusor muscle to relax while stimulation of the α receptors of the urethra causes the urethra to contract.[6-8]

Parasympathetic innervation occurs via the pelvic nerve, which originates from the sacral spinal cord (S1 to S3). Stimulation of the parasym-

Originally published in Volume 7, Number 7, July 1985

TABLE I
Classification of Clinical Signs and Causes of Urinary Incontinence

Type of Incontinence	Pathophysiology	Common Causes
Stress	Urethral incompetence resulting in incontinence whenever there is an increase in intraabdominal pressure; occurs in the absence of detrusor contraction	Usually refers to a human condition in which there is an anatomic defect that causes weakening of the urethral sphincter; term applicable to any situation in which there is urethral incompetence
Urge	Involuntary loss of urine linked to a strong uncontrollable urge to void	Cystitis, urethritis, urolithiasis, trauma, cystic, or urethral neoplasia
Paradoxical	A result of organic or functional partial urethral obstruction; linked to involuntary contraction of the detrusor muscle or overdistention of the bladder causing pressures that overcome urethral resistance	Reflex dyssynergia, obstructing urethral calculi, neoplasia, and pressure applied on the urethra from masses in the periurethral tissue
Overflow	Detrusor areflexia resulting in maximum filling of the bladder; occurs when bladder pressures are greater than urethral resistance	Lower motor neuronal lesions affecting sacral cord or roots; destruction of detrusor muscles because of chronic overdistention of the bladder
Reflex	No cortical perception by the patient of either bladder filling or emptying; occurs because the bladder empties independent of the desire to void	Upper motor neuronal lesion; usually occurs secondary to severe brain stem or upper motor neuronal spinal cord lesions

pathetic receptors of the lower urinary tract causes contraction of the detrusor muscle. The striated muscle of the urethra is also innervated by the somatic nervous system via somatic nerves.[6-8]

Micturition has two phases: storage and emptying. The storage phase is characterized by relaxation of the detrusor muscle (β-adrenergic stimulation) and sphincter contraction (α-adrenergic stimulation). When the bladder reaches the filling point, impulses are sent from the bladder to the brain stem. Impulses are then sent from the brain stem to the sacral parasympathetic nervous system. Parasympathetic stimulation causes the bladder to contract at the same time sympathetic stimulation of the urethra is inhibited; relaxation of the urethral sphincter results. When the bladder is empty, parasympathetic discharges end, sympathetic stimulation of α- and β-adrenergic receptors is no longer inhibited, and the storage phase begins again. Under normal circumstances, sphincter tone increases during sudden increases in intraabdominal pressure (e.g., coughing or barking).[6-8]

Voluntary control of micturition comes from the cerebral cortex and is mediated by the pudendal nerve and the external urethral sphincter.

Normally, an animal can hold its urine voluntarily even when the bladder is full. Voluntary control of micturition comes from the cerebral cortex and is mediated by the pudendal nerve and the external urethral sphincter.[6-8]

Causes of Urinary Incontinence in Elderly Dogs

In geriatric dogs, urinary incontinence can occur secondary to a number of pathologic processes (Table II). Inability to control micturition can result from behavior problems, neurologic dysfunction, alterations in bladder and urethral tone, urinary tract infection and obstruction, prostatic disease, bladder and urethral neoplasia, and administration of certain drugs.[2,3,6-10] All of these causes are possible in young animals but the risk of their occurrence increases with age. Older animals are more susceptible to pathologic processes and are more likely to have multiple episodes of illness.[9,11-12] Small insults may be serious in older animals, and older animals fail to respond to therapy as well as younger animals do.[12-15] Age-related problems of impaired vision, diminished mobility, impaired balance, senility, decreased muscle tone, decreased bladder capacity, decreased ability to concentrate urine, and increased urine volume contribute to and aggravate an incontinence problem.[5,9,13-15]

Behavior Problems Associated with Urinary Incontinence

One review of canine geriatric medicine states that an early sign of senility is the lack of fastidiousness in

TABLE II
Age-Related Causes of Urinary Incontinence

Clinical Problem	Effect on Continence
Neurologic defects	Decreased cortical awareness of appropriate voiding behavior patterns, detrusor areflexia, reflex dyssynergia, reflex incontinence
Diminished vision and mobility, impaired balance, weakness	Decreased ability to get to appropriate voiding areas
Increased restlessness at night	Nocturia
Decreased urethral sphincter tone	Stress incontinence
Abnormalities in bladder tone	Overflow incontinence; detrusor hyperreflexia resulting in frequent voiding of small volumes
Decreased bladder capacity	Urgency, frequency, nocturia, frequent voiding of small volumes
Polyuria/polydipsia	Increased urine volume
Urinary tract infection	Irritation, urgency, frequency
Obstruction (urolithiasis, neoplasia)	Paradoxical incontinence, overflow incontinence, detrusor atony
Bladder and urethral neoplasia	Damage to sphincter or obstruction
Prostatic disease	Urethral impairment or obstruction; urethral discharge of prostatic fluid
Drug-related	
Diuretics and corticosteroids	Increased urine formation
Tranquilizers	Decreased cortical awareness of appropriate voiding habits
α- and β-adrenergic drugs	Increased urinary retention; overflow incontinence

excretory habits.[15] Old age may expedite undesirable changes in behavior patterns.[16] Puppies are house-trained when they are very young. Older animals may simply forget to go outside to urinate and may have to be retrained. Older dogs may also suddenly urinate when greeting an owner or when excited. The problem is controlled by avoiding placing the animal in stressful situations.

Certain problems of incontinence that appear to be behavioral may be the result of real pathologic processes;

other behavioral urinary problems may not justifiably be called *incontinence* because they are not involuntary. These abnormal urinary behavior patterns are discussed in this article because of their importance in geriatric medicine. An animal may be too lethargic or in too much pain to make it outside, especially if there are obstacles, such as stairs, to overcome. Loss of sight and equilibrium also might cause an animal to forget old behavior patterns of urination. Older animals are also more restless in their sleeping habits, and an awake animal may be more reluctant to wait until morning to urinate. Understanding the problem and retraining may be all that is required to make the animal an acceptable pet.[16]

Effects of Aging on Bladder and Urethral Tone

Aging is associated with a decrease in total muscle mass. These changes can be the result of muscle cell atrophy and/or replacement of muscle with fibrous connective tissue.[2,9,13-15] Muscular changes in the lower urinary tract can result in decreased bladder capacity, decreased urethral sphincter tone, or urethral stricture, any of which can result in incontinence.

Scarring of the bladder and urethra secondary to chronic urinary tract infection, urolithiasis, or prostate problems can also result in a small nondistensible bladder and/or a constricted or ineffective urethral sphincter.[2,3,9] Age-related neurologic disorders can also affect bladder and urethral tone.[6,7]

One of the common diagnosed incontinence problems is hormone-responsive (estrogen or testosterone) urinary incontinence.[3,8,10] This problem may be caused by a decrease in urethral sphincter tone or a urethral incompetence[3,8,10] and occurs primarily in females but has been described in males.[3,10,17] An affected animal will be continent when awake but will involuntarily void urine when relaxed or when asleep. No physical or laboratory abnormalities can be found in these patients. Affected animals are usually neutered.[3,8,10,17] The exact cause of the syndrome is unclear; however, one theory states that testosterone and estrogen are required for maintenance of normal urethral tone.[3,8]

Increased Production of Urine

Increased output of urine can be a factor in an incontinent animal, especially an elderly patient.[2,9,13-16] An expanded bladder resulting from increased formation of urine places additional pressure on the urethral sphincter. Older animals with decreased bladder capacity and urethral tone have a difficult time retaining the increased volume of urine for even short periods, and incontinence may result. There are many causes for polyuria and polydipsia, including diabetes insipidus, renal failure, renal tubular disease, hypercalcemia, hypokalemia, hyperadrenocorticism, hypoadrenocorticism, hepatic failure, pyometra, drugs (lithium carbonate, methoxyflurane, and α-adrenergic agents), and primary polydipsia.[18,19] Any of these conditions might lead to incontinence, and many of them are more common in older animals.[12-15]

Chronic renal insufficiency is seen often in geriatric medicine.[13-16,20,21] In studies of experimental animals and humans, aging is associated with a loss of 20% to 30% of kidney weight and a decrease in glomerular filtration rate of 60% to 70% from peak early adult weights and function.[20] Although there is little experimental evidence implicating age-related progressive renal dysfunction in dogs, clinical data indicate that the onset of chronic renal failure occurs more often in middle-aged and elderly dogs than in young dogs.[20] One survey suggests that the mean age of diagnosis of renal failure in dogs is 6.95 years.[20] Renal failure can occur in any age group, but the risk of occurrence seems to increase with age. One of the initial signs of renal failure in dogs is an inability to concentrate urine, which results in increased water intake and urine output, nocturia, and incontinence.[21-23]

Urinary Tract Infections

The age of the animal greatly affects the immune system's ability to withstand infection.[11,14,15] The immune system is at its functional peak at puberty and slowly declines thereafter.[11] An older animal is more likely to be susceptible to urinary tract infection because of impaired defense mechanisms and is more likely to have suffered multiple infections.[9,15,24] Urinary tract infection causes bladder irritation, damage, and scarring. These can result in bladder spasticity, decreased bladder capacity, and an uncontrollable urge to void (urge incontinence).[3,8,9] Urethral inflammation can result in loss of control or obstruction because of stricture.[8,9] Urinary tract infections can occur in animals of any age; but when they occur in older animals with other predisposing problems, the risk of secondary incontinence is greater than it is in younger animals.

Urolithiasis

Phosphate, oxalate, urate, cystine, and silica uroliths reportedly occur between five and eight years of age.[25] Urolithiasis results in bladder irritation and urge incontinence. Multiple persistent episodes result in scarring, thickening, and decreased capacity of the bladder. Urethral calculi can also result in obstruction and paradoxical incontinence (Table I).

Neurologic Causes

Aging in animals is generally associated with a chronic, slowly progressive decrease in neural function.[13-16] Neuronal changes that occur secondary to aging are altered receptor sites, neurotransmitter changes, and decreases in the number of cells of various parts of the nervous system.[15] Intervertebral disk disease, which is a degenerative process, can also occur secondary to aging.[26] Neurologic causes of incontinence can be linked to dysfunction of lower urinary tract neuroreceptors, smooth muscle fibers, peripheral innervation, afferent

and efferent spinal tracts, and upper neural centers.[6,7] Specific disorders occurring either alone or in combination and associated with neurogenic incontinence are detrusor areflexia, sphincter hypertonia, spastic or neuropathic bladder, sphincter areflexia, detrusor hyperreflexia, and reflex dyssynergia.[6,7]

Detrusor areflexia, sphincter hypertonia, and reflex or automatic neuropathic bladder occur secondary to lesions from the pons to spinal cord segment L7. These upper motor neuronal lesions cause a lack of cortical awareness of micturition, increased sphincter tone, and reflex incontinence (Table I). The increased sphincter tone results in interrupted and incomplete voiding.[6,7]

Detrusor areflexia and normal sphincter tone also can result from lesions of the brain to spinal cord segment L7. Reflex incontinence still results in these cases, but the stream of urine is normal and the bladder will empty completely.[6,7]

Detrusor areflexia and sphincter areflexia usually occur secondary to lower motor neuronal lesions involving the sacral spinal cord or roots. Overflow incontinence usually results from this type of problem (Table I). Detrusor hyperreflexia can occur secondary to long tract or cerebellar lesion and will result in frequent voiding of small amounts of urine.[6,7]

Reflex dyssynergia is caused by a partial nervous system lesion cranial to the sacral spinal cord. Dogs with this lesion have the ability to contract their detrusor muscle, but there is no simultaneous relaxation of the urethra. Reflex dyssynergia results in frequent urges to micturate. The micturition is characterized by short spurts of urine and straining. The dog will eventually stop straining but will still have a partially full bladder.[6,7]

Bladder and Urethral Neoplasia

Age-related cellular and immune-system events increase the susceptibility of older animals to cancer.[27] As with most neoplastic problems, bladder and urethral tumors are primarily diseases of older animals. In one study, Osborne et al found the mean age of dogs with bladder tumors to be 9.1 years.[28] The reported average age of dogs with urethral tumors is greater than 10.0 years.[29] The most common clinical signs of bladder tumors are unresponsive hematuria, frequent urination, tenesmus, and incontinence.[30] The incontinence is usually due to tumor damage to the trigonal area of the bladder and urethra. Clinical signs associated with urethral tumors are hematuria and strangury, but incontinence is also seen.[30]

Diseases of the Prostate

Prostatic diseases are common problems in older male dogs.[31] In one study involving 140 cases of prostatic disease, over 90% of the confirmed cases were in dogs older than five years of age. The mean age of this group of dogs was 9.3 years.[31]

A number of pathologic processes occurs in the prostate, including acute and chronic prostatitis, prostatic abscesses, benign hyperplasia, cysts, neoplasia, and calculi.[31,32] The presenting signs of these conditions vary with the cause. Incontinence, however, may be a presenting complaint for any of these prostatic disorders.[31,32] Any intact male presenting with a complaint of incontinence or dripping fluid from the penis should be evaluated for a possible prostatic problem. Urethral discharges of prostatic origin are a common finding in prostatic disease and may be mistaken for incontinence.

Diagnosis

A good history will identify incontinence; however, diagnosis of the precise cause of incontinence requires not only a history but a physical examination and appropriate clinical pathologic and radiographic evaluations. The minimum data base for an elderly patient with an initial presenting complaint of incontinence should include an accurate history, a thorough physical examination, a urinalysis, and a urine culture. The clinician should carefully question the owner about previous illnesses, surgical procedures performed, and medication the animal is receiving that may affect renal-concentrating mechanisms and urethral and bladder tone. The β-adrenergic–blocking agents, diuretics, glucocorticoids, and tranquilizers all can aggravate or initiate an animal's problem with incontinence. The animal's water intake and urine output should be quantitated, and night and day and sleeping and waking voiding patterns should be assessed. The owner should be questioned as to when and under what circumstances the problem occurs. The chronologic progression of the problem should also be assessed.

A complete neurologic examination should be performed, especially assessment of the patient's mental alertness, coordination, physical strength, and anal tone. The physical examination should include abdominal palpation to evaluate the following: bladder distention, tenderness, and wall thickness as well as the presence of growths in the bladder; prostatic size; and kidney size, shape, and consistency. The penis should be inspected and palpated, and the external genitalia should be inspected and palpated in the female for abnormalities. Vaginoscopy should be performed to assess the urethral orifice. A digital rectal examination should be conducted to identify urethral irregularities and growths in animals of both sexes and to assess prostatic size, shape, and consistency in males.

If the history, physical examination, and urinalysis fail to uncover the cause of incontinence, the patient should be evaluated further . . . .

The pattern of urination should be observed to assess the adequacy of the stream of urine, and the stream should be interrupted to assess urethral sphincter tone. A sustained stream of urine is an indication of a functioning detrusor muscle. The ability to stop urinating with a partially full bladder is an indication of a functioning urethral sphincter. The patient should be allowed to finish urinating, and residual urine should be measured by catheterization to assess the ability of the detrusor muscle to empty the bladder completely. Volumes of residual urine greater than 0.2 to 0.4 ml/kg have been reported as being abnormal.[7]

A urinalysis is mandatory on any geriatric patient with incontinence to rule out the possibility of urinary tract infection. If the results of the urinalysis are consistent with infection, a urine culture and antibiotic sensitivity testing should be performed.

If the history, physical examination, and urinalysis fail to uncover the cause of incontinence, the patient should be evaluated further by performing a complete blood count and serum chemistry analysis and taking survey abdominal radiographs. These procedures can help detect occult disease. If the initial workup implicates a specific organ system (e.g., prostate or nervous system), a more detailed evaluation of that organ system is indicated.

Other diagnostic tests include contrast cystography and urethrography, electromyography, cystometrography, and urethral pressure profiles.[4,6-8,32] Contrast radiography of the lower urinary tract could reveal important information about the cause of incontinence that might not be obvious from survey radiographs. Contrast cystograms might identify nonradiopaque cystic calculi, masses, patent urachus, or other causes of recurrent urinary tract infection and incontinence. Contrast urethrograms also allow visualization of calculi and neoplasia as well as strictures, all of which can be associated with incontinence.[32]

The electromyogram helps in the evaluation of areas of partial or complete denervation and may help localize a suspected neurologic lesion.[6-8] With cystometrography, pressure within the lumen of the bladder can be measured during a micturition reflex. This test provides quantitative information about bladder function, including the micturition reflex function, threshold and maximum volumes of urine, and vesicular pressure.[6-8] For the urethral pressure profile, a fluid-filled catheter can be placed in the bladder and withdrawn through the urethra. As it is being withdrawn, luminal pressure should be evaluated and recorded along the length of the urethra. Urethral pressure profiles can detect areas of obstruction or increased resistance and incompetence or decreased resistance.[7,8] Urethral incompetence is a major cause of incontinence in dogs.[2,3,6-10,17] By using these three tests, which are available at specialized practices and university veterinary hospitals, the clinician can have objective data concerning bladder and urethral function and thus determine the location of the problem and select the most appropriate therapeutic agent accordingly.

Treatment

The key to successful treatment of an elderly animal with urinary incontinence is to make an accurate diagnosis. If a specific problem can be defined, a specific therapeutic regimen may be instituted.

Older dogs with behavior problems or that are senile may have to be retrained to urinate outdoors or indoors on paper as well as before being left alone for a long period of time[6,16] (an empty bladder reduces the pressure placed on a weak sphincter). In some cases, behavior-modifying drugs (i.e., anticonvulsants or tranquilizers) may help a hyperexcitable animal that has a problem with incontinence.[6]

A weak urethral sphincter (urethral incompetence) in both sexes can be treated hormonally or with drugs that specifically increase urethral tone.[3,8,10] Females are usually treated with estrogens, which apparently help to increase urethral tone by increasing the sensitivity of the urethra to α-adrenergic stimulation.[3,8,10] Testosterone-responsive urinary incontinence has been reported in male dogs and may have a therapeutic basis similar to that of estrogen-responsive incontinence.[10,17] Diethylstilbestrol at a dosage of 0.1 to 1.0 mg/day for three to five days followed by a maintenance dosage of 1 mg/week has been recommended for estrogen-responsive incontinence, and testosterone propionate at a dose of 2.2 mg/kg intramuscularly has reportedly been effective in treating incontinence in neutered males.[3,10]

One drug that is particularly effective in treating the clinical signs of urethral incompetence in elderly patients is ephedrine. Ephedrine is an α-adrenergic agent that stimulates α receptors in the urethra and thereby results in increased urethral tone. Both male and female dogs respond equally to ephedrine, and prolonged use has not been demonstrated to cause any drug resistance. The maximum dosage of ephedrine is reported to be 4 mg/kg body weight given orally three times a day. Published side effects of ephedrine are hypertension, restlessness, hyperexcitability, anxiety, and increased heart rate. The authors have not noticed any adverse effects to date when this drug is used at the appropriate dosage and usually start large breeds on 25 mg three times a day, increasing the dose to 50 mg if there is no clinical response at the lower dosage. After the incontinence is controlled, the frequency of the drug can be reduced until the minimum amount of drug that main-

---

Urinary tract infections . . . should be treated with an appropriate antibiotic for at least six weeks.

---

tains the patient free of clinical signs is being given. Other α-adrenergic agents that can be substituted for ephedrine are phenylpropanolamine and phenylephrine.

Urinary tract infections in the elderly should be treated with an appropriate antibiotic for at least six weeks. A urine culture and sensitivity testing should be evaluated before selecting the antibiotic; the culture should be repeated 72 hours and three weeks after therapy has been initiated as well as one week, one month, and six months after therapy is discontinued. Urinalysis should be performed every 6 to 12 months to check for infectious inflammation of the urinary tract.

If polyuria and polydipsia are contributing factors, treating the underlying condition may help ameliorate the incontinence. The authors have found moderately restricted salt diets (e.g., Prescription Diet k/d® and u/d®—Hill's Pet Products) to be very effective in reducing or eliminating incontinence in dogs with chronic renal failure. Restricted salt diets probably are beneficial because they reduce water intake and urinary output and thereby reduce bladder distention and pressure on the urethral sphincter. Salt supplementation to these diets has been observed by the authors to result in a relapse of incontinence in dogs with chronic renal failure.

Therapy for neurologic incontinence varies depending on the cause. In all types of incontinence, treatment should be directed at correcting the specific cause of the disease. Therapy to alleviate clinical signs includes intermittent manual expression and/or aseptic catheterization of the bladder to remove urine from an areflexic bladder. Animals with partial or complete inability to empty the bladder should be monitored very closely for urinary tract infection.

Neurogenic incontinence can be treated with pharmacologic agents that either increase or decrease bladder or urethral tone as needed.[6,7] Reflex dyssynergia has been treated with neuromuscular relaxants and α-adrenergic–blocking agents. The diagnosis and treatment of neurologic urinary incontinence have been described in the veterinary literature.[6,7]

Four classes of drugs can be used to treat urinary incontinence (Table III): (1) cholinergic agents, which increase bladder contractibility; (2) anticholinergic agents, which decrease bladder contractibility; (3) α-adrenergic agents, which increase sphincter tone; and (4) α-adrenergic–blocking agents, which decrease sphincter tone.[8,9]

Therapeutic approaches to prostatic disease, lower urinary tract neoplasia, and urolithiasis should be followed as outlined in the veterinary literature.[25,27-32]

Some patients fail to respond to treatment either initiated for a specific cause or directed at alleviating clinical signs. In these cases, both the patient and the owner should be managed with compassion and intelligence. Euthanasia is always an alternative, but it is unacceptable to some clients. The authors have many

TABLE III
Drugs Used to Treat Urinary Incontinence

Class	Action and Uses	Specific Drugs and Dosages
Cholinergic agents	Increase the tone of the detrusor muscle; used to induce bladder contraction and micturition	Bethanechol: 2.5–10 mg subcutaneously 3 times/day
Anticholinergic agents	Decrease the tone of the detrusor muscle; used in certain types of urge incontinence to decrease spastic bladder contraction	Propantheline: 15 mg 3 times/day initially Oxybutynin: 5 mg 2–3 times/day Dicyclomine: 10 mg 3–4 times/day Flavoxate: 100–200 mg 3–4 times/day
α-adrenergic agents	Increase urethral sphincter tone; used in urethral incompetence	Ephedrine: 15–50 mg (no more than 4 mg/kg) orally 3 times/day Phenylpropanolamine: 12.5–50 mg orally 3 times/day
α-adrenergic-blocking agents	Decrease urethral sphincter tone; used for functional urethral obstruction	Phenoxybenzamine: 2.5–30 mg/day in divided doses

incontinent patients that require a diaper while in the house. Owners can also be taught to express and even catheterize the bladder as needed. These alternatives may be quite acceptable if they are presented with a positive, concerned approach.

REFERENCES

1. International Continence Society Standardization Committee: The standardization of terminology related to lower urinary tract function. *Scand J Urol Nephrol* 11:193-196,1977.
2. Hald T, Bradley WE: Urinary incontinence, in: *The Urinary Bladder*. Baltimore, The Williams & Wilkins Co, 1982, pp 175-201.
3. Osborne CA, Oliver JE, Polzin DE: Non-neurogenic urinary incontinence, in Kirk RW (ed): *Current Veterinary Therapy VII*. Philadelphia, WB Saunders Co, 1980, pp 1128-1136.
4. Rosin AE, Barsanti JA: Diagnosis of urinary incontinence in dogs: Role of the urethral pressure profile. *JAVMA* 178(8):814-822, 1981.
5. DiBartola SP, Adams WM: Urinary incontinence associated with malposition of the urinary bladder, in Kirk RW (ed): *Current Veterinary Therapy VIII*. Philadelphia, WB Saunders Co, 1983, pp 1089-1092.
6. Oliver JE, Osborne CA: Neurogenic urinary incontinence, in Kirk RW (ed): *Current Veterinary Therapy VII*. Philadelphia, WB Saunders Co, 1980, pp 1122-1127.
7. Moreau PM: Neurogenic disorders of micturition in the dog and cat. *Compend Contin Educ Pract Vet* 4(1):12-21, 1982.
8. Rosin AH, Ross L: Diagnosis and pharmacological management of disorders of urinary continence in the dog. *Compend Contin Educ Pract Vet* 3(7):601-609, 1981.
9. Freed SE: Urinary incontinence in the elderly. *Hosp Pract* 17:81-94, 1982.
10. Barsanti JA, Finco DR: Hormonal responses to urinary incontinence, in Kirk RW (ed): *Current Veterinary Therapy VIII*. Philadelphia, WB Saunders Co, 1983, pp 1086-1087.
11. Banks KL: Changes in the immune response related to age. *Vet Clin North Am* 11(4):683-688, 1981.
12. Brunson DB, Short CE: Anesthesia for the small animal geriatric patient. *Cornell Vet* 68(7):15-21, 1978.
13. Kirk RW: Small animal geriatric and pediatric medicine. *Cornell Vet* 68(7):268-275, 1978.
14. Mosier JE: Canine and feline geriatrics. *AAHA Proc* 45:153-160, 1978.
15. Mosier JE: Canine geriatrics. *AAHA Proc* 48:137-145, 1981.
16. Houpt KA, Beaver B: Behavioral problems of geriatric dogs and cats. *Vet Clin North Am* 11(4):643-652, 1981.
17. Barsanti JA, Edwards PD, Losonsky J: Testosterone responsive urinary incontinence in a castrated male dog. *JAAHA* 17:117-119, 1981.
18. Hardy RM, Osborne CA: Water deprivation and vasopression concentration tests in the differentiation of polyuric syndromes, in Kirk RW (ed): *Current Veterinary Therapy VII*. Philadelphia, WB Saunders Co, 1980, pp 1080-1085.
19. Hardy RM: Disorders of water metabolism. *Vet Clin North Am* 12(3):353-373, 1982.
20. Cowgill LD, Spangler WL: Renal insufficiency in geriatric dogs. *Vet Clin North Am* 11(4):727-748, 1981.
21. Guttman PH: Renal pathology, in Anderson AC (ed): *The Beagle as an Experimental Dog*. Ames, IA, Iowa State University Press, 1970, pp 546-557.
22. Osborne CA, Finco DR, Low DG: Pathophysiology of renal disease, renal failure and uremia, in Ettinger SJ (ed): *Textbook of Veterinary Internal Medicine*. Philadelphia, WB Saunders Co, 1983, pp 1733-1792.
23. Cowgill LD: Diseases of the kidney, in Ettinger SJ (ed): *Textbook of Veterinary Internal Medicine*. Philadelphia, WB Saunders Co, 1983, pp 1793-1879.
24. Osborne CA, Klausner JS, Lees GE: Urinary tract infections: Normal and abnormal host defense mechanisms. *Vet Clin North Am* 9(4):587-609, 1979.
25. Osborne CA, Klausner JS: War on canine urolithiasis: Problems and solutions. *AAHA Proc* 45:569-637, 1978.
26. Walker TL, Gage ED, Selcer RR: Disorders of the spinal cord and spine of the geriatric patient. *Vet Clin North Am* 11(4):765-786, 1981.
27. Morrison WB, Ott RL: Cancer and the aging process. *Vet Clin North Am* 11(4):677-682, 1981.
28. Osborne CA, Low DG, Perman V: Neoplasms of the canine and feline urinary bladder: Incidence, etiology, occurrence and pathology. *Am J Vet Res* 29:2041-2055, 1968.
29. Tarvin G, Patnaiki A, Green RW: Primary urethral tumors in dogs. *JAVMA* 172:931-933, 1978.
30. Green RW, Scott RC: Diseases of the bladder and urethra, in Ettinger SJ (ed): *Textbook of Veterinary Internal Medicine*. Philadelphia, WB Saunders Co, 1983, pp 1890-1936.
31. Hornbuckle WE, MacCoy DM, Allan GA, et al: Prostatic disease in the dog. *Cornell Vet* 68(7):284-305, 1978.
32. Greiner TP, Johnson RG: Diseases of the prostate gland, in Ettinger SJ (ed): *Textbook of Veterinary Internal Medicine*. Philadelphia, WB Saunders Co, 1983, pp 1459-1492.

UPDATE

FURTHER READING

Moreau PM, Lappin MR: Pharmacologic management of urinary incontinence, in Kirk RW (ed): *Current Veterinary Therapy, X*. Philadelphia, WB Saunders Co, 1989, pp 1214–1222.

Azotemia: A Review of What's Old and What's New Part I. Definition of Terms and Concepts

Carl A. Osborne, DVM, PhD
David J. Polzin, DVM, PhD

Department of Small Animal
Clinical Sciences
College of Veterinary Medicine
University of Minnesota
St. Paul, Minnesota

Dr. Carl A. Osborne has updated both parts of this series on azotemia. The update appears as an addendum to Part II. Asterisks (*) throughout both articles mark the passages for which Dr. Osborne has included changes in the addendum.

Definition of Terms and Concepts Related to Azotemia

Confusion and misunderstanding often occur when two people attempt to communicate using two different languages. More commonly, confusion arises between individuals using the same language but attaching different meanings or different definitions to what appears to be a universally accepted term (such as *renal disease*). Confusion caused by use of the terms *renal disease, renal failure, azotemia,* and *uremia* as synonyms may result in misdiagnosis and formulation of inappropriate or even contraindicated therapy.

Renal Disease

Renal disease should not be used synonymously with *renal failure* or *uremia* unless it is described as generalized renal disease because of the functional reserve capacity of the kidneys. Depending on the quantity of renal parenchyma affected and the severity and duration of lesions, renal disease(s) may or may not cause renal failure or uremia. The clinical relevance of the difference between renal disease and renal failure is emphasized by the fact that symptomatic and supportive therapies designed to correct fluid, electrolyte, acid-base, nutrient, and endocrine imbalances in patients with renal failure typically are not appropriate for patients with renal disease without renal dysfunction. Patients with adequate renal function have no need for dietary modification, anabolic agents, alkalinizing agents, and supplemental vitamins.

Renal disease may affect glomeruli, tubules, interstitial tissue, and/or vessels. Some renal diseases may be associated with dysfunction (e.g., some forms of nephrogenic diabetes insipidus and some forms of renal tubular acidosis) or biochemical abnormalities (e.g., cystinuria) without detectable morphologic alterations. Others may be associated with morphologic renal disease (anomalies, infections, endogenous or exogenous toxin-induced lesions, damage caused by obstruction to urine outflow, neoplasia, ischemic lesions, immune-mediated lesions, damage caused by hypercalcemia and other mineral imbalances, traumatic lesions) that affects one or both kidneys. The specific cause(s) of renal disease(s) may or may not be known; however, quantitative information about renal function (or dysfunction) is not defined. Renal disease(s) may regress, persist, or advance. Unfortunately, many renal diseases escape detection until they become so generalized that they induce clinical signs as a result of serious impairment of renal function.

Renal Failure (Insufficiency)

Failure is defined as an inability to perform. The term *renal failure* (or renal insufficiency) has been typically used to imply that two-thirds or three-quarters or more of the functional capacity of the nephrons of both kidneys have been impaired. It often is used to connote a less severe state of renal dysfunction (or renal insufficiency) that is not (yet) associated with polysystemic clinical manifestations (i.e., uremia). Studies in dogs revealed that impaired ability to concentrate and dilute urine caused by primary renal disease was not detected by evaluation of urine specific gravity (SG) until about two-thirds of the nephrons of both kidneys were surgically extirpated.[1,2] Although the serum concentrations of urea nitrogen and creatinine vary inversely with glomerular filtration rate, primary renal azotemia and retention of other metabolites normally excreted by the kidneys are usually not recognized until the functional capacity of 70 to 75% of the nephrons is affected (Table I).

Renal function *adequate* for homeostasis does not require that *all* nephrons be functional. The concept that adequate renal function is not synonymous with total renal function is of importance in understanding the difference between renal disease and renal failure; formulating meaningful prognoses; and formulating specific, supportive, and symptomatic therapy.[3]

The term *renal failure* is analogous to liver failure or heart failure in that a level organ dysfunction is described rather than a specific disease entity. The kidneys perform multiple functions including selective elimination of waste products of metabolism from the body, synthesis of a variety of hormones, and degradation of a variety of hormones. Failure to perform these functions may not be an *all or none phenomenon* (Table I). For example, in slowly progressive renal diseases, failure to appropriately concentrate or dilute urine according to body need typically precedes failure to eliminate waste products of metabolism of such magnitude that it causes azotemia. In turn, laboratory detection of impaired ability to eliminate waste products of metabolism (such as urea and creatinine) and to maintain electrolyte and nonelectrolyte solute balance within normal limits typically precedes the onset of polysystemic signs of renal dysfunction.

Clinical signs of polysystemic disorders caused by abnormalities of water, electrolyte, acid-base, endocrine, and nutrient balance are not invariably present in patients with primary renal failure (i.e., not all patients with primary renal failure are uremic). This is related, at least in part, to the reserve capacity of the kidneys and the ability of unaffected nephrons to undergo compensatory hypertrophy and hyperplasia. Polysystemic signs of renal failure (i.e., uremia), including vomiting, diarrhea, depression, anorexia, dehydration, and weight loss, usually do not occur until more than three-quarters of the total nephron population has been functionally impaired.

Although compensatory mechanisms of the body maintain a state of biochemical homeostasis despite significant renal dysfunction, a price is paid for loss of functional renal reserve capacity. Patients with presymptomatic primary renal failure have reduced capacity to respond to physiologic and pathologic stresses. A uremic crisis may be suddenly precipitated by decreased intake of water or nutrients, development of concomitant but unrelated diseases in other body systems, and/or administration of certain drugs.

Azotemia

Azotemia is defined as an abnormal concentration of urea, creatinine, and other nonprotein nitrogenous

TABLE I

COMPARISON OF LEVEL OF NEPHRON FUNCTION ASSOCIATED WITH TYPICAL MANIFESTATIONS OF RENAL DYSFUNCTION

Type of Impaired Function	Nephron Dysfunction (%)
Altered glomerular capillary permeability to plasma proteins	Variable[a]
Impaired tubular concentration or dilution of glomerular filtrate	≥ 2/3
Azotemia and hyperphosphatemia due to impaired glomerular filtration rate	≥ 3/4
Impaired synthesis of erythropoietin and 1,25-vitamin D	> 3/4
Polysystemic signs of uremia	> 3/4

[a] Glomerular proteinuria may occur in patients with normal glomerular filtration rate, normal tubular reabsorption, and normal tubular secretion. It may also occur when these functions are mildly or severely altered.

substances in blood, plasma, or serum. Azotemia is a laboratory finding with several fundamentally different causes. Since nonprotein nitrogenous compounds (including urea and creatinine) are endogenous substances, abnormally elevated concentrations in serum may be caused by an increased rate of production (by the liver for urea; by muscles for creatinine), or by a decreased rate of loss (primarily by the kidneys).

Because azotemia may be caused by factors that are not directly related to the urinary system and by abnormalities of the lower urinary tract not directly related to the kidney, *azotemia* should not be used as a synonym for renal failure or uremia. Although the concentrations of serum urea nitrogen and creatinine are commonly used as crude indices of glomerular filtration rate, meaningful interpretation of these parameters depends on recognition and evaluation of prerenal, primary renal, and postrenal factors that may reduce glomerular filtration rate (Tables II and III).

Uremia

Uremia is defined as (1) abnormal quantities of urine constituents in blood caused by primary generalized renal disease *and* (2) the polysystemic toxic syndrome which occurs as a result of abnormal renal function. When the structural and functional integrity of both kidneys has been compromised to such a degree that polysystemic signs of renal failure are clinically manifested, the relatively predictable symptom complex called *uremia* appears, regardless of underlying cause. In some

TABLE II

LOCALIZATION OF AZOTEMIA CAUSED BY
REDUCED GLOMERULAR FILTRATION

Causes of Reduced Glomerular Filtration	Localization of Azotemia
Decreased blood volume	Prerenal
Decreased blood pressure	Prerenal
Decreased colloidal osmotic pressure[a]	Prerenal
Decreased number of patent vessels	Primary renal
Decreased glomerular permeability	Primary renal
Increased renal interstitial pressure	Primary renal (tubular obstruction)
Increased intratubular pressure	Postrenal (obstruction of ureters, bladder, and/or urethra)
Combinations of causes	Prerenal and primary renal, postrenal and primary renal, or prerenal and postrenal

[a]Reduction in plasma colloidal osmotic pressure as a result of severe hypoalbuminemia is actually a mechanism of decreased blood volume. It is listed separately for emphasis.

instances, uremic crises may suddenly be precipitated by prerenal disorders (e.g., congestive heart failure, acute pancreatitis, hypoadrenocorticism), or, less commonly, postrenal disorders (urethral obstruction, displacement of the urinary bladder into a perineal hernia, etc.) in patients with previously compensated primary renal failure (Table II).

Uremia is characterized by multiple physiologic and metabolic alterations that result from renal insufficiency. Renal insufficiency may be caused by a large number of disease processes which have in common impairment of at least three-quarters of the function of both kidneys. Depending on the biological behavior of the disease in question, primary renal failure may be reversible or irreversible, acute or chronic, and oliguric and/or polyuric.

To recapitulate, renal disease may precede renal failure, and likewise, renal failure may precede uremia. In some situations renal disease may not progress to a state of renal failure. In others prerenal events may precipitate a uremic crisis in patients with chronic renal failure. In untreated patients, uremia is always accompanied by renal disease, renal failure, and azotemia.

Differentiation of Renal Disease from Renal Failure

Differentiation between renal disease and renal failure (with or without uremia) may be facilitated by knowledge that not all diagnostic procedures used to detect disorders of the urinary system provide information about renal functional capacity, nor is it always possible to differentiate inflammatory diseases of the lower urinary tract from those affecting the upper urinary tract (Table IV). For example, detection of a significant number of casts in urine sediment provides reliable evidence of renal tubular involvement because casts form in the loops of Henle, distal tubules, and collection ducts. One cannot infer that detection of large numbers of casts is indicative of renal failure, however, because their presence or absence cannot be correlated with the degree of renal dysfunction (if any).

Differentiation between renal disease and renal failure is of great clinical significance when gastrointestinal, endocrine, pancreatic, and hepatic diseases causing clinical signs similar to those associated with uremia (i.e., vomiting, diarrhea, polydipsia, dehydration, depression, anorexia, and weight loss) secondarily induce prerenal azotemia and/or ischemic tubular disease characterized by formation of variable numbers of epithelial, granular, and waxy casts (Table IV). Although extrarenal fluid loss and subsequent reduction in renal perfusion may be of sufficient magnitude to damage some nephrons and cause prerenal azotemia, detection of concentrated urine (specific gravity > 1.030 in dogs or > 1.035 in cats) indicates a population of functioning nephrons adequate to prevent signs caused by primary renal failure (Tables III and IV).* Every effort should be made to restore renal perfusion, however,

TABLE III

EXAMPLES OF DIFFERENT CAUSES OF AZOTEMIA IN DOGS

Factors	Prerenal Causes		Postrenal Causes	Primary Renal Causes			
	Pancreatitis (Boston Terrier, 7-yr-old, Male)	Hypoadreno-corticism (Greyhound, 3-yr-old, Female)	Urethral Obstruction (Miniature Poodle, 9-yr-old, Male)	Hypercalcemic Nephropathy (Mixed-Breed, 5-yr-old, Female)	Ischemic Renal Failure (Beagle, 11-yr-old, Female)	Early Glomerular with Glomerulotubular Imbalance Amyloidosis (Great Dane, 7-yr-old, Female)	Advanced Glomerular Amyloidosis (Beagle, 5-yr-old, Male)
S urea nitrogen (mg/dl)	65	75	54	75	207	50	148
S creatinine (mg/dl)	2.1	2.5	2.0	4.5	16.2	2.0	5.1
U volume	Decreased	Decreased	Absent	Increased	Decreased	Normal	Increased
U SG	1.047	1.017	1.021	1.014	1.010	1.024	1.011
U protein	Negative	Negative	2^a4+	Negative	1+^{a}	3+	4+
U casts	Moderately granular	Few granular	Negative	Negative	Negative	Occasional hyaline	Rare hyaline
S sodium (mEq/L)	147	136	151	159	133	144	146
S potassium (mEq/L)	4.9	7.1	4.1	4.4	6.0	3.1	3.8
S Na:K ratio	> 25:1	< 25:1	> 25:1	> 25:1	< 25:1	> 25:1	> 25:1
S calcium (mg/dl)	10.0	11.5	9.0	14.7	9.1	9.8	7.0^b
S amylase (DiAmyl units)	12,800	2130	ND	2900	ND	3200	540

Key: S = serum; U = urine; ND = not determined.
^{a}Associated with red and white blood cells in sediment and attributable to hemorrhage or an inflammatory response.
^{b}Associated with a marked reduction in the total concentration of serum protein, and the serum concentration of albumin.[33]

since progressive destruction of nephrons may induce primary ischemic renal failure.

Definition of Terms and Concepts Related to Urine Osmolality and Specific Gravity
Osmolality

Dissolution of one or more substances (or solutes) in a solvent (water) changes four mathematically interrelated physical characteristics (known as *colligative properties*): osmotic pressure, freezing point, vapor pressure, and boiling point. These properties are all directly related to the total number of solute particles within the solution and are independent of the homogenicity or nonhomogenicity of molecular species, molecular weight, and molecular size. As solute is added to solvent, osmotic pressure increases, freezing point decreases, vapor pressure decreases, and boiling point increases.[3] Changes in these colligative properties depend on the number of particles of solute in solution and not on other particle characteristics such as molecular weight, electrical charge, chemical nature, or shape. In clinical medicine, the osmotic concentration of solutions is usually measured with instruments that determine freezing point (freezing point osmometer) or vapor pressure (vapor pressure osmometer).

The unit of osmotic concentration is the osmole. Since the osmole represents a large mass of solute, the milliosmole (mOsm) has been developed for clinical use. One milliosmole = 0.001 osmole. Sodium, chloride, and bicarbonate account for approximately 300 mOsm/kg of water. Sodium, chloride, and urea account for the majority of osmotic activity in urine. The osmotic concentration of glomerular filtrate is about 300 mOsm/kg of water. Normally, the osmotic concentration of urine is variable, being dependent on the fluid and electrolyte balance of the body and the nitrogen content of the diet. Species differences in the ability to concentrate urine are significant (Table V).[3]

The ratio of urine osmolality (U_{osm}) to plasma osmolality (P_{osm}) is a good clinical index of the ability of the

TABLE IV

DIAGNOSTIC PROCEDURES COMMONLY USED TO DETECT AND LOCALIZE
DISORDERS OF THE URINARY SYSTEM[a]

Method	Renal Function	Localize to Kidney	Localize to Urinary System
Urea nitrogen (serum or plasma)	GFR	No[a]	No
Creatinine (serum or plasma)	GFR	No[a]	No
Specific gravity (urine)	Tubular reabsorption	No[a]	No
Osmolality (urine)	Tubular reabsorption	No[a]	No
Phenolsulfonphthalein (urine excretion)	RBF; tubular secretion	No[a]	No
Sodium sulfanilate (plasma retention)	GFR	No[a]	No
Intravenous urography	Crude index of RBF and GFR	Yes	Yes
Ultrasonography	No	Yes	Yes
Water deprivation and vasopressin response tests	Tubular function	No[a]	No
Renal tubular epithelial cells	No	No[b]	No
Urinary casts	No	Yes	–
Renal biopsy	No	Yes	–
Significant bacteriuria	No	No	Yes[c]
Proteinuria	No	No[d]	No
Pyuria	No	No[e]	Yes[c]
Hematuria	No	No[e]	Yes[c]

[a]From Osborne CA, Finco DR, Low DG: Pathophysiology of renal disease, renal failure and uremia, in Ettinger SG (ed): *Textbook of Veterinary Internal Medicine*, vol 2, ed 2. Philadelphia, WB Saunders Co, 1982, p 1755. Modified with permission.
[b]Alterations in renal function are not always caused by diseases localized to the kidneys.
[c]Unless present in urinary casts
[d]Assuming urine not contaminated by genital tract
[e]Large quantities of protein in absence of RBC and WBC suggest glomerular disease.

kidneys to concentrate or dilute glomerular filtrate.[4] A $U_{osm}:P_{osm}$ ratio above 1 indicates that the kidneys are concentrating urine above plasma and glomerular filtrate. Following water deprivation, the $U_{osm}:P_{osm}$ of normal dogs may be 7 or higher.[5] A $U_{osm}:P_{osm}$ ratio of approximately 1 indicates that water and solute are being excreted in a state that is isoosmotic with plasma. A $U_{osm}:P_{osm}$ ratio significantly below 1 indicates that the tubules are capable of reabsorbing solute in excess of water (i.e., they are diluting glomerular filtrate).

Specific Gravity

Specific gravity is the ratio of the density of a liquid to the density of water under standard conditions of temperature and pressure. The *density* of a liquid is defined as the mass of a unit volume of the liquid at standard temperature and pressure.

Urine specific gravity is a measurement of the density of urine compared with pure water. Stated in another way, urine specific gravity is the ratio of the weight of urine to the weight of an equal volume of water, both

TABLE V

APPROXIMATE URINE OSMOLALITY AND SPECIFIC GRAVITY VALUES
FOR ADULT DOGS, CATS, AND HUMANS

Factor	Species		
	Dog	Cat	Human
Range of normal SG	1.001 to ~1.065+	1.001 to ~1.080+	1.001 to ~1.035+
Usual SG, normal hydration	1.015 to ~1.045	1.035 to ~1.060	1.015 to ~1.025
Range of normal osmolality (mOsm/kg)	50 to ~2500+	50 to ~3000	50 to ~1500+

measured at the same temperature and pressure (SG = weight of urine/weight of water).[6] The specific gravity of water is 1.000. Urine is denser than water because it is composed of water and various solutes of different densities.

There is only an approximate relationship between specific gravity and osmolality (total solute concentration). In addition to the number of molecules of solute, specific gravity is influenced by other factors including molecular size and molecular weight of solutes. Since each species of solute has its own characteristic effect on the specific gravity of urine, urine samples having equivalent numbers of solute molecules per unit volume may have different specific gravity values if different mixtures of solutes are present. For example, equal numbers of molecules of urea, sodium, chloride, albumin, globulin, fibrinogen, and glucose all have a different quantitative effect on specific gravity. Thus urine specific gravity is a direct, but not necessarily proportional, index of the number of solute particles in urine. It provides only an estimate of osmolality because of the variability in quantity of heterogenous solutes in urine. Measurement of urine specific gravity is useful as a screening procedure, but it may be unsuitable in some circumstances requiring more precise evaluation of the renal tubular concentrating and diluting capacity.

Interpretation of urine specific gravity values of randomly obtained samples depends on knowledge of the patient's hydration status, the plasma or serum concentration of urea nitrogen or creatinine, and knowledge of drugs or fluids that have been administered to the patient. Knowledge of urine volume and water consumption may also be helpful. In some instances, interpretation may require knowledge of urine and plasma osmolality.

Hypersthenuria, Isosthenuria, and Hyposthenuria

Hypersthenuria, isosthenuria, and *hyposthenuria* are terms that depict the solute and water composition of urine compared with glomerular filtrate. Hypersthenuria (also called *baruria*) depicts urine of high specific gravity and osmolality compared with glomerular filtrate. Isosthenuria depicts urine with a specific gravity and osmolality similar to that of plasma and glomerular filtrate. Complete loss of ability to concentrate or dilute glomerular filtrate according to body need is sometimes referred to as *fixed specific gravity.* Hyposthenuria depicts formation of dilute urine with a specific gravity and osmolality that are significantly lower than that of plasma and glomerular filtrate.

The specific gravity of urine of normal dogs and cats is variable, being dependent on the fluid and electrolyte balance of the body, the nitrogen content of the diet, and other variables related to species and individuals (Table V). The urine specific gravity often fluctuates widely from day to day and within the same day. Urine specific gravity may range from 1.001 to 1.060 or greater

in adult normal dogs and from 1.001 to 1.080 or greater in adult normal cats. Depending on the requirements of the body for water and/or solutes, any specific gravity value within these ranges may be normal. Therefore the concept of an average normal specific gravity is misleading because it implies that values above or below the average may not be normal. Randomly collected urine samples from normal adult dogs and cats often have a specific gravity that encompasses a narrower range than that just mentioned (approximately 1.015 to ~1.045 for dogs and 1.035 to ~1.060 for cats) (Table V), but an individual urine sample with a specific gravity outside these values is not reliable evidence of renal dysfunction.

Maximum, minimum, and typical urine specific gravity values for infant and immature dogs and cats have not been extensively evaluated. In one study, the measurement of urine specific gravity of canine fetuses 10 days prior to birth revealed values that ranged from 1.008 to ~1.025.[7] Randomly collected urine samples from dogs that were 2 days old had an osmolality approximately twice that of plasma, but the ratio was approximately 7 times that of plasma when the pups were 77 days old.[8] These observations have been interpreted to suggest that the kidneys of newborn puppies can concentrate urine to some degree and that concentrating capacity improves with age.[9] This parallels tubular function in human infants who are able to concentrate urine to a maximum of 700 to 800 mOsm/kg of water at the time of birth.[10] Newborn human infants can dilute urine to values as low as 40 mOsm/kg of water.[11] It is emphasized that appropriate caution must be used when interpreting urine specific gravity and osmolality values of immature animals since they probably have different average, minimum, and maximum values than those of mature animals. Similar caution is appropriate when comparing normal adult and infant levels of glomerular filtration and tubular reabsorption.[11,12]

A urine specific gravity that is similar to that of glomerular filtrate (1.008 to 1.012) may be observed in individuals with normal renal function since the ability of normal kidneys to influence specific gravity encompasses these values. Since such values may be normal or abnormal, they should be viewed as presumptive evidence of an abnormality. Further data are required, however, to prove or disprove this presumption.

Significance of USG = 1.025 in Humans, Dogs, and Cats*

The ability of patients to excrete urine with a specific gravity significantly above that of glomerular filtrate (1.008 to 1.012) depends on an intact system for production and release of antidiuretic hormone, a sufficient population of functional nephrons to generate and maintain a high-solute concentration in the renal medulla, and a sufficient population of functional tubules to respond to antidiuretic hormone. Data obtained from experimental studies in dogs suggest that only about one-third of normal renal function is required to concentrate urine to 1.025 or greater.[2] Stated another way, significant impairment of the kidneys' ability to concentrate (or dilute) urine is usually not detected until at least two-thirds of the total renal functional parenchyma has been impaired.

The ability of dogs to concentrate urine to a specific gravity of 1.025 has been generally accepted as evidence of *adequate* renal concentrating capacity to maintain homeostasis and to prevent clinical signs of primary renal failure. It appears that the urine specific gravity end point of 1.025 previously used by many veterinarians has been extrapolated from human data. Since humans can concentrate their urine to a maximum of 1.035 to 1.040, whereas values for dogs may reach 1.060 or more and values for cats may reach 1.080 or more, concentration of urine to 1.025 probably implies better renal tubular function in humans than in cats or dogs (Table V).

Uncontrolled clinical observations in dogs indicate that detection of a urine specific gravity ≥1.025 indicates a population of nephrons adequate to prevent clinical signs associated with primary renal failure. A significant degree of renal disease may exist in dogs able to concentrate their urine to a specific gravity of 1.025, though. In one study, the maximal urine specific gravities of three partially nephrectomized dogs (two-thirds of total nephrons removed) subjected to 48 hours of water deprivation were 1.023, 1.018, and 1.027.[2]

Experimental studies recently performed on cats at the University of Georgia revealed that animals with less than 25% functional nephrons could concentrate their urine significantly higher than a specific gravity of 1.025.[13] Further studies in cats are required to determine the urine specific gravity value that indicates an adequate population of functional nephrons to prevent clinical signs associated with primary renal failure.

Since metabolic work is required to dilute glomerular filtrate by removing solute in excess of water, a urine specific gravity significantly below 1.007 (1.001 to 1.005) indicates that a sufficient number of functional nephrons is present to prevent clinical signs associated with primary renal failure. Although the minimum number of nephrons required to dilute canine or feline urine to a specific gravity of ≤ 1.005 has not been determined, it has been assumed to be similar to that required for urine concentration (i.e., about one-third of the total nephron mass). However, normal diluting ability may be maintained with fewer functional nephrons than normal concentrating ability.[14,15]

Abnormal Values

The section on definitions of terms and concepts related to azotemia should be consulted for information on renal disease, renal function, azotemia, and uremia.

Relationship to Renal Failure

Varying degrees of impaired ability to concentrate or dilute glomerular filtrate is a consistent finding in all forms of primary renal failure. Because the kidneys have tremendous reserve capacity, impairment of their ability to concentrate or dilute urine may not be detected until at least two-thirds (dogs) or more (cats) of the total population of nephrons has been damaged. Complete inability of the nephrons to modify glomerular filtrate typically results in formation of urine with a specific gravity that is similar to that of glomerular filtrate. Total loss of the ability to concentrate and dilute urine (SG = 1.008 to 1.012) often does not occur as a sudden event but may develop gradually. For this reason urine specific gravity values between approximately 1.006 to 1.029 in dogs and 1.006 to 1.034 in cats associated with clinical dehydration and/or azotemia are highly suggestive of primary renal failure (Tables III and VI).* Contrary to statements widely publicized at one time, acute renal diseases of severity sufficient to cause primary renal failure are not associated with marked elevation in urine specific gravity values. Azotemia associated with hypersthenuria should prompt a high index of suspicion of prerenal azotemia.

Once urine specific gravity reflects impaired ability to concentrate or dilute urine (1.006 to 1.029 in dogs), it is more of a general index of nephron function than a specific index of distal tubular and collecting duct function since, in addition to generalized tubular lesions, this abnormality is related to other factors. These factors include (1) increased clearance and decreased fractional tubular reabsorption of solutes retained in plasma (urea, creatinine, phosphorus, sodium, etc.) by viable nephrons. These phenomena induce an obligatory osmotic diuresis; and (2) reduction in the number of functioning nephrons, resulting in impaired ability to maintain the high medullary osmotic gradient required for a functional countercurrent system.

Once the ability to concentrate or dilute urine has been permanently destroyed, repeated evaluation of specific gravity will not be helpful in evaluation of progressive deterioration of renal function. Therefore, serial evaluation of urine specific gravity is of greatest help in detecting functional changes earlier during the course of primary renal failure or in monitoring functional recovery associated with reversible renal diseases.

If sufficient clinical evidence is present to warrant examination of the patient's renal function by determining the serum concentration of creatinine or blood urea nitrogen, the urine specific gravity (or osmolality) should be evaluated at the same time. As emphasized above, a concentrated urine sample associated with an abnormal elevation in serum creatinine or urea nitrogen concentration suggests the probability of *prerenal azotemia* (Tables III and VI). Azotemia associated with a specific gravity of 1.006 to ∼1.029 (dogs) or 1.034 (cats) indicates the probability of primary renal failure, although on occasion hypoadrenocorticism may induce

TABLE VI

Characteristic Urine Volumes and Urine Specific Gravity Associated with Different Types of Azotemia in Dogs and Cats[a],*

Prerenal azotemia
Physiologic oliguria
  Dogs: $U_{SG} > 1.030$
  Cats: $U_{SG} > 1.035$

Primary acute ischemic or nephrotoxic azotemia
Initial oliguria
  Dogs: $U_{SG} = 1.006$ to ~1.029
  Cats: $U_{SG} = 1.006$ to ~1.034

Subsequent polyuric phase
  Dogs: $U_{SG} = 1.006$ to ~1.029
  Cats: $U_{SG} = 1.006$ to ~1.034

Obstructive postrenal azotemia
Initial oliguria or anuria
Diuresis and polyuria following relief of obstruction

Primary chronic azotemia
Polyuria
  Dogs: 1.006 to ~1.029
  Cats: 1.006 to ~1.034[b]

Terminal oliguric phase
  $U_{SG} = 1.007$ to ~1.013

Reversible oliguria may be caused by onset of nonrenal disorder that induces prerenal azotemia.
  Dogs: $U_{SG} = 1.006$ to ~1.029
  Cats: $U_{SG} = 1.006$ to ~1.034

---

[a]From Osborne CA, et al: Pathophysiology of renal disease, renal failure, and uremia, in Ettinger SG (ed): *Textbook of Veterinary Internal Medicine*, vol 2, ed 2. Philadelphia, WB Saunders Co, 1982, p 1758. Modified with permission.

[b]Urine specific gravity may become fixed between approximately 1.007 and 1.013 if sufficient nephron function is altered. The specific gravity of glomerular filtrate is approximately 1.008 to 1.012.

---

similar findings (Table VII).* If nonazotemic patients have impaired ability to concentrate urine, causes of pathologic polyuria should be explored. Determination of urine specific gravity or osmolality may allow one to determine whether a disorder characterized by water (0.001 to ~1.006) or solute (~1.008 or greater) diuresis is probable.[16] Water deprivation and vasopressin response tests may also be required.[5,9,17–20]

Applied Biochemistry and Clinical Pathology
Blood Urea Nitrogen*

Urea is a nonprotein nitrogenous substance that is formed primarily by the liver as a mechanism for excretion of ammonia generated by catabolism of nitrogen-containing compounds (i.e., endogenous and dietary amino acids).[9] Normally, an insignificant quantity of urea per se is consumed in the diets of dogs and cats. Therefore, the rate of urea formation depends on the rate at which amino acids are delivered to the liver for catabolism.

Urea is a small molecule (molecular weight = 60 daltons) that diffuses readily throughout all body fluid compartments (Table VIII). Because its concentration is equal in intracellular (including red cells) and extra-cellular fluid, its concentration is similar in whole blood, plasma, and serum.[21] As currently used, the acronym *BUN* (blood urea nitrogen) is a misnomer since most laboratories use serum (SUN) or plasma (PUN) rather than blood to measure the concentration of urea.

Although some urea synthesized by the liver normally diffuses into the intestinal lumen (estimated to be approximately 25% of hepatic production), it is catabolized by enteric bacteria to ammonia, which is reabsorbed and resynthesized by the liver into urea. This hepatic-enteric cycle prevents significant fecal loss of urea from the body.

The kidneys are the primary route of excretion of urea from the body. Because urea freely passes through glomerular capillary walls into Bowman's spaces, its concentration in glomerular filtrate is similar to its concentration in plasma. Urea is both passively reabsorbed and secreted by the renal tubules.[22] However, the net effect of these two opposing mechanisms is renal tubular reabsorption. Less than 50% of the urea filtered by glomeruli appears in urine excreted from the body. Urea reabsorbed by the tubules plays an important role in renal medullary hyperosmolality and function of the countercurrent system. The rate of tubular reabsorption of urea is influenced by the volume of tubular filtrate. More urea is absorbed during periods of reduced (about 35 to 40%) than increased urine flow.[23]

Because the kidneys are the primary route of excretion of urea from the body, the serum or plasma concentration of urea is commonly used as an index of renal function. The relationship between SUN and glomerular filtration rate (GFR) is sufficiently predictable that, *providing that urea production is relatively constant* and a relatively high rate of urine flow exists, their product remains constant (GFR × SUN = constant) (Figure 1). Thus measurement of the concentration of SUN provides a crude index of GFR.

Any abnormality (prerenal, primary renal, and/or postrenal) that decreases GFR will cause an increase in the concentration of SUN (Tables II and III). Unfortunately, abnormal elevations in the concentration of SUN that occur as a result of impaired renal function are not detectable until approximately 75% (or more in patients with chronic progressive renal disease in which viable nephrons have undergone compensatory adaptation) of the nephrons of both kidneys become nonfunctional. In other words, detection of a normal concentration of urea nitrogen in serum or plasma does not rule out a substantial reduction in GFR. Although the concentration of SUN increases during early stages of progressive reduction in GFR, the increase is so gradual at first that it is hidden within the normal limits of SUN concentration (7 to 30 mg/dl in dogs and 20 to 35 mg/dl in cats). Stated another way, early stages of progressive renal diseases are accompanied by only a minor increase in the concentration in SUN, even though there has been destruction of a large quantity of renal parenchyma. As the disease progresses, a stage is eventually reached

TABLE VII

DIFFERENTIATION OF ACUTE PRIMARY OLIGURIC RENAL FAILURE FROM HYPOADRENOCORTICISM

Factor	Acute Oliguric Renal Failure[a]	Acute Hypoadrenocorticism[b]
Vomiting	+++	++
Diarrhea	+	+
Weakness	++	++
Depression	+++	++
Anorexia	+	++
Collapse	+	++
Bradycardia	+	+
Arrhythmia	+	+
Electrocardiogram	Typical of hyperkalemia	Typical of hyperkalemia
Hypotension	+	+
Shock	+	+
Packed-cell volume	Variable	Variable
Total serum proteins	Variable	Variable
Blood eosinophils	Sometimes decreased	Variable
Blood lymphocytes	Sometimes decreased	Variable
Serum urea nitrogen	Increased	Increased
Serum creatinine	Increased	Increased
Urine volume	Decreased	Variable
Urine specific gravity	1.007–1.029	< 1.030
Serum sodium	Variable	Typically decreased
Serum potassium	Increased	Typically increased
Na:K (serum ratio)	< 1:25	< 1:25
Serum calcium	Variable	Sometimes increased
Blood pH	Decreased	Decreased
Plasma bicarbonate	Decreased	Decreased
Blood glucose	Variable	Sometimes increased
Plasma cortisol	?	Decreased
Response to ACTH stimulation	?	Abnormal
Response to treatment with glucocorticoids	Variable to poor	Often dramatic improvement

[a] Additional factors that support a diagnosis of acute primary oliguric renal failure include a history of exposure to nephrotoxic agents and recent occurrence of disorders likely to cause profound renal ischemia.
[b] An additional factor that supports a diagnosis of hypoadrenocorticism is previous response of gastrointestinal signs to symptomatic treatment with glucocorticoids.

when destruction of a relatively small number of nephrons is accompanied by a relatively large increase in the concentration of SUN (Figure 1).

Several nonrenal factors that have no direct relationship to the kidneys may substantially affect the concentration of SUN. These factors are related to the rate of production of urea or to body fluid balance (or both).

Although several factors tend to limit the specificity of SUN as an index of renal function, the test is of clinical value provided it is properly interpreted. Determination of SUN is technically easy and economical. It is not a good test of GFR before three-quarters of

the functional capacity of the nephrons has been impaired, but it may be used to confirm the presence of renal failure. When performed serially, it provides a good index of response to certain forms of therapy for renal failure. If performed serially and interpreted in association with other clinical, laboratory, and biopsy findings, it provides information that is useful in establishing a prognosis.

Creatinine*

Creatinine is another form of nonprotein nitrogen that is irreversibly formed as a result of nonenzymatic

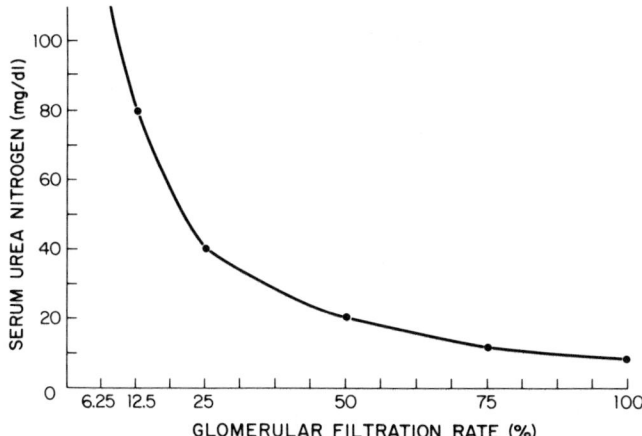

Figure 1—Approximate graphic relationship between GFR and SUN concentration. The same approximate relationship applies to GFR and serum creatinine concentration.

TABLE VIII

COMPARISON OF MOLECULAR WEIGHTS OF SUBSTANCES INCLUDED IN AND EXCLUDED FROM GLOMERULAR FILTRATE

Substance	Molecular Weight	Presence in Glomerular Filtrate
Water	18	+
Potassium	19	+
Urea	60	+
Phosphate	96	+
Creatinine	113	+
Glucose	180	+
Lysozyme	14,000	+
Myoglobin	17,000	+
Bence Jones monomers	22,000	+
Bence Jones dimers	44,000	+
Amylase	50,000	+
Hemoglobin[a]	68,000	±
Albumin	69,000	±
Immunoglobulin-G	160,000	−
Immunoglobulin-A (dimer)	300,000	−
Fibrinogen	400,000	−
Alpha-2-macroglobulin	840,000	−
Immunoglobulin-M	900,000	−

[a] Probably excreted as a dimer with a molecular weight of approximately 32,000.

metabolism of creatine and phosphocreatine in muscle.[9] It is an end product of muscle metabolism. Creatinine is a larger molecule than urea (molecular weight = 113 daltons), and it therefore diffuses throughout fluid compartments more slowly than urea (Table VIII).

Creatinine is not reutilized by the body like urea. Creatinine may diffuse into the intestinal lumen, where a portion is degraded by bacteria.[9,24] Products of enteric creatinine catabolism are not reutilized to reform creatinine but apparently are lost in the feces. Thus, some creatinine may be eliminated from the body by nonrenal routes.

The kidneys are a major route of excretion of creatinine from the body. Because creatinine freely passes through glomerular capillary walls into Bowman's spaces, its concentration in glomerular filtrate is similar to its concentration in plasma. Although creatinine is not reabsorbed by the renal tubules of dogs or cats, an extremely weak proximal tubular secretory mechanism has been identified in normal dogs.[25,26] Creatinine is not secreted by the tubules in cats.[27,28] Although the renal excretion of creatinine is apparently independent of urine flow rate, the amount secreted by canine renal tubules is influenced by serum creatinine concentration. Abnormal elevations in plasma creatinine caused by reduction in renal function are associated with an increase in tubular secretion of creatinine.[29,30] However, provided its rate of production is constant, measurement of the serum creatinine concentration provides a crude index of GFR (GFR × creatinine = constant).

As with SUN, any abnormality (prerenal, primary renal, and/or postrenal) that decreases GFR will cause an increase in the serum concentration of creatinine (Tables II and III). In addition, like SUN, abnormal elevations in the concentration of creatinine that occur as a result of impairment of renal function are not detectable until approximately three-quarters or more of the nephrons of both kidneys become nonfunctional. Therefore, detection of normal concentrations of creat-

inine in serum do not rule out substantial reductions in glomerular filtration.

The concentration of serum creatinine is affected by fewer variables than is the concentration of SUN. Creatinine concentration is not substantially affected by diet or protein catabolic factors such as fever, infection, administration of corticosteroids, and so forth.[31,*] Normal daily production of creatinine is relatively constant within the same individual, but it may vary among individuals. Theoretically, diseases characterized by active destruction of muscle could cause an increase in production and serum concentration of creatinine that is unrelated to renal function. We have not knowingly encountered such diseases in dogs or cats.

Several techniques have been advocated for determining the serum concentration of creatinine. Because the alkaline picrate method (Jaffé's) of creatinine determination measures noncreatinine chromogens present in serum as well as creatinine, this method gives erroneously high creatinine values.[9] The use of Lloyd's reagent (fuller's earth) has been reported to allow the measurement of *true* creatinine concentration by excluding noncreatinine chromogens. When the concentration of creatinine exceeds 1.2 to 2.0 mg/100 ml of plasma or serum (depending on whether or not noncreatinine chromogens were measured), GFR is reduced. As with SUN, the reduction in GFR may be caused by prerenal, primary, and/or postrenal uremia.

Choice of Tests

Serum concentrations of urea and creatinine are commonly used as a crude index of GFR. The basis for this statement is related to the fact that abnormal concentrations caused by damage to renal parenchyma cannot be detected until approximately three-quarters of the functional capacity of the nephrons has been impaired. In addition, the concentration of serum or plasma urea and creatinine may be affected by variables other than those associated with GFR.

Despite the relative insensitivity of SUN and creatinine as indices of GFR, the ease with which they can be measured in plasma or serum and the difficulty associated with more precise measurements of GFR have resulted in their widespread clinical use. Meaningful interpretation of urea nitrogen and creatinine values, however, is dependent on recognition of variables that influence GFR (Table II).

Evaluation of SUN or creatinine concentrations in conjunction with other clinical and laboratory data (especially urine osmolality or specific gravity) is of far greater significance than choice of one or the other (Table III). As will be discussed in Part II, there may be some value in determination of both parameters. Irrespective of which test is chosen, the same test should be selected if it is to be performed serially. When utilizing either test as an index of response to dietary management of primary renal failure, it is important to recognize that restriction of dietary protein may reduce the concentration of SUN without any substantial improvement in GFR. Therefore, it is recommended that both SUN and creatinine concentrations be evaluated as indices of dietary adherence and therapeutic response.

There is often significant variability between the serum concentration of urea nitrogen or creatinine and the severity of clinical signs of uremia. The latter may be related, at least in part, to the duration of the renal disease. Patients with acute renal failure often have severe polysystemic illness even though their serum concentration of urea and creatinine is lower than that observed in asymptomatic patients with polyuric chronic renal failure. Progressive renal diseases that destroy renal parenchyma at a relatively slow rate allow the body to compensate for progressive but gradually developing alterations in fluid, acid-base, and electrolyte balance and to minimize life-threatening imbalances. Because patients with acute renal failure survive for a longer period in a state of renal dysfunction, though,

TABLE IX

Method for Performing Endogenous Creatinine Clearance Studies in Dogs

1. Catheterize and empty the urinary bladder. Rinse the bladder with several milliliters of sterile saline. Discard urine and saline.

2. Collect *all* urine produced during a timed period. If an extended collection period is used, place the patient in a metabolism cage or frequently collect voluntarily voided urine.

3. At the midpoint of the timed urine collection, obtain a blood sample for determination of serum creatinine concentration (S_c).

4. At the end of the timed urine collection, catheterize and empty the bladder. Rinse the bladder with several milliliters of sterile saline. Urine *and* saline should be added to urine already collected. Record the total time elapsed during urine collection (T). The total urine volume produced (including the final saline rinse) should be measured (V). A well-mixed aliquot of urine should be submitted for determination of urine creatinine concentration (U_c).

5. Accurately determine the dog's body weight (BW).

6. Calculate clearance of creatinine (C_{cr}) using the following formula:

$$C_{cr} = \frac{U_c V}{S_c \cdot T \cdot BW}$$

Where C_{cr} = ml/minute/kg; U_c and S_c = mg/dl; V = milliliters; T = minutes; and BW = kilograms.

changes in other body systems are often much severer in patients with chronic progressive primary renal failure.

Because it is affected by fewer nonrenal variables, creatinine has gained the false reputation of being a much more specific index of the severity of renal damage and a more reliable index of prognosis than SUN. The assumption that recovery from renal failure cannot occur if creatinine levels exceed 5 mg/100 ml is completely erroneous. Although a marked elevation in serum creatinine concentration does indicate severe functional or organic impairment of nephron function, it is not of significantly greater value than SUN concentration in indicating the degree of reversibility or irreversibility of the underlying disease process since it does not permit establishment of the underlying cause and its biologic behavior.

In the event that a more sensitive index of glomerular filtration is desired, consideration should be given to endogenous or exogenous creatinine clearance tests (Table IX).[29] Recently, a simplified test of exogenous creatinine clearance which encompasses subcutaneous injection of creatinine has been validated for use in dogs.[32]

REFERENCES

1. Bradford JR: The results following partial nephrectomy and the influence of the kidney on metabolism. *J Physiol* 23:415-496, 1899.
2. Haymann JM, Shumway NP, Dunke P, et al: Experimental hyposthenuria. *J Clin Invest* 18:195-211, 1939.
3. Osborne CA, Finco DR, Low DG: Pathophysiology of renal disease, renal failure, and uremia, in Ettinger SJ (ed): *Textbook of Veterinary Internal Medicine,* ed 2. Philadelphia, WB Saunders Co, 1983, pp 1751-1759.
4. Bovee KC: Urine osmolality as a definitive indicator of renal concentrating ability. *JAVMA* 155:30-35, 1969.
5. Hardy RM, Osborne CA: Water deprivation test in the dog: Maximal normal values. *JAVMA* 174:479-484, 1979.
6. Osborne CA, Stevens JB: *Handbook of Canine and Feline Urinalysis.* St. Louis, Ralston Purina Co, 1981, p 44.
7. Rahill WH, Subramanian S: Use of fetal animals to investigate renal development. *Lab Anim Sci* 23:92-96, 1973.
8. Horster M, Valtin H: Postnatal development of renal function: Micropuncture and clearance studies in the dog. *J Clin Invest* 50:779-795, 1971.
9. Finco DR: Kidney function, in Kaneko JJ (ed): *Clinical Biochemistry of Domestic Animals,* ed 3. New York, Academic Press, 1980.
10. Edelmann CM Jr, Barnett HL, Troupkov V: Renal concentrating mechanisms in newborn infants: Effect of dietary protein and water content, role of urea, and responsiveness to antidiuretic hormone. *J Clin Invest* 39:1062, 1960.
11. Guignard JP: Renal function in the newborn infant. *Ped Clin North Am* 29:777-790, 1982.
12. Nash MA, Edelmann CM Jr: The developing kidney. Immature function of appropriate standard. *Nephron* 11:81-90, 1973.
13. Ross LA, Finco DR: Relationship of selected clinical renal function tests to glomerular filtration rate and renal blood flow in cats. *Am J Vet Res* 42:1704-1710, 1981.
14. Johnson WJ: Evaluation of renal function in far advanced renal failure and in intermittent dialysis, in Duarte CG (ed): *Renal Function Tests.* Boston, Little, Brown & Co, 1980.
15. Papper S: *Clinical Nephrology,* ed 2. Boston, Little, Brown & Co, 1980.
16. Osborne CA, Finco DR, Scott RC: Problem oriented diagnosis of diseases of the urinary system: I. The kidney. *Scientific Proc, 42nd AAHA Annu Meet, South Bend, IN:*1975.
17. Brietschwerdt EB: Clinical abnormalities of urinary concentration and dilution. *Compend Contin Educ Pract Vet* 3:414-421, 1981.
18. Hardy RM, Osborne CA: Water deprivation and vasopressin concentration tests in the differentiation of polyuric syndromes, in Kirk RW (ed): *Current Veterinary Therapy,* vol 7. Philadelphia, WB Saunders Co, 1980.
19. Hardy RM, Osborne CA: Aqueous vasopressin response test in clinically normal dogs undergoing water diuresis: Technique and results. *Am J Vet Res* 43:1987-1990, 1982.
20. Hardy RM, Osborne CA: Repositol vasopressin response test in clinically normal dogs undergoing water diuresis: Technique and results. *Am J Vet Res* 43:1991-1993, 1982.
21. Dunegan LJ, Knight DC, Brennan MF, Moore FD: Urea distribution in renal failure. *J Surg Res* 24:401-403, 1978.
22. Baum N, Dichosis CC, Carlton CE: Blood urea nitrogen and serum creatinine. Physiology and interpretations. *Urology* 5:583-588, 1975.
23. Austin JH, Stillman NE, Van Slyke DD: Factors governing excretion rate of urea. *J Biol Chem* 46:91, 1921.
24. Finco DR, Duncan JR: Evaluation of blood urea nitrogen and serum creatinine as indicators of renal dysfunction: A study of 111 cases and a review of related literature. *JAVMA* 168:593-601, 1976.
25. O'Connell JMB, Romeo JA, Mudge GH: Renal tubular secretion of creatinine in the dog. *Am J Physiol* 203:985-990, 1962.
26. Swanson RE, Hakim AA: Stop-flow analysis of creatinine excretion in the dog. *Am J Physiol* 203:980-984, 1962.
27. Eggleton MG, Habib YA: The mode of excretion of creatinine and insulin by the kidney of the cat. *J Physiol* 112:191-200, 1951.
28. Finco DR: Mechanism of urinary creatinine excretion by the cat. *Am J Vet Res* 43:2207-2209, 1982.
29. Bovee KC, Joyce T: Clinical evaluation of glomerular function: 24-hour creatinine clearance in dogs. *JAVMA* 174:488-491, 1979.
30. Robinson T, Harbison M, Bovee KC: Influence of reduced renal mass on tubular secretion of creatinine in the dog. *Am J Vet Res* 35:487-491, 1974.
31. Watson ADJ, Church DB, Fairburn AJ: Postprandial changes in plasma urea and creatinine concentrations in dogs. *Am J Vet Res* 42:1878-1880, 1981.
32. Finco DR, Coulter DB, Barsanti JA: Simple accurate method for clinical estimation of glomerular filtration rate in the dog. *Am J Vet Res* 42:1874-1877, 1981.
33. Osborne CA, Hammer RF, Stevens JB, Resnick JS, Michael AF: The glomerulus in health and disease: Review of domestic animals and man. *Adv Vet Sci Comp Med* 21:207-285, 1977.

Azotemia: A Review of What's Old and What's New. Part II. Localization*

Carl A. Osborne, DVM, PhD
David J. Polzin, DVM, PhD

Department of Small Animal Clinical Sciences
College of Veterinary Medicine
University of Minnesota
St. Paul, Minnesota

Dr. Carl A. Osborne has updated both parts of this series on azotemia. The update appears as an addendum to Part II. Asterisks (*) throughout both articles mark the passages for which Dr. Osborne has included changes in the addendum.

I. Priority of clinical investigation and its application to localization of problems
II. Significance of localization of azotemia
III. Prerenal azotemia
  A. Dietary and miscellaneous factors
  B. Perfusion factors
    1. Etiopathogenesis
    2. Diagnosis
    3. Diagnostic dilemmas
    4. Prognosis
IV. Postrenal azotemia
  A. Obstructive uropathy
    1. Etiopathogenesis
    2. Diagnosis
    3. Prognosis
  B. Rupture of the excretory pathway
    1. Pathogenesis
    2. Diagnosis
V. Primary renal function
  A. Generalized nephron dysfunction
    1. Etiopathogenesis
    2. Diagnosis
  B. Glomerulotubular imbalance
    1. Etiopathogenesis
    2. Diagnosis
VI. Primary renal azotemia plus prerenal or postrenal azotemia
  A. Etiopathogenesis
  B. Diagnosis
VII. Problem-specific data base for azotemia

Priority of Clinical Investigation and Its Application to Localization of Problems

The first step in the azotemia diagnostic process is to define and verify

---

*Due to the length of this article, the editors of *The Compendium* felt that the outline above would be helpful to the reader.

Originally published in Volume 5, Number 7, July 1983

TABLE I

GENERAL PRIORITIES OF CLINICAL INVESTIGATION

I. Collect information (data base)
   A. Define data to be collected
     1. Minimum data base
     2. Problem-specific data base
II. Define problem(s) (problem list)
   A. Refine to highest degree of refinement
   B. Do not overstate problems
III. Formulate plan
   A. Diagnostic plans
     1. Verification of problem(s) is first priority
       a. Especially important for historical problems such as hematuria, polyuria, dysuria
       b. Also of significance for transient or intermittent problems
     2. Localization of problem(s) to body system(s) or organ(s) is second priority
     3. Consider probable cause(s) as third priority
       a. Pathophysiology first (DAMN IT)
       b. Specific cause(s) next
   B. Prognostic plans
   C. Therapeutic plans
     1. Specific
     2. Supportive
     3. Symptomatic
     4. Palliative
   D. Client education
IV. Formulative follow-up plans (progress notes)

clinical problems (Table I). Problem definition is essential because one must be able to define problems before they can be solved. It is often necessary to verify problems detected by clinical evaluation, especially those identified by clients. Errors in identification and verification of clinical problems are among the most common and fundamental causes of misdiagnosis. Such errors not only lead to fruitless pursuit of nonexistent disorders, but they may result in a costly and time-consuming series of diagnostic and therapeutic plans before errors are identified.

Following accurate definition and verification of problems from data collected from the history, physical examination, and laboratory or radiographic procedures when appropriate, a complete problem list should be constructed.[1] Problems should be stated at their highest level of refinement and defined in such a way that their refinement can be defended with reasonable certainty on the basis of current knowledge about the patient. Listed from the lowest to the highest level of refinement, problems may be defined as:

1. An unquantified clinical finding (vomiting, polydipsia, depression, etc.). Further information is often required to verify the existence of such problems.
2. A reproducible diagnostic finding (palpable abdominal mass, proteinuria, leukocytosis, azotemia, hypercalcemia, etc.).
3. A pathophysiologic syndrome (renal failure, nephrotic syndrome, malabsorption syndrome, congestive heart failure, etc.). Problem refinement of

this degree requires integration of diagnostic information.
4. A diagnostic entity (pyelonephritis caused by staphylococci, congestive heart failure caused by *Dirofilaria immitis*, hematuria and dysuria caused by a transitional cell carcinoma of the urinary bladder). In many instances, it is not possible to obtain this level of problem refinement. In such instances, the problems should not be overstated by guessing their causes.

The following example illustrates definition of problems at an appropriate degree of refinement. Instead of listing vomiting, depression, dehydration, azotemia, an inappropriately low urine specific gravity (1.018), and numerous granular casts in urine sediment as individual problems, they are grouped under the problem of primary renal failure (a pathophysiologic syndrome) (Table II). In contrast, if a patient has a disorder characterized by vomiting, depression, dehydration, azotemia, concentrated urine (SG = 1.040), and numerous granular casts in urine sediment, these problems should not be refined to a diagnosis of primary renal failure. Grouping them together under the problem of primary renal failure would be an overstatement since there is no evidence of intrinsic failure of renal function (Table III). Although detection of numerous granular casts in urine sediment is a reliable index of renal disease, the fact that the urine is concentrated to a specific gravity of 1.040 indicates that the patient has adequate renal function to prevent vomiting, dehydration, depression, and azotemia. The azotemia is probably associated with lack of renal perfusion caused by hypovolemia induced by vomiting. Clinical dehydration of the patient supports this conclusion.

Disciplined thought is required to construct a meaningful problem list (Tables II and III). When integrating problems to their highest degree of refinement, it is important to consider that clinical manifestations of disease are usually a combination of signs induced by disease (such as bacteriuria associated with infection of

TABLE II

PROPERLY DEFINED VERSUS OVERSTATED CAUSES OF VOMITING

Proper Definition	*Overstated*
Secondary gastrointestinal disease associated with	Oliguric primary renal failure[a] characterized by
1. Vomiting	1. Vomiting
2. Dehydration	2. Dehydration
3. Impaired ability to concentrate urine (SG = 1.018)	3. Impaired ability to concentrate urine
4. Azotemia	4. Azotemia
5. Hyperkalemia	5. Hyperkalemia
6. Increased packed-cell volume	6. Hemoconcentration

[a]Similar signs may be caused by hypoadrenocorticism.

TABLE III

DEFINING PROBLEMS AT AN APPROPRIATE LEVEL OF REFINEMENT

Unrefined	*Refined*
1. Polyuria	Dysfunction of the kidney associated with
2. Polydipsia	1. Impaired ability to concentrate urine (SG = 1.015), polyuria, and compensatory polydipsia
3. Dehydration	
4. Inappropriate urine specific gravity (1.015)	2. Reduced glomerular filtration rate (azotemia)
5. Proteinuria	3. Primary or secondary infection of the urinary tract (significant bacteriuria), associated with inflammation (pyuria and proteinuria)
6. Pyuria	
7. Significant bacteriuria	4. Dehydration
8. Azotemia	

the urinary tract) and the body's compensatory response to these problems (such as pyuria and perhaps proteinuria and hematuria caused by inflammation to eradicate bacteriuria and repair damaged tissues).

Localization of problems should follow their definition and verification (see Part I of this article, Table IX). For example, if a patient is examined because of gross hematuria but no other abnormalities are initially identified, the problem should be listed as gross hematuria. Additional information is required to determine its location(s) (kidneys, ureters, urinary bladder, urethra, or genital tract) and cause(s) (anomalies, neoplasia, infection, uroliths, exogenous or endogenous toxins, coagulopathies, and so forth). In contrast, if hematuria occurs independently of micturition and is associated with a palpable lesion of the urethra, the problem might be defined as a urethral lesion associated with gross hematuria.

Following localization of problems to a body system or organ, it is useful to think of basic pathophysiologic mechanisms when trying to determine probable (rather than possible) causes of each problem (Table I).[1] The acronym *DAMN IT* may be useful for this purpose (Table IV). One of the most frequent errors made by

TABLE IV

"DAMN IT" ACRONYM OF PATHOPHYSIOLOGIC CAUSES OF DISEASE

D	Degenerative disorders Dementia (i.e., psychologic) disorders
A	Anomalies Autoimmunity
M	Metabolic disorders
N	Neoplasia (benign or malignant) Nutritional disorders
I	Inflammation (infectious or noninfectious) Immune disorders Iatrogenic disorders Idiopathic disorders
T	Toxicity (endogenous or exogenous) Trauma (external or internal)

inexperienced diagnosticians is the premature consideration of specific disease entities without verifying the existence of problems (especially those identified by owners), without localizing problems to the appropriate body system or organ, and without considering basic pathophysiologic disease mechanisms that might be involved. If one habitually bypasses these important components of problem solving, one will become overly dependent on establishing diagnoses on the basis of previous experience rather than developing the ability to diagnose disease processes that one has never encountered.

Following the establishment of the most probable causes (tentative diagnosis) of a problem, appropriate diagnostic tests and procedures should be performed to prove (rule in) or disprove (rule out) them.

Significance of Localization of Azotemia

Azotemia is defined as an abnormal elevation in the concentration of urea, creatinine, or other nonprotein metabolites in blood, serum, or plasma. Unlike uremia, which is a clinical syndrome, azotemia is a laboratory finding. The value of a clinical laboratory test result depends on its ability to answer a clinical question. In the context of this discussion, the question that usually prompts a request for determination of the serum concentration of urea or creatinine is "Does the patient have evidence of renal dysfunction?" Unfortunately, azotemia is a laboratory finding with several fundamentally different causes (Figure 1). Azotemia may occur when (1) renal structure and function are normal, (2) renal structure is normal but renal function is abnormal, and/or (3) renal structure and function are abnormal. Determination of the underlying cause(s) of azotemia is of great clinical significance since this information will significantly influence prognosis and therapy. Failure to do so may lead to formulation of ineffective and even contraindicated therapy.

Because by definition in azotemia there is an accumulation of nonprotein nitrogenous substances produced by the body in blood, plasma, or serum, the underlying mechanisms of azotemia must be related to (1) an

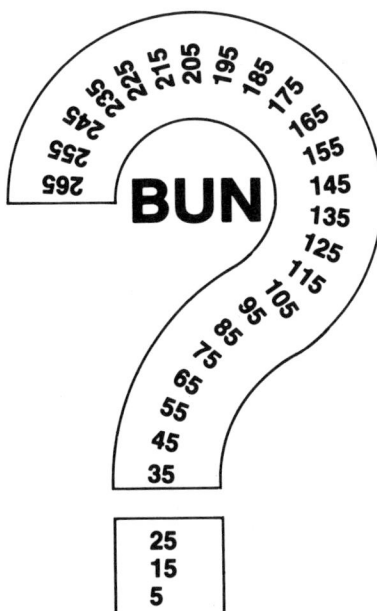

Figure 1—Azotemia is not pathognomonic of primary renal failure. The cause of azotemia should be localized to prerenal, primary renal, and/or postrenal factors. The numbers represent the serum concentration of urea nitrogen.

increased rate of production, (2) a decreased rate of excretion, or (3) both of these mechanisms. As will be discussed, increased rates of production of urea may cause a mild degree of azotemia. If the endogenous rates of production of urea nitrogen and creatinine are constant, however, azotemia occurs as a result of reduction in glomerular filtration rate. Reduction in glomerular filtration may be caused by alterations in blood volume, blood pressure, colloidal osmotic pressure, the number of patent renal arteries and glomerular capillaries, the permeability of glomerular capillaries, renal interstitial pressure, and/or renal intratubular pressure (Part I, Table II). Thus glomerular filtration depends on prerenal components (blood volume, blood pressure, colloidal osmotic pressure), renal components (patency of renal arteries and glomerular capillaries, permeability of glomerular capillaries, renal interstitial pressure, renal intratubular pressure), and postrenal components (influence of patency of ureters, bladder, and urethra on renal functions, and influence of the integrity of the excretory pathway on elimination of urine from the body). Therefore the cause(s) of reduction in glomerular filtration may be categorized as prerenal, primary renal, and/or postrenal. Because of clinically significant differences in pathogenesis, prognosis, and treatment, it is recommended that causes of decreased glomerular filtration associated with azotemia always be localized according to this classification (Part I, Tables II and III). The fact that different forms of azotemia may coexist should also be considered.

The section in Part I of this article, entitled "Definition of Terms and Concepts Related to Azotemia" should be consulted for a review of important conceptual differences between renal disease, renal failure, azotemia, and uremia. The section called "Terms and Concepts Related to Urine Osmolality and Specific Gravity" (Part I) can also be checked for information on normal and abnormal values. Knowledge of urine specific gravity is extremely helpful in localization of the underlying cause of azotemia. A basic understanding of the metabolism of urea and creatinine is also of fundamental importance.

Prerenal Azotemia
Dietary and Miscellaneous Factors

An increase in the serum concentration of urea nitrogen may occur in response to acceleration in the rate of protein catabolism rather than as a result of decreased renal excretion. The increase is usually, but not invariably, mild ($\leq$ 50 mg/dl). In such a situation, renal structure and function are normal. Urine specific gravity may vary over a wide range to help maintain body fluid balance. The effect of dietary protein on serum urea nitrogen (SUN) concentration is illustrated by the results of one study in which the mean SUN concentrations of normal beagle dogs were 18.8 ± 6.7 mg/dl during consumption of a commercially prepared nonprescription diet (10.0% protein), 9.0 ± 3.2 mg/dl during consumption of a restricted protein diet (5.4% protein), and 6.2 ± 1.7 mg/dl during consumption of an ultra-low-protein diet (2.4% protein).[2] The mean SUN concentration of six normal beagle dogs consuming a restricted protein diet (1.5% protein) designed to induce dissolution of magnesium ammonium phosphate uroliths was 3.5 ± 2.4 mg/dl. In a study of normal beagle dogs, the SUN concentration was elevated 10 to 18 hours following food consumption, with peak effects occurring two to three hours following eating.[3] In some dogs, postprandial SUN exceeded 40 mg/dl. In another study of various breeds of dogs consuming raw or boiled meat, postprandial urea nitrogen concentrations between 70 and 80 mg/dl were common.[4]

In those circumstances in which the significance of a mildly elevated SUN concentration (i.e., approximately 35 to 60 mg/dl) cannot be determined because of the variable of diet, withholding all protein-containing foods from the patient for 12 to 18 hours and reevaluation of SUN concentration may be of value. Nonprotein calories can be given to minimize production of urea by catabolism of body proteins for energy during the protein-fasting period. If the concentration of SUN remains elevated, dietary protein must not have been an important component of the azotemia. If the SUN concentration returns to normal values, however, a significant component of the azotemia can be attributed to dietary protein. In assessing the significance of such findings, however, consideration should be given to the fact that a patient with marginal renal dysfunction is more likely to develop prerenal azotemia by consuming a high-protein diet than is a patient with normal renal function.[5]

Endogenous sources of protein including gastrointestinal hemorrhage and rapid catabolism of body tissue (from infection, trauma, fever, or burns) may also increase the concentration of SUN. Starvation and sustained strenuous exercise have been cited as causes of prerenal azotemia in human beings.[6,7] Drugs that increase protein catabolism (glucocorticoids) or decrease protein anabolism (tetracyclines) have also been incriminated as causes of prerenal azotemia.[8-10] The significance of tetracycline as a cause of prerenal azotemia in dogs requires further study, because results of preliminary studies have provided conflicting results.[8,11]

Perfusion Factors

Etiopathogenesis

Nonurinary diseases may cause varying degrees of alteration of renal blood flow and glomerular filtration without damaging nephrons. Because urea nitrogen and creatinine are endogenous substances that continue to be produced, inadequate perfusion of normal glomeruli with blood, regardless of cause (dehydration, cardiac dysfunction, shock, hypoadrenocorticism, reduction in plasma colloidal osmotic pressure due to severe hypoalbuminemia) will (if persistent) reduce their rate of filtration by glomeruli and predispose to prerenal azotemia (Part I, Tables II and III). Dehydration will cause a minor increase in the serum concentration of urea nitrogen and creatinine as a result of a decrease in the percentage of water in serum. Reduction in blood volume and pressure as a result of dehydration, hypoadrenocorticism, hypovolemic shock, or severe heart failure may result in azotemia as a result of altered renal function. Since blood pressure provides the force necessary for glomerular filtration, a decrease in blood pressure below a critical level (approximately 70 mm Hg) will result in cessation of glomerular filtration and anuria. Less severe reductions in renal perfusion pressure and glomerular filtration rate may result in oliguria. In addition to reduction in volume and pressure of blood perfusing glomeruli, an increase in colloidal osmotic pressure (relative hyperalbuminemia) in dehydrated patients may significantly counteract hydrostatic pressure–induced filtration at the level of glomeruli.

Prerenal azotemia is initially associated with structurally normal kidneys that are capable of quantitatively normal renal function providing that compromised renal perfusion is corrected prior to the onset of ischemic nephron damage. Development of primary renal failure due to ischemia may occur, however, and will prolong and reduce the likelihood of recovery.

Diagnosis

In dogs, prerenal azotemia associated with altered perfusion should be considered if azotemia is associated with appropriately concentrated urine (SG ≥ 1.030) in patients with no specific evidence of glomerular disease (Part I, Table VI). The same generality applies to azotemic cats with a urine specific gravity ≥ 1.035. Such patients do not have a history of polyuria because they have compensatory physiologic oliguria. Care must be taken to differentiate physiologic from pathologic oli-

guria. Detection of urine specific gravity values greater than these approximate values in association with azotemia indicates that a sufficient quantity of functional nephrons is present to concentrate urine (estimated to be at least one-third of the total nephron population). Significant elevations in the serum concentration of urea nitrogen or creatinine due solely to primary renal failure (primary renal azotemia) cannot be detected in dogs and cats until approximately three-quarters of the nephron population is functionally impaired.

Concentration of urine (indicated by production of a relatively small volume of urine with high specific gravity and osmolality) associated with prerenal azotemia probably reflects compensatory response by the body to combat low perfusion pressure and blood volume by secreting aldosterone (and possibly other substances) to conserve filtered sodium (and thus water) throughout nephrons, and antidiuretic hormone to conserve water by distal nephrons. The relatively small volume of urine produced during prerenal azotemia caused by reduced renal perfusion will be low in sodium (estimated to be less than approximately 10 mEq/L in humans) in addition to being concentrated. Restoration of renal perfusion by appropriate volume-replacement therapy is typically followed by a dramatic reduction in the concentration of serum urea and creatinine to normal in approximately one to three days.

In humans with prerenal azotemia, increased renal tubular reabsorption of urea during a period of decreased formation of glomerular ultrafiltrate results in a disproportionate elevation in serum urea concentration compared with serum creatinine concentration. The SUN:creatinine ratio is often greater than 10:1, compared with a ratio of 10:1 in primary renal azotemia.[12,13] SUN:creatinine ratios were compared in a retrospective evaluation of dogs and cats with known prerenal or primary renal azotemia.[5] When patients were matched according to serum creatinine concentration, no difference was detected between the prerenal (36.8:1) and primary (36.0:1) renal azotemia groups. Results of the investigation indicate that measuring SUN:creatinine ratios is an unreliable method of localizing azotemia in dogs and cats.[a]

In summary, prerenal azotemia should be suspected in patients with (Part I, Table V) (1) azotemia; (2) physiologic oliguria characterized by production of urine with a high specific gravity (≥ 1.030 in dogs, ≥ 1.035 in cats)* and low sodium concentration (<10 mEq/L); (3) disorders capable of altering renal perfusion; and (4) dramatic correction of azotemia following administration of appropriate therapy to restore renal perfusion.

---

[a]Empirical clinical observations made of dogs evaluated at the University Teaching Hospital, University of Minnesota, indicate that the SUN:creatinine ratio in hypercalcemic azotemic dogs is often less than normal. The authors hypothesize that this change may be related to impaired renal tubular reabsorption of urea mediated by detrimental effects of excessive calcium on renal tubules.

Diagnostic Dilemmas

Primary diseases of the urinary system may secondarily affect other body systems, and vice versa. In both situations, clinical signs and laboratory findings may be similar. Severe hypoalbuminemia mediated by primary glomerular disease, acute pancreatitis, and hypoadrenocorticism are deserving of further discussion.

Potentially reversible prerenal azotemia may develop in patients with glomerulonephropathy and severe hypoproteinemia. This form of azotemia may be considered to be prerenal even though the initiating event occurs because of altered selective permeability of glomerular capillaries to plasma proteins. Such patients may or may not have impairment of glomerular perfusion caused by renal lesions which encroach upon glomerular capillary lumens. They do have marked damage to glomerular capillary walls, however, which interferes with their ability to prevent loss of proteins from plasma. The resultant reduction in colloidal osmotic pressure due to hypoalbuminemia initiates two opposite influences on glomerular hydrostatic pressure. Reduction in colloidal osmotic pressure at the level of glomeruli favors filtration because it provides less antagonism to hydrostatic forces. This effect is usually more than offset by a reduction in systemic vascular volume as a consequence of hypoalbuminemia. When hypoalbuminemia is severe, fluid leaving the vascular spaces may result in dependent, nonpainful, pitting edema. The net effect of severe hypoalbuminemia (reduction in systemic vascular volume vs. reduced opposition of hydrostatic pressure at the level of glomeruli) is often reduction in glomerular filtration which may be of a magnitude sufficient to cause azotemia. Therefore, the significance of azotemia must be carefully defined in patients with glomerulonephropathy and severe hypoalbuminemia.

Prerenal azotemia caused by hypoalbuminemia in patients with glomerulonephropathy should be suspected when the disorder is characterized by azotemia, ability to significantly concentrate (or dilute) glomerular filtrate, severe proteinuria, and marked hypoalbuminemia (approximately 1.0 g/dl or lower).[14] Patients may or may not have hypoproteinemic edema (i.e., nonpainful pitting subcutaneous edema, ascites, and/or hydrothorax). Renal biopsy specimens will be characterized by generalized patency of glomerular capillaries but minimal to mild light microscopic alterations in glomerular capillary walls. Reduction in the magnitude of azotemia that occurs concomitantly with a spontaneous or therapeutically induced increase in serum albumin concentration lends strong support to this diagnosis.

Elevated serum amylase and lipase activities are not pathognomonic of acute pancreatitis since it may also be associated with primary renal failure.[15-18] Knowledge of the serum concentration of urea or creatinine may not permit differentiation of pancreatitis from primary renal failure since vomiting induced by pancreatitis may result in fluid loss of sufficient magnitude to cause prerenal azotemia. Evaluation of the ability of the kidneys to concentrate urine is very helpful in distinguishing between acute pancreatitis and primary renal failure, however, providing that both diseases are not present simultaneously (Table V). Acute pancreatitis in dogs is typically associated with severe hyperamylasemia (up to seven times normal values), severe hyperlipasemia, occasionally azotemia, and ability of kidneys to significantly concentrate urine (SG > 1.030). Primary renal failure is typically associated with mild to severe azotemia, impaired ability to concentrate or dilute urine (SG = 1.006 to 1.029), and frequently moderate hyperamylasemia (two to three times normal values) and moderate hyperlipasemia (two to four times normal values). Since occurrence of chronic renal failure in dogs without acute pancreatitis would be expected to have approximately a two and one-half-fold increase in serum amylase activity and a two- to fourfold increase in serum lipase activity, detection of greater increases in serum amylase or lipase activity in dogs with chronic renal failure should prompt consideration of concurrent acute pancreatitis. Although it has been suggested that the uremic syndrome may be causally related to pancreatitis, the authors' studies failed to reveal morphologic

TABLE V

DIFFERENTIATION OF ACUTE PANCREATITIS AND
PRERENAL AZOTEMIA FROM PRIMARY RENAL AZOTEMIA

Factor	Disorder	
	Acute Pancreatitis and Prerenal Azotemia	Primary Renal Azotemia
Serum amylase activity	Elevated	Sometimes elevated
Serum lipase activity	Elevated	Sometimes elevated
Serum urea concentration	Elevated	Elevated
Serum creatinine concentration	Elevated	Elevated
Urine volume	Physiologic oliguria	Pathologic oliguria or pathologic polyuria
Urine specific gravity*	> 1.030 (dog)	1.006 to ~1.029 (dog)

changes in the pancreas of dogs with confirmed chronic renal failure.[17] Whether or not uremia causes dysfunction of the pancreas in the absence of light microscopic *changes remains an unanswered question.

Hypoadrenocorticism in dogs is associated with signs referable to the gastrointestinal system (vomiting; polydipsia; dark, tarry feces), urinary system (prerenal azotemia, variable specific gravity of urine), and cardiovascular system (cardiac conduction defects), in addition to nonlocalizing signs (anorexia, depression, dehydration, weight loss, weakness, and collapse). Decreased production and release of mineralocorticoids caused by destruction of the adrenal glands is associated with impaired renal conservation of sodium and chloride and subnormal renal tubular secretion of potassium. Loss of abnormal quantities of sodium in urine results in depletion of extracellular fluid volume, reduction in blood volume and pressure, and ultimately peripheral vascular collapse. Hyperkalemia caused by impaired renal secretion of potassium induces multiple cardiac arrhythmias and bradycardia, which further impair perfusion of organs and tissues. In addition to hemoconcentration, reduction in vascular volume is associated with reduced renal perfusion and prerenal azotemia. Unlike most diseases associated with prerenal azotemia, the urine specific gravity of dogs with hypoadrenocorticism is often below 1.030 (Part I, Table VII). The authors have commonly observed values between 1.015 and 1.020, as have others.[19] Impaired release of antidiuretic hormone from the posterior pituitary gland as a result of hypoosmolality of plasma is not a tenable explanation of this observation since maximum output of antidiuretic hormone (ADH) would be expected as a result of marked reduction in vascular volume. Impaired ability to concentrate urine may be caused by solute diuresis induced by natriuresis, and reduction in medullary hyperosmolality. The magnitude of diuresis is usually not sufficient to produce clinically evident polyuria; however, polyuria has been observed in a minority of cases.[19] A high index of suspicion is required to prevent confusion of hypoadrenocorticism and prerenal azotemia with primary oliguric renal failure.[20,21]

Prognosis

The prognosis for maintenance of adequate renal function is favorable providing that renal perfusion is rapidly restored to adequate levels. Persistent reduction in renal perfusion may result in a variable degree of structural and functional damage, though. There is no sharp clinical dividing line that indicates the period of transition from a state of prerenal uremia to a state of organic renal failure. Even after organic renal failure develops, it is not an all-or-nothing phenomenon. The severity of renal damage caused by ischemia increases in proportion to the duration of the state of renal hypoperfusion. For this reason, timely administration of renal protective therapy may reduce or prevent the development of a functional state of acute ischemic nephrosis.

Despite the potential for occurrence, most patients do not develop significant azotemia following surgery, trauma, or shock. Hypotension must be severe and prolonged in order to cause irreversible damage to previously normal kidneys. The sensitivity of the kidneys to ischemia appears to be intermediate between the skin and skeletal muscles (which can withstand long periods of ischemia without detrimental effects) and the central nervous system (which cannot withstand ischemia for more than a few minutes). In experimental dogs, renal ischemia produced by complete occlusion of the renal pedicle for 30 minutes was not associated with development of significant renal lesions.[22] Complete occlusion of the renal pedicle for two hours usually, but not invariably, produced a significant degree of reversible functional and morphologic renal damage.[23,24] Gradual recovery of renal function usually occurred in the latter dogs over a period of two to three weeks. Complete renal ischemia for more than four hours consistently caused irreversible renal injury leading to death due to renal failure in four to eight days. It is important to note that the above data were collected under circumstances of total lack of renal perfusion. It is doubtful that a complete shutdown of renal perfusion is a common clinical occurrence. Experimental dogs in which renal perfusion at a pressure of less than 30 mm Hg (which is less than that required to produce irreversible shock) was allowed to persist for as long as three hours following partial occlusion of the renal pedicle did not develop significant functional impairment.[25] This experimental data is of clinical value in that it provides some perspective regarding the amount of time that can elapse before the kidneys are irreversibly damaged by renal ischemia. If adequate blood volume is restored and maintained in patients known to or suspected of having renal hypoperfusion, renal failure may be corrected or prevented.

Postrenal Azotemia
Obstructive Uropathy
Etiopathogenesis

Diseases that obstruct urine outflow from both kidneys may rapidly induce metabolic disturbances characterized by azotemia, hyperosmolality, hyperkalemia, hyperphosphatemia, hypermagnesemia, and severe acidosis. Dehydration and retention of metabolic waste products also occur. The exact sequence of events involved in obstructive injury has not been precisely defined, but a combination of abnormal pressure and ischemia appears to be involved. Back pressure transmitted to the kidneys as a result of obstruction to outflow impairs tubular function (reabsorption and secretion), renal blood flow, and glomerular filtration.[26-28] Azotemia can usually be detected 24 hours following complete obstruction of outflow to both ureters, the urinary bladder, or the urethra. Damage to the integrity of the bladder may enhance the onset of azotemia.[29] Serum creatinine concentrations in excess of 5 mg/dl are common and may be as high as 15 to 20 mg/dl in severe cases. Renal dysfunction caused by unilateral ureteral obstruction will not be associated with azotemia (unless generalized disease of the nonobstructed kidney is also present), since the remaining kidney has a population of functional nephrons adequate to prevent retention of significant quantities of urea and creatinine in serum. The affected kidney may be completely destroyed if the patient survives for a sufficient period of time, though.

Following correction of bilateral obstruction to urine outflow, postobstructive diuresis which lasts for hours to days may develop. Postobstructive diuresis may be caused by (1) elimination of urea, creatinine, phosphorus, and other osmotically active solutes that have accumulated in the body as a result of impaired renal function caused by obstruction, (2) varying degrees of functional and/or morphologic alterations in tubular reabsorptive and renal concentrating mechanisms initiated by abnormal back pressure, and (3) elimination of excessive quantities of parenteral fluids administered immediately following relief of obstruction.[28] Knowledge of postobstructive diuresis is of importance when assessing the patient's renal functional capacity following relief of obstruction and in formulating fluid therapy designed to minimize water and electrolyte imbalances.

If partial obstruction to urine outflow allows survival for a longer time, obstruction to urine outflow will initiate a sequence of changes that have the potential to cause primary structural and functional damage to the kidneys. Constant back pressure and alteration in hemodynamics induced by obstruction to urine outflow cause tubular cell atrophy and necrosis. Bacterial infection of the urinary tract is a common complication of obstructive uropathy and may significantly enhance the severity of renal lesions and nephron dysfunction.[30] In fact, bacterial infection associated with complete obstruction may cause the onset of acute primary renal failure.

The severity of structural damage to the kidneys is related to the degree and duration of the obstruction. Studies performed in dogs in which total obstruction of one ureter was induced by ligation revealed that, in the presence of a normally functioning contralateral kidney, permanent structural and functional alteration did not occur provided that the obstruction was removed within six to seven days.[31-34] If the obstruction was allowed to persist for two weeks prior to removal, the affected kidney regained only 50 to 60% of its preobstruction functional capacity. Functional damage was irreversible after six to eight weeks of obstruction.

Diagnosis
Obstructive postrenal azotemia should be considered in patients with (1) azotemia; (2) oliguria or anuria, dysuria or tenesmus; and (3) obstructive lesions (urethral plugs or calculi, herniated urinary bladders, etc.) detected by physical examination and/or radiography (Part I, Table VI). Because of its variability, the urine specific gravity of patients with postrenal azotemia due to obstruction to outflow is not as reliable an index of renal function as it is in patients with prerenal or primary renal azotemia (Part I, Table III). Although a complete urinalysis should always be performed in such patients, azotemia associated with characteristic findings of obstruction provides the best criteria with which to establish postrenal azotemia. Radiography and/or ultrasonography are often required to confirm a diagnosis of urine outflow obstruction and to localize the site(s) of mechanical or functional abnormalities.

Prognosis
Untreated patients with complete obstruction to urine outflow usually die within three to six days, prior to development of significant structural alterations.[35,36] Damage to the mucosal surface of the urinary bladder may shorten survival time.[29] Death is related to severe fluid, electrolyte, and acid-base imbalances and retention of metabolic waste products. Superimposition of urinary tract infection during obstruction to outflow may significantly decrease the chance for recovery.[30]

Although the metabolic disturbances associated with acute bilateral obstruction of the kidneys are potentially lethal (especially hyperkalemia, metabolic acidosis, and severe dehydration), they are potentially reversible. If the obstructive lesion(s) is rapidly removed, and if the patient is given appropriate supportive and symptomatic therapy, the short-term prognosis for survival and recovery of normal renal function is favorable. The long-term prognosis depends on the reversibility of the underlying cause of obstruction.

Rupture of Excretory Pathway
Pathogenesis
Traumatic rupture of the urinary bladder is typically associated with a sudden increase in intravesical pressure in a bladder distended with urine. Traumatic rupture of the bladder in animals with no predisposing abnormalities of the urinary system has been most commonly encountered in male dogs. Traumatic rupture of the urinary bladder may occur in dogs or cats with partial or total obstruction of the urethra, especially if the integrity of the urinary bladder wall has been altered by concomitant infection or neoplasia. Bladder rupture occasionally occurs as a sequela of urethral obstruction in male cats; less frequently, it occurs in female dogs with urethral calculi.

Because of the anatomic location of the urinary bladder in dogs and cats, rents in the bladder wall usually communicate with the peritoneal cavity. Extravasation of urine from the excretory pathway of the urinary system into the peritoneal cavity is usually associated with marked ascites and peritonitis. Following accumulation of hyperosmolal urine in the peritoneal cavity, isoosmolal fluid from the extravascular spaces moves into the peritoneal cavity to establish osmotic equilibrium. At the same time, high concentrations of solutes (including urea and creatinine) excreted in urine diffuse back into the body to establish solute equilibrium. The magnitude of these changes depends on urine osmolality and the rate of urine formation. If patients with ruptured urinary bladders are oliguric because of renal hypoperfusion associated with traumatic shock and/or loss of fluid into the peritoneal cavity, the onset of significant shifts in fluid balance may require more time to develop than would be the situation in patients with good renal function.

Azotemia that occurs as a sequela to rupture of the excretory pathway is primarily related to absorption of urine from the peritoneal cavity. Unless the kidneys are damaged as a result of hypovolemic shock or trauma secondary to the underlying cause of rupture of the excretory pathway, they are structurally normal.

Because concentrated urine is irritating to tissues, peritonitis may develop. The severity of peritonitis may be aggravated by contamination with bacterial pathogens present in the urinary tract. Depending on the presence or absence of bacteria in urine at the time of rupture, cytologic evaluation of peritoneal fluid will reveal that it is an exudate (septic) or a modified transudate (nonseptic).

Diagnosis

Clinical findings associated with rupture of the urinary bladder vary depending on the precipitating cause, the size of the rent, and the duration of urine leakage. Significant findings in the history may include recent trauma, attempts to manually express a bladder distended with urine, improper use of catheters, or recent retrograde contrast radiography. Depression, vomiting, a stiff gait, and abdominal pain are indicative of a severe problem. Physical examination may reveal abdominal pain, spasm of abdominal musculature, ascites, inability to palpate the urinary bladder, and partial or total obstruction of the urethra. However, small rents may be asymptomatic.

Postrenal azotemia caused by rupture of the urinary bladder is usually associated with hyperphosphatemia, hemoconcentration, hyponatremia, and eventually hyperkalemia.[37] Microscopic evaluation of ascitic fluid removed by paracentesis typically reveals polymorphonuclear leukocytes, red cells, macrophages, degenerate mesothelial cells, and occasionally bacteria. The concentration of urea nitrogen in plasma and ascitic fluid is usually elevated to a similar degree. The concentration of creatinine in ascitic fluid is often higher than it is in serum or plasma. This may be related, at least in part, to the fact that creatinine has a larger molecular weight than urea (Part I, Table VIII).

Diagnosis of exudative ascites caused by rupture of the urinary bladder is best confirmed by positive-contrast cystography.[38]

Prognosis

The short-term prognosis for survival of patients with postrenal azotemia due to rupture of the excretory pathway is favorable, providing that the rent is rapidly repaired and appropriate supportive therapy is provided. The long-term prognosis depends on the reversibility of the underlying cause.

Primary Renal Azotemia
Generalized Nephron Dysfunction
Etiopathogenesis

Primary renal azotemia (primary renal failure) may be caused by *any disorder* that damages the functional capacity of approximately 70 to 75% or more of the nephrons. Primary renal azotemia in dogs and cats may be caused by a variety of different causal agents that damage nephrons rapidly (acute) or slowly (chronic) (Table VI). The fact that an indistinguishable degree of azotemia is a manifestation of a variety of different causal agents is related to the fact that functional (and morphologic) abnormalities of the kidneys can be manifested clinically in only a limited number of ways. Depending on the biologic behavior of the disease in question, it may be (1) reversible, (2) irreversible and nonprogressive, or (3) irreversible and progressive (Table VII). Primary renal azotemia may be acute or chronic and may be associated with oliguria and/or polyuria. The observation of reduced urine volume per se cannot be used to localize azotemia since prerenal azotemia may be associated with physiologic oliguria, primary renal azotemia may be associated with pathologic oliguria, and postrenal azotemia may be associated with oliguria or anuria. On the other hand, concomitant occurrence of azotemia and polyuria should arouse a high index of suspicion of primary renal failure.

Azotemia may be induced by a primary disease of glomeruli (amyloidosis, immune-mediated disorders, congenital hypoplasia, etc.) that impairs glomerular filtration rate. Reduction in glomerular perfusion alters the microcirculation in remaining portions of the nephron and secondarily alters renal tubular function (reabsorption and secretion). Impaired ability to concentrate glomerular filtrate results, at least in part, from loss of the functional capacity of a population of nephrons sufficient to interfere with the function of the countercurrent system. Increased clearance of solutes retained in plasma (urea, creatinine, sodium, phosphorus, etc.) by remaining functioning nephrons induces an osmotic diuresis which also contributes to obligatory polyuria.

In addition to primary glomerular disorders, primary diseases of tubules (ischemic tubular nephrosis, nephrotoxic nephrosis, etc.), interstitial tissue (pyelonephritis, leptospirosis, etc.), and/or vessels may hinder one or more functional mechanisms of the kidney. Because various components of nephrons function intra- and interdependently, these disorders often initiate changes that secondarily reduce glomerular filtration rate and cause azotemia.

TABLE VI

CAUSES OF RENAL DISEASE ACCORDING TO PRIMARY SITE OF INVOLVEMENT[a]

Glomeruli	*Tubules*	*Interstitium*	*Vessels*
1. Amyloidosis	1. Congenital disorders	1. Amyloid (cats)	1. Atherosclerosis (uncommon)
2. Diabetic glomerulopathy (?)	2. Hypercalcemia	2. Drugs	2. Thrombotic and embolic disorders
3. Disseminated intravascular coagulation	3. Immune-complex and anti-tubular basement membrane disorders (?)	3. Heavy metals	
4. Thrombotic or embolic disorders	4. Ischemia	4. Immune disorders (?)	3. Polyarteritis nodosa (uncommon)

5. Immune-complex disorders
  a. Bacterial endocarditis (?)
  b. *Dirofilaria immitis*
  c. Drugs (haptens)
  d. Feline leukemia
  e. Lupus erythematosus
  f. Neoplasia
  g. Pyometra (?)
  h. Idiopathic forms
  i. Others
	5. Nephrotoxins
	  a. Drugs
	  b. Heavy metals
	  c. Organic toxins
	  d. Hemoglobin, myoglobin (?)
	
	6. Neoplasia
	  a. Benign
	  b. Malignant
		5. Leptospirosis
		6. Pyelonephritis
		7. Systemic mycoses
		8. Others
			4. Others

6. Antiglomerular basement membrane disorders
  a. *Dirofilaria immitis* (?)
  b. Idiopathic forms
	7. Obstructive disorders
	
	8. Tubular transport disorders
	  a. Fanconi's syndrome
	  b. Renal tubular acidosis
	  c. Primary renal glucosuria		

7. Hypertension (?) 8. Others	9. Others		

[a]From Osborne CA, Finco DR, Low DG: Pathophysiology of renal disease, renal failure, and uremia, in Ettinger SJ (ed): *Textbook of Veterinary Internal Medicine*, vol 2, ed 2. Philadelphia, WB Saunders Co, 1982. Adapted with permission.

Diagnosis

Because of the kidneys' functional reserve capacity, impairment of their ability to concentrate or dilute urine cannot be readily detected until at least two-thirds of the normal renal function has been impaired. Significant elevations in the serum or plasma concentrations of urea nitrogen or creatinine that occur as a result of disorders localized to the kidney cannot be readily detected until 70 to 75% of normal renal function has been impaired. Thus impairment in urine concentration and dilution (one type of renal dysfunction) may precede the onset of azotemia (another type of renal dysfunction) (Part I, Table I). This might be viewed as a form of *tubuloglomerular* functional imbalance in contrast to primary renal failure caused by *glomerulotubular* functional imbalance (to be discussed). This phenomenon is common in dogs with bacterial pyelonephritis. Therefore, lack of azotemia does not rule out the possibility of generalized renal disease which affects approximately two-thirds but less than three-quarters of the nephrons.

Total loss of ability to concentrate or dilute urine does not always occur suddenly, but often develops gradually. Empirical clinical observations and experimental evaluation of normal dogs indicate that canine patients with an *adequate* population of functional nephrons should be able to concentrate urine to a specific gravity ≥ 1.030.[39] In the event of generalized nephron impairment that is severe enough to prevent *adequate* urine concentration but not of sufficient severity to prevent some degree of urine concentration, a specific gravity value between approximately 1.006 and 1.029 (1.006 to 1.034 in cats) would be expected (Part I, Table V).* For this reason, canine and feline urine specific gravity values within this range in the face of dehydration (and therefore release of endogenous antidiuretic hormone) and/or azotemia should prompt consideration of abnormal renal water conservation caused by primary renal failure. The total inability of nephrons to concentrate urine (isosthenuria) as a result of intrinsic renal disease results in formation of urine that is similar to that of glomerular filtrate (1.007 to 1.013).

In contrast to renal conservation of sodium in patients with prerenal azotemia caused by decreased renal perfusion, primary renal azotemia is associated with production of oliguria or polyuria and natriuresis. In humans with acute renal failure, the urine sodium concentration is often greater than 30 mEq/L.[40] The magnitude of natriuresis in dogs with acute and chronic renal failure has not been well documented in a large series of cases, but empirical clinical observations indicate that it is similar to that in humans.

If nondehydrated, nonazotemic patients with a history of polyuria and polydipsia do not have urine specific gravities that indicate that kidneys can definitely concentrate urine, further tests are required before meaningful conclusions can be established about the kidneys' capacity to concentrate urine. Water deprivation and/or vasopressin response tests may help in differentiating

TABLE VII
CHECKLIST OF SOME POTENTIALLY REVERSIBLE CAUSES OF AZOTEMIA[a,b]

Prerenal	*Primary Renal*	*Postrenal*
Catabolic states	Acute tubular necrosis	Rent in excretory pathway

1. Catabolic drugs
  a. Glucocorticoids
  b. Tetracyclines (?)
  c. Thyroid preps
	1. Ischemia	Obstruction
		1. Uroliths

2. Anorexia	2. Nephrotoxins
	  a. Ethylene glycol
	  b. Arsenicals
	  c. Amphotericin B
	  d. Aminoglycoside antibiotics
	  e. Others
		2. Operable neoplasms

3. Extensive tissue necrosis		3. Herniated bladder
		4. Blood clots
	Immune disorders	5. Spay granuloma
Decreased renal perfusion	Hypercalcemia	

1. Dehydration due to
  a. Vomiting
  b. Diarrhea
  c. Diuretics
  d. Limited water consumption
	Pyelonephritis	

	Drug reactions	
2. Hypovolemia due to hemorrhage	Heatstroke	
3. Heart failure	Leptospirosis	
4. Severe hypoalbuminemia	Some forms of glomerulonephropathy	
5. Hypoadrenocorticism		
6. Anesthetics		
Increased nonprotein nitrogen		
1. High-protein diets		
2. Gastrointestinal hemorrhage		

[a]Combinations of prerenal and primary renal factors are common. Correction of a reversible prerenal cause of azotemia in a patient with concomitant primary renal dysfunction may result in remission of the azotemia.
[b]From Osborne CA, Finco DR, Low DG: Pathophysiology of renal disease, renal failure and uremia, in Ettinger SJ (ed): *Textbook of Veterinary Internal Medicine*, vol 2, ed 2. Philadelphia, WB Saunders Co, 1982. Adapted with permission.

obligatory polyuria from compensatory polyuria. Following appropriate water-deprivation tests, patients with adequate renal function will excrete urine with an elevated specific gravity (> 1.030 in dogs, >1.035 in cats), high osmolality, and relatively small volume.[8,41,*] Patients that are still unable to concentrate urine following abrupt and/or gradual water deprivation may be given an exogenous source of ADH to prove or disprove the presence of pituitary diabetes insipidus.[42–44]

Production of dilute urine requires removal of more solute than water from nephrons. Since this is an energy-requiring process, significant dilution of urine provides an index of adequate renal function in much the same fashion that production of concentrated urine does. Most dogs with pathologic polyuria characterized by production of dilute urine (U_{SG} = 1.001 to approximately 1.005) have nonrenal disorders associated with water diuresis.[41,45] The most common forms are pituitary diabetes insipidus, renal diabetes insipidus (i.e., pyometra), and psychogenic water consumption.

For reasons that are not completely understood, some dogs and humans with primary polyuric renal failure may also form dilute urine.[8,46] It has been suggested that this phenomenon may be associated with the fact that urine that flows from the ascending limb of Henle's loop into the distal tubules is hypotonic to glomerular filtrate in dogs[47] and humans.[46] When large quantities of hypotonic urine enter the collecting ducts, osmotic equilibrium with the adjacent interstitial tissue may not be achieved. Alternatively, medullary solute concentration may be less than that of plasma and glomerular filtrate.

Clinical data that indicate that primary renal disorders are the probable cause of azotemia are helpful, but they fall short of allowing consistently accurate forecasts of the reversibility of the underlying cause or permitting formulation of effective specific, supportive, and symptomatic therapy. Knowledge of circulating red cell mass, kidney size, electrolyte and acid-base status, and in some instances data obtained by biopsy is needed to provide consistently meaningful prognoses and formulation of effective therapy.[38,48,49]

Glomerulotubular Imbalance
Etiopathogenesis
Abnormal elevation in the serum concentration of urea nitrogen or creatinine may also occur in association with an elevated urine specific gravity (± 1.025) in some

patients with primary renal failure caused by generalized glomerular disease.[14] A conceptual understanding of azotemia associated with primary renal failure and glomerulotubular imbalance is essential to differentiate this syndrome from prerenal azotemia.

Caution should be used not to overinterpret the absolute value of urine specific gravity of proteinuric patients with glomerular disease because it may be falsely elevated by the effect of protein. Addition of 400 mg of protein per 100 ml of urine will increase the urine specific gravity by approximately 0.001.[50]

The renal lesion in patients with primary azotemia and glomerulotubular imbalance must be characterized by glomerular damage that is sufficiently severe to impair renal clearance of urea and creatinine but that has not yet induced a degree of ischemic atrophy and necrosis of renal tubular cells sufficient to prevent urine concentration. Thus glomerular filtrate that is formed can be concentrated, at least to some degree. The specific gravity rarely exceeds 1.025 to 1.030, though, possibly as a result of obligatory solute diuresis.

Diagnosis

This group of patients may be differentiated from patients with prerenal azotemia by (1) failure of a search for one of the extrarenal causes of poor renal perfusion, (2) detection of persistent proteinuria, and (3) lack of significant reduction in the magnitude of azotemia by therapy designed to restore vascular volume and renal perfusion (Table VIII).

Primary Renal Azotemia Plus Prerenal or Postrenal Azotemia
Etiopathogenesis

Because kidneys with generalized disease have diminished ability to compensate for stresses imposed by concomitant diseases of other body systems, uremic crises may be abruptly precipitated by a variety of prerenal, and less commonly postrenal, disorders which develop in patients with previously compensated chronic renal failure. For example, factors that accelerate endogenous protein catabolism (anorexia, infection, and extensive tissue necrosis) may significantly increase the quantity of metabolic by-products in the body since the kidneys have impaired capacity to excrete them. Stress states (fever, infection, and change in environment) are associated with release of glucocorticoids from the adrenal glands. Glucocorticoids stimulate conversion of proteins to carbohydrates (gluconeogenesis) and thus increase the quantity of protein metabolic by-products in the body. In these situations, uremic crises may be precipitated since protein by-products contribute significantly to the production of uremic signs in patients with renal failure.[20] Any nonrenal abnormality that decreases renal perfusion (vomiting, diarrhea, decreased water consumption, shock, and cardiac decompensation) may also result in decomposition of primary renal failure.

Diagnosis

Precipitation of uremic crises by nonrenal diseases in patients with previously compensated primary renal failure may be difficult to detect, especially if both disorders are associated with vomiting, polydipsia, dehydration, anorexia, and weight loss. A high index of suspicion and diagnosis by therapeutic trial are often necessary. Whereas patients with uremic crises precipitated by reversible extrarenal disorders (pancreatic disease, gastroenteritis, Addison's disease, hepatic disease) may rapidly respond to specific, supportive, and symptomatic therapy, patients with uremic crises caused by progressive irreversible destruction of nephrons will not respond as dramatically, if at all.

Problem-Specific Diagnostic Data Base[b] for Azotemia
   I. History
      A. Current diet? Appetite?
      B. Water availability?
      C. Water intake? Changes?

[b]Further diagnostic procedures may be required to determine the specific cause(s) of prerenal, primary renal, or postrenal azotemia.

TABLE VIII
DIFFERENTIATION OF PRERENAL AZOTEMIA FROM PRIMARY RENAL AZOTEMIA ASSOCIATED WITH GLOMEROLOTUBULAR IMBALANCE

Factor	Prerenal Azotemia	Glomerulotubular Imbalance and Primary Renal Azotemia
SUN	Increased	Increased
Serum creatinine	Increased	Increased
Urine specific gravity	Dogs > 1.030 Cats > 1.035	± 1.020 to 1.030
Proteinuria	Usually negative	Positive
Prerenal cause	Present	Absent
Response to correction of renal perfusion	Usually within 1 to 3 days	Usually minimal

D. Urine output? Changes?

E. Pollakiuria (frequency, dysuria, tenesmus)?

F. Changes in urine color and/or odor?

G. Duration of current problem?

H. Exposure to nephrotoxins? (environment? drugs? etc.)

I. Recent traumatic or hypovolemic episodes? (including hit by car, fractures, shock, anesthesia, surgery, snake or insect bites, vomiting, diarrhea, others)

J. Recent illnesses?

K. Chronic illnesses? (including kidney or heart disease, endocrine diseases, urinary tract infection, or urolithiasis)

L. Current medications or treatments?

II. Physical examination

A. Body weight

B. Hydration status

C. Presence of ascites and/or dependent subcutaneous edema

D. Cardiovascular system (heart rate and rhythm, heart sounds, heart murmurs, pulse rate and character, membrane color, capillary refill time, blood pressure)

E. Kidneys (size, shape, location, surface contour, consistency, pain, masses, uroliths)

F. Urinary bladder (size, shape, location, surface contour, consistency, pain, masses, uroliths)

G. Urethra (size, shape, location, surface contour, consistency, pain, masses, uroliths)

H. Prostate (size, shape, location, surface contour, consistency, pain, masses, uroliths)

III. Laboratory and special examination data

A. Confirm vomiting, diarrhea, and other subjective historical problems. Initial data base: urinalysis, complete blood count, SUN, and serum creatinine concentrations.

B. Determine urine production rate (i.e., confirm polyuria, oliguria, etc.). If substantially proteinuric, consider a 24-hour urine protein determination.

C. Consider serum electrolytes (Na^+, K^+, Ca^{+2}).

D. If oliguric, consider urine sodium concentration or urine/serum creatinine ratios.

E. Based on history and physical examination findings, consider tests that may confirm the causal basis of prerenal azotemia (e.g., amylase, pancreatitis; SGPT, hepatic disease; toxicology studies, suspected intoxication, etc.).

F. Consider radiography or ultrasonography

1. Survey radiographs of entire urinary system, including urethra

2. Intravenous urogram and/or renal ultrasound for patients with suspected renal and/or ureteral diseases

3. Contrast cystography or intravenous urography for patients with suspected bladder disease

4. Contrast urethrocystography for patients with urethral disease; contrast urethrocystography and/or ultrasound for patients with prostate disease.

G. Consider renal biopsy.

REFERENCES

1. Osborne CA: The problem oriented medical system: Improved knowledge, wisdom, and understanding of patient care. *Vet Clin North Am.* In press, 1983.

2. Polzin DJ, Osborne CA, Hayden DW, Stevens JB: Experimental evaluation of reduced protein diets in the management of primary polyuria renal failure. Preliminary findings and their clinical significance. *Minn Vet* 21:16-29, 1981.

3. Street AE, Chesterman H, Smith GAA, Quinton RM: Prolonged blood urea elevation in the beagle after feeding. *Toxicol Appl Pharmacol* 13:363-371, 1968.

4. Watson ADJ, Church DB, Fairburn AJ: Postprandial changes in plasma urea and creatinine concentrations in dogs. *Am J Vet Res* 42:1878-1880, 1981.

5. Finco DR, Duncan JR: Evaluation of blood urea nitrogen and serum creatinine as indicators of renal dysfunction: A study of 111 cases and a review of related literature. *JAVMA* 168:593-601, 1976.

6. Kumar R, Steen P, McGrown MG: Chronic renal failure or simple starvation. *Lancet* 2:1005, 1972.

7. Refsum HE, Stromme SB: Urea and creatinine production and excretion in urine during prolonged and heavy exercise. *Scand J Clin Lab Invest* 33:247-254, 1974.

8. Finco DR: Kidney function, in Kaneko JJ (ed): *Clinical Biochemistry of Domestic Animals,* ed 3. New York, Academic Press, 1980.

9. Kopple JD, Coburn JW: Evaluation of chronic uremia. Importance of serum urea nitrogen, serum creatinine, and their ratio. *JAMA* 227:41-44, 1974.

10. Osborne CA, Stevens JB, McClean R, Vernier RL: Membranous lupus glomerulonephritis in a dog. *JAAHA* 9:295-300, 1973.

11. Osborne CA, Klausner JS: Adverse drug reactions in the uremic patient, in Kirk RW (ed): *Current Veterinary Therapy,* vol 6. Philadelphia, WB Saunders Co, 1977.

12. Austin JH, Stillman NE, Van Slyke DD: Factors governing excretion rate of urea. *J Biol Chem* 46:91, 1921.

13. Dossetor JB: Creatinine versus uremia. The relative significance of blood urea nitrogen and serum creatinine concentrations in azotemia. *Ann Int Med* 65:1287-1299, 1966.

14. Osborne CA, Hammer RF, Stevens JB, Resnick JS, Michael AF: The glomerulus in health and disease: Review of domestic animals and man. *Adv Vet Sci Comp Med* 21:207-285, 1977.

15. Finco DR, Stevens JB: Clinical significance of serum amylase activity in the dog. *JAVMA* 155:1686-1691, 1969.

16. Osborne CA, Stevens JB, Polzin DJ: Gastrointestinal manifestations of urinary diseases, in Anderson NV (ed): *Veterinary Gastroenterology.* Philadelphia, Lea & Febiger, 1980.

17. Polzin DJ, Osborne CA, Stevens JB, Hayden DW: Serum amylase and lipase activities in dogs with chronic polyuric renal failure. *Am J Vet Res* 44:404-410, 1983.

18. Wagner AG, Macy DW: Nephelometric determination of serum amylase and lipase in naturally occurring azotemia in the dog. *Am J Vet Res* 43:697-699, 1982.

19. Willard MD, Schall WD, McCaw DE, Nachreiner RF: Canine hypoadrenocorticism: Report of 37 cases and review of 39 previously reported cases. *JAVMA* 180:59-62, 1982.

20. Osborne CA, Finco DR, Low DG: Pathophysiology of renal disease, renal failure, and uremia, in Ettinger SJ (ed): *Textbook of Veterinary Internal Medicine,* ed 2. Philadelphia, WB Saunders Co, 1983, pp 1751-1759.

21. Rahill WH, Subramanian S: The use of fetal animals to investigate renal development. *Lab Anim Sci* 23:92-96, 1973.

22. Bernardini R, Bruttini GP, Giglio C: Sensitivity to ischemia of dog kidney. *Gass Int Med Chir* 74:1520, 1969.

23. Hamilton PB, Phillips RA, Hiller A: Duration of renal ischemia required to produce uremia. *Am J Physiol* 152:517, 1948.

24. Roof BS, et al: Recovery of glomerular and tubular function,

including p-aminohippurate extraction, following two hours of renal artery occlusion in the dog. *Am J Physiol* 166:666, 1951.

25. Moyer JH, et al: Renal failure. I. The effect of complete renal artery occlusion for variable periods of time as compared to exposure to subfiltration arterial pressures below 30 mm Hg for similar periods. *Ann Surg* 145:41, 1957.

26. Chisholm GD, Osborn DE: Pathophysiology of obstructive uropathy, in Williams DI, Chisholm CD (eds): *Scientific Foundations of Urology*, vol 1. *Renal Disorders, Infection, and Calculi.* London, W Heinemann Med Books, 1976.

27. Klahr S, Buerkert J, Purkerson ML: The kidney in obstructive uropathy. *Contrib Nephrol* 7:220-249, 1977.

28. Wright FS, Howards SS: Obstructive injury, in Brenner BM, Rector FC (eds): *The Kidney*, vol 2, ed 2. Philadelphia, WB Saunders Co, 1981.

29. Finco DR, Kneller SK, Crowell WA: Diseases of the urinary system, in Catcott EJ (ed): *Feline Medicine and Surgery*, ed 2. Santa Barbara, CA, American Vet Publ Inc, 1975.

30. Osborne CA, Klausner JS, Lees GE: Urinary tract infections: Normal and abnormal host defense mechanisms. *Vet Clin North Am* 9:587-609, 1979.

31. Katul MJ, Wax SH: Evaluation of renal function during experimental hydronephrosis by means of the radioisotope renogram. *Surg Gynecol Obstet* 126:563, 1968.

32. Kerr WS: Effect of complete ureteral obstruction for one week on kidney function. *J Appl Physiol* 6:672, 1954.

33. Pridgen WR, Woodhead DM, Younger RK: Alterations in renal function produced by ureteral occlusion. *JAMA* 178:149, 1963.

34. Vaughn ED, Sorenson EJ, Gillenwater JY: The renal hemodynamic response to chronic unilateral complete ureteral occlusion. *Invest Urol* 8:78, 1970.

35. Finco DR, Cornelius LM: Characterization and treatment of water, electrolyte, and acid-base imbalances of induced urethral obstruction in the cat. *Am J Vet Res* 38:823-830, 1977.

36. Osborne CA, Lees GE: Feline cystitis, urethritis, urethral obstruction syndrome. *Mod Vet Pract* 59:173-180, 349-357, 513-520, 669-673, 1978.

37. Burrows CF, Bovee KC: Metabolic changes due to experimentally induced rupture of the canine urinary bladder. *Am J Vet Res* 35:1083-1088, 1974.

38. Osborne CA, Low DC, Finco DR: *Canine and Feline Urology.* Philadelphia, WB Saunders Co, 1972.

39. Hardy RM, Osborne CA: Water deprivation test in the dog: Maximal normal values. *JAVMA* 174:479-484, 1979.

40. Levinsky NG, Alexander EA, Venkatachalam MA: Acute renal failure, in Brenner BM, Rector FC (eds): *The Kidney*, vol 1, ed 2. Philadelphia, WB Saunders Co, 1981.

41. Hardy RM, Osborne CA: Water deprivation and vasopressin concentration tests in the differentiation of polyuric syndromes, in Kirk RW (ed): *Current Veterinary Therapy*, vol 7. Philadelphia, WB Saunders Co, 1980.

42. Brietschwerdt EB: Clinical abnormalities of urinary concentration and dilution. *Compend Contin Educ Pract Vet* 3:414-421, 1981.

43. Hardy RM, Osborne CA: Aqueous vasopressin response test in clinically normal dogs undergoing water diuresis: Technique and results. *Am J Vet Res* 43:1987-1990, 1982.

44. Hardy RM, Osborne CA: Repositol vasopressin response test in clinically normal dogs undergoing water diuresis: Technique and results. *Am J Vet Res* 43:1991-1993, 1982.

45. Osborne CA, Finco DR, Scott RC: Problem oriented diagnosis of diseases of the urinary system: I. The kidney. *Sci Proc 42nd AAHA Annu Meet, South Bend, IN:*1975.

46. Bricker NS, Schultze RG: Renal function: General concepts, in Maxwell MH, Kleenan CR (eds): *Clinical Disorders of Fluid and Electrolyte Metabolism*, ed 2. New York, McGraw-Hill Book Co, 1972.

47. Clapp JR, Robinson RR: Osmolality of distal tubular fluid in the dog. *J Clin Invest* 45:1847-1853, 1966.

48. Cowgill LD: Disease of the kidney, in Ettinger SJ (ed): *Textbook of Veterinary Internal Medicine*, vol 2, ed 2. Philadelphia, WB Saunders Co, 1982.

49. Osborne CA, Polzin DJ: Strategy in the diagnosis, prognosis and management of renal disease, renal failure, and uremia. *Proc 46th Annu Meet AAHA, South Bend, IN:*559-630, 1979.

50. Osborne CA, Stevens JB: *Handbook of Canine and Feline Urinalysis.* St. Louis, Ralston Purina Co, 1981, p 44.

UPDATE

Experimental studies have revealed that cats with less than 25% of nephrons functional could concentrate their urine at a specific gravity (SG) significantly higher than 1.040.[1-3] Although we commonly use a SG value of 1.035 to 1.040 to indicate adequate urine concentrating capacity in cats, further studies are required to determine the urine SG value that best indicates a population of functional nephrons adequate to prevent the clinical signs associated with primary renal failure.

Dietary protein intake or parenteral administration of amino acids may profoundly affect the glomerular filtration rate. High protein intake enhances glomerular filtration and renal blood flow, whereas dietary protein restriction minimizes these hemodynamic effects. The mechanism(s) by which dietary protein enhances renal hemodynamics is not understood, but it is likely that the activation of some circulating or humoral effector system is involved. Proposed circulating or humoral effectors of this phenomenon include glucagon, growth hormone, prostaglandins, the renin-angiotensin system, biogenic amines and a hepatic-derived vasodilator known as glomerulopressin. The point is that normal glomerular filtration rate, clearance values, and serum urea nitrogen and creatinine concentrations are influenced by the quantity of protein being consumed.

References

1. Adams LG, Polzin DJ, Osborne CA, O'Brien TD: Effects of dietary protein restriction in clinically normal cats and cats with surgically induced chronic renal failure. *Am J Vet Res* 54:1643–1662, 1993.

2. Lulich JP, Osborne CA, O'Brien TD, Polzin DJ: Feline renal failure: Questions, answers, questions. *Compend Contin Educ Pract Vet* 14:127–152, 1992.

3. Ross LA, Finco DR: Relationship of selected renal function tests to glomerular filtration rate and renal blood flow in cats. *Am J Vet Res* 42:1704–1710, 1981.

Polyuria and Polydipsia

KEY FACTS

- Polyuria and polydipsia are common in small animal patients.
- Although polyuria and polydipsia may be signs of many disease states, the list of common diagnostic differentials is quite short, especially in cats.
- Appreciation of the prevalence of polyuria and polydipsia in a particular disease state as well as the relative incidence of diagnostic differentials ensures an appropriate evaluation.
- Most causes of polyuria and polydipsia are diagnosed by integrating the history, physical examination, complete blood count, chemistry screen, and urinalysis findings; the ease and success of the diagnostic workup are facilitated by a problem-solving approach.

University of Pennsylvania
Dez Hughes, BVSc, MRCVS

POLYURIA and polydipsia are common in small animal patients. Polyuria (i.e., excretion of an abnormally large amount of urine) is specifically defined as a daily output of urine in excess of 50 ml/kg/day.[1] Polydipsia (i.e., excessive ingestion of fluid) has been estimated as a fluid intake that exceeds 100 ml/kg/day.[1] This estimate of the amount of fluid intake to denote polydipsia may be too high, however (especially for cats), and may cause some animals with polyuria and polydipsia to be overlooked. It therefore is prudent to investigate any significant increase in fluid intake or urine production, regardless of the estimated volumes.

Two distinct, intertwined feedback loops function to control extracellular fluid homeostasis (Figure 1). These loops maintain osmolality and volume of the extracellular fluid within relatively narrow limits. Osmolality is controlled by osmoreceptors in the hypothalamus that stimulate thirst and release of antidiuretic hormone.[2–4] Extracellular volume primarily depends on total body sodium content, which is principally determined by the renin–angiotensin–aldosterone system and probably modulated by atrial natriuretic peptide.[5] A schematic representation of extracellular fluid homeostasis is shown in Figure 1.

If water loss from the body exceeds water intake, plasma osmolality rises. Hypothalamic osmoreceptors then stimulate thirst and release of antidiuretic hormone from the neurohypophysis. Antidiuretic hormone increases passive osmotic water reabsorption from the collecting tubule into the hypertonic medullary interstitium. Augmented water intake and reabsorption by the kidneys combine to decrease plasma osmolality. Fluctuations in plasma osmolality necessary to stimulate thirst and antidiuretic hormone release are very small (approximately 4 mOsm/kg).

In addition to stimulating a compensatory response to maintain systemic blood pressure, hypovolemia initiates a series of events leading to extracellular volume expansion. Sympathetic outflow and decreased stretch of renal afferent arterioles stimulate renin release from the juxtaglomerular cells. Renin activates angiotensinogen to angiotensin I, which is then converted to angiotensin II. Sodium and water reabsorption is increased by angiotensin II in the proximal tubule. Angiotensin II–mediated aldosterone release also promotes distal tubular sodium reabsorption. The feedback loops controlling extracellular volume and osmolality overlap with the hypovolemic stimulus for antidiuretic hormone release and thirst. Thirst is mediated, at least partially, by angiotensin II. The renin–angiotensin–aldosterone system, antidiuretic hormone, and the mechanisms of thirst thereby increase retention of sodium and water to expand extracellular volume.

Most animals presented for polyuria and polydipsia are inappropriately polyuric with a compensatory, appropriate polydipsia. Because of the obligatory fluid loss, these animals (when deprived of adequate access to water) are extremely prone to rapid dehydration. The temptation to provide short-term symptomatic relief by water restriction

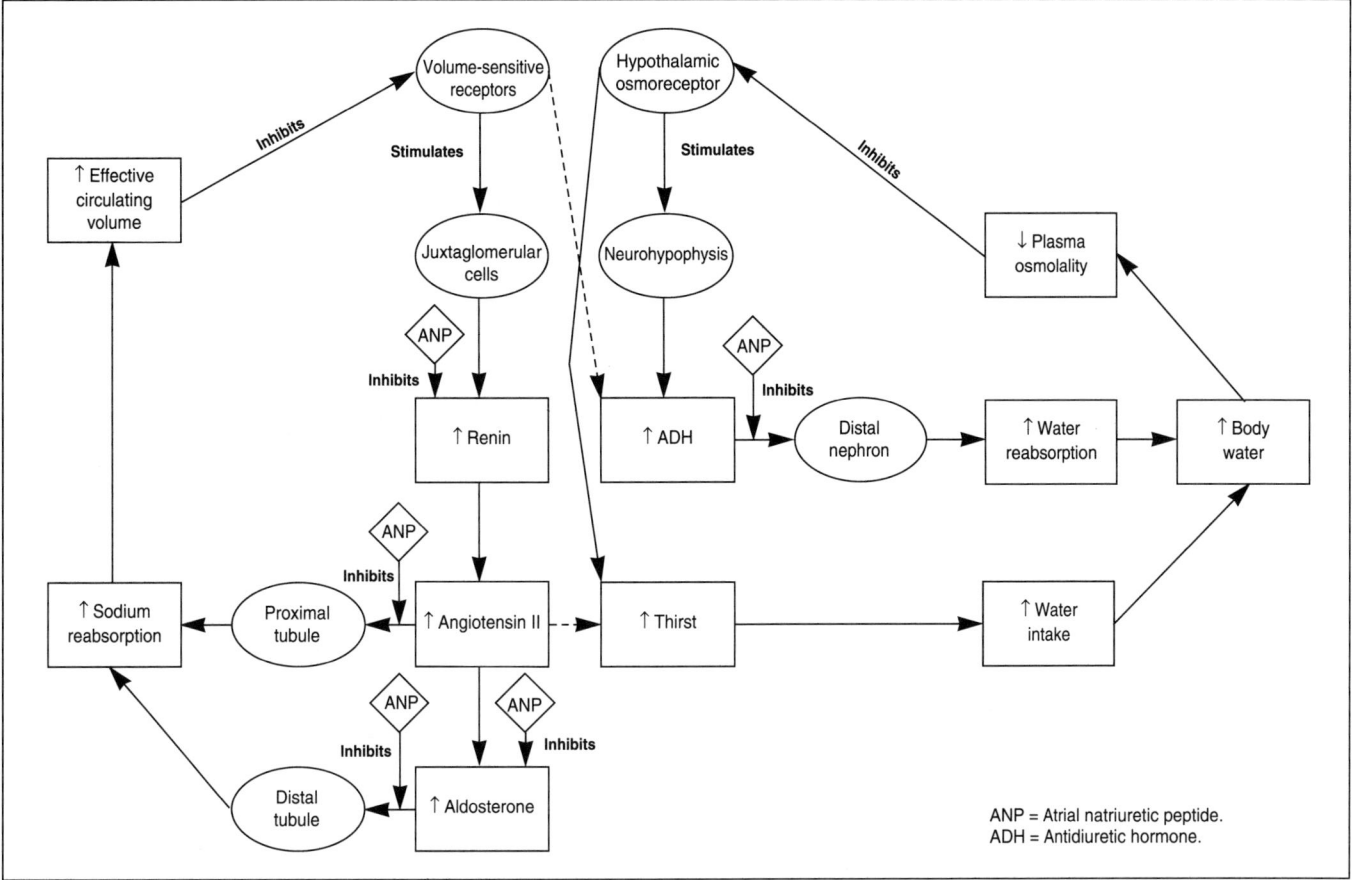

Figure 1—Extracellular fluid homeostasis.

should therefore be strenuously avoided. On rare occasions, an animal may exhibit primary polydipsia with an appropriately increased urine output. Such an animal would have a physiologic reduction in antidiuretic hormone release, thereby allowing water diuresis to prevent overhydration. Certain conditions may cause primary polyuria and primary polydipsia.

MANY DISEASE STATES involve more than one mechanism of polyuria and polydipsia in the same animal. Primary polyuria may result from osmotic diuresis, reduced renal responsiveness to antidiuretic hormone, or antidiuretic hormone deficiency (central diabetes insipidus). The most common solutes that cause osmotic diuresis are glucose in cases of diabetes mellitus and sodium (and others) in cases of renal failure. Reduced renal responsiveness to antidiuretic hormone, also referred to as nephrogenic diabetes insipidus, is a common pathophysiologic mechanism for polyuria and polydipsia. Reduced renal responsiveness usually is secondary to an underlying disease process. Antidiuretic hormone deficiency rarely occurs and usually results from intracranial neoplasia. Primary polydipsia may

result from psychogenic or behavioral causes or be associated with such disease conditions as hyperthyroidism or hypokalemia (see Pathophysiologic Mechanisms of Polyuria and Polydipsia).

HISTORY

The goal of initial anamnesis should be to verify polyuria and polydipsia. The propensity of owners to report polydipsia but not polyuria is widely recognized. If excessive amounts of fluid have not been lost as a result of such factors as panting or exercise, this situation is physiologically implausible and is almost always an inaccurate observation by the owner.

As with any animal presenting with an abnormality related to micturition, the clinician should attempt to distinguish between polyuria (excretion of an abnormally large volume of urine), incontinence (inability to control urination voluntarily), dysuria (difficult urination), pollakiuria (abnormally frequent urination), and behaviorally inappropriate micturition. Nocturia or urinating in the house may suggest polyuria. Polydipsia may be variably reported as a constant refilling of the animal's water bowl, the animal drinking from puddles or toilets, eating snow, or (in severe cases) drinking urine.

Pathophysiologic Mechanisms of Polyuria and Polydipsia

Primary polyuria

Osmotic diuresis (e.g., natriuresis, glucose, mannitol)

Reduced renal responsiveness to antidiuretic hormone, which may result from:
- Abnormal antidiuretic hormone structure
- Ineffective antidiuretic hormone and/or tubular cell membrane receptor interaction
- Dysfunction of the adenylate cyclase second messenger system
- Changes in permeability in the distal nephron
- Reduction in renal medullary interstitial hypertonicity (medullary washout)[a]

Antidiuretic hormone deficiency (central diabetes insipidus)

Primary polydipsia

Conditions causing abnormal stimulation of thirst
Behavioral and/or psychogenic factors

---

[a]Medullary washout can result from either decreased sodium chloride or urea reabsorption or increased solute loss from the medullary interstitium, which usually is a consequence of increased blood flow leaving the medulla. Animals with polyuria and polydipsia usually develop renal unresponsiveness to antidiuretic hormone from medullary washout to some degree.

Although polyuria and polydipsia may be the only historical complaint, owners may report other signs indicative of the underlying disease process. For example, weight loss may suggest renal disease, liver disease, hyperthyroidism, or diabetes mellitus. Polyphagia may be associated with hyperthyroidism or diabetes mellitus, whereas anorexia occurs in many other diagnostic differentials. Many dogs with hyperadrenocorticism are reported to pant or tremble. Hepatic disease may cause neurologic signs. History taking also should include any current medications and the possibility of exposure to toxins.

THE SPECIES, age, sex, and breed may indicate an underlying cause. Most cats with spontaneous polyuria and polydipsia have renal disease, diabetes mellitus, or hyperthyroidism.[6] Congenital or hereditary abnormalities usually manifest at an early age, whereas older animals are more at risk of neoplasia or chronic renal disease. An older, intact bitch with a vaginal discharge beginning two months after cessation of estrus is very likely to have pyometra. Hypoadrenocorticism tends to affect young to middle-aged bitches, and diabetes mellitus is overrepresented in older bitches. It also is important to be aware of breed predispositions to

certain disorders, such as hyperadrenocorticism in toy poodles, liver disease in Doberman pinschers, and renal tubular transport defects in basenjis and Norwegian elkhounds.

PHYSICAL EXAMINATION

Although some animals with polyuria and polydipsia seem normal, the physical examination can provide valuable information. Small, irregular kidneys often are associated with chronic renal disease. Most cats with hyperthyroidism have a thyroid nodule revealed by careful palpation. Examining a dog with pyometra often reveals a vaginal discharge and a distended, tubular, fluid-filled viscus on abdominal palpation. A panting, potbellied, small-breed dog with appendicular muscle wasting, truncal obesity, and alopecia may have hyperadrenocorticism. Hepatomegaly may be found in conjunction with hyperadrenocorticism, diabetes mellitus, or lymphoma. Moderate to severe, firm, nonpainful peripheral lymphadenopathy usually indicates lymphoma. More subtle physical findings include small, perirectal, anal sac adenocarcinomas or the broad, bulky features of patients with acromegaly.

DIAGNOSTIC DIFFERENTIALS

In compiling a list of diagnostic differentials, an appreciation of the relative incidence of possible underlying causes is essential. For example, the most common cause of polyuria and polydipsia in dogs and cats is chronic renal failure. Most polyuric and polydipsic cats without renal disease have hyperthyroidism or diabetes mellitus.[6] Table I lists the diagnostic differentials for polyuria and polydipsia in dogs and cats according to the relative incidence in the general animal population. In this article, the discussion of diagnostic differentials of polyuria and polydipsia is biased toward those of relative clinical importance. Rare or less significant causes of polyuria and polydipsia are discussed only briefly.

Common Causes of Polyuria and Polydipsia
Chronic Renal Insufficiency or Failure

Chronic renal disease is the most common cause of polyuria and polydipsia in dogs and cats. In animals with chronic renal disease, polyuria and polydipsia are reported to occur less frequently in cats.[7] Loss of 66% or more of the functioning renal mass results in an inability of the kidneys to concentrate urine.[8,9] Before this stage is reached, nephron loss is offset by a compensatory increase in the glomerular filtration rate of the remaining nephrons. As the single-nephron glomerular filtration rate continues to increase because of progressive nephron loss, increasing quantities of glomerular filtrate are presented to each functioning nephron. Eventually, the augmented distal nephron flow overwhelms the reduced reabsorptive capabilities; osmotic diuresis occurs and is further complicated by medullary washout.[10]

TABLE I
Diagnostic Differentials of Polyuria and Polydipsia in Dogs and Cats

Dogs	*Cats*
Common causes of polyuria and polydipsia	
Chronic renal insufficiency or failure	Chronic renal insufficiency or failure
Pyometra	Postobstructive diuresis
Diabetes mellitus	Hyperthyroidism
Hyperadrenocorticism	Diabetes mellitus
Liver disease	Iatrogenic causes
Iatrogenic causes	
Uncommon causes of polyuria and polydipsia	
Hypercalcemia	Liver disease
Hypoadrenocorticism	Pyometra
Pyelonephritis	
Rare or less significant causes of polyuria and polydipsia	
Central diabetes insipidus	Pheochromocytoma
Psychogenic polydipsia	Polycythemia
Acromegaly	Hyperadrenocorticism
Hypokalemia	Hypoadrenocorticism
Renal glycosuria	Hypercalcemia
Fanconi syndrome	Pyelonephritis
Primary nephrogenic diabetes insipidus	Central diabetes insipidus
	Acromegaly

Animals presenting with chronic renal insufficiency or failure usually are older. Azotemic animals usually present for weight loss, inappetence, lethargy, and vomiting with varying degrees of dehydration. Blood chemistry analysis shows azotemia, and urinalysis reveals insufficient concentrating ability, often in conjunction with dehydration. Urine specific gravity will be in the isosthenuric range (1.008 to 1.012) or minimally concentrated (up to 1.025). Animals without azotemia but with reduced renal concentrating ability as a result of nephron loss (i.e., animals with 66% to 75% nephron loss) should have diminished urinary concentrating ability. Documentation of reduced glomerular filtration rate may be obtained by measuring creatinine clearance,[11] and histopathologic evidence of renal disease can be obtained by renal biopsy. It should be noted that not all animals with acute renal failure have oliguria or anuria. Because of the large quantity of plasma filtered by the kidneys each day, animals with nephron loss sufficient to cause azotemia may still be polyuric because of reduced tubular reabsorption.

Pyometra

Approximately two thirds of bitches with pyometra are noted to have polydipsia.[12] The polydipsia is believed to be secondary to primary polyuria resulting from reduced renal responsiveness to antidiuretic hormone with medullary washout.[13] Studies suggest that uterine bacterial infection is required for polyuria and polydipsia to develop,[14] although the specific mechanism has not been identified. The concentrating defect often is reversible in two to eight weeks after ovariohysterectomy.[13]

A history of anorexia, lethargy, polyuria and polydipsia, and vomiting in an older, intact bitch two to three months after cessation of estrus strongly indicates pyometra. Physical findings of an enlarged uterus, especially with purulent or sanguinous vaginal discharge, are virtually pathognomonic for the disorder. A blood smear commonly reveals moderate to severe neutrophilia with a left shift. Urine specific gravity is variable, with one study reporting 20% of cases less than 1.007 and 27% of cases greater than 1.024.[12] Vaginal cytology, abdominal radiography, and abdominal ultrasonography may be helpful in confirming the diagnosis.

Diabetes Mellitus

Almost all diabetic animals have polyuria and polydipsia. Polydipsia is secondary to primary osmotic diuresis resulting from glycosuria. Persistent hyperglycemia eventually exceeds the tubular transport maximum for glucose reabsorption (180 to 220 mg/dl in dogs and a mean of 290 mg/dl in normal cats[15]; diabetic cats may, however, have a lower renal threshold for glucose of roughly 200 mg/dl[16]). Polyuria and polydipsia resolve as diabetes mellitus is adequately regulated and blood glucose no longer exceeds the renal threshold.

A MIDDLE-AGED to old, overweight bitch with a history of polyuria and polydipsia, polyphagia, and weight loss is the classic diabetes mellitus patient. The physical examination usually is unrewarding; obesity and hepatomegaly are common but are nonspecific findings. Clinical signs referable to concurrent disease may be identified (e.g., urinary tract infection and pancreatitis are frequently seen with diabetes mellitus). Urinalysis and blood glucose measurement reveal glycosuria with or without ketonuria and hyperglycemia. Diagnosis of feline diabetes mellitus should be based on repeated blood glucose measurements if hyperglycemia is in the range of 200 to 400 mg/dl. Stress hyperglycemia, which is extremely common in cats, may fall within this range. Glycosuria does not sufficiently indicate diabetes mellitus in cats—14% of cats with chronic renal failure have normoglycemic glycosuria.[7]

Hyperadrenocorticism

Hyperadrenocorticism is common in dogs but rare in cats. In animals with hyperadrenocorticism, polyuria and polydipsia are seen in 85% to 97% of dogs[16] and approximately 90% of cats.[17] The cause of the concentrating defect in hyperadrenocorticism is controversial, but primary polyuria resulting from reduced antidiuretic hormone secretion[18] and interference with antidiuretic hormone and tubular cell interaction[19,20] have been proposed. The polyuria and polydipsia respond if treatment to reduce cortisol levels is successful.

Affected dogs usually are middle-aged to older. Clinical signs range from only polyuria and polydipsia or skin disease to the full-blown presentation of alopecia with potbelly, hepatomegaly, panting, truncal obesity, and appendicular muscle wasting. A complete blood count may reveal mature neutrophilia with eosinopenia and lymphopenia. Blood chemistry analysis commonly shows elevated serum alkaline phosphatase, alanine transaminase, and cholesterol. Urinalysis may reveal a urinary tract infection. Some investigators report urine specific gravity less than 1.007 in as many as 85% of cases.[16] A low-dose dexamethasone suppression test or corticotropin-stimulation test may be done to confirm the diagnosis of hyperadrenocorticism.

Liver Disease

The term *liver disease* encompasses a spectrum of disease entities. The severity and chronicity of hepatic dysfunction therefore varies widely, and it is predictable that the prevalence of polyuria and polydipsia in liver disease also varies. Polyuria and polydipsia seem to be most common in cases of cirrhosis and portosystemic shunts.[21] One third of dogs with portosystemic shunts may have polyuria and polydipsia.[22] The pathophysiology of polyuria and polydipsia in liver disease is poorly understood. Suggested mechanisms include medullary washout, portal osmoreceptor effects, hypokalemia, elevated endogenous corticosteroids, and primary polydipsia.[21] Reversibility of polyuria and polydipsia in liver disease depends on the success of treatment of the underlying disease process.

ALTHOUGH certain breeds are predisposed to liver disease (e.g., Doberman pinschers and Bedlington terriers), signalment and history usually are nonspecific. Icterus, ascites, or changes in liver size may provide additional evidence of liver disease. Diagnosis is based on critical assessment of biochemical parameters and physical findings. Hepatic enzymes and indicators of hepatic function, such as albumin, urea, ammonia, glucose, bilirubin, bile acids, coagulation factors, and sulfobromophthalein retention, may be useful. Ultimately, hepatic biopsy is required for a definitive diagnosis.

Hyperthyroidism

Hyperthyroidism is common in cats but rare in dogs. Approximately 50% of hyperthyroid cats exhibit polyuria and polydipsia.[23] Canine thyroid tumors are nonfunctional in 80% to 95% of patients; however, approximately 95% of

TABLE II
Iatrogenic Causes of Polyuria and Polydipsia

Common Causes	Less Common Causes
Diuretics	Radiographic contrast agents
Corticosteroids	Thyroid hormones
Parenteral fluid therapy	Amphotericin B
Anticonvulsants	Methoxyflurane

dogs with functional thyroid tumors exhibit polyuria and polydipsia.[16]

The pathophysiologic mechanism for polyuria and polydipsia in cases of hyperthyroidism remains ill-defined. The proposed theories involve thyrotoxicosis-induced primary polydipsia[24] or medullary washout resulting from increased medullary blood flow.[25] Feline hyperthyroidism affects middle-aged to old cats. A history compatible with feline hyperthyroidism includes polyphagia, polyuria and polydipsia, hyperactivity, and weight loss. Some cats with hyperthyroidism, however, present with vague gastrointestinal signs (such as vomiting and diarrhea) or signs attributable to secondary thyrotoxic cardiomyopathy. Fortunately, from a diagnostic standpoint, up to 90% of hyperthyroid cats have a thyroid nodule that can be detected on careful palpation.[26] Mild to moderate elevation of hepatic enzymes, which normalizes with treatment, is an incidental finding in 50% to 75% of affected cats.[26] Urine specific gravity varies over a wide range; one study reported values from 1.006 to 1.060.[16] Definitive diagnosis is most often made on the basis of an elevated resting T_4 level.

Postobstructive Diuresis

Postobstructive diuresis is a phenomenon most frequently encountered after relief of urethral obstruction in cats. Primary polyuria occurs and may be severe. Early theories regarding the pathogenesis of the condition were based on solute retention and volume expansion during obstruction and subsequent osmotic diuresis. More recent studies, however, have suggested that humoral factors (such as atrial natriuretic peptide) accumulate or are released during or after complete postrenal obstruction.[27,28] Decreased solute reabsorption, medullary washout, and reduced water reabsorption in the cortical collecting tubule all may contribute to postobstructive diuresis.[28] Signs usually are reversible two to five days after relief of the obstruction. Diagnosis of the syndrome usually is easy. The important issue in affected cats is to provide a sufficiently high fluid rate to compensate for urinary fluid losses as well as to replace any preexisting fluid deficits.

Iatrogenic Causes of Polyuria and Polydipsia

Major iatrogenic causes of polyuria and polydipsia are listed in Table II. Among these causes, corticosteroids and diuretics are the most clinically important. The owner should be carefully questioned about current drug administration.

Uncommon Causes of Polyuria and Polydipsia
Hypercalcemia

Polyuria and polydipsia are common in animals with hypercalcemia. In one study, 64% of dogs with hypercalcemia resulting from primary hyperparathyroidism had mild to moderate polyuria and polydipsia.[16] Hypercalcemia is rarely seen in cats. Primary polyuria results from depletion of active adenylate cyclase[29] and reduced sodium chloride reabsorption into the medullary interstitium, resulting in medullary washout.[30]

RENAL INSUFFICIENCY or failure may also result from the nephrotoxic effects of elevated serum calcium. Reversibility of polyuria and polydipsia after successful resolution of hypercalcemia depends on the severity of the secondary renal damage. The underlying cause of hypercalcemia in most dogs is neoplasia resulting from lymphoma, anal sac adenocarcinoma, or primary hyperparathyroidism. Hypercalcemia resulting from cholecalciferol rodenticide intoxication also is becoming more common.

Urine specific gravity may be hyposthenuric, isosthenuric, or minimally concentrated. In the series of dogs with primary hyperparathyroidism discussed previously, all dogs had urine specific gravity less than 1.028.

Hypoadrenocorticism

Retrospective analyses have shown that roughly 20% to 40% of dogs with hypoadrenocorticism exhibit polyuria and polydipsia.[31,32] Hypoadrenocorticism is very rare in cats, but approximately 30% of cats with the disorder have polyuria and polydipsia.[17] Hypoaldosteronemic natriuresis,[16] medullary washout,[19] and reduced permeability of the collecting duct to water[33] are suggested mechanisms for the primary polyuria. Polyuria and polydipsia usually resolve after successful treatment of hyperadrenocorticism. Seventy percent of affected dogs are female, and most are young or middle-aged.

The history usually reveals vague signs, including anorexia, weakness, and gastrointestinal disorders or acute collapse. Physical examination often reveals no definitive clues; therefore, a high index of suspicion is necessary to pursue a diagnosis. Hyperkalemia and hyponatremia suggest the disorder; however, definitive diagnosis requires a corticotropin-stimulation test. Urinalysis often reveals inadequate urinary concentration in conjunction with azotemia. Urine specific gravity, although often less than 1.025, is reported to vary from 1.006 to 1.056.[31]

Pyelonephritis

Bacterial pyelonephritis is poorly documented in dogs and especially in cats. The prevalence of polyuria and polydipsia in pyelonephritis is unknown. A primary polyuria occurs, which may result from medullary washout[34] and/or active renal bacterial infection itself.[35] Ultimately, renal insufficiency or failure may ensue. Reversibility of the polyuria and polydipsia depends on the degree of damage incurred and the success of treatment of pyelonephritis.

Signalment, history, and physical examination only suggest the disorder. Urinalysis may reveal bacteriuria and casts, thereby providing support for the diagnosis. Urine specific gravity often is in the minimally concentrated range. Dogs with experimentally induced pyelonephritis exhibited a mean urine specific gravity of 1.017 10 days after renal inoculation with *Staphylococcus aureus*.[36] Excretory urography and ultrasonography can be used to demonstrate renal abnormalities but are unable to provide a definitive diagnosis.

Rare or Less Significant Causes of Polyuria and Polydipsia

The previously mentioned causes of polyuria and polydipsia should be ruled out before testing for more rare causes is begun. Rare or less significant causes of polyuria and polydipsia are listed in Table I.

All animals with central diabetes insipidus have primary polyuria as a result of antidiuretic hormone deficiency, which may be partial or complete. Most canine cases result from primary or metastatic intracranial neoplasia and are seen in middle-aged to old dogs.[37] Physical examination may be unremarkable or reveal neurologic signs referable to an intracranial space-occupying lesion. Central diabetes insipidus tends to affect young cats; however, few feline cases have been reported. Definitive diagnosis is based on results of a modified water deprivation–antidiuretic hormone response test.

THERE IS A PAUCITY of adequately documented cases of psychogenic polydipsia in the literature. It has been stated that psychogenic polydipsia occurs most commonly in large-breed dogs, especially German shepherds. Large-breed dogs with hyperadrenocorticism often present for polyuria and polydipsia only and may concentrate their urine in response to a water deprivation test. Most investigators therefore emphasize that diagnosis of psychogenic polydipsia requires exclusion of all other possibilities, including hyperadrenocorticism, and a compatible modified water deprivation–antidiuretic hormone response test.

In cats, the most common cause of glycosuria without hyperglycemia is renal failure. Hereditary tubular transport defects causing euglycemic glycosuria also have been reported in dogs. Basenjis and Norwegian elkhounds are most frequently affected.[38–40]

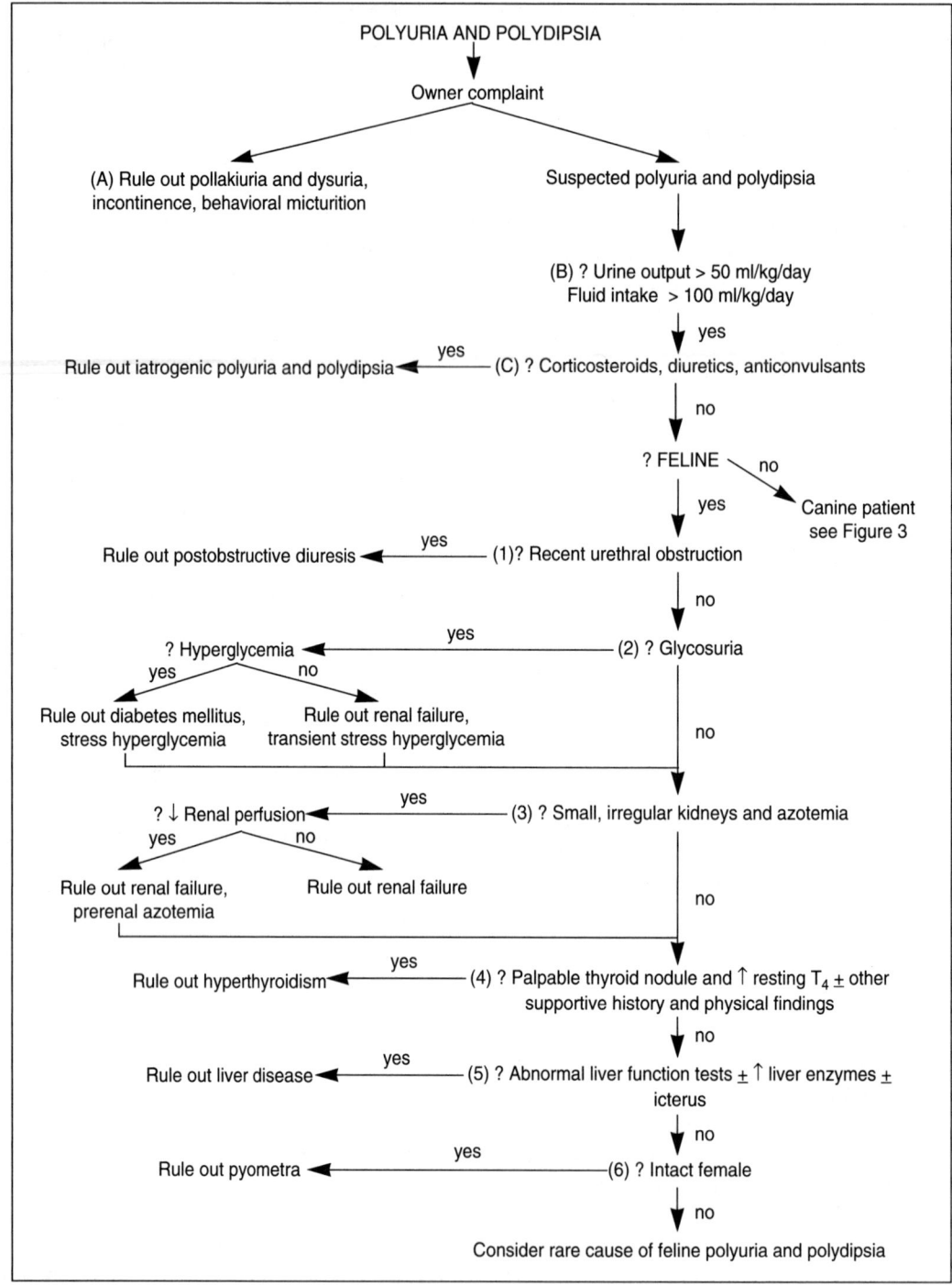

POLYURIA AND POLYDIPSIA

Owner complaint

(A) Rule out pollakiuria and dysuria, incontinence, behavioral micturition

Suspected polyuria and polydipsia

(B) ? Urine output > 50 ml/kg/day
Fluid intake > 100 ml/kg/day

yes

Rule out iatrogenic polyuria and polydipsia ← yes — (C) ? Corticosteroids, diuretics, anticonvulsants

no

? FELINE → no → Canine patient see Figure 3

yes

Rule out postobstructive diuresis ← yes — (1)? Recent urethral obstruction

no

? Hyperglycemia ← yes — (2) ? Glycosuria

yes / no

Rule out diabetes mellitus, stress hyperglycemia   Rule out renal failure, transient stress hyperglycemia

no

? ↓ Renal perfusion ← yes — (3) ? Small, irregular kidneys and azotemia

yes / no

Rule out renal failure, prerenal azotemia   Rule out renal failure

no

Rule out hyperthyroidism ← yes — (4) ? Palpable thyroid nodule and ↑ resting T_4 ± other supportive history and physical findings

no

Rule out liver disease ← yes — (5) ? Abnormal liver function tests ± ↑ liver enzymes ± icterus

no

Rule out pyometra ← yes — (6) ? Intact female

no

Consider rare cause of feline polyuria and polydipsia

Figure 2—Algorithm outlining the initial approach to patients with polyuria and polydipsia as well as the diagnostic evaluation of cats with polyuria and polydipsia.

Canine acromegaly is almost exclusively a condition of intact bitches as a result of progestogen-induced growth hormone secretion.[41] The progestogen is either endogenous (released during the luteal phase of the estrus cycle) or exogenous (resulting from veterinary progestogen administration). Feline acromegaly usually affects male cats and is caused by a functioning hypophyseal tumor.[42] Primary polyuria occurs

because of hyperglycemia and subsequent glycosuria from growth hormone–induced insulin resistance.

Hypokalemia as a cause of polyuria and polydipsia is documented in humans and experimentally in animals.[43] The clinical significance in small animals is questionable. Primary congenital or hereditary nephrogenic diabetes insipidus is an extremely rare phenomenon reported only in

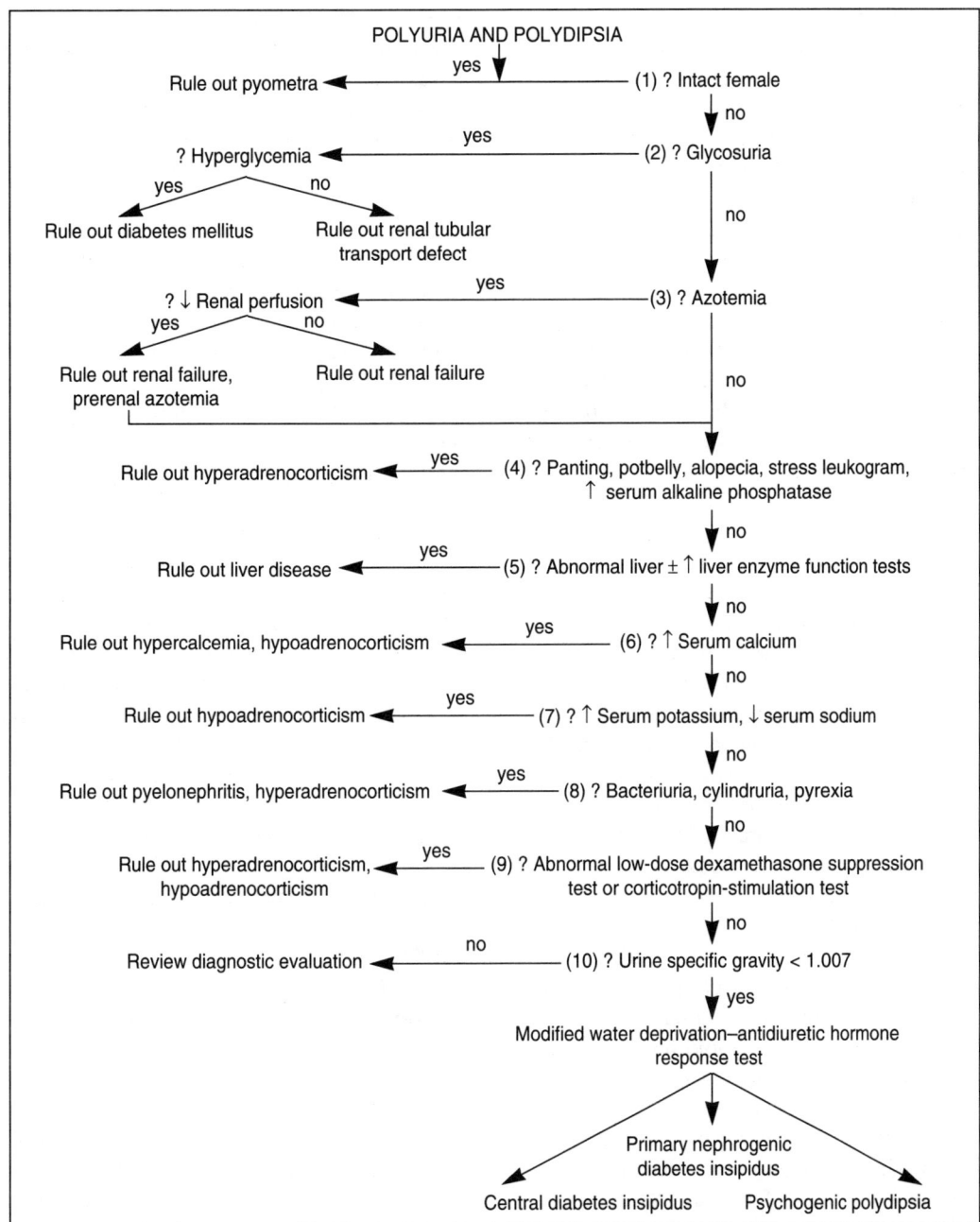

Figure 3—Algorithm outlining the diagnostic evaluation of dogs with polyuria and polydipsia.

dogs.[44,45] Pheochromocytoma is often diagnosed after death.[46] Polyuria and polydipsia have also been reported in dogs with polycythemia.[47]

DIAGNOSTIC WORKUP

Preliminary evaluation after signalment, history, and physical examination should (in most cases) comprise a complete blood count, blood chemistry screen, and complete urinalysis. These modalities reveal the major diagnostic differentials as well as allow screening for any concurrent disease processes. Urinalysis should include dipstick analysis, urine specific gravity, and sediment evaluation.

Because of wide variations within disease states and the relative incidence of the diseases involved, urine specific gravity is more helpful in excluding diagnostic differentials than in suggesting specific causes. Urine specific gravity greater than 1.030 usually contradicts the presence of polyuria and polydipsia unless large amounts of solute are present. Urine specific gravity less than 1.007 indicates successful dilution of urine by the kidneys and therefore rules out renal failure and complete medullary washout. Urine specific gravity less than 1.007 more commonly indicates hyperadrenocorticism or pyometra than diabetes insipidus or psychogenic polydipsia.

When planning the diagnostic investigation of an animal with polyuria and polydipsia, the clinician should interpret information gleaned from the history and physical examination in light of the relative incidence of possible causes. In cats, this approach has only three major diagnostic rule-outs. The evaluation of feline and canine patients is therefore considered separately.

Algorithms outlining the initial approach to polyuria and polydipsia in cats and dogs are presented in Figures 2 and 3, respectively. Clinical features used in the algorithms are not pathognomonic or mutually exclusive; instead, they direct further investigation of specific body systems. The discussion of the diagnostic workup of polyuria and polydipsia supplements the clinical algorithms, which should be followed concurrently. Letters and numbers in the text refer to decision points in the algorithms.

INITIALLY (Figure 2, letter A), polyuria and polydipsia should be differentiated from pollakiuria and dysuria, incontinence, or behaviorally inappropriate micturition. Quantitation of water intake and/or urine output (Figure 2, letter B) is justified if the history remains inconclusive or suspect. Standard guidelines of fluid intake greater than 100 ml/kg/day and urine output of more than 50 ml/kg/day in dogs and cats are widely accepted but infrequently documented.[1,48,49] Because many owners are unable to quantitate these parameters accurately, any noticeable increase must be viewed with suspicion. Iatrogenic causes (Figure 2, letter C) should be ruled out first.

The diagnostic approach for cats is substantially less complicated than for dogs. After ruling out postobstructive diuresis (Figure 2, No. 1), the presence or absence of glycosuria with or without hyperglycemia should be determined (Figure 2, No. 2). Stress hyperglycemia is probably the most common cause of glycosuria in cats. Urine retention in the bladder may result in persistence of glycosuria after return to euglycemia. The owner may be instructed to measure urine glucose at home to differentiate stress hyperglycemia from diabetes mellitus. Stress hyperglycemia does not result in persistent polyuria and polydipsia; thus, an alternative diagnosis should be sought. Cats with chronic renal disease may exhibit euglycemic glycosuria.[7]

When evaluating azotemic cats (Figure 2, No. 3), prerenal azotemia and coexistent renal disease should be considered before identifying renal disease as the sole causative factor of polyuria and polydipsia. Polyuria and polydipsia resulting from nonazotemic renal insufficiency require a creatinine clearance study to document reduced glomerular filtration rate. It is now recognized that animals with acute renal failure may be polyuric and not oliguric or anuric.

A resting T_4 level (Figure 2, No. 4) may be considered part of the minimum data base for the polyuric and polydipsic cat. The clinician should maintain a high index of suspicion to facilitate diagnosis of atypical presentations of feline hyperthyroidism. Mild liver disease (Figure 2, No. 5) in cats can present a diagnostic challenge. Elevated hepatic enzymes and abnormal liver function parameters, such as urea, albumin, coagulation factors, ammonia, bile acids, or sulfobromophthalein retention, may be supportive; however, hepatic biopsy often is necessary for a definitive diagnosis.

Pyometra (Figure 2, No. 6) should be considered in an intact queen. After exploring the major diagnostic differentials, the diagnostic workup should be reviewed before the clinician begins searching for rare causes of feline polyuria and polydipsia.

Polyuria and polydipsia in dogs require a more extensive assessment than in cats; however, the most common causes are relatively easy to identify (Figure 3). Pyometra (Figure 3, No. 1) may be tentatively ruled out on the basis of history and physical examination. Canine glycosuria (Figure 3, No. 2) with polyuria and polydipsia usually is caused by diabetes mellitus, although urinary tract hemorrhage or inflammation may cause a positive urine glucose test. Renal tubular transport defects are extremely rare and require urinary excretion studies for definitive diagnosis. Evaluation of azotemic dogs (Figure 3, No. 3) is similar to evaluation of azotemic cats. The main difference between polyuria and polydipsia in dogs and cats (Figure 3, No. 4) is the more common incidence of hyperadrenocorticism and, to a lesser extent, hypoadrenocorticism in dogs. Some dogs with hyperadrenocorticism may exhibit polyuria and polydipsia with no other physical examination findings.

OCCULT LIVER DISEASE as a cause of polyuria and polydipsia (Figure 3, No. 5) is probably more common in dogs than cats. Scrutiny of serum electrolytes may reveal hypercalcemia (Figure 3, No. 6); hyperkalemia (Figure 3, No. 7) and hyponatremia occur in most, but not all, dogs with hypoadrenocorticism. Bacterial pyelonephritis (Figure 3, No. 8) may be extremely difficult to diagnose because of variable, intermittent clinical signs; the difficulty of localizing a urinary tract infection; and the lack of a specific diagnostic test. Because of atypical clinical presentations of adrenocortical dysfunction (Figure 3, No. 9), all animals should be assessed for normal hypothalamic–hypophyseal–adrenal axis function before the modified water deprivation–antidiuretic hormone response test is done.

Failure to identify an underlying cause (Figure 3, No. 10) for polyuria and polydipsia in an animal with urine specific gravity greater than 1.007 after a complete evaluation should prompt review of the diagnostic evaluation. Urine specific gravity of less than 1.007 warrants consideration of a modified water deprivation–antidiuretic hormone response test. The technicalities and interpretation of the modified water deprivation–antidiuretic hormone response

TABLE III
Results of Hematology and Chemistry Organ Panels for Case Example

Parameter	Patient	Canine Reference Range
Hematology		
White blood cells (/μl)	25,300	6,000–7,000
Neutrophils (/μl)	23,000	5,000–14,000
Bands (/μl)	250	0–300
Lymphocytes (/μl)	2,020	1,200–5,000
Red blood cells (10^6/μl)	5.95	5.0–8.0
Hematocrit (%)	41%	37%–55%
Platelets	Adequate	NA
Chemistry Organ Panels		
Glucose (mg/dl)	91	65–135
Urea nitrogen (mg/dl)	4	7–27
Creatinine (mg/dl)	0.7	0.1–1.2
Phosphorus (mg/dl)	4.0	2.0–4.5
Calcium (mg/dl)	10.5	8.0–11.0
Sodium (mMol/L)	165→147	135–155
Potassium (mMol/L)	4.9	3.5–5.5
Chloride (mMol/L)	115	113–123
Albumin (g/dl)	3.2	2.7–3.6
Globulin (g/dl)	3.0	2.1–4.3
Alanine transaminase (U/L)	174	13–57
Alkaline phosphatase (U/L)	417	35–169
Total bilirubin (mg/dl)	0.4	0–1.0
Cholesterol (mg/dl)	192	150–250
Urine specific gravity	1.001–1.003	1.001–1.060
Urine sediment	No abnormality	NA

test have been described[49,50] and reviewed[37,51] elsewhere; readers are encouraged to consult this literature for a complete discussion. In order for the clinician to glean as much information as possible, water should gradually be restricted over two to three days and then a modified water deprivation–antidiuretic hormone response test should be done. The test must be conducted meticulously, or the diagnostic value of the test will be greatly compromised.

CASE EXAMPLE
History

An 11-year-old, spayed, 32-kg, mixed-breed female dog presented with a one-year history of progressive polyuria and polydipsia. A mucopurulent, unilateral nasal discharge began one week before presentation. The dog had received no previous medication and was otherwise normal according to the owners.

Physical Examination

Physical examination revealed a depressed, overweight, German shepherd–type mixed-breed dog with a mucopurulent nasal discharge from the left nostril. Body temperature was 103.4°F (39.6°C). The only other abnormalities revealed by the examination were moderate dental disease, mildly enlarged submandibular lymph nodes, and a slightly dull haircoat.

Clinical Pathology

Because of the relatively nonspecific nature of the history and physical examination, a complete blood count, chemistry screen, and urinalysis were done (the results of which are shown in Table III). A problem list was then constructed based on problems identified from history, physical examination, and laboratory data.

Obesity	Neutrophilia
Polyuria and polydipsia	↓ Blood urea nitrogen
Nasal discharge	Hypernatremia
Fever	↑ Alanine transaminase
Dental disease	↑ Serum alkaline
Submandibular	phosphatase
lymphadenopathy	Hyposthenuria
Dull haircoat	

Hypernatremia, polyuria and polydipsia with hyposthenuria, nasal discharge, neutrophilia, and fever were considered the problems most worthy of initial investigation. After the patient was given free access to water for five hours, serum sodium normalized, thereby suggesting a free-water deficit from urinary losses greater than water intake.

Daily water intake (Figure 2, letter B) was estimated to be 4800 ml (150 ml/kg), thereby confirming the presence of polydipsia. The dog had received no medications (Figure 2, letter C). The remainder of the diagnostic evaluation of this patient can be followed through the algorithm in Figure 3.

This dog was a spayed female, thereby reducing the likelihood of pyometra (Figure 3, No. 1); the dog was euglycemic (Figure 3, No. 2) and nonazotemic (Figure 3, No. 3). Blood urea nitrogen was low, probably because of increased urinary losses resulting from polyuria and polydipsia. The physical examination did not overtly reveal hyperadrenocorticism (Figure 3, No. 4). In addition to blood urea nitrogen being low, alanine transaminase and alkaline phosphatase were mildly elevated (Figure 3, No. 5); however, there was no other evidence of hepatic dysfunction. Serum calcium (Figure 3, No. 6) as well as potassium and sodium (Figure 3, No. 7) were now normal. Hyposthenuria was the only abnormality revealed by urinalysis (Figure 3, No. 8).

Many of the problems (i.e., dull haircoat, polyuria and polydipsia, hyposthenuria, elevated serum alkaline phosphatase and alanine transaminase, neutrophilia) could be directly attributable to hyperadrenocorticism. A low-dose dexamethasone suppression (LDDS) test was done (Figure 3, No. 9) followed by a high-dose dexamethasone suppression (HDDS) test the next day. Cortisol levels were measured at zero, three, and eight hours after administration of dexamethasone. The results of the tests were:

Resting Cortisol		
(μg/dl)	*Three Hours Later*	*Eight Hours Later*
LDDS 2.3	1.0	1.6
HDDS 2.7	0.7	0.6

The results were consistent with hypophysis-dependent hyperadrenocorticism. Although the nasal discharge and fever could have resulted from rhinitis secondary to increased susceptibility to infection associated with hyperadrenocorticism, a definitive diagnosis was pursued.

Preanesthetic chest and abdominal radiographs were within normal limits. Skull radiographs were normal, and rhinoscopy and nasal biopsy revealed mild suppurative rhinitis. *Staphylococcus aureus* was cultured from the nasal biopsy specimen. Submandibular lymphadenopathy was attributed to dental disease.

The dog was treated successfully with o,p'-DDD and antibiotic nasal drops. Polyuria and polydipsia resolved after 10 days of induction therapy with o,p'-DDD.

SUMMARY

When a patient is presented with polyuria and polydipsia, the clinician may use a standardized approach to ensure consideration of all possible diagnostic differentials. After the presence of polyuria and polydipsia is confirmed, a thorough workup intended to rule out the most common problems first is recommended. This diagnostic approach eliminates unnecessary testing and reduces the time involved in arriving at a diagnosis, thereby benefiting both the veterinarian and the client.

About the Author
Dr. Hughes is affiliated with the Center for Veterinary Clinical Care, Department of Clinical Studies, School of Veterinary Medicine, University of Pennsylvania, Philadelphia, Pennsylvania.

REFERENCES

1. Osborne CA, Low DG, Finco DR: *Canine and Feline Urology.* Philadelphia, WB Saunders Co, 1972.
2. Rose BD: Regulation of plasma osmolality, in Rose BD (ed): *Clinical Physiology of Acid-Base and Electrolyte Disorders,* ed 3. New York, McGraw-Hill Book Co, 1989, pp 248–260.
3. Thrasher TN: Osmoreceptor mediation of thirst and vasopressin secretion in the dog. *Fed Proc* 41(9):2528–2532, 1982.
4. Wade CE, Bie P, Keil LC, Ramsay DJ: Osmotic control of plasma vasopressin in the dog. *Am J Physiol (Endocrinol Metab)* 243:E287–E292, 1982.
5. Rose BD: Regulation of the effective circulating volume, in Rose BD (ed): *Clinical Physiology of Acid-Base and Electrolyte Disorders,* ed 3. New York, McGraw-Hill Book Co, 1989, pp 225–247.
6. Atkins CE: Polyuria and polydipsia, in Ettinger SJ (ed): *Textbook of Veterinary Internal Medicine,* ed 3. Philadelphia, WB Saunders Co, 1989, pp 139–147.
7. DiBartola SP, Rutgers HC, Zack PM, Tarr MJ: Clinicopathologic findings associated with chronic renal disease in cats (1973–1984). *JAVMA* 190(9):1196–1202, 1987.
8. Bradford JR: The results following partial nephrectomy and the influence of the kidney upon metabolism. *J Physiol* 23:415–496, 1898.
9. Nayman JM, Shumway NP, Dumke R, Miller M: Experimental hyposthenuria. *J Clin Invest* 18:195–212, 1939.
10. Meyer TW, Scholey JW, Brenner BM: Nephron adaptation to renal injury, in Brenner BM, Rector FC (eds): *The Kidney,* ed 4. Philadelphia, WB Saunders Co, 1991, pp 1871–1908.
11. Bovee KC, Joyce T: Clinical evaluation of glomerular function: 24 hour creatinine clearance in dogs. *JAVMA* 174:488–491, 1979.
12. Hardy RM, Osborne CA: Canine pyometra: Pathophysiology, diagnosis and treatment of uterine and extra-uterine lesions. *JAVMA* 165:245–268, 1974.
13. Asheim A: Pathogenesis of renal damage and polydipsia in dogs with pyometra. *JAVMA* 147:736–745, 1965.
14. Asheim A: Renal function in dogs with pyometra. Part 8. Uterine infection and the pathogenesis of the renal dysfunction. *Acta Pathol Microbiol Scand* 60:99–107, 1964.
15. Kruth SA, Cowgill LD: Renal glucose transport in the cat. *ACVIM Scientific Proceedings,* Salt Lake City, 1982, p 78.
16. Feldman EC, Nelson RW: *Canine and Feline Endocrinology and Reproduction.* Philadelphia, WB Saunders Co, 1987.
17. Peterson ME: Endocrine disorders in cats: Four emerging diseases. *Compend Contin Educ Pract Vet* 10(12):1353–1362, 1988.
18. Raff H: Glucocorticoid inhibition of neurohypophyseal vasopressin secretion. *Am J Physiol (Reg Integr Comp Physiol)* 252:R635–R644, 1987.
19. Cooke RA, Steenburg RW: Effects of aldosterone and cortisol on the renal concentrating mechanism. *J Lab Clin Med* 82(5):784–792, 1973.
20. Joles JA, Rijnberk WE, van den Brom WE: Studies on the mechanism of polyuria induced by cortisol excess in the dog. *Vet Q* 2:199–205, 1980.
21. Grauer GF, Nichols CER: Ascites, renal abnormalities, electrolyte and acid-base disorders associated with liver disease. *Vet Clin North Am [Small Anim Pract]* 15:197–214,1987.
22. Grauer GF, Pitts RP: Primary polydipsia in three dogs with portosystemic shunts. *JAAHA* 23:197–200, 1987.
23. Peterson ME: Feline hyperthyroidism. *Vet Clin North Am [Small Anim Pract]* 14(4):809–826, 1984.
24. Evered DC, Hayter CJ, Surveyor I: Primary polydipsia in thyrotoxicosis. *Metabolism* 21:393–404, 1972.
25. Cutler RE, Glatte H, Dowling JT: Effect of hyperthyroidism on the renal concentrating mechanisms in humans. *J Clin Endocrinol Metab* 27:453–460, 1967.

26. Peterson ME, Kintzer PP, Cavanagh PG, et al: Feline hyperthyroidism pretreatment clinical and laboratory evaluation of 131 cases. *JAVMA* 183(1):103–110, 1983.

27. Purkerson ML, Blaine EN, Stokes TJ, Klahr S: Role of atrial peptide in the natriuresis and diuresis that follows relief of obstruction in the rat. *Am J Physiol (Renal Fluid Electrolyte Physiol)* 256:F583–F589, 1989.

28. Klahr S: New insights into the consequences and mechanisms of renal impairment in obstructive nephropathy. *Am J Kidney Dis* 18(6):689–699, 1991.

29. Beck N, Singh H, Reed SW, et al: Pathogenic role of cyclic AMP in the impairment of renal concentrating ability in acute hypercalcemia. *J Clin Invest* 54:1049–1055, 1974.

30. Sejersted OM, Steen PA, Kiil F: Inhibition of transcellular NaCl reabsorption in dog kidneys during hypercalcemia. *Acta Physiol Scand* 120:543–549, 1984.

31. Rakich PM, Lorenz MD: Clinical signs and laboratory abnormalities in 23 dogs with spontaneous hypoadrenocorticism. *JAAHA* 20:647–649, 1984.

32. Willard MD, Schall WD, McCaw DE, Nachreiner RF: Canine hypoadrenocorticism: Report of 37 cases and review of 39 previously reported cases. *JAVMA* 180(1):59–62, 1982.

33. Schwartz MJ, Kokko JP: Urinary concentrating defect of adrenal insufficiency permissive role of adrenal steroids on the hydroosmotic response across the rabbit cortical collecting tubule. *J Clin Invest* 66:234–242, 1980.

34. Finco DR, Barsanti JA: Bacterial pyelonephritis. *Vet Clin North Am [Small Anim Pract]* 9(4):645–666, 1979.

35. Miller TE, Layzell D, Stewart E: Experimental pyelonephritis: The effect of chronic active pyelonephritis on renal function. *Kidney Int* 9:23–29, 1976.

36. Finco DR, Schotts EB, Crowell WA: Evaluation of methods of localization of urinary tract infection in the female dog. *Am J Vet Res* 40(5):707–712, 1979.

37. Madewell BA, Osborne CA, Norrdin RA, et al: Clinicopathologic aspects of diabetes insipidus in the dog. *JAAHA* 11:497–506, 1975.

38. Easley JR, Breitschwerdt EB: Glucosuria associated with renal tubular dysfunction in three Basenji dogs. *JAVMA* 168(10):938–942, 1976.

39. Noonan CHB, Kay JM: Prevalence and geographic distribution of Fanconi syndrome in Basenjis in the United States. *JAVMA* 197:345–349, 1990.

40. Finco DR, Kurtz HJ, Low DG, Perman V: Familial renal disease in Norwegian elkhound dogs. *JAVMA* 156(6):747–760, 1970.

41. Eigenman JE: Acromegaly in the dog. *Vet Clin North Am [Small Anim Pract]* 14(4):827–836, 1984.

42. Peterson ME, Taylor S, Greco DS, et al: Acromegaly in 14 cats. *J Vet Intern Med* 4(4):192–200, 1991.

43. Rutecki GW, Cox JW, Robertson GW, Ferris TF: Urinary concentrating ability and antidiuretic hormone responsiveness in the potassium depleted dog. *J Lab Clin Med* 100(1):53–60, 1982.

44. Lage AL: Nephrogenic diabetes insipidus in a dog. *JAVMA* 163(3):251–253, 1973.

45. Breitschwerdt EB, Verlander JW, Hribernik TN: Nephrogenic diabetes insipidus in three dogs. *JAVMA* 179(3):235–238, 1981.

46. Bouayad H, Feeney DA, Caywood DD, Hayden DW: Pheochromocytoma in dogs: 13 cases (1980–1985). *JAVMA* 191(12):1610–1614, 1987.

47. Peterson ME, Randolph JF: Diagnosis of canine primary polycythemia and management with hydroxyurea. *JAVMA* 180(4):415–418, 1982.

48. O'Connor WJ, Potts DJ: The external water exchanges of normal laboratory dogs. *Q J Exp Physiol* 54:244–265, 1969.

49. Mulnix JA, Rijnberk A, Hendricks HJ: Evaluation of a modified water deprivation test for diagnosis of polyuric disorders in dogs. *JAVMA* 169(12):1327–1330, 1976.

50. Hardy RM, Osborne CA: Water deprivation test in the dog: Maximal normal values. *JAVMA* 174(5):479–483, 1979.

51. Hardy RM, Osborne CA: Water deprivation and vasopressin concentration tests in the differentiation of polyuric syndromes, in Kirk RW (ed): *Current Veterinary Therapy. VII.* Philadelphia, WB Saunders Co, 1980.

Feline Urologic Signs (*continued from page 159*)

versus dietary management in prevention of recurrent lower urinary tract disease in male cats. *J Small Anim Pract* 32:296-305, 1991.

14. Osborne CA, Kruger JP, Lulich JP, et al: Feline matrix crystalline urethral plugs. A unifying hypothesis of causes. *J Small Anim Pract*, 33:172–177, 1992.

15. Lulich JP, Osborne CA: Fungal urinary tract infections, in Bonagura JD, Kirk RW (eds): *Current Veterinary Therapy*, XI. Philadelphia, WB Saunders Co, 1992, pp 914–919.

16. Osborne CA, Johnston GR, Polzin DJ, Kruger JM, et al: Redefinition of the feline urologic syndrome: Feline lower urinary tract disease with heterogeneous causes. *Vet Clin North Am Small Anim Pract* 14:409-438, 1984.

17. Jones DC, Rhodes JA, Hawkins EC, Hinsman EJ: Development of an Elisa to quantify Tamm-Horsfall glycoprotein in cats with feline urinary syndrome. *J Cell Biology* 109 (No. 4 Part 2):37a, 1989.

18. Cornelius CE, Mia AS, Rosenfeld S: Ruminant urolithiasis VII. Studies on the origin of Tamm-Horsfall urinary mucoprotein and its presence in ovine calculous matrix. *Investigative Urology* 2:453-457, 1965.

19. Grant AM, Baker LRI, Neuberger A: Urinary Tamm-Horsfall glycoprotein in certain kidney diseases and its content in renal and bladder calculi. *Clinica Scientifica* 44:377-384, 1973.

20. Bjugn R, Flood RR: Scanning electron microscopy of human urine and purified Tamm-Horsfall's glycoprotein. *Scandanavian Journal of Urology and Nephrology* 22:313-315, 1988.

21. Hoyer JR, Seiler MW: Pathophysiology of Tamm-Horsfall protein. *Kidney International* 16:279-289, 1979.

22. Rutecki GJ, Goldsmith C, Schreiner GE: Characterization of proteins in urinary casts. Fluorescent-antibody identification of Tamm-Horsfall mucoprotein in matrix and serum proteins in granules. *N Engl J Med* 284:1049-1052, 1971.

23. Barsanti JA, et al: Effect of therapy on susceptibility of urinary tract infection in male cats with indwelling urethral catheters. *J Vet Int Med* 6:64-70, 1992.

The Pathophysiology of Uremic Bleeding

KEY FACTS

- A bleeding time is a valuable test in the evaluation of platelet function, factor VIII-von Willebrand factor activity, platelet count, and vascular contractility for primary hemostasis.
- Platelet aggregation, in response to exogenous adenosine phosphate, epinephrine, ristocetin, and collagen is often defective in human chronic renal failure patients.
- In uremic individuals, changes in coagulation factors (especially factor VIII-von Willebrand complex and platelet factor 3 release), content, and activity play a role in the bleeding diathesis.
- Eicosonoid synthesis might be altered in glomerular disease and result in a disorder in fatty acid metabolism; the cyclooxygenase pathway might play a role in uremic bleeding.
- The difficulty in assessing the etiology of the bleeding diathesis is largely because of the lack of complete understanding of the defects that occur during renal failure.

University of Illinois, Urbana-Champaign
Cheryl L. Harris, DVM   Donald R. Krawiec, DVM, PhD

Little is known about the pathophysiology of uremic bleeding in dogs, and much of the available data is based on studies of human subjects. The incidence of bleeding in human patients is chronic, and acute renal failure has been reported to be as high as 75% in these patients.[1] In dogs, the reports vary. Polzin et al, in a study of 18 dogs with experimentally induced renal failure, found only slight prolongation of the bleeding time. They determined that the prolongation was not statistically significant.[2] In a study by Jergens et al, however, the use of buccal mucosa bleeding times to assess primary hemostasis was evaluated. The study indicated that five of six uremic dogs had bleeding times significantly higher than normal dogs. The degree of uremia of these dogs was greater than those studied by Polzin et al.[3]

The incidence of thrombocytopenia in renal failure is controversial. Many reports have stated that it is not uncommon to find thrombocytopenia in human patients with chronic renal failure; however, the reported incidence varies from 0% to 50%.[1] Decreased platelet counts are believed to be a result of insufficient thrombogenesis.[4] This hypothesis was based on finding normal numbers of megakaryocytes in bone marrow aspirates of thrombocytopenic individuals with end-stage renal disease; decreased

thrombopoietic activity in their plasma was also determined in these patients by a thrombopoietin bioassay. In humans and dogs, thrombopoietin is believed to be produced by kidney cells and renal disease might preclude adequate production of this substance; however, inhibition rather than decreased stimulation is a possibility.[4] Regardless of the cause, thrombocytopenia in canine and human uremia patients is usually mild and does not correlate with the incidence of bleeding.[1,4-6]

Primary hemostasis is initiated when circulating platelets are exposed to the elements of the vascular wall, such as collagen, basement membranes, and microfibrils associated with elastin. Adhesion can induce the release reaction, which results in the secretion of platelet granules that contain adenosine phosphate, adenosine triphosphate, calcium, serotonin, acid hydrolases, fibrinogen, von Willebrand factor, and factor V.[7,8] Adenosine phosphate changes the shape of the platelets, causes them to adhere to each other (platelet aggregation), and stimulates further release of platelet granules. The adhesion causes activation of platelet membrane phospholipase and transforms arachidonic acid to thromboxane A_2. Both adenosine phosphate and thromboxane A_2 are required for optimum amplification of the release reaction. The von Willebrand factor is required to bind platelets fully to the subendothelial collagen; it is then synthesized by endothelial cells and megakaryocytes. There appears to be a greater quantity of the larger protein molecules intracellularly than in the plasma. The von Willebrand molecules serve as transport proteins for factor VIII.[4]

The most valuable diagnostic tool to assess the tendency for hemorrhagic episodes in dogs is the bleeding time. The bleeding time is evaluated by determining the time required for bleeding to cease from an incision made by a standardized cut. This test reflects the combined roles of platelet function, factor VIII-von Willebrand factor activity, platelet count, and vascular contractility for primary hemostasis.[3]

THE FIRST reported abnormality of human uremic platelet function was decreased clot-promoting activity of platelet membrane phospholipids.[9] This factor is considered to be a function of the platelet membrane and not a specific platelet membrane phospholipid. Platelet factor 3 is required for the conversion of prothrombin to thrombin by the intrinsic mechanism of blood coagulation.[8] Rabiner found that 75% of human uremia patients had both defective release and diminished content or activity of platelet factor 3. They also found that dialysis corrected these abnormalities.[1] Hemodialysis might reduce the frequency and severity of the bleeding in humans, but it does not always alleviate the bleeding completely.[10-12]

PLATELET AGGREGATION IN UREMIA

Platelet aggregation can be evaluated in response to adenosine diphosphate, epinephrine, ristocetin, and collagen; therefore, in an attempt to elucidate the etiology of the defective primary hemostasis of human chronic renal failure patients, the response of the platelets to these agents was measured after exposure to various compounds.[7,13] Adenosine phosphate results in direct aggregation of platelets. At higher concentrations, adenosine phosphate can induce even greater aggregation by means of the release of platelet contents and endogenous adenosine phosphate. Epinephrine, collagen, and ristocetin can cause platelet aggregation both directly and by stimulation of the release reaction.[1]

Di Minno et al documented repeatedly that platelets in human uremia patients required larger concentrations of these compounds for aggregation. This observation has been supported by others.[5,13-15] Jorgensen and Ingeberg, however, found platelet aggregation in human uremia patients to be normal and ascribed the defect found by others to the use of drugs that affect platelet function. They evaluated platelets from uremic patients, but these individuals all had normal bleeding times.[16] Di Minno found that even after washing the platelets and removing them from the uremic plasma, there was still an abnormal response to the aggregating agents.[14]

Whole-blood platelet aggregation was assessed in 22 uremic dogs, six of which were bleeding actively. The investigators did not find abnormal platelet aggregation using collagen, arachidonic acid, and adenosine phosphate. The investigators were uncertain if an aggregation defect, undetected by the whole blood system, would result in clinical bleeding.[17]

Exogenous arachidonic acid is metabolized by cyclooxygenase to cyclic endoperoxides. The cyclic endoperoxides are acted on by thromboxane synthetase to become thromboxane A_2. This effect causes platelet aggregation and platelet secretion. Di Minno et al demonstrated that the platelets of the blood of human uremia patients responded normally to exogenous arachidonic acid. It was therefore presumed that cyclooxygenase and thromboxane synthetase is uninhibited by the acid. DiMinno et al stated that because adenosine phosphate and epinephrine act by the initiation of endogenous arachidonic acid release, which is abnormal in uremic individuals, that an inhibitor to arachidonic acid release exists. This inhibition factor is dialyzable because it is resolved following hemodialysis.[13] In contrast, Remuzzi et al found that human thromboxane A_2 synthesis was abnormal in response to exogenous arachidonic acid; DiMinno and Remuzzi agreed, however, that this abnormality is consistent with a functional cyclooxygenase defect. The subsequent decrease in thromboxane A_2 is responsible for abnormal platelet function.[15]

Other studies, however, indicated conflicting results regarding the potential cyclooxygenase defect. Bloom et al found normal activity of the enzyme in human patients.[18] Rao had findings similar to Remuzzi, but could not eliminate the possibility that a defect more proximal in the cascade might result in the abnormal release of arachidonic acid from phospholipids.[19]

THE ROLE OF COMPOUNDS

The compounds in human uremic serum that are responsible for the platelet dysfunction have not been identified conclusively. Urea was implicated initially, but many investigators disagree. No detectable defect was found even when the urea content of the plasma of normal human volunteers was experimentally increased to 200 mg/dl. Still other investigators found a transient inhibition followed by enhanced aggregation.[1] Davis et al proposed that the discrepancy existed because the other studies were based on the use of changes of optical density for determination of platelet aggregation and that the platelets were not adequately incubated with urea. They also suggested that because of the initial osmotic changes in solution, other investigators might have interpreted an increase in the optical density of the test solutions to be a result of platelet aggregation when, in fact, it was a result of osmotic shrinkage. According to their own platelet aggregation studies, Davis et al found urea to inhibit human platelet aggregation in vitro, and they believed that the platelet aggregation inhibition would correlate with conditions in vivo.[20]

Guanidinosuccinic acid, a metabolite of urea, is often elevated in human uremic serum. When this compound was added to human platelet-rich plasma in vitro, it inhibited adenosine phosphate-induced platelet factor 3 activation. This inhibition was reversible with the addition of calcium, according to Horowitz et al. Rabiner and Hrodek, however, did not find this to be true.[1] Davis et al found no inhibition of adenosine phosphate-induced platelet factor 3 activation. He found slight inhibition of collagen-induced activation but only at levels higher than those found in uremic serum.[20]

PHENYLIC ACIDS have also been implicated as a cause of uremic bleeding. Phenolic acids are enzyme inhibitors that affect glycolysis, but the mechanism by which they interfere with platelet function is unknown.[1] Fractionation of the serum of uremic humans has been accomplished by chromatography, and compounds located in the middle molecular range were postulated to be involved in the platelet defects. The findings have shown that considerable inhibition does occur, but the inhibition is inconsistent and does not correlate consistently with the degree of uremia.[21] Parathyroid hormone has been suggested as a possible uremic toxin that contributes to the hemostatic defect. No correlation existed between platelet aggregation and the degree of secondary hyperparathyroidism.[22] When human patients with hyperparathyroidism were treated effectively, they did not show an associated improvement in their uremic thrombocytopathy.[22]

THE ROLE OF COAGULATION FACTORS

Abnormalities in the factor VIII-von Willebrand complex have been reported by many authors. The complex is responsible for the conversion of factor X to its activated form, X_a, and by binding to a specific platelet receptor, the complex mediates the adhesion of platelets to subendothelial collagen.[9] Many authors believe that the larger multimeric forms are associated with biologic activity.[11,12,23,24] There are varied reports of the plasma concentrations of factor VIII-related antigen (VIII:ra), factor VIII-procoagulant activity (VIII:c), and factor VII-von Willebrand factor activity (VIII:vWf) in humans. Factor VII-related antigen, factor VIII-procoagulant activity, and factor VIII-von Willebrand factor have all been found in increased levels in the plasma except by Kazatchkine et al who found decreased levels of factor VIII-von Willebrand factor.[9,12,22,24-26]

Kazatchkine interpreted this data by proposing that uremic individuals have a functional abnormality of the von Willebrand factor because of the disproportionate ratio of factor VIII-related antigen to factor VIII-von Willebrand factor.[25] Because additional studies have shown an elevation of factor VIII-related antigen in relation to factor VIII-von Willebrand factor and the structure of the von Willebrand multimers in the plasma of human patients in chronic renal failure to be normal, many authors disagree with Kazatchkine et al.[12,23,24,26] Juhl suggested, based on his own data, that there might be a von Willebrand factor receptor defect in uremia.[23]

Recently, it has been discovered that cryoprecipitate and deamino-8-d-arginine vasopressin (DDAVP) are useful in treating the hemorrhagic tendencies in human uremia patients. The mechanism of action is believed to be related to these compounds causing an increase in the plasma of the larger factor VIII:von Willebrand factor multimers. These larger multimers, however, have not been proven to be more effective than smaller ones in promoting platelet adhesion to the subendothelial collagen in the initiation of hemostasis.[26]

Weinstein, with the use of ^{125}I-labeled antibody, found that the coagulant portion of factor VIII is degraded and a large fraction of the circulating factor VIII-procoagulant exists in a lower molecular weight form in the plasma of patients with severe uremia and prolonged bleeding times than in the plasma of normal individuals. This coagulant piece circulates attached to the von Willebrand multimers; therefore, it is assumed that the factor complex must be subject to degradation by proteolytic enzymes.[23]

THE ROLE OF EICOSANOID SYNTHESIS

Greenland Eskimos have prolonged bleeding times and abnormal platelet function, which is related to their marine diet. Their dietary protein is high in omega 3 and low in omega 6 fatty acids.[28] The alteration in platelet function has been attributed to the use of eicosapentaenoic acid (an omega 3 fatty acid), instead of arachidonic acid. Because eicosapentaenoic acid is not a good substrate for the cyclooxygenase enzyme, the resulting prostaglandins and thromboxanes do not have normal activity. Evidence suggests that glomerular disease causes alteration of eicosanoid synthesis.[29] The dysfunction in fatty acid metabolism has not yet been evaluated as a possible etiology of uremic bleeding. Because dietary manipulations can increase or inhibit the production of specific eicosanoids, they could be useful therapeutically.

SUMMARY

The lack of complete understanding of the defects that occur in humans and dogs with renal failure results in the difficulty of assessing the etiology of the bleeding diathesis. There is a consensus that a platelet factor 3 abnormality exists; however, the defect or defects that cause the decrease in platelet aggregation is unknown. Investigations of certain compounds, such as phenol, found in the plasma of human uremia patients could be implicated as the cause of these imperfections, but the manner in which they cause the imperfections has not been determined. Changes in coagulation factors, especially the changes in the factor VIII-von Willebrand complex, have been demonstrated, but their relationship to the bleeding disorder also has not been established completely. The understanding of eicosanoids and their role in renal disease is just beginning.

CURRENT treatment of uremic bleeding, if available, is generally expensive and temporary. Hemodialysis

Wait! You've just scratched the surface of

VLS BOOKS
VETERINARY LEARNING SYSTEMS

Take time to review the complete array of valuable resources for veterinary practitioner, staff, and student from the respected publishers of *Compendium*.

See page 277 for ordering information and Order Form.

(and, more effectively, peritoneal dialysis), cryoprecipitates, and deamino-8-d-arginine vasopressin have been shown to be useful in human medicine, although these therapies are currently not practical in veterinary medicine. When the bleeding disorder of uremia is completely understood, therapeutic modalities might also become accessible for use in animals.

About the Authors

When this article was submitted for publication, Dr. Harris was affiliated with the Department of Small Animal Clinical Sciences, College of Veterinary Medicine, University of Illinois, Urbana-Champaign. She is currently in private practice in Ohio. Dr. Krawiec is affiliated with the Department of Small Animal Clinical Sciences, College of Veterinary Medicine, University of Illinois, Urbana-Champaign.

REFERENCES

1. Rabiner SF: Bleeding in uremia. *Med Clin North Am* 56:221–233, 1972.
2. Polzin D, Osborne CA, Hayden D, et al: Influence of reduced protein diets on morbidity, mortality, and renal function in dogs with induced chronic renal failure. *Am J Vet Res* 45:506–517, 1983.
3. Jergens A, Turrentine M, Krause K, et al: Buccal mucosa bleeding times of healthy dogs and of dogs in various pathologic states, including thrombocytopenia, uremia, and von Willebrand's disease. *Am J Vet Res* 48:1337–1342, 1987.
4. Gafter U, Bessler H, Mallachi T, et al: Platelet count and thrombopoietic activity in patients with chronic renal failure. *Nephron* 45:207–210, 1987.
5. Evans KP, Branch RA, Bloom AL: A clinical and experimental study of platelet function in chronic renal failure. *J Clin Path* 25:745–753, 1972.
6. Nenci GG, Berrettini M, Agnelli G, et al: Effect of peritoneal dialysis, haemodialysis, and kidney transplantation on blood platelet function. *Nephron* 23:287–292, 1979.
7. Weiss HJ: Platelet physiology and abnormalities of platelet function. Part I. *N Engl J Med* 293:531–541, 1973.
8. Jackson M: Platelet physiology and platelet function: Inhibition by aspirin. *Compend Contin Educ Pract Vet* 9:627–635, 1987.
9. Carvalho A: Bleeding in uremia: A clinical challenge. *N Engl J Med* 308:38–39, 1983.
10. Hakim R, Schafer A: Hemodialysis-associated platelet activation and thrombocytopenia. *Am J Med* 78:575–579, 1985.
11. Watson A, Whelton A: Therapeutic manipulations in uremic bleeding. *J Clin Pharmacol* 25:315–317, 1985.
12. Mannucci P, Remuzzi G, Pusineri F, et al: Deamino-8-D-arginine vasopressin shortens the bleeding time in uremia. *N Engl J Med* 308:8–12, 1983.
13. DiMinno G, Martinez J, McKean M, et al: Platelet dysfunction in uremia. *Am J Med* 79:552–559, 1985.
14. DiMinno G, Cervone A, Usberti M, et al: Platelet dysfunction in uremia II. *J Lab Clin Med* 108:246–252, 1986.
15. Remuzzi G, Benigni A, Dodesini P, et al: Reduced platelet thromboxane formation in uremia. *J Clin Invest* 71:762–768, 1983.
16. Jorgensen K, Ingeberg S: Platelets and platelet function in patients with chronic uremia on maintenance hemodialysis. *Nephron* 23:233–236, 1979.
17. Forsythe L, Jackson M, Meric S: Whole blood platelet aggregation in uremic dogs. *Am J Vet Res* 50:1754–1757, 1989.
18. Bloom A, Greaves M, Preston FE, et al: Evidence against a platelet cyclooxygenase defect in uremic subjects on chronic hemodialysis. *Br J Haematol* 62:143–149, 1986.
19. Rao AK: Uremic platelets. *Lancet* i:913–914, 1986.
20. Davis J, McField J, Phillips P, et al: Guanidinosuccinic acid on human platelet effects of exogenous urea, creatinine, and aggregation in vitro. *Blood* 39:388–397, 1972.
21. Bazilinski N, Shaykh M, Dunea G, et al: Inhibition of platelet function by uremic middle molecules. *Nephron* 43:28–32, 1985.
22. Docci D, Turci F, Delvecchio C, et al: Lack of evidence for the role of secondary hyperparathyroidism in the pathogenesis of uremic thrombocytopathy. *Nephron* 43:28–32, 1986.
23. Deykin D: Uremic bleeding. *Kidney Int* 24:698–705, 1983.
24. Juhl A: DDAVP, cryoprecipitate, and highly "purified" factor VIII concentrate in uremia. *Nephron* 43:305–306, 1986.
25. Kazatchkine M, Sultan Y, Caen JP, et al: Bleeding in renal failure: A possible cause. *Br Med J* 2:612–615, 1976.
26. Warrell R, Hultin M, Coller B: Increased factor VIII/von Willebrand factor antigen and von Willebrand factor activity in renal failure. *Am J Med* 66:226–228, 1979.
27. Remuzzi G, Livio M, Roncaglioni MC, et al: Bleeding in renal failure: Is von Willebrand factor implicated? *Br Med J* 2:359–361, 1977.
28. Sinclair HM: The relative importance of essential fatty acids of the linoleic and linolenic families: Studies with an eskimo diet. *Prog Lipid Res* 20:897–899, 1981.
29. Rahman MA, Stork JE, Dunn MJ: The roles of eicosanoids in experimental glomerulonephritis. *Kidney Int* 32:s40–48, 1987.

Hematuria: An Algorithm for Differential Diagnosis

Steven E. Crow, DVM
Diplomate, ACVIM
Assistant Professor
Department of Small Animal Surgery
and Medicine
College of Veterinary Medicine
Michigan State University
East Lansing, Michigan

Hematuria, the presence of blood in the urine, may indicate serious disease of the urinary tract.[1] This commonly observed clinical sign presents two diagnostic challenges for the veterinarian in small animal practice. The first of these tasks is to identify the site (or sites) of origin of bleeding in the urinary tract or associated organs. Localization of hemorrhage to kidneys, ureters, bladder, urethra, or reproductive organs is important in establishing a diagnosis. History taking, physical examination, observation of micturition, and catheterization usually provide adequate clues for localizing the bleeding. The second task is to identify the cause of the bleeding. This may be aided by hematologic, cytologic, and radiographic studies, but bacterial cultures or biopsy is frequently required for a definitive diagnosis.

Because there are many potential causes for hematuria[2-4] (Table I and Figs 1 through 7), a logical, systematic, problem-oriented approach is suggested for differentiating between these causes. In this article a step-by-step outline, or algorithm, for localizing the origin of hematuria will be presented, followed by detailed diagnostic plans to define the cause of urogenital bleeding. Several case histories will also be presented to demonstrate the usefulness of this algorithm.

The Data Base

The *problem-specific data base* is the information that is gathered on all animals presented for a specific problem. The recommended data base for hematuria includes a medical history, physical examination, observation of micturition, and analysis of voided urine.

Historical information obtained from the owner should include the duration, severity, and progression of hematuria. In addition, the owner's observations of when blood appears during urination (e.g., only at the end of the stream) may be helpful. The amount of urine passed, presence of straining, and response to any previous treatment should be noted. The owner's account of these characteristics should be confirmed by direct observation. The possibility of bleeding from sources other than the urinary tract, i.e., spurious hematuria, should be explored. The owner may interpret bloody vaginal or preputial discharge as urine dribbling. The passage of

TABLE I

CAUSES OF HEMATURIA IN DOGS AND CATS

Infection

Calculi

Neoplasm, benign or malignant

Trauma, accidental or iatrogenic
  Urethral prolapse

Parasites
  Dioctophyma renale
  Capillaria plica
  Microfilariae of *Dirofilaria immitis*

Chronic passive congestion of kidney

Renal infarcts

Glomerular disease

Strenuous exercise[2]

Systemic diseases with hemorrhagic tendencies
  Hemophilia and related disorders
  Thrombocytopenia
  Warfarin poisoning
  Leptospirosis
  Systemic lupus erythematosus

Drug-related causes
  Sulfonamides
  Cyclophosphamide

Anomalies
  Welsh corgi renal hematuria (other breeds also)
  Fistulae—renal, vesicular

Extraurinary causes
  Estrus
  Subinvolution of placental sites
  Trauma to genital tract
  Inflammation or neoplasm of genital tract

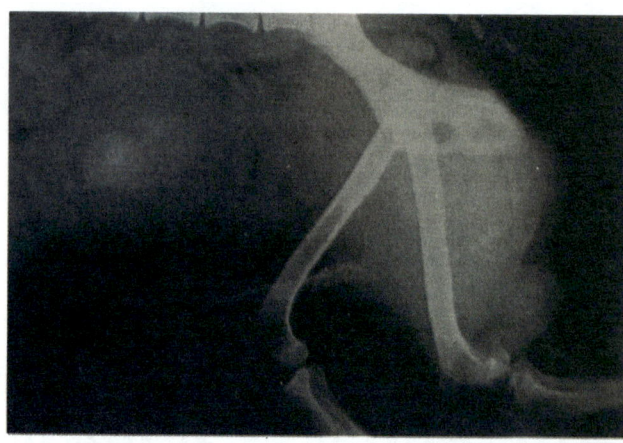

Fig 2—Lateral radiograph of the pelvic region of the dog in Fig 1. Note presence of many calculi in the penile urethra. (Courtesy of Dr. R. Walshaw)

blood-tinged fluid indoors by a housebroken pet should cue the clinician to look for lower-urinary-tract or extraurinary causes for hematuria.

A complete physical examination should be performed, with special attention given to the urinary tract and external genitalia. A rectal examination is extremely useful in evaluating the prostate and vagina.

Differentiation of hemoglobinuria and myoglobinuria from hematuria can be determined by examination of the urine sediment. When hematuria has been present for more than one week, a complete blood count and blood urea nitrogen determination should be performed.

Identifying the Source

Occult hematuria is often an incidental finding in animals with stranguria, pollakiuria, or other signs of urinary tract disease.[1,5,6] An animal with several episodes of occult hematuria should be investigated as if overt hematuria were present. Single occurrences of overt or occult hematuria usually do not represent serious urinary tract disease and may not warrant further evaluation. When occult hematuria is detected, the plan for investigating hematuria that occurs throughout micturition should be used, since the time of appearance of blood during micturition cannot be determined in occult hematuria.

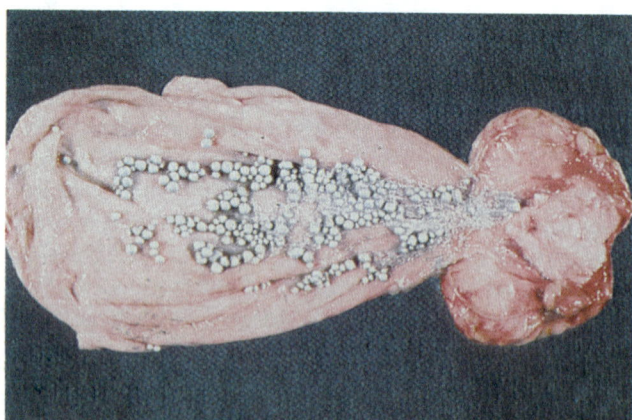

Fig 1—A dog's urinary bladder containing many triple phosphate calculi. The dog had marked, intermittent stranguria and mild hematuria. (Courtesy of Dr. R. Walshaw)

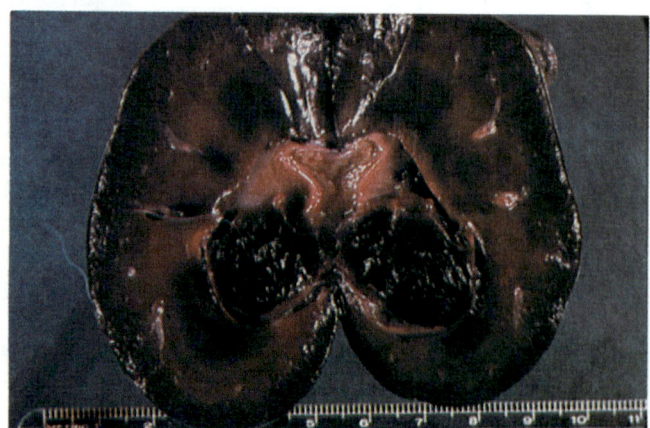

Fig 3—Hemangiosarcoma of renal pelvis resulting in severe hematuria, anemia, and lumbar pain in the eight-year-old German shepherd of Case 1.

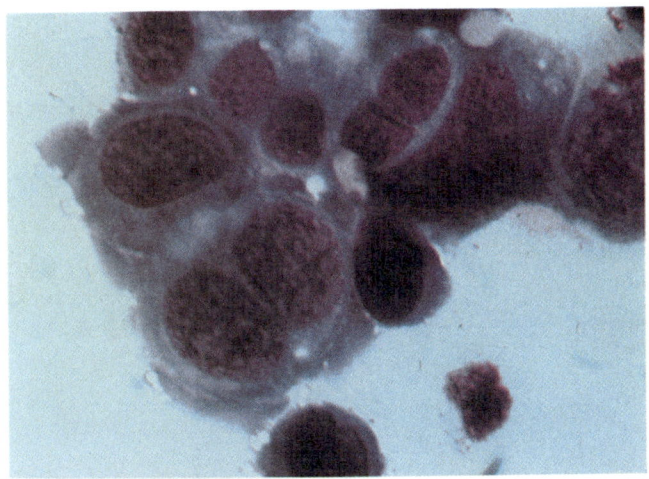

Fig 4—Clusters of malignant epithelial cells from urine, suggestive of transitional cell carcinoma.

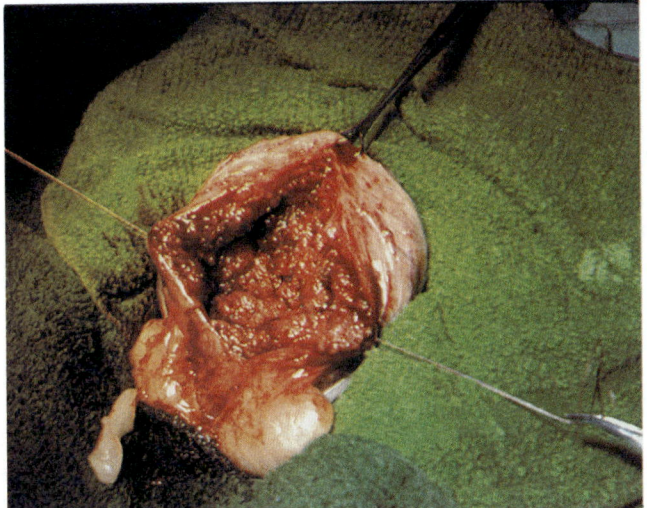

Fig 5—Transitional cell carcinoma of urinary bladder of an 11-year-old miniature poodle (Case 2). Note typical diffuse nature of the neoplasm.

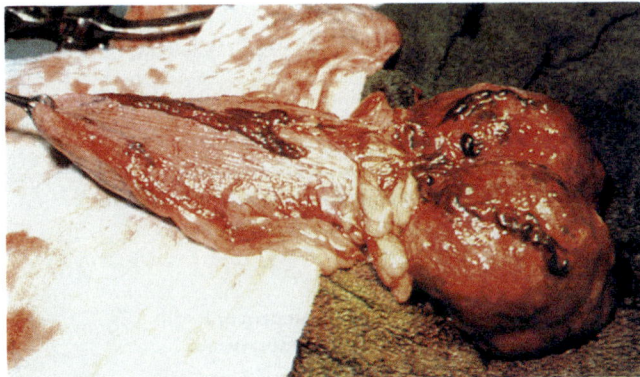

Fig 6—Enlarged prostate gland of a seven-year-old borzoi. Infection of the gland led to necrosis and resultant hematuria. Prostatectomy was required for resolution of disease.

Micturition should be observed when obtaining urine because the time of appearance of blood during micturition forms the major basis of stratification in the algorithm. Other segregations made in the algorithm are based on historical and physical data; no sophisticated clinical tests are needed to identify the affected organ (or organs) and derive an appropriate diagnostic plan (Table II).

The most frequent clinical presentation is hematuria that occurs throughout micturition. Localizing the site of bleeding is often difficult in animals with this presentation because of the possibilities of prostatic fluid reflux into the bladder and an ascending urinary tract infection. Signs of systemic illness (including fever, dehydration, anorexia, emesis, diarrhea, and abdominal pain) associated with hematuria are strong indications for careful evaluation of the animal. If anemia, leukocytosis, or azotemia is documented, then renal function should be evaluated by determining

urine output, specific gravity, ad serum creatinine concentration. In such cases, water intake should be measured, serum electrolyte concentrations should be determined, and the patency of the urinary outflow tract should be assured (see Table III, Diagnostic Plan A). If an animal's condition is deteriorating, supportive therapy should be initiated.

Animals with hematuria throughout micturition but without signs of serious systemic illness are

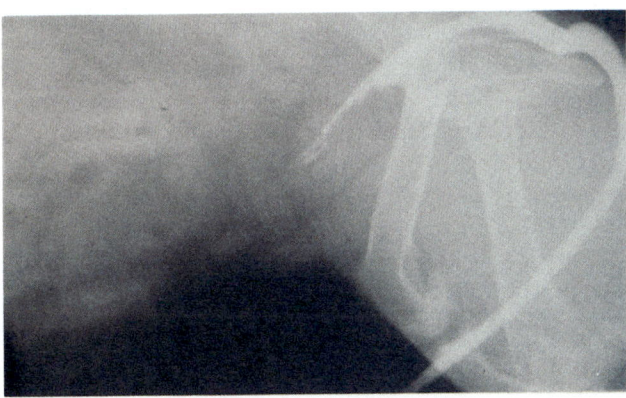

Fig 7—Positive contrast urethrocystogram of a nine-year-old Scottish terrier with cyclophosphamide-induced cystitis. Note thickened bladder wall and small lumen.

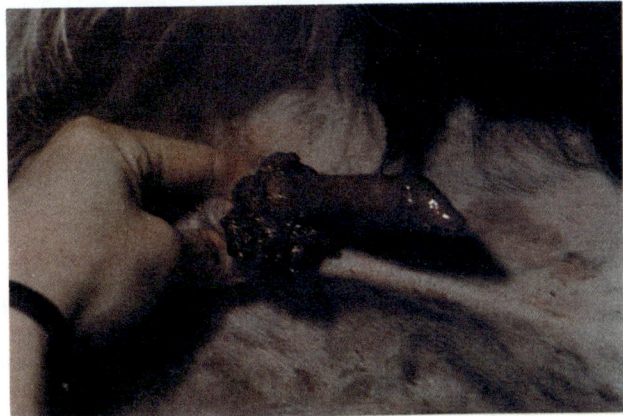

Fig 8—Transmissible venereal tumor on the penis of a dog presented because of "bloody urine dripping from prepuce." Physical examination revealed cause of this spurious "hematuria."

TABLE II

ALGORITHM FOR HEMATURIA OF DOGS AND CATS
PART 1

Presentation		Probable Organs of Origin	Differential Diagnoses	Refer to
Repeated episodes	Occurring throughout micturition (including occult hematuria)	Kidneys Ureters Bladder Prostate	(delay)	Part 2
	Spurious or hematuria at the beginning of micturition	Prostate Urethra Penis Uterus Vagina	(delay)	Part 3
	At the end of micturition	Bladder	Cystitis Cystic calculi Bladder neoplasia	Diagnostic Plan B
		Prostate	Prostatic hyperplasia Prostatic cyst(s) Prostatic neoplasia Prostatitis	
Single episodes		Any urinary genital organ	Trauma, accidental or iatrogenic Physiologic (exercise) Extraurinary causes	History and physical examination

conveniently divided into two groups; those show-ing dysuria (straining, discomfort, and increased frequency) and those without dysuria. Dysuria usu-ally indicates disease of the lower urinary or genital tract (bladder, prostate, vagina, or urethra), and its presence requires expansion of the data base (see Table III, Diagnostic Plan B). When dysuria is not reported, the kidneys or ureters are the most likely sources of hematuria. A variety of disorders can cause blood loss from the kidneys (see Table I and Table II, Part 2). Careful recapitulation of data base information is essential in selecting appropriate additional tests (Table III, Diagnostic Plan C).

Spurious hematuria is the presence in urine of red blood cells that do not originate from one of the organs of the urinary tract. Sources of spurious hematuria include the uterus, vagina, vulva, penis, prostate, and other genital organs. The prostate is a common cause of spurious hematuria, and palpa-tion and massage of the prostate, followed by cytol-ogy of the exfoliated cells may help in determining the cause of prostatic bleeding. Abdominal and rectal palpation of a pelvic or abdominal mass may similarly lead to a diagnosis. In the absence of a demonstrable mass, vaginal swabs and digital or visual examination should be performed. Urethritis may cause hematuria at the beginning of the urine stream and thereby mimic spurious hematuria.

When the diagnostic plans presented in Table III do not achieve a definitive diagnosis, laparoscopy or laparotomy may be indicated. Review of the historical and physical data and their application to the algorithm will guide the clinician in further investigation.

Case Histories

The following abstracts are presented to demon-strate the usefulness of the algorithm in deriving an appropriate diagnostic plan. Case 1 is an exam-ple of improper use of the problem-solving scheme. Proper use of the scheme in the management of Cases 2, 3, 4, and 5 led to definitive diagnosis.

Case 1

An eight-year-old male German shepherd was presented because of persistent hematuria and a reluctance to sit that lasted for 2 weeks. Eighteen months previously, a bloody preputial discharge not associated with micturition in this dog was diagnosed clinically as urethral trauma. One week before presentation, the referring veterinarian noted prostatic enlargement. A hemogram and survey thoracolumbar radiograms were normal.

At the time of presentation, the owners reported that the dog had not eaten for several days and was inactive. Physical examination revealed slight pros-tatomegaly and a 1 cm nodule in the skin of the right flank. The hematuria was erroneously classi-fied as spurious, i.e., not associated with micturi-tion, because of the previous presentation one and one-half years earlier. Consequently, the prostate

TABLE II
PART 2
ALGORITHM FOR HEMATURIA THAT OCCURS THROUGHOUT MICTURITION
(INCLUDING OCCULT HEMATURIA)

Presentation			Probable Organs of Origin	Differential Diagnoses	Refer to
Severe, generalized or systemic illness			Kidney Ureter	Pyelonephritis	Diagnostic Plan A
			Bladder Urethra	Obstructive uropathy	
			Prostate	Severe prostatitis	
Mild, or no generalized or systemic illness	Dysuria	Female	Bladder	Cystitis Cystic calculi Neoplasia	Diagnostic Plan B
		Male dog with normal prostate, or male cat	Bladder Prostate	Cystitis Cystic calculi Neoplasia Prostatic cyst(s)	
		Male dog, enlarged or painful prostate	Prostate Bladder	Prostatic cyst(s) Prostatic hyperplasia Prostatic neoplasia Prostatitis Cystitis Cystic calculi Neoplasia	
	No dysuria		Kidney	Chronic passive congestion Renal parasites Hemorrhagic diatheses Trauma/violent exercise Anomalies Renal infarction Renal neoplasia	Diagnostic Plan C

was considered the most likely diseased organ. In following the algorithm (Table II, Part 3) prostatic massage was performed. Cytology and bacterial culture were negative. A positive contrast urethrogram identified an anomalous duplicate urethra but did not show a cause for hematuria. The complete blood count revealed a blood-loss anemia and thrombocytopenia. Cytologic examination of an aspirate of the flank nodule was consistent with sarcoma. The dog was euthanatized; necropsy revealed metastatic hemangiosarcoma, with a large tumor present in the medulla and pelvis of the right kidney (Fig 3).

Considerable delay in diagnosis resulted from the improper attention to historical data. The presence of hematuria occurring throughout micturition, general malaise, and anemia should have directed the diagnostic approach. Since there were signs suggestive of systemic illness and no dysuria, the kidney should have been identified as the probable organ. In this case, an excretory urogram would have identified a large lesion in the renal pelvis; and correlation with cytologic information

from the cutaneous aspirate would have permitted a tentative diagnosis of metastatic sarcoma.

Case 2

An 11-year-old spayed female miniature poodle was presented for persistent dysuria and mild hematuria of five weeks duration. Transient improvement was observed following treatment with urinary antiseptics, acidifiers, and antibiotics. The owners reported vulvar licking, occasional incontinence, and frequent micturition. Physical examination identified four small (1 to 2 mm) nodules in the mammae and a thickened bladder. On inspection, hematuria was not observed, but urine analysis revealed many red blood cells. Even without a confirming physical finding, the bladder was the suspected organ (Table II, Part 2). Urine obtained by percutaneous cystocentesis was sterile but contained many clusters of abnormal epithelial cells (see Fig 4). Positive contrast cystography revealed a thickening of the posteroventral wall of the bladder. A tentative diagnosis of transitional cell carcinoma was made. The owners requested eu-

TABLE II

PART 3

ALGORITHM FOR SPURIOUS HEMATURIA AND HEMATURIA THAT OCCURS
AT THE BEGINNING OF MICTURITION

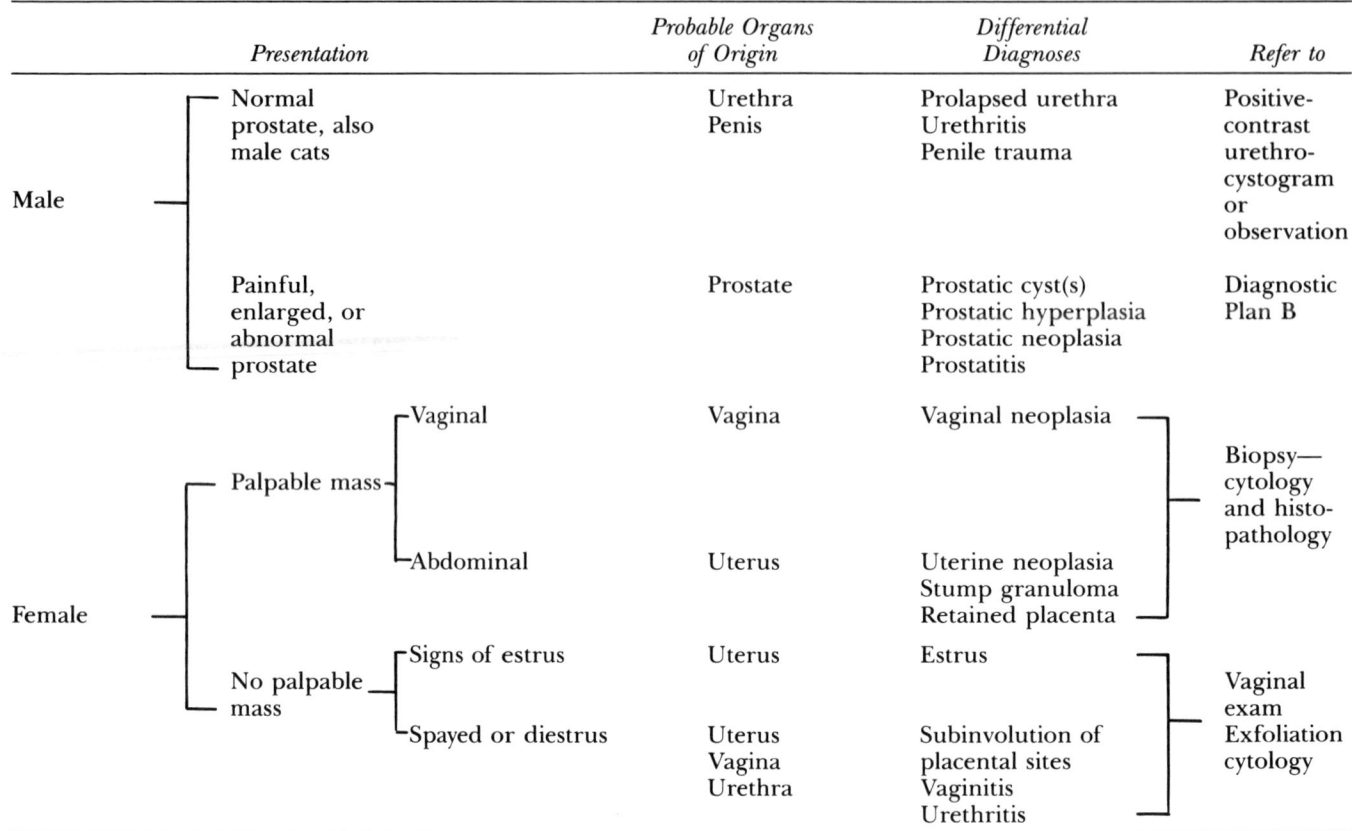

	Presentation		Probable Organs of Origin	Differential Diagnoses	Refer to
Male	Normal prostate, also male cats		Urethra Penis	Prolapsed urethra Urethritis Penile trauma	Positive-contrast urethro-cystogram or observation
	Painful, enlarged, or abnormal prostate		Prostate	Prostatic cyst(s) Prostatic hyperplasia Prostatic neoplasia Prostatitis	Diagnostic Plan B
Female	Palpable mass	Vaginal	Vagina	Vaginal neoplasia	Biopsy—cytology and histo-pathology
		Abdominal	Uterus	Uterine neoplasia Stump granuloma Retained placenta	
	No palpable mass	Signs of estrus	Uterus	Estrus	Vaginal exam Exfoliation cytology
		Spayed or diestrus	Uterus Vagina Urethra	Subinvolution of placental sites Vaginitis Urethritis	

thanasia; necropsy confirmed the clinical diagnosis.

Case 3

A four-year-old male Great Dane was presented because of hematuria of eight months duration. Previous attempts to identify the cause had been unsuccessful. Treatment with antibiotics resulted in temporary remission on two occasions. Careful questioning of the owner revealed that bleeding from the preputial orifice was exacerbated by exercise or excitement. The urine was occasionally blood stained. Neither pollakiuria or stranguria was observed. Physical examination revealed no abnormality. Rectal palpation revealed a slightly enlarged prostate gland.

The prostate gland was identified as the most likely source of the bleeding (Table II, Part 3). Prostatic massage was unrewarding. Prostatic fluid was sterile and showed no evidence of inflammation or neoplasia. Positive contrast urethrocystography was normal. Castration was recommended, but the owners were reluctant to accede. Consequently, an open biopsy was performed. Several intraprostatic cysts containing serosanguineous fluid were observed. Bilateral orchiectomy was per-

formed. Histopathology revealed benign, cystic hypertrophy of the prostate gland. Complete and permanent resolution of clinical signs occurred within three weeks.

Case 4

A seven-year-old spayed female domestic shorthair cat was referred because of hematuria of five weeks duration. Mild stranguria was occasionally noted and observed mainly at the end of micturition. Prolonged treatment with antibiotics and urinary acidifiers did not produce improvement. Seven days after the withdrawal of treatment, urine obtained by cystocentesis was sterile. No evidence of urinary calculi was obtained by radiography or urine analysis. When micturition was observed in the hospital, blood was noticed only at the end. Repeat urine culture and cytology were negative. Double contrast cystography revealed diffuse thickening of the bladder wall. A cystotomy and bladder wall biopsy resulted in a diagnosis of subacute edematous cystitis. A pure culture of *Escherichia coli* was isolated from a biopsy sample from the bladder wall. Prolonged treatment with a combination of antibacterial drugs resulted in remission of hematuria.

TABLE III

DIAGNOSTIC PLANS FOR HEMATURIA IN DOGS AND CATS

Diagnostic Plan A*

1. Monitor H_2O intake and urine output.
   a. In male: Catheterize aseptically to ascertain patency of urethra. Collect urine for analysis, culture/sensitivity, and cytology. Perform prostatic massage and washing, or ejaculation.
   b. In female: Collect urine by percutaneous cystocentesis. Submit for analysis, culture/sensitivity, and cytology.
2. Radiograph abdomen.
3. Repeat urine specific gravity, serum creatinine, Ca, P, Na, K, and Cl determinations.
4. Perform serum chemistries, e.g., alanine aminotransferase (SGPT), serum alkaline phosphatase (SAP), and creatinine.
5. Repeat urinalysis for cytology (concentration technique); do darkfield for spirochetes.

Diagnostic Plan B

1. Obtain urine for analysis, culture, and cytology via aseptic catheterization or percutaneous cystocentesis. In male dog, do prostatic massage, cytology, and culture/sensitivity.
2. Radiograph abdomen; follow with positive contrast urethrocystogram if indicated.†

Diagnostic Plan C

1. Collect urine for culture/sensitivity and cytology; do flotation for parasite ova.
2. Reevaluate history and physical findings.
3. Perform platelet count, activated clotting time, or one-state prothrombin time and activated partial thromboplastin time.
4. Perform serum chemistries, e.g., alanine aminotransferase (SGPT), serum alkaline phosphatase (SAP), and creatinine.
5. Do an excretory urogram.†

*These procedures should be delayed in favor of supportive therapy, e.g., parenteral fluids, whole blood, and rapid-acting corticosteroids, if the animal's condition is unstable.
†Positive contrast radiography is recommended because of the potential for fatal air embolism following pneumocystography when overt hematuria is present.

Case 5

An 11-year-old male standard poodle was presented because of severe hematuria of five days duration. The dog was noted to pass large clots of blood and dark red urine. Neither urgency nor increased frequency of urination was noted. Anorexia and vomiting had been observed for three days. Physical examination revealed pallor and weakness. Rectal palpation disclosed an enlarged but smooth and symmetrical prostate gland; digital compression of the gland caused no apparent discomfort.

Because of the severity of hematuria and weakness, Diagnostic Plan A to expand the data base was immediately implemented (Table II, Part 2). The dog's hydration was satisfactory. A hemogram revealed a mild anemia. The blood chemistry profile (Table III, Diagnostic Plan A) was normal. Urine was obtained for bacterial culture. Survey abdominal radiographs were normal. While awaiting these results, the dog's pallor became more pronounced. A second hemogram revealed a regenerative anemia (PCV, 19%; reticulocytes, 22.5%). Prostatic massage and attempts to obtain an ejaculate were unsuccessful. An excretory urogram was normal. Repeat urinalyses consistently contained blood

clots but the source of the blood remained obscure.

Following whole-blood transfusion, exploratory surgery of the urinary tract disclosed a swollen cystic and hemorrhagic prostate gland. Bilateral orchiectomy was performed. Histopathologic examination of the biopsy specimens revealed an interstitial cell tumor in one testis and severe, chronic prostatitis. Severe hematuria continued during the first 10 days following surgery. After a nearly fatal hemorrhagic episode, whole-blood transfusion was repeated and a prostatectomy was performed. This treatment resulted in immediate and permanent resolution of signs. Sections of prostate gland confirmed the diagnosis of severe, chronic prostatitis (see Fig 6).

Conclusion

Use of the algorithm presented for differential diagnosis of causes of hematuria will not lead to definitive diagnosis in every case, because the presentation of hematuria does not always determine the organ of origin. However, the algorithm, relying on the clinical skills of observation and interview, provides a logical and practical scheme for obtaining a diagnosis.

REFERENCES

1. Archibald J, Owen R: Urinary system, in Archibald J (ed): *Canine Surgery*, ed Archibald 2. Santa Barbara, CA, American Veterinary Publications, Inc, 1974, pp 673-701.
2. Osborne CA, Low DG, Finco DR: Diseases of the urethra, in *Canine and Feline Urology*. Philadelphia, WB Saunders Co, 1972, pp 51, 400.
3. Ling GV: Personal communication, 1976.
4. Cabaluna C, Eisinger RP: Gross hematuria as a manifestation of advanced glomerular disease. *Nephron* 12:59-62, 1973.
5. Greene RW, Scott RC: Diseases of the urethra, in Kirk RW (ed): *Current Veterinary Therapy, VI*. Philadelphia, WB Saunders Co, 1977, pp 1180-1184.
6. Sanders JK: Clinical forum: Management of hematuria. *Canine Pract* (March-April): 5, 8, 53, 1975.

Interpretation of Urine Protein-Creatinine Ratios in Dogs with Glomerular and Nonglomerular Disorders

KEY FACTS

- The urine protein-creatinine ratio is a sensitive, rapid, and convenient test for the detection and quantification of clinically significant proteinuria.
- Ratios greater than one are considered abnormal.
- In the absence of hyperproteinemia and abnormal cells in the urine sediment, an elevated ratio is strong evidence of glomerular disease.

University of Minnesota

Jody P. Lulich, DVM   Carl A. Osborne, DVM, PhD

PROTEINURIA (abnormally high concentrations of protein in urine) is a common laboratory finding in dogs evaluated for various illnesses. Determining its clinical significance requires knowledge of its magnitude and persistence. Qualitative tests (e.g., dipstick dye test and sulfosalicylic acid turbidimetric test) used to screen patients for urine proteins are very sensitive. Qualitative tests, however, are affected by urine concentration and volume; estimating the magnitude of proteinuria is therefore often difficult even with a timed collection of urine.

Q. WHAT ARE URINE PROTEIN-CREATININE RATIOS?

A. The urine protein–creatinine ratio (UP/UC) is a sensitive, rapid, and convenient test for the detection and quantification of significant proteinuria in randomly collected urine samples. Unlike the qualitative tests, the ratio is not affected by urine concentration and volume.

Urine protein–creatinine ratios of single, randomly collected urine samples have excellent correlation with the protein content of 24-hour urine samples obtained from normal dogs and from dogs with glomerular dysfunction.[1-5] These observations indicate that when renal function is stable, glomerular filtration and tubular concentration mechanisms affect protein and creatinine similarly. Consequently, urine protein–creatinine ratios offer the accuracy of 24-hour urine protein measurements without the need to perform a 24-hour urine collection.

Urine samples submitted for analysis should be collected by cystocentesis or during midstream voiding. The sample should then be centrifuged to separate particulate matter (cells) from dissolved substances (protein). The supernatant is saved for determination of protein and creatinine concentrations. The sediment and remaining supernatant should be used for routine urinalysis. The urine protein-creatinine ratio is obtained by dividing the protein concentration (mg/dl) by the creatinine concentration (mg/dl). The result is a unitless ratio.

Terms Related to Proteinuria

Bence Jones proteinuria is the presence of Bence Jones proteins in urine. These proteins are named after the English physician Henry Bence Jones, who described their ability to precipitate when urine is gradually warmed (45° to 70°C) and subsequently to redissolve as urine is heated near boiling. Bence Jones proteins are identical to immunoglobulin light chains (compare with paraproteinuria) and may be observed in urine of patients with neoplastic disorders of plasma cells (multiple myeloma).

Clinically significant proteinuria warrants further investigation of its cause and biological behavior. It is persistent and exceeds that associated with normal excretion.

Functional proteinuria may occur in association with stress, exercise, fever, seizures, exposure to extremes of temperature, and venous congestion in the kidneys. Although glomerular function is temporarily altered, the process is rapidly reversible. The exact mechanisms are not clear but may be related to changes in glomerular blood flow or in the permeability of capillary walls of glomeruli. Although it must be differentiated from other forms of proteinuria, functional proteinuria has no apparent clinical significance.

Glomerular proteinuria results from pathologic damage to various components of glomerular capillary walls. Glomerular proteinuria is typically persistent and usually involves albumin (66,000 daltons) and other proteins of high molecular weight.

Glomerular-overload proteinuria (also called protein-overload proteinuria) has been experimentally induced in dogs by parenteral administration of large quantities of plasma proteins. As serum protein concentrations rise, large quantities of albumin and other proteins of high molecular weight are excreted in urine. Glomerular morphology is reversibly altered during abnormal protein excretion. Glomerular-overload proteinuria should be considered as a cause of proteinuria in dogs with severe hyperproteinemia (greater than 9 g/dl).

Paraproteinuria is a form of overload proteinuria that may occur when complete immunoglobulins, immunoglobulin fragments, macroglobulins, or cryoglobulins produced by neoplastic plasma cells reach abnormally high concentrations in plasma. If readily filtered through glomerular capillary walls, these proteins attain abnormally high concentrations in the urine.

Postglomerular proteinuria results from protein loss arising within the urogenital tract but below the level of the glomerulus. Protein exudation is commonly the result of inflammatory, neoplastic, ischemic, or traumatic diseases. Examples include pyelonephritis, urocystitis, prostatitis, urolithiasis, acute tubular necrosis, and transitional cell carcinomas. Tubular proteinuria may also be considered to be a form of postglomerular proteinuria.

Preglomerular proteinuria refers to proteinuria resulting from abnormalities in systems other than the urogenital tract. Examples include functional proteinuria and overload proteinuria.

Proteinuria is a laboratory finding of urine protein excretion in excess of normal (i.e., greater than 20 mg/kg/day). It is a common manifestation of renal disease but also commonly occurs in association with nonrenal disorders.

Selective proteinuria may occur in association with mild to moderate glomerular pathology. Minimally damaged glomerular capillary walls allow passage of plasma proteins within a narrow range of molecular weights (approximately 60,000 to 80,000 daltons). If glomerular lesions worsen, however, plasma proteins of all sizes and weights easily pass through the capillary walls (i.e., nonselective proteinuria).

Tubular proteinuria is characterized by excretion of plasma proteins of low molecular weight (1500 to 45,000 daltons) as a result of defective resorption by proximal tubules. Protein electrophoresis may reveal prominent alpha and beta bands, which are characteristic of tubular proteinuria. In humans, excreted proteins typically include β_2-microglobulin (11,800 daltons), lysozyme (14,500 daltons), α_1-microglobulin (27,000 daltons), and α_1-acid glycoprotein (40,000 daltons) in addition to many amino acids.

Tubular-overload proteinuria may be associated with excessive production of serum proteins of low molecular weight (less than 45,000 daltons). Such proteins easily pass through glomerular capillary walls and overload tubular resorptive mechanisms. The result is protein loss through the kidneys. Examples of this condition include hemoglobinuria, myoglobinuria, and paraproteinuria.

TABLE I
Urine Protein-Creatinine Ratios of Normal Dogs

Range of Ratio	Number of Dogs Evaluated	Method of Analysis
0.02–0.14	16	Coomassie brilliant blue[3]
0.00–0.31	14	Coomassie brilliant blue[4]
0.08–1.02[a]	9	Coomassie brilliant blue[5]
0.01–0.38	19	Trichloroacetic acid Ponceau-S[1]
0.08–0.54	8	Trichloroacetic acid Ponceau-S[2]

[a]Values were determined from eight collections from each dog. One dog was eliminated from the original published study because the influence of proestrus was unknown. When the results from this dog are included, the range is 0.08 to 1.62.

 **WHAT PROTEIN-CREATININE RATIO VALUES ARE NORMAL FOR CANINE URINE?**

On the basis of reported values (Table I), empirical observations, and extrapolation from data on normal protein excretion in dogs, the following criteria have been established:

- Less than 0.5 is normal.
- Between 0.5 and 1.0 is questionable.
- Greater than 1.0 is abnormal.

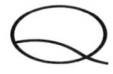 **WHAT MECHANISMS NORMALLY INFLUENCE RENAL EXCRETION OF PROTEIN?**

The capillary walls of glomeruli are semipermeable filters that retain most of the plasma proteins in the vascular compartment. Glomerular capillary walls are composed of the following three layers: capillary endothelial cells, noncellular basement membranes, and cytoplasmic processes (extensions) of renal epithelial cells (podocytes). The processes wrap around portions of capillary loops. Collectively, these three layers form the functional units (the so-called filtration barrier) of glomeruli.

As blood flows through a glomerulus, a large quantity of an acellular, low-protein ultrafiltrate is formed. The degree to which individual proteins are normally filtered through glomerular capillary walls is a function of their plasma concentration and their molecular size, shape, and charge.[6] In other words, the primary factors that influence the movement of proteins across glomerular capillaries are the size-selective properties of glomeruli, the charge-selective properties of glomeruli, and hemodynamic forces operating across glomerular capillary walls.

In general, transport of protein molecules through glomerular capillary walls progressively diminishes as protein size (as estimated from molecular weight) increases (Table II). Normally, proteins of high molecular weight (e.g., immunoglobulin M, which has a molecular weight of 900,000 daltons) do not appear in glomerular ultrafiltrate in detectable amounts.

Even though plasma contains high concentrations of albumin, small quantities of albumin are normally present in glomerular ultrafiltrate partly because albumin has a molecular weight of approximately 66,000 daltons. In addition, fixed negative charges on glomerular capillary walls impede the passage of negatively charged plasma molecules, such as albumin. Plasma proteins with molecular weights of 1500 to 45,000 daltons pass through more readily but appear in urine in lower concentrations because of their relatively low concentrations in plasma.

Although hemoglobin has a small molecular size, it rarely enters glomerular ultrafiltrate because it is usually bound to haptoglobin, which is a larger plasma protein. This phenomenon is called protein binding.

The proportion of filtered plasma proteins ultimately excreted in urine depends on the extent of resorption by renal tubules. Albumin constitutes approximately 40% to 60% of the total protein excreted in urine because it is not completely resorbed by renal tubule cells.[7,8] In contrast, plasma

TABLE II
Comparison of Molecular Weights of Plasma Proteins Included in and Excluded from Glomerular Ultrafiltrate

Plasma Protein	Approximate Molecular Weight (daltons)	Presence in Glomerular Ultrafiltrate
β_2-microglobulin	11,800	Present
Lysozyme (muramidase)	14,400	Present
Myoglobin	17,600	Present
Bence Jones (monomer)	22,000	Present
α_1-microglobulin	27,000	Present
α_1-acid glycoprotein	40,000	Present
Bence Jones (dimer)	44,000	Present
Amylase	50,000	Present
Hemoglobin (tetramer)[a]	64,500	Sometimes present
Albumin	66,000	Sometimes present
Haptoglobin (monomer)	120,000	Absent
Immunoglobulin G	160,000	Absent
Immunoglobulin A (dimer)	300,000	Absent
Fibrinogen	400,000	Absent
α_2-macroglobulin	840,000	Absent
Immunoglobulin M	900,000	Absent

[a]Plasma hemoglobin is normally bound to haptoglobin. Once this binding capacity is saturated, dissociated hemoglobin readily passes through glomerular capillary walls as low-molecular-weight (32,000 daltons) dimers.[12]

proteins of low molecular weight are actively resorbed from tubular filtrate, catabolized by proximal tubular cells, and returned to the blood as amino acids. Distal renal tubule cells secrete small amounts of protein (Tamm-Horsfall mucoprotein and possibly secretory immunoglobulin A), which add to the final urine protein concentration.

Small amounts of protein are normal in canine urine[9]; however, the quantity is often below the level of sensitivity of qualitative tests commonly used to screen for proteinuria. On occasion, a positive test result may be obtained from normal dogs that have formed highly concentrated urine.

Q. WHAT TYPES OF CONDITIONS ARE ASSOCIATED WITH PROTEINURIA IN DOGS?

A. Proteinuria can be classified as preglomerular, glomerular, or postglomerular. Preglomerular proteinuria results from abnormalities of systems other than the urogenital tract. Preglomerular proteinuria can be further subdivided into functional proteinuria and overload proteinuria. Functional proteinuria is sometimes associated with strenuous exercise, extremes of heat or cold, stress, fever, seizures, or venous congestion.

In humans, functional proteinuria apparently results from alterations in glomerular blood flow or in permeability of glomerular capillary walls.[10] Decreased tubular resorption of filtered proteins also can occur.[11] Although glomerular function is temporarily altered, the process is rapidly reversible. Functional proteinuria typically consists of mild, transient albuminuria.

Tubular-overload proteinuria is associated with excessive production of plasma proteins of low molecular weight (e.g., immunoglobulin fragments, myoglobin, or hemoglobin) or the reduction in available binding sites on carrier molecules (e.g., haptoglobin for hemoglobin).[12-15] When plasma concentrations of proteins that weigh less than 45,000 daltons (and that therefore easily pass through glomerular capillary walls) are increased, the resorptive mechanisms of the tubules become overloaded. Detectable quantities of protein then appear in urine.

Glomerular-overload proteinuria (also called protein-overload proteinuria) has been experimentally induced in dogs and rats by parenteral administration of large quantities of plasma proteins.[16-18] When plasma protein concentrations were above 9 g/dl, large quantities of albumin and other proteins of high molecular weight were excreted in urine. Alterations in glomerular morphology were detected in rats during episodes of hyperproteinemia and proteinuria.[19,20] Glomerular abnormalities consisted of numerous protein resorption droplets as well as swelling and obliteration of the foot processes of epithelial cells. These changes completely reversed after resolution of hyperproteinemia and proteinuria. Glomerular-overload proteinuria should be considered to be a cause of proteinuria in animals with severe hyperproteinemia (e.g., in patients with multiple myeloma or ehrlichiosis or after overzealous administration of plasma).[21-26]

Glomerular proteinuria is the most commonly recognized and potentially most severe form of canine proteinuria. Glomerular proteinuria results from disease-induced alterations of glomerular capillary barriers, which normally prevent loss of larger plasma proteins into glomerular ultrafiltrate. Damage can be characterized by loss of the fixed negative charges of glomerular capillaries. In addition, structural changes in the filtration barrier may result from primary disorders (e.g., antiglomerular basement membrane disease, inflammation, or neoplasia) or secondary disorders (e.g., immune complex deposition, amyloidosis, hyperfiltration, or hyperadrenocorticism). Protein in the urine of patients with these forms of glomerular dysfunction primarily consists of albumin and varying quantities of proteins of high molecular weight (e.g., immunoglobulins and coagulation proteins).

In postglomerular proteinuria, plasma or tissue proteins gain access to urine after it has passed through the glomeruli. Postglomerular proteinuria can result from normal genital secretions. It may also result if the epithelial linings of the urogenital tract are disrupted by inflammation, neoplasia, ischemia, or trauma. Postglomerular proteinuria can usually be differentiated from glomerular proteinuria by evaluating clinical signs and urine sediment. Postglomerular proteinuria is often associated with leukocyturia or erythrocyturia or both; in the urine of patients with glomerular proteinuria, these cells are typically absent.

It may be difficult to recognize a combination of glomerular proteinuria and postglomerular proteinuria. The combination may have been present if cell-free proteinuria persists after successful treatment of postglomerular inflammation or hemorrhage. If successful treatment of postglomerular proteinuria is not possible, detection of high concentrations of albumin in urine should prompt consideration of concurrent glomerular dysfunction, especially if hypoalbuminemia is also detected.

Postglomerular proteinuria occasionally results from defects in proximal tubular resorption of proteins of between 1500 and 45,000 daltons; this condition is called tubular proteinuria.[27] This form of proteinuria is typically mild and may not be detected by qualitative screening tests for proteinuria. Familial (e.g., Fanconi's syndrome) and acquired (e.g., gentamicin toxicity) causes of tubular proteinuria have occurred in dogs.[28-31]

Q. WHAT IS THE CLINICAL VALUE OF URINE PROTEIN-CREATININE RATIOS?

Do Urine Protein-Creatinine Ratios Help Confirm Significant Proteinuria?

A. Urine protein concentrations that persistently exceed normal limits are clinically significant. Screening tests (dipstick dye or sulfosalicylic acid) used to detect urine protein are sensitive to protein concentrations between 5 and 30 mg/dl.[32] In dilute urine, significant concentrations of protein may remain undetectable by these procedures or may appear to be so low that they are misinterpreted as insignificant. Because urine protein–creatinine ratios are unaffected by urine concentration and volume, they aid in the accurate assessment of urine protein loss in patients with urine of low specific gravity.

Can Urine Protein-Creatinine Ratios Aid Localization of Protein Loss?

Do Increased Urine Protein-Creatinine Ratios Indicate Glomerular Disease?

A. A retrospective evaluation of proteinuria in 45 dogs admitted to the University of Minnesota Veterinary Teaching Hospital (Figure 1) suggests that mildly elevated urine protein–creatinine ratios may be associated with preglomerular, glomerular, or postglomerular proteinuria. Diagnoses of preglomerular (n = 2) and postglomerular (n = 7) proteinuria were established on the basis of rapid and persistent resolution of proteinuria after appropriate therapy. Diagnoses of primary glomerular proteinuria (n = 6) were established on the basis of persistent proteinuria in addition to light-, immunofluorescent-, and electron-microscope evaluation of renal biopsy specimens. The protein–creatinine ratios were relatively low in urine of patients with pre- and postglomerular proteinuria and of some patients with primary glomerular disease. Most of the patients with urine protein–creatinine ratios greater than 5.0 had primary glomerular disease.

These findings emphasize that urine protein–creatinine ratios cannot differentiate the proteinuria associated with glomerular dysfunction from increases in plasma concentrations of proteins of low molecular weight (e.g., hemoglobin, myoglobin, and Bence Jones proteins) or postglomerular exudation of tissue or plasma proteins. In addition to urine protein–creatinine ratios, other tests may be required to rule out preglomerular proteinuria (e.g., tests for hemoglobinemia, increased serum globulin concentration, or increased serum creatine phosphokinase concentration) and postglomerular proteinuria (e.g., urine sediment analysis or urine culture) and confirm glomerular proteinuria (e.g., serum albumin, serum creatinine, and urine albumin concentrations). If hyperproteinemia is not present and there are no abnormal cells in urine sediment, an elevated urine protein–creatinine ratio is strong evidence of glomerular dysfunction.

Do Urine Protein-Creatinine Ratios Aid Prediction of the Underlying Cause of Protein-Losing Glomerulopathy?

A. At the University of Minnesota Veterinary Teaching

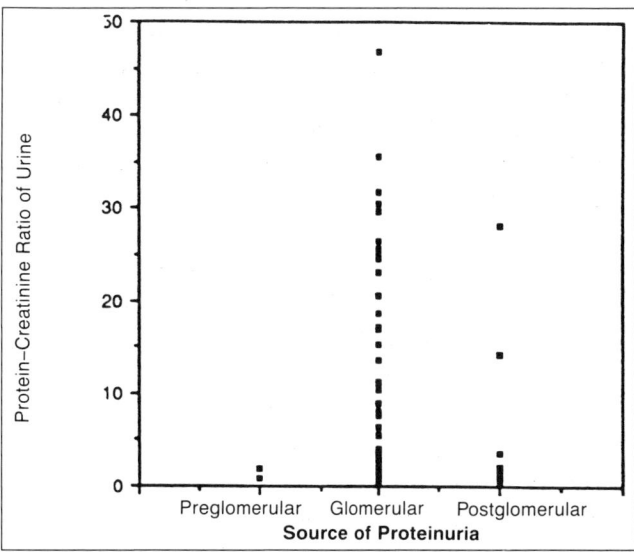

Figure 1—Distribution of urine protein–creatinine ratios in dogs with preglomerular (n = 2), glomerular (n = 36), and postglomerular (n = 7) proteinuria.

Hospital, a retrospective study of 36 dogs with glomerular dysfunction indicated that urine protein–creatinine ratios overlapped considerably (Table III). The dogs had diagnoses of glomerulosclerosis (n = 13), nonamyloid glomerulopathy (n = 22), or glomerular amyloidosis (n = 11) as determined by light, immunofluorescent, and electron microscopy. The highest mean urine protein–creatinine ratios, however, were observed in dogs with glomerular amyloidosis. This finding has also been reported by other investigators.[1] Although the association of high urine protein–creatinine ratios with canine renal amyloidosis is useful in formulating diagnostic probabilities, we emphasize that urine protein–creatinine ratios are not sensitive enough to detect the underlying cause consistently.

In the evaluation of clinical cases of glomerular disease, the following guidelines should be considered:

- In dogs with microscopic evidence of glomerulosclerosis or atrophy from various causes, urine protein–creatinine ratios are often less than 5.0.

TABLE III
Magnitude of Urine Protein-Creatinine Ratios[a] in Dogs with Morphologic Evidence of Glomerular Dysfunction

Morphologic Classification	Number Evaluated	Mean Ratio	Range of Ratio
Sclerosis	13	2.34	0.28–8.05
Glomerulopathy	22	12.66	0.65–31.88
Amyloidosis	11	24.38	8.9–46.85

[a]Protein values were determined by the Coomassie brilliant blue method.

- Urine protein–creatinine ratios from 5 to 13 are often associated with nonamyloid glomerulopathy.
- Renal lesions consistent with severe glomerulopathy or glomerular amyloidosis commonly occurred in patients with urine protein–creatinine ratios greater than 13.
- In general, dogs with generalized glomerular amyloidosis have the highest urine protein–creatinine ratios.

Are Urine Protein-Creatinine Ratios of Diagnostic Value for Dogs with Evidence of Leukocyturia, Erythrocyturia, or Urinary Tract Infection?

A. In most cases of postglomerular disease, urine protein–creatinine ratios offer no advantage over complete urinalysis results. Interpretation of urine protein–creatinine ratios is based on the assumption that creatinine and protein are both handled similarly by glomerular filtration and tubular concentration mechanisms. In patients with postglomerular proteinuria, however, the excess protein is not filtered through glomeruli or associated with tubular defects in protein resorption. In cases of postglomerular inflammation or hemorrhage, the rate of creatinine excretion is different from that of protein excretion (Table IV).

High urine protein–creatinine ratios in patients with postglomerular diseases should prompt consideration of glomerular proteinuria; however, additional studies are required to confirm this combination of disorders. For example, we have observed protein–creatinine ratios greater than 10 in urine of dogs with staphylococcal infection of the lower urinary tract.

Can Urine Protein-Creatinine Ratios Be Used to Calculate Daily Urine Protein Losses?

. Urine protein–creatinine ratios can be used to estimate urine protein losses. In turn, knowledge of the magnitude of daily protein loss may aid in estimating the quantity of dietary protein needed to maintain albumin homeostasis. The advisability of replacing persistent and severe renal protein loss in dogs through oral protein supplementation, however, has been questioned. Investigations in humans and laboratory animals indicate that provision of supplemental dietary protein to patients with protein-losing glomerulopathy may augment progression of glomerular disease and proteinuria.[33-36] At present, our recommendations for dietary management of dogs with protein-losing glomerulopathy incorporate a stepwise assessment of response by evaluation of body weight, serum albumin concentration, and urine protein excretion following each successive increase in dietary protein supplementation.

How Can Urine Protein Loss Be Calculated From Urine Protein-Creatinine Ratios?

A. Equations used to determine daily protein loss (mg/kg) in urine were constructed from previously reported values by designating the urine protein–creatinine ratio as the dependent variable in a linear regression analysis (Table V).[2,3,37] Daily protein loss in urine can be calculated by solving the equation once the urine protein–creatinine ratio has been determined. Knowledge of the laboratory method used to determine urine protein concentration is essential for selection of the correct equation.

Consider a 13.6-kg (30-lb), six-year-old, male water spaniel being evaluated because of lethargy and weight loss of four months duration. Urinalysis reveals a specific gravity of 1.011 and a 2+ dipstick dye test for protein. No cells are found during microscopic examination of urine sediment. The protein concentration of a urine sample is 1000 mg/dl, and the creatinine concentration is 76 mg/dl. The urine protein–creatinine ratio is therefore 1080 ÷ 76 or 14.2.

TABLE IV
Urinalysis Values and Urine Protein-Creatinine Ratios of a Seven-Year-Old Labrador Retriever[a]

Parameter	Before Therapy	After Therapy
Color	Red	Yellow
Specific gravity	1.013	1.016
Occult blood	2+	Negative
Red blood cells per high-power field	Too numerous to count	10
White blood cells per high-power field	5	3
Bacterial colony-forming units per milliliter	$>10^5$	7.0×10^2
Urine protein	788	13
Urine creatinine[b]	28	61
Protein–creatinine ratio of urine	28.1	0.21

[a]This dog had bilateral hindlimb paralysis, urine retention, and *Escherichia coli* urinary tract infection. Parameters were evaluated at the time of diagnosis and three days after initiation of antimicrobial therapy with trimethroprim/sulfamethazine (15 mg/kg every eight hours). Note the rapid resolution of the urine protein–creatinine ratio after therapy. This illustration emphasizes that postglomerular proteinuria can affect urine protein–creatinine ratios.
[b]Determined by Coomassie brilliant blue method.

TABLE V
Equations[a] for Calculation of
Daily Urine Protein Excretion

Method of Analysis		Regression Equation (protein mg/kg/day)
Coomassie brilliant blue[3]	=	$3.1 + (19.2 \times UP/UC^b)$
Trichloroacetic acid Ponceau-S[2]	=	$2.8 + (28.72 \times UP/UC)$

[a]Equations used to determine urine protein loss were constructed from previously reported values by designating the urine protein–creatinine ratio as the dependent variable in a linear regression analysis.
[b]UP/UC = protein–creatinine ratio of urine.

According to the equation based on the Coomassie brilliant blue method for protein determination, the daily protein excretion is $3.1 + (19.2 \times 14.2) = 275.7$ mg/kg/day or 13.6 kg $\times$ 275.7 mg/kg/day = 3.75 g/day. The daily urine protein loss may also be interpolated from published charts.[2,3]

How Much Protein Do Normal Dogs Excrete in Urine?

A. Few investigators have performed controlled studies of large numbers of dogs to assess normal daily excretion of protein in urine (Table VI). Additional confusion concerning normal protein excretion exists because various methods used for protein determination give significantly different results.[38] In one study, for example, the Coomassie brilliant blue method consistently yielded higher protein concentrations than were obtained by use of the trichloroacetic acid Ponceau-S method on identical samples.[8] Differences were greater with higher protein concentrations.

Likewise, two groups of investigators using the same method to determine urine protein concentration (Coomassie brilliant blue method) reported different values for normal dogs. Grauer et al[3] reported that young adult beagles excreted 0.6 to 5.1 mg/kg/day of protein. This value is lower than that reported by McCaw et al, who determined that normal canine outpatients ranging in age from 0.5 to 10 years excreted 1.8 to 22.4 mg/kg/day of protein.[4] Using the trichloroacetic acid Ponceau-S method for urine protein determination, Center et al and White et al found similar results (maximum protein excretion was 11.7 mg/kg/day).[1,2]

Biewenga et al evaluated 29 clinically normal dogs of various breeds, sexes, and ages and reported a range of 2.7 to 23.2 mg/kg for daily protein excretion.[39] Although the subjects were clinically and biochemically normal, immunofluorescent staining methodology revealed immune deposits in glomeruli of about half of the dogs. The significance of glomerular immune deposits in clinically normal dogs was not determined.[39]

Seventeen dogs (six males and 11 females) evaluated by DiBartola et al had urine protein excretion of 4.55 to 28.3 mg/kg/day.[40] Dogs with active urine sediment (more than five white blood cells per high-power field or more than five red blood cells per high-power field or both), however, were included in this group; their inclusion may account for higher protein excretion values than that reported by other investigators. The 24-hour urine protein excretion by male dogs (16.5 ± 10 mg/kg/day) was not significantly different from that of female dogs (12.4 ± 6.1 mg/kg/day) in the small sample of dogs evaluated.[40]

On the basis of these observations, we concluded that a urine protein concentration in excess of 20 mg/kg/day evaluated by either the Coomassie brilliant blue method or trichloroacetic acid Ponceau-S is abnormal. This value corresponds to a urine protein–creatinine ratio between 0.67 to 0.96 according to the linear regression equations established for dogs.[2-4]

Can Urine Protein-Creatinine Ratios Be Used to Monitor Therapeutic Response?

A. If the cause of the patient's proteinuria (e.g., dirofilariasis, neoplasia, or hyperadrenocorticism) has been identified or if some forms of therapy (e.g., diet, aspirin, or antimicrobials) have been initiated, urine protein–creatinine ratios can be used to monitor response to therapy. Decreases in urine protein concentrations, however, may not always be associated with improvement in the underlying glomerular dysfunction. If accompanied by increases in serum creatinine concentration, decreases in

TABLE VI
Daily Urine Protein Excretion in Normal Dogs

Protein (mg/kg/day)		Method of Analysis	Number of Dogs Evaluated
Range	*Mean*		
0.6–5.1	2.3	Coomassie brilliant blue[3]	16
1.8–22.4	7.66	Coomassie brilliant blue[4]	14
0.2–7.7	2.45	Trichloroacetic acid Ponceau-S[1]	19
1.9–11.7	4.76	Trichloroacetic acid Ponceau-S[2]	8
2.7–23.2	6.6	Trichloroacetic acid Ponceau-S[39]	29
4.55–28.3	13.9	Trichloroacetic acid Ponceau-S[40]	17

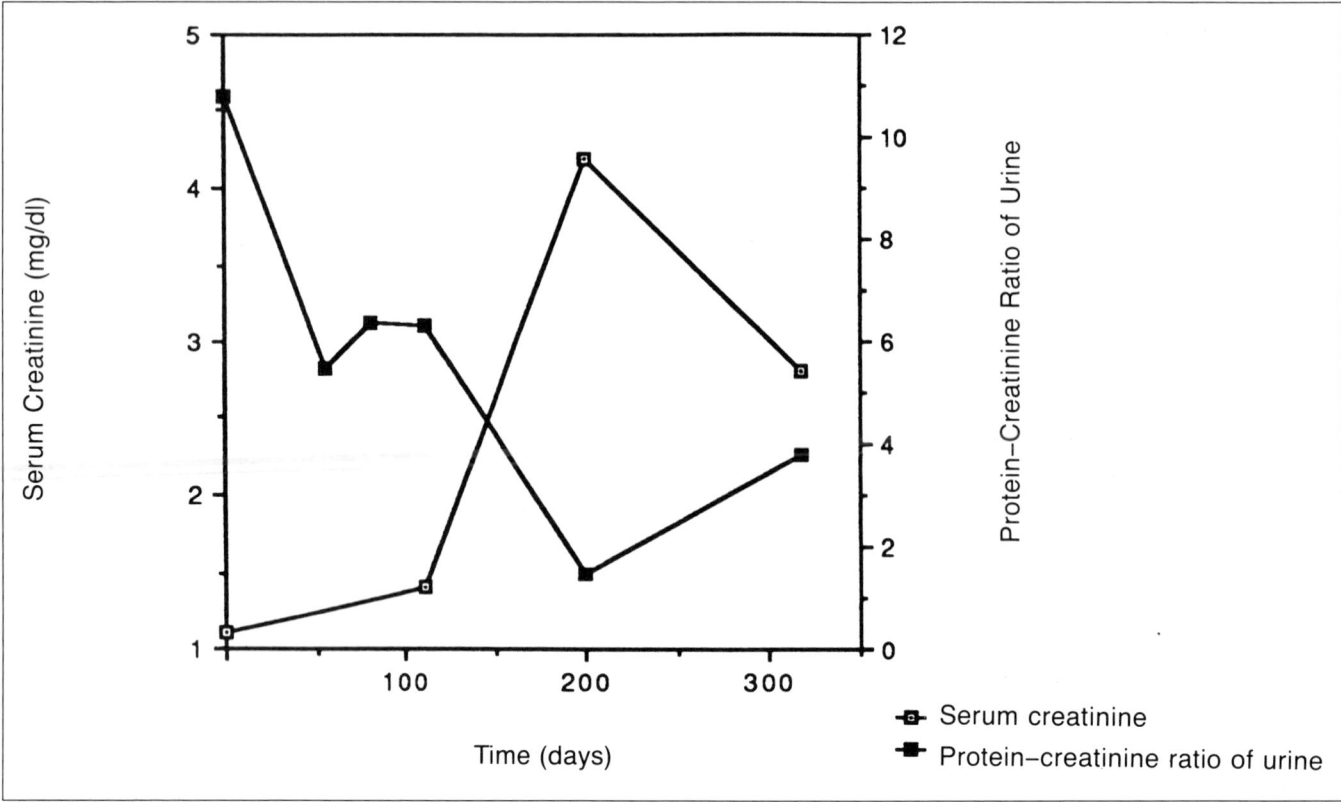

Figure 2—Serum creatinine concentrations and urine protein–creatinine ratios of an 11-year-old springer spaniel with glomerular amyloidosis and splenic hemangiosarcoma. Note the decline in the ratio after splenectomy (Day 1) and the inverse relationship between serum creatinine concentration and urine protein–creatinine ratio with time.

urine protein reflect progressive changes in glomerular dysfunction (Figure 2).[41]

Can Urine Protein-Creatinine Ratios Aid Prediction of Outcome?

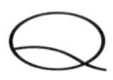. Retrospective analysis of 45 dogs evaluated at the University of Minnesota Veterinary Teaching Hospital because of protein-losing glomerulopathy revealed that those with urine protein–creatinine ratios greater than 13 had hypoalbuminemia (Figure 3). This correlation is important because hypoalbuminemic dogs are at high risk for protein malnutrition, edema, thromboembolic disorders, and renal failure—if these conditions are not already present.[1,42,43]

Q. WHEN SHOULD URINE PROTEIN-CREATININE RATIOS BE EVALUATED?

A. We utilize a diagnostic algorithm (see the flowchart on pages 246 and 247) to aid in localization of proteinuria. We emphasize that the algorithm may be misleading if two or more causes of clinically significant proteinuria coexist.

Q. WHAT FACTORS MAY ALTER THE RELIABILITY OF URINE PROTEIN-CREATININE RATIOS?

A. The method and time of collection, the sex of the animal, whether the animal is confined to a cage, and the protein content of the diet reportedly have little effect on the protein–creatinine ratio of urine.[4,5] These variables currently are not important in the clinical interpretation of protein–creatinine ratios of urine.

Accurate interpretations of urine protein–creatinine ratios are based on the following assumptions:

- Glomerular filtration rate is stable.
- Protein loss during a 24-hour period is constant.
- Glomerular filtration and tubular concentration of urine affect protein and creatinine similarly.

These assumptions may not be tenable for some diseases. For example, acute renal failure may be associated with rapid and significant changes in glomerular filtration rate. In this situation, urine protein–creatinine ratios may aid in determination of glomerular involvement. Because of rapid changes in glomerular filtration rate, however, calculations of daily protein loss are likely to be in error.

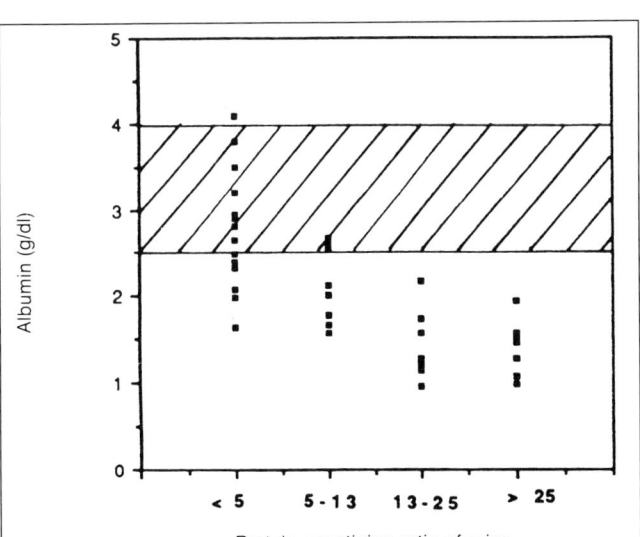

Figure 3—Distribution of serum albumin concentrations in dogs with urine protein–creatinine ratios less than 5 (n = 19), 5 to 13 (n = 6), 13 to 25 (n = 10), and greater than 25 (n = 8). The *shaded area* represents the normal range.

Cats excrete creatinine solely by glomerular filtration[44]; tubular secretion and glomerular filtration are involved in the elimination of creatinine in male dogs.[45] Tubular secretion of creatinine is normally minimal, but it increases as serum creatinine concentration rises.[46] Consequently, ratios may be lower than expected in male dogs with moderate to advanced azotemic renal failure.

The size-selective and charge-selective properties of glomeruli and the hemodynamic forces operating across glomerular capillary walls are the primary features that influence the movement of proteins across glomerular capillaries. Hemodynamic forces are important for at least two reasons: normal perfusion maintains a negative charge across glomerular capillary walls, and the quantity of protein lost in urine is related to its rate of delivery to glomeruli. In patients with hypoalbuminemia, vascular volume may be decreased because of reduced colloidal osmotic pressure. In such cases, there is a corresponding reduction in the rate and quantity of protein passing through glomerular capillaries and glomerular loss of proteins is consequently reduced. Urine protein–creatinine ratios may therefore be lower than when normal vascular volume is restored.

Errors in estimating daily urine protein loss can occur with urine protein–creatinine values that require extrapolation beyond established ranges. For example, the highest ratio used in the construction of one linear regression equation was 15.1.[3] Estimations of the nature of the regression line beyond this level are speculative.

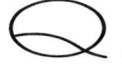 **HAVE NORMAL PROTEIN-CREATININE RATIOS BEEN ESTABLISHED FOR FELINE URINE?**

A. The 24-hour urine protein excretion and urine protein–creatinine ratios from random urine samples of 12 healthy adult cats (six males and six females)[47] were evaluated. Urine protein concentrations were determined by the Coomassie brilliant blue method. Mean daily protein excretion was lower in females (8.69 mg/kg) than in males (16.62 mg/kg). The range of the urine protein–creatinine ratio in all cats was 0.096 to 0.472, and the ratio was highly correlated with 24-hour protein determinations ($r^2 = 0.945$). Although protein-losing glomerulopathy in cats is not commonly reported, urine protein–creatinine ratios should be evaluated for cats with hypoalbuminemia, lymphosarcoma, feline infectious peritonitis, or feline leukemia virus infection.[48-51]

About the Authors
Dr. Lulich and Dr. Osborne are affiliated with the Department of Clinical Sciences, College of Veterinary Medicine, University of Minnesota, St. Paul, Minnesota.

REFERENCES

1. Center SA, Wilkinson E, Smith CA, et al: 24 hour urine protein/creatinine ratio in dogs with protein-losing nephropathies. *JAVMA* 187:820–823, 1985.
2. White JV, Olivier NB, Reimann K, et al: Use of protein-to-creatinine ratio in a single urine specimen for quantitative estimation of canine proteinuria. *JAVMA* 185:882–885, 1984.
3. Grauer GF, Thomas CB, Eicker SW, et al: Estimation of quantitative proteinuria in the dog using the urine protein-to-creatinine ratio from a random, voided sample. *Am J Vet Res* 46:2216–2119, 1985.
4. McCaw DL, Knapp DW, Hewett JE: Effect of collection time and exercise restriction on the prediction of urine protein excretion using urine protein/creatinine ratio in dogs. *Am J Vet Res* 46:1665–1669, 1985.
5. Jergens AE, McCaw DL, Hewett JE: Effects of collection time and food consumption on the urine protein/creatinine ratio in the dog. *Am J Vet Res* 48:1106–1109, 1987.
6. Deen WM, Satvat B: Determinants of the glomerular filtration of proteins. *Am J Physiol* 241:F162–F170, 1981.
7. Porter P: Comparative study of the macromolecular components excreted in the urine of dog and man. *J Comp Pathol Ther* 74:108–118, 1964.
8. Harvey DG, Hou CM: The use of paper electrophoresis for the routine identification of urinary proteins in the dog. *J Small Anim Pract* 7:431–440, 1966.
9. Barsanti JA, Finco DR: Protein concentration in urine of normal dogs. *Am J Vet Res* 40:1583–1588, 1979.
10. Dennis VW, Robinson RR: Proteinuria, in Seldon DW, Giebisch G (eds): *The Kidney: Physiology and Pathophysiology*. New York, Raven Press, 1985, pp 1805–1816.
11. Poortman JR: Postexercise proteinuria in humans. *JAMA* 253:236–240, 1985.
12. Fairbanks VF, Klee GG: Biochemical aspects of hematology, in Tietz NW (ed): *Textbook of Clinical Chemistry*. Philadelphia, WB Saunders Co, 1986, pp 1495–1588.
13. Nelson DA, Davey FR: Erythrocyte disorders, in Henry JB (ed): *Clinical Diagnosis and Management by Laboratory Methods*, ed 17. Philadelphia, WB Saunders Co, 1984, pp 652–703.
14. Torrance AG, Fulton RB: Zinc-induced hemolytic anemia in a dog. *JAVMA* 191:443–444, 1987.
15. Giger U, Harvey JW: Hemolysis caused by phosphofructokinase deficiency in English springer spaniels: Seven cases (1983–1986). *JAVMA* 191:453–459, 1987.
16. Terry R, Hawkins DR, Church EH, et al: Proteinuria related to hyperproteinemia in dogs following plasma given parenterally. *J Exp Med* 87:561–573, 1948.
17. Vernier RL, Papermaster BW, Olness K, et al: Morphologic studies

PROTEINURIA LOCALIZATION

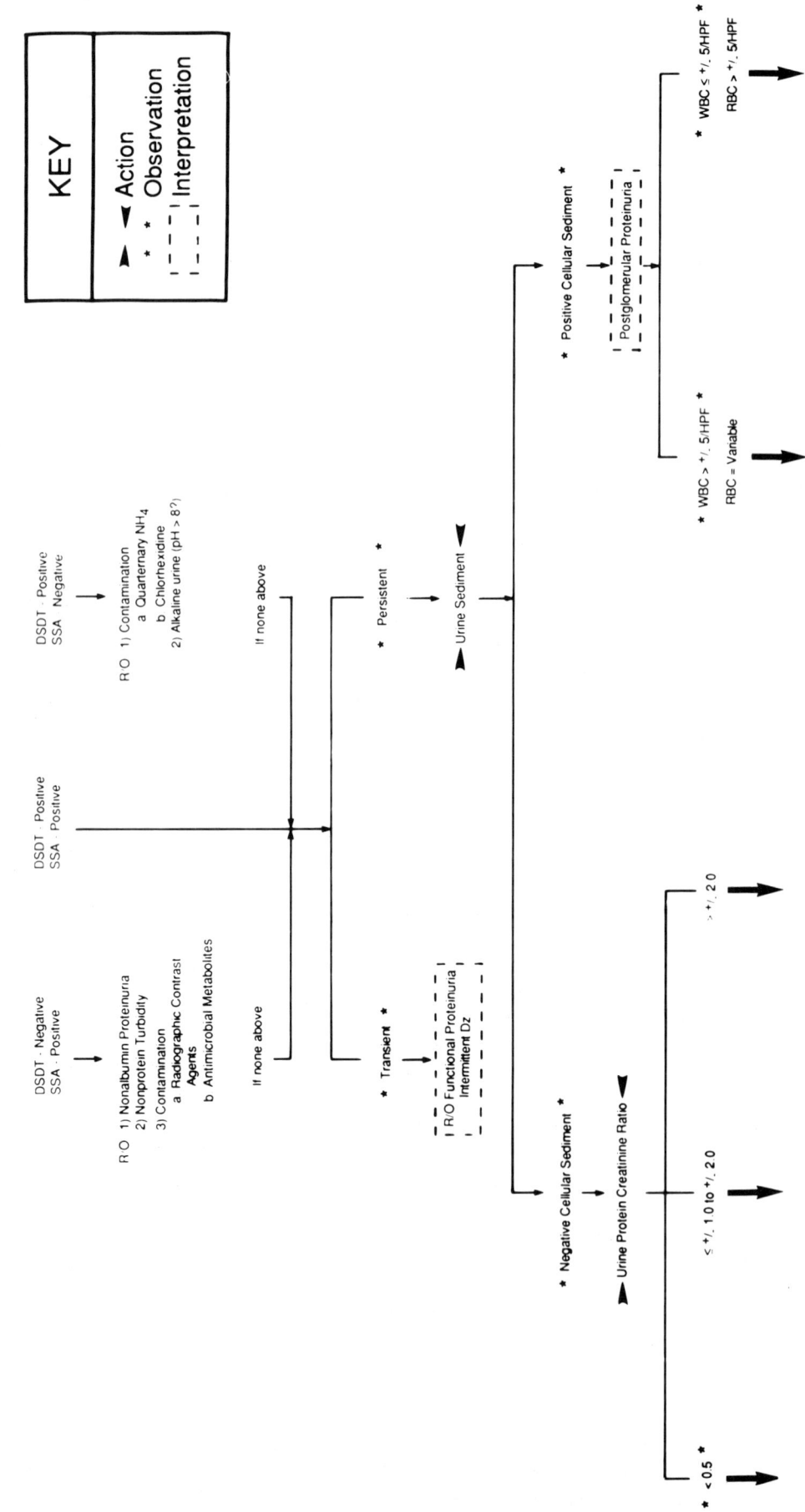

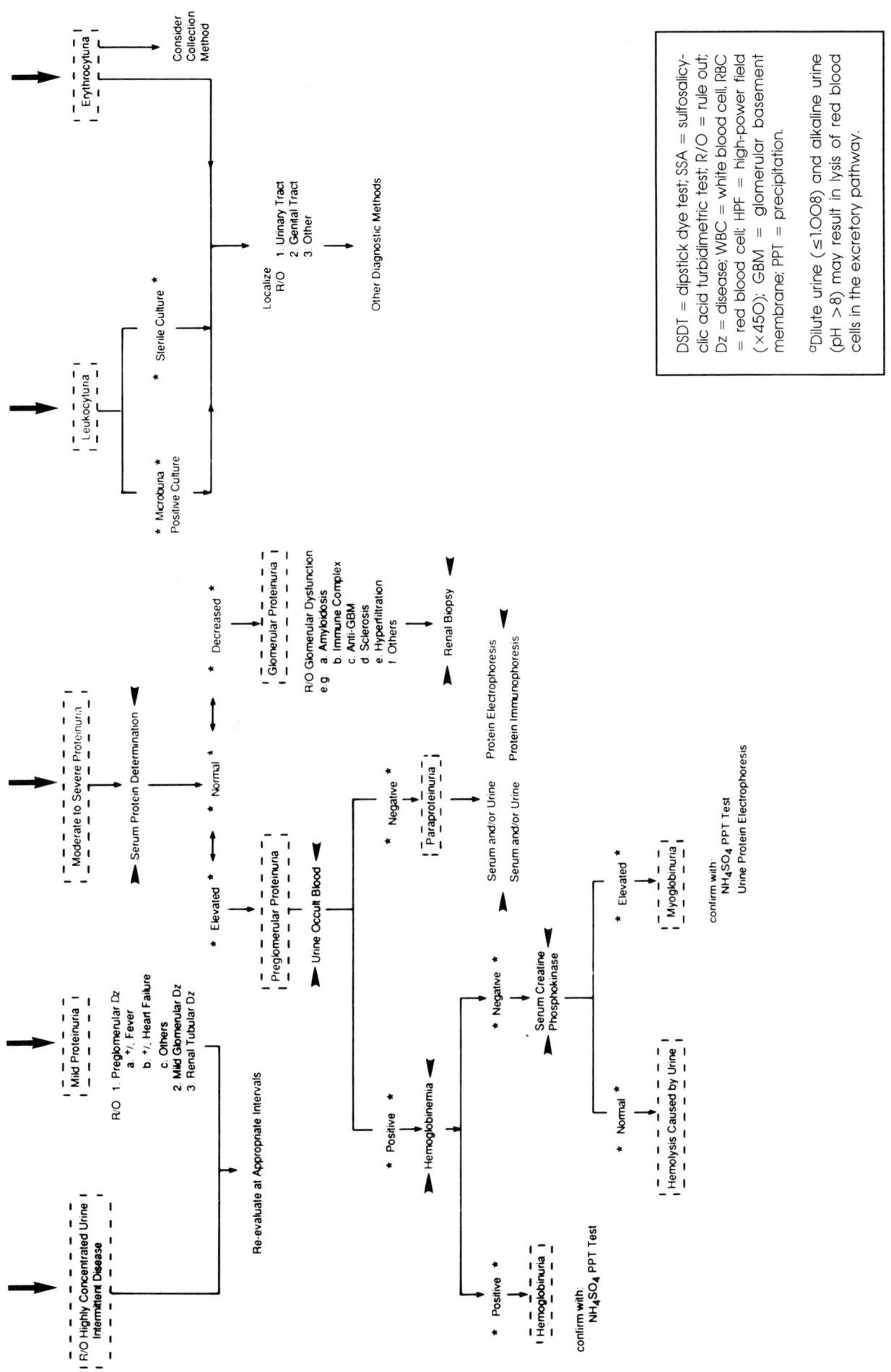

DSDT = dipstick dye test; SSA = sulfosalicyclic acid turbidimetric test; R/O = rule out; Dz = disease; WBC = white blood cell; RBC = red blood cell; HPF = high-power field (×450); GBM = glomerular basement membrane; PPT = precipitation.

^aDilute urine (≤1.008) and alkaline urine (pH >8) may result in lysis of red blood cells in the excretory pathway.

of the mechanism of proteinuria. *Am J Dis Child* 100:476–478, 1960.

18. Lambert PP, Gassee JP, Askenasi R: Physiologic basis of protein excretion, in Manuel Y, Revillard JP, Betuel H (eds): *Proteins in Normal and Pathological Urine*. Basel, Switzerland, S Kager, 1970, pp 67–82.

19. Weening JJ, Van Guildener C, Daha MR, et al: The pathophysiology of protein-overload proteinuria. *Am J Pathol* 129:64–73, 1987.

20. Mori H, Yamasshita H, Nakanishi C, et al: Proteinuria induced by transplantable rat pituitary tumor MtT SA5. *Lab Invest* 54:636–644, 1986.

21. Schull RM, Osborne CA, Barrett RE, et al: Serum hyperviscosity syndrome associated with IgA multiple myeloma in two dogs. *JAAHA* 14:58–70, 1978.

22. Miller C, Fish MB, Danelski TF: IgA multiple myeloma with multisystem manifestations in the dog: A case report. *JAAHA* 18:53–56, 1982.

23. Matus RE, Leifer CE, Gordon BR, et al: Plasmapheresis and chemotherapy of hyperviscosity syndrome associated with monoclonal gammopathy in the dog. *JAVMA* 183:215–218, 1983.

24. Center SA, Smith JF: Ocular lesions in a dog with serum hyperviscosity secondary to an IgA myeloma. *JAVMA* 181:811–813, 1982.

25. Matus RE, Leifer CE, MacEwen EG, et al: Prognostic factors for multiple myeloma in the dog. *JAVMA* 188:1288–1292, 1986.

26. Breitschwerdt EB, Woody BJ, Zerbe CA, et al: Monoclonal gammopathy associated with naturally occurring canine ehrlichiosis. *J Vet Intern Med* 1:2–9, 1987.

27. Hall PW, Chung-Park M, Vacca CV, et al: The renal handling of beta 2-microglobulin in the dog. *Kidney Int* 22:156–161, 1982.

28. Finco DR: Familial renal disease in Norwegian elkhound dogs: Physiologic and biochemical examinations. *Am J Vet Res* 37:87–91, 1976.

29. Easley JR, Breitschwerdt EB: Glucosuria associated with renal tubular dysfunction in three basenji dogs. *JAVMA* 168:938–943, 1976.

30. Bovee KC, Joyce T, Blazer-Yost B, et al: Characterization of renal defects in dogs with a syndrome similar to the Fanconi syndrome in man. *JAVMA* 174:1094–1099, 1979.

31. Brown SA, Rakich PM, Barsanti JA, et al: Fanconi syndrome and acute renal failure associated with gentamicin therapy in a dog. *JAAHA* 22:635–640, 1986.

32. Osborne CA, Stevens JB: *Handbook of Canine and Feline Urinalysis*. St Louis, Mo, Ralston Purina Co, 1981, pp 76–85.

33. Scott RC: Immune-mediated renal disease, in Kirk RW (ed): *Current Veterinary Therapy VIII. Small Animal Practice*. Philadelphia, WB Saunders Co, 1983, p 968.

34. Rosenberg ME, Swanson JE, Thomas BL, et al: Glomerular and hormonal responses to dietary protein intake in human renal disease. *Am J Physiol* 253:F1083–F1090, 1987.

35. Kaysen GA, Gambertoglio J, Jimenez I, et al: Effect of dietary protein intake on albumin homeostasis in nephrotic patients. *Kidney Int* 29:572–577, 1986.

36. Meyer TW, Lawrence WE, Brenner BM: Dietary protein and the progression of renal disease. *Kidney Int* 24:S243–S247, 1983.

37. Ott L: *An Introduction to Statistical Methods and Data Analysis*, ed 2. Boston, Duxbury Press, 1984, pp 242–324.

38. Dilena BA, Penberthy LA, Fraser CG: Six methods for determining urinary protein compared. *Clin Chem* 29:553–557, 1983.

39. Biewenga WJ, Gruys E, Hendricks HJ: Urinary protein loss in the dog: Nephrological study of 29 dogs without signs of renal disease. *Res Vet Sci* 33:366, 1982.

40. DiBartola SP, Chew DJ, Jacobs G: Quantitative urinalysis including 24-hour protein excretion in the dog. *JAAHA* 16:537–546, 1980.

41. Jaenke RS, Allen TA: Membranous nephropathy in the dog. *Vet Pathol* 23:718–733, 1986.

42. Polzin DP: Diagnosis of renal dysfunction: Reading the signs. *Proc AAHA*:134, 1987.

43. Green RA, Russo EA, Greene RT, et al: Hypoalbuminemia-related platelet hypersensitivity in two dogs with nephrotic syndrome. *JAVMA* 186:485–488, 1985.

44. Finco DR, Barsanti JA: Mechanism of urinary excretion of creatinine by the cat. *Am J Vet Res* 12:2207–2209, 1982.

45. O'Connell JMB, Romeo JA, Mudge GH: Renal tubular secretion of creatinine in the dog. *Am J Physiol* 203:985–990, 1962.

46. Swanson RE, Hakim AA: Stop-flow analysis of creatinine excretion in the dog. *Am J Physiol* 203:980–984, 1962.

47. Monroe WE, Davenport DJ, Saunders GK: Twenty-four hour urine protein loss in normal cats and the urinary protein-creatinine ratio as an estimate. *Proc ACVIM* 6:765, 1988.

48. Jeraj KP, Hardy R, O'Leary TP, et al: Immune complex glomerulonephritis in a cat with renal lymphosarcoma. *Vet Pathol* 22:287–290, 1985.

49. DiBartola SP, Rutgers HC, Zack PM, et al: Clinicopathological findings with chronic renal disease in cats: 74 cases (1973–1984). *JAVMA* 190:1196–1202, 1987.

50. Mooney SC, Hayes AA, Matus RE, et al: Renal lymphosarcoma in cats: 28 cases (1977–1984). *JAVMA* 191:1473–1477, 1987.

51. Hayashi T, Ishida T, Fujiwara K: Glomerulonephritis associated with feline infectious peritonitis. *Jpn J Vet Sci* 44:909–916, 1982.

The Excretory Urogram: Part I Techniques, Normal Radiographic Appearance, and Misinterpretation

D. A. Feeney, DVM, MS
Assistant Professor
Department of Small Animal
Clinical Sciences
College of Veterinary Medicine
University of Minnesota
St. Paul, Minnesota

D. L. Barber, DVM, MS
Assistant Professor
Department of Anatomy and
Radiology
College of Veterinary Medicine
University of Georgia
Athens, Georgia

G. R. Johnston, DVM, MS
Assistant Professor

C. A. Osborne, DVM, PhD
Professor and Chairman

Department of Small Animal
Clinical Sciences
College of Veterinary Medicine
University of Minnesota
St. Paul, Minnesota

As excretory urography evolved in veterinary medicine over the years two major shortcomings persisted: (1) a standardized technique for excretory urography was not widely adopted, and (2) quantitation of parameters of normal excretory urography and factors affecting these parameters for each of the various techniques were not available. Comparison of results of serial studies performed in the same patient or comparison of findings of one group of investigators with those of another is significantly hindered if a standardized technique is not used. This article presents (1) a standardized method of excretory urography for use in dogs and cats, (2) the normal radiographic appearance of the canine and feline urinary tract based on this technique, and (3) radiographic findings that may be misinterpreted. Adoption of a standardized technique by the veterinary profession will facilitate recognition of disease entities and a better understanding of the pathophysiology of various disorders of the urinary system by allowing meaningful comparison of results obtained by different investigators.

Use of the excretory urogram as a diagnostic modality in small-animal practice was first documented in 1953.[1,2] Five years later, some recommendations for standardizing technique and analysis of some variables (i.e., contrast medium dose, exposure sequence, abdominal compression) affecting the appearance of the normal canine excretory urogram were reported.[3] Since that time numerous authors have described variations of the technique and interpretation of the excretory urogram in dogs and cats.[4-13]

The primary use of the excretory urogram is to evaluate portions of the urinary tract that cannot be adequately visualized by survey radiography. Evaluation of the size, shape, position, and surface contours of the kidneys, ureters, and urinary bladder plays an important role in localizing and diagnosing various disorders of the urinary tract.[4,14] Because there are many variables that affect the appearance of the excretory urogram, it should not be used as a quantitative index of renal function.

Technique

Preparation of the patient for excretory urography has been addressed previously.[4,5,10,12-14] In general, food should be withheld for 24 hours and cleansing enemas and/or laxatives should be administered to ensure that the gastrointestinal tract is empty. Water should be available at all times. Preliminary dehydration is not advised.[3,4,8-10,15] Sedation or anesthesia has been recommended[1,2,5,11] but should be avoided if the procedure can be performed satisfactorily without it. Commonly used sedative and anesthetic compounds may have variable effects on blood pressure and ureteral motility, and these effects may alter radiographic appearance.

Survey radiographs should always be made before contrast medium is administered. A wide range of contrast media and doses have been recommended.[1,4,5,9,13] Various methods of administration of contrast media also have been recommended, including rapid intravenous bolus injection,[9,15,16] slow intravenous injection,[1,5] and drip infusion of the diluted contrast material.[6,7,10-12] The authors' recommendation is bolus intravenous injection of 400 mg of iodine per lb (0.45 kg) of body weight of either ionic or nonionic agents.[15,16] Quantification of the normal appearance of the excretory urogram in dogs has been evaluated by the authors using this dosage.[15,16]

Recommendations for sequence of exposing radiographs following administration of contrast medium have varied widely.[1-12] Since the appearance of the normal excretory urogram varies predictably with the length of time after injection, the authors recommend a definitive filming sequence.[15,16] Table I is a general summary of the recommended technique for excretory urography in the dog and cat.

TABLE I
TECHNIQUE FOR INTRAVENOUS UROGRAPHY*

1. Routine patient preparation
   a. 24 hours without food; water ad libitum
   b. Cleansing enema at least 2 hours before radiography

2. Assess hydration status; proceed only if it is normal

3. Obtain survey radiographs

4. Infuse contrast medium intravenously via the cephalic or jugular vein as rapidly as possible (bolus injection)
   a. Dose: 400 mg of iodine/lb body weight†
   b. Contrast medium: sodium iothalamate, sodium diatrizoate, or nonionic agents (expensive)

5. Make abdominal radiographs in the following sequence:
   a. Ventrodorsal views at 5 to 20 seconds, 5 minutes, 20 minutes, and 40 minutes postinjection for general assessment
   b. Lateral view at 5 minutes postinjection for general assessment
   c. Oblique views at 3 to 5 minutes postinjection for ureteral termination in urinary bladder
   d. Lateral and ventrodorsal views at 30 to 40 minutes postinjection to observe urinary bladder if retrograde cystography is contraindicated or impossible

*From Feeney DA, Barber DL, Osborne CA: Advances in canine excretory urography, in *30th Gaines Veterinary Symposium (1981)*. White Plains, NY, 1981, pp 8-22. Adapted with permission.
†If renal function is extremely poor, use 800 mg of iodine/lb body weight.

Currently available radiographic contrast media are either ionic or nonionic, triiodinated benzoic acid derivatives. The anionic component is usually iothalamate or diatrizoate; the cationic component is usually sodium or methylglucamine. The anionic portions of the contrast agent are excreted almost exclusively by glomerular filtration.[17] In the authors' experience, ionic sodium compounds give a denser opacification of the renal pelves and ureters.

Abdominal compression has been recommended to improve visualization of the renal pelves and pelvic diverticula by causing temporary ureteral compression which impedes urine outflow.[1,3,5,10,12-14] Provided the ureters can be compressed, increased pressure may distend the renal pelvis and its diverticula with urine containing contrast material. The authors do not recommend this procedure because it induces unpredictable effects on glomerular filtration and often does not uniformly compress both ureters.[4,8,17] Although abdominal compression has been advocated as an important technique to detect the early stages of pyelonephritis, this disorder can be diagnosed radiographically without abdominal compression using the technique described herein.[18]

Normal Appearance

The excretory urogram has two basic phases: the nephrogram and the pyelogram. The nephrogram represents opacification of the kidney by accumulation of contrast medium in the renal vessels (vascular nephrogram), which occurs within 10 to 15 seconds after bolus intravenous injection, and/or subsequent accumulation of contrast medium within renal tubules (tubular nephrogram). During the early vascular phase, the cortex is denser than the medulla (Figure 1). Nephrographic opacity rapidly becomes uniform in normal kidneys and becomes most dense 10 to 20 seconds after injection. Renal opacity decreases progressively for one to three hours following injection of contrast medium until it is no denser than that observed on survey radiographs (Figure 1).[16]

The pyelogram represents opacification of the renal pelves, pelvic diverticula, and ureters. Opacity of the pyelogram is much greater than that of the nephrogram since contrast medium has been concentrated by obligatory and facultative resorption of water as glomerular filtrate passed through the renal tubules. The pyelogram is normally visualized one to three minutes following intravenous injection of contrast material, and it persists for several hours after injection. The pyelogram is best visualized within one hour after contrast medium injection (Figure 1).[16]

Studies of the effects of dose, time, and individual dog variations on the canine excretory urogram have been reported.[16] Quantitative parameters of canine and feline excretory urography are summarized in Table II. The radiographic appearance of the normal canine and feline excretory urograms is shown in Figures 2 and 3.

Although excretory urography is not the optimal

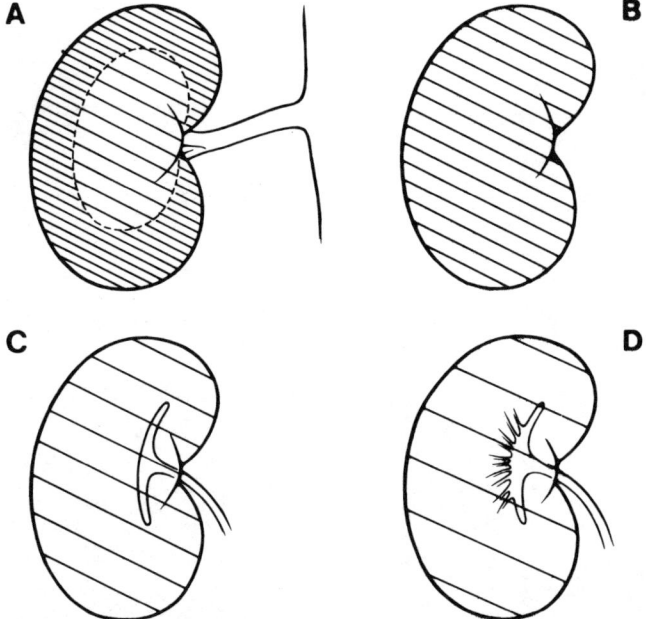

Figure 1—Diagram of a normal canine urogram. **(A)** Early vascular nephrogram; **(B)** tubular nephrogram; **(C)** 5-minute postinjection nephrogram and pyelogram; **(D)** 20- or 40-minute postinjection nephrogram and pyelogram. (From Feeney DA, Barber DL, Osborne CA: Advances in canine excretory urography, in *30th Gaines Veterinary Symposium (1981)*. White Plains, NY, Gaines Dog Research Center, 1981, pp 8-22. Reprinted with permission.)

contrast study for evaluation of the urinary bladder, it can be used for this purpose. On occasion, catheterization required for positive contrast cystography may be impossible or contraindicated. Provided renal function is adequate, satisfactory opacification and adequate distention of the urinary bladder may be obtained 30 to 40 minutes following injection of contrast medium as described for excretory urography. The urinary bladder is normally ovoid; its caudal aspect is more pointed in the region of the trigone. The mucosal surface is smooth and the bladder wall is of uniform thickness, provided nearly complete distention is achieved. The ureters commonly curve anteriorly and ventrally just prior to their entry into the trigone of the bladder.

Common Misinterpretations

The excretory urogram, as is true of any procedure performed on a living organism, has effects and variables that must be recognized to ensure accurate interpretation. For example, the end-on view of the deep circumflex iliac arteries visualized by survey radiography should not be mistaken for ureteral calculi in the caudal lumbar area of the abdomen in the lateral projection.[8] The following discussion summarizes interpretive pitfalls; the technical pitfalls have been described elsewhere in detail.[21]

The radiographic appearance of the normal pyelogram is somewhat variable. Pelvic diverticula often cannot be visualized in the normal dog without abdominal compression.[16] This is of no consequence, provided the renal pelves and proximal ureters are normal in size

and the renal pelvis has a uniform shape (Figure 2). Absence of detectable pelvic diverticula following excretory urography without abdominal compression is therefore not a reliable index of early pyelonephritis if the renal pelvis is normal.

Ureters propel urine containing contrast medium from the kidney to the bladder via rhythmic peristaltic contractions. Filling defects within the ureters caused by these contraction waves should not be misinterpreted as obstructive lesions (e.g., calculi, blood clots, or strictures). Peristaltic contractions of various portions of the ureters may be readily distinguished from obstructive disorders because they do not remain at the same site on serially obtained views.

On occasion, administration of radiographic contrast media may be followed by systemic hypotension and collapse. This may result in persistence of the nephrographic opacity and delay in pyelographic opacity. This is not the normal appearance of an excretory urogram, and it should arouse suspicion of contrast medium–in-

TABLE II

QUANTITATIVE APPEARANCE OF NORMAL CANINE AND FELINE EXCRETORY UROGRAMS

Structure	Measure-ment*	Value†	Reference
Kidney	Length	Dog	
		3.00 ± 0.25 × L-2	16
		2.50 to 3.50 × L-2	19
		2.25 to 3.00 vertebrae	9
		Cat	
		2.4 to 3.0 × L-2	20
		4.0 to 4.5 cm	5
	Width	Dog	
		2.00 ± 0.20 × L-2	16
		Cat	
		3.0 to 3.5 cm	5
Renal pelvis	Width	Dog	
		0.03 ± 0.017 × L-2	16
		(generally ≤ 1.0 mm)	
		Cat	
		Not reported	
Pelvic diverticula	Width	Dog	
		0.02 ± 0.005 × L-2	16
		(generally ≤ 1.0 mm)	
		Cat	
		Not reported	
Proximal ureter	Width	Dog	
		0.07 ± 0.018 × L-2	16
		(generally ≤ 1.0 mm)	
		Cat	
		Not reported	
Distal ureter	Width	Not reported	
		in dogs or cats	

*Measurements apply only to the VD view.
†L-2 = the length of the body of the second lumbar vertebral body as visualized on the ventrodorsal view.

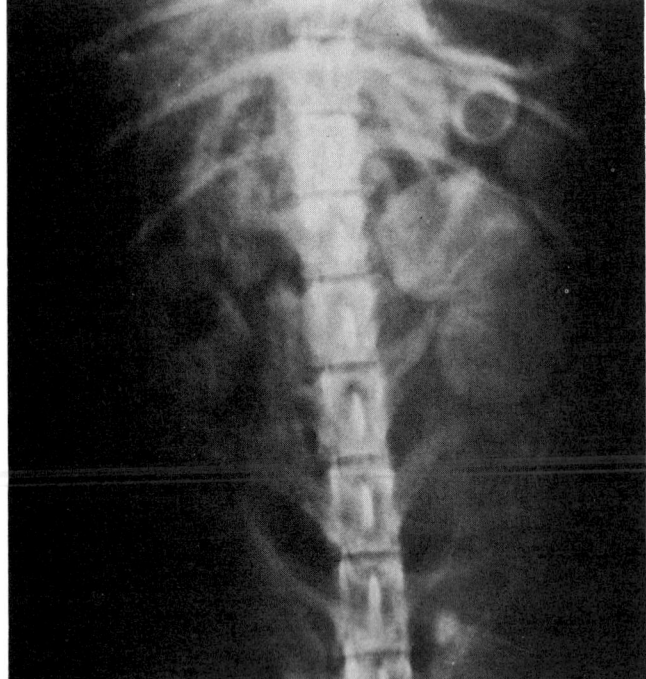

Figure 2A

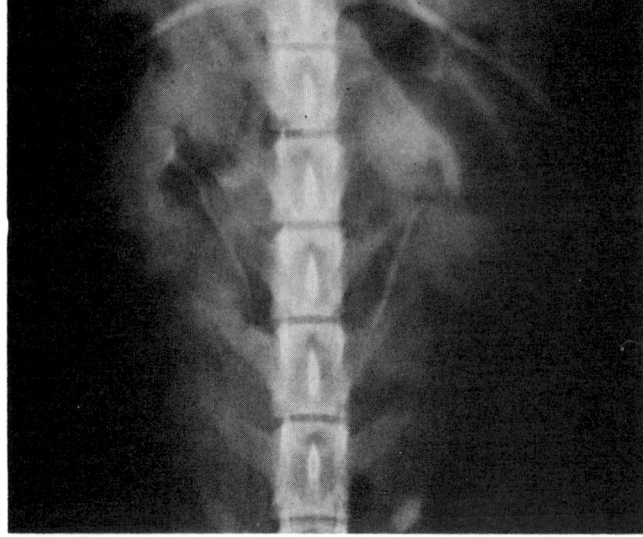

Figure 2B

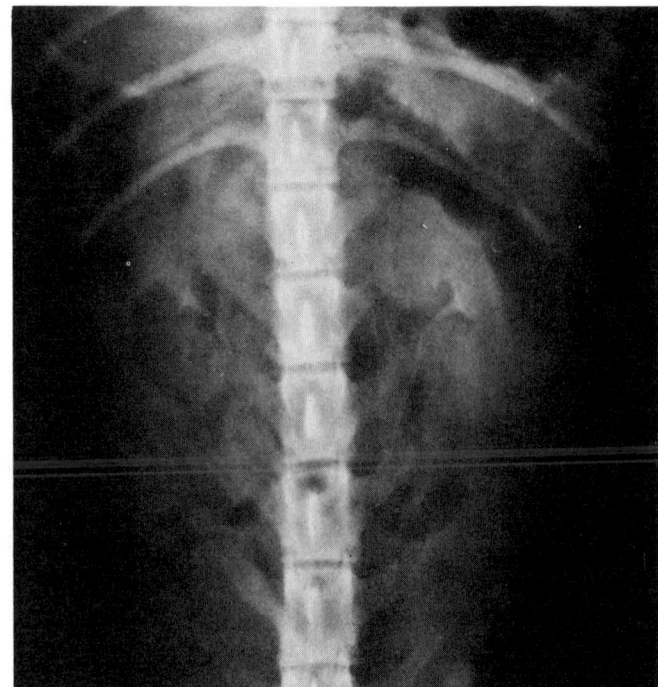

Figure 2C

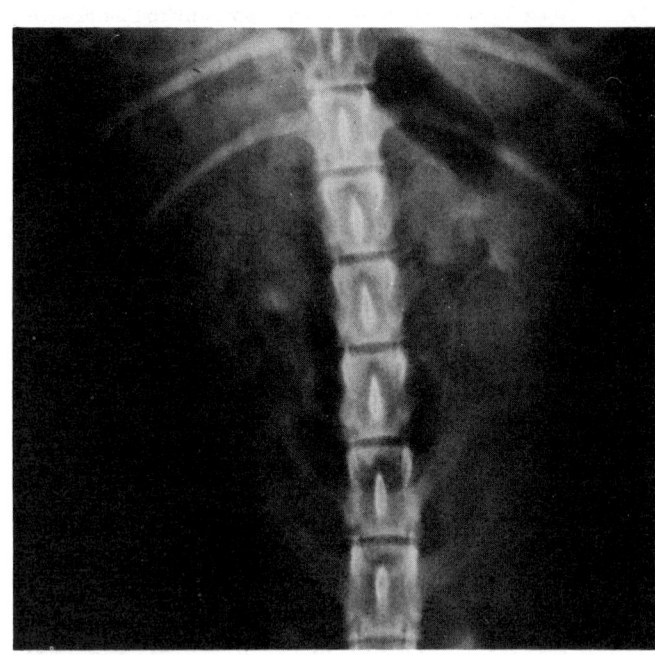

Figure 2D

Figure 2—Normal canine excretory urogram. Ventrodorsal radiographs made at **(A)** 10 seconds, **(B)** 5 minutes, **(C)** 20 minutes, and **(D)** 40 minutes following contrast medium administration.

duced systemic hypotension and should be treated in the same manner as hypovolemic shock. Intravenous administration of atropine (routine preanesthetic dose) should also be considered since parenterally administered contrast media may cause bradycardia despite systemic hypotension. A persistent nephrogram has also been associated with urine outflow obstruction, contrast medium–induced renal failure, glomerular disease, and renal tubular necrosis.[17,22]

Radiopaque contrast medium may cause a false-positive reaction for protein and alter specific gravity values determined during routine urinalyses.[23] False-positive protein reactions have most commonly been observed when sulfosalicylic acid is used. However, radiographic contrast medium does not interfere with tests that incorporate indicator dyes (bromphenol blue[a] and tetra-

[a] Albutest®, Ames Co., Elkhart, IN 46515.

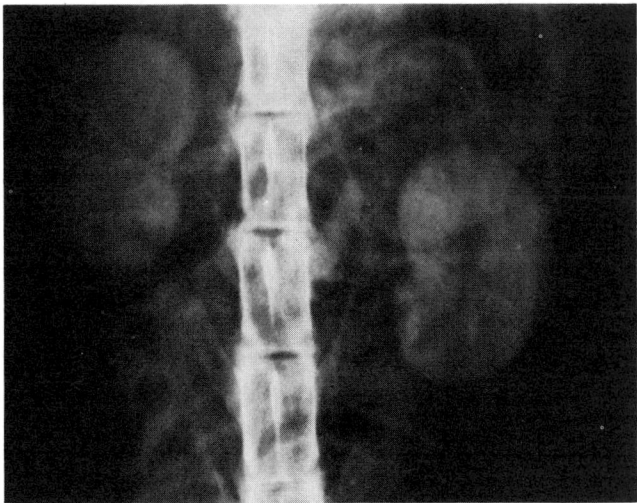

Figure 3A

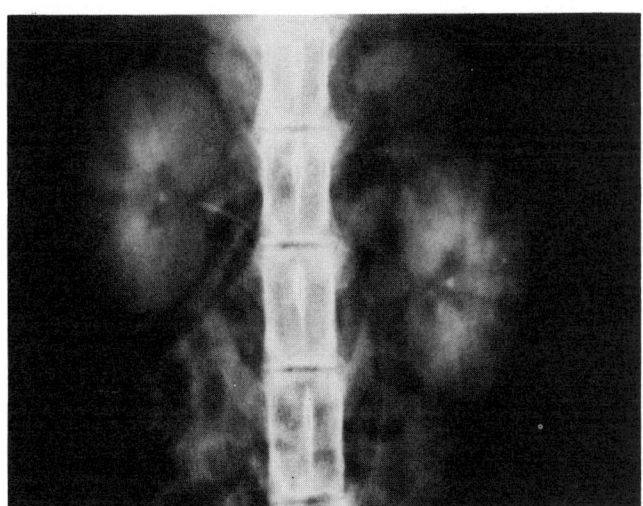

Figure 3B

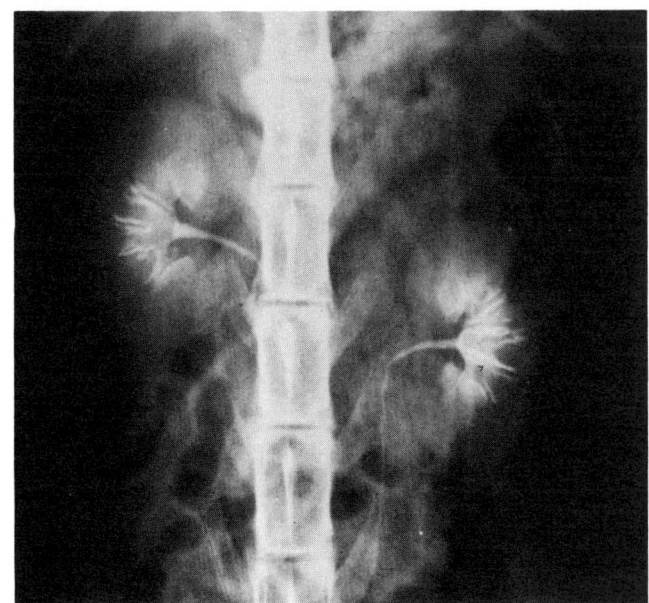

Figure 3C

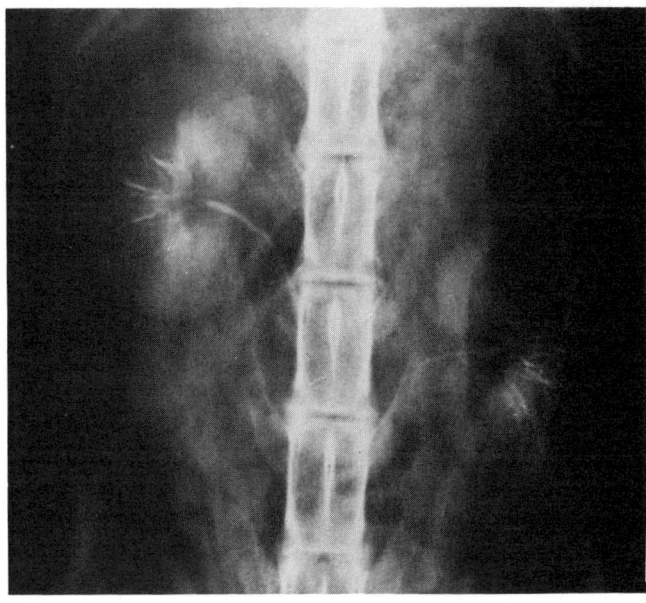

Figure 3D

Figure 3—Normal feline excretory urogram. Ventrodorsal radiographs made at **(A)** 10 seconds, **(B)** 5 minutes, **(C)** 20 minutes, and **(D)** 40 minutes following contrast medium administration.

bromphenol blue[b]).[23] Changes in urine specific gravity following excretory urography in dogs have been reported.[23] In dogs, the direction and magnitude of change in urine specific gravity are dependent on the degree of urine concentration prior to administration of the contrast agent.[23] If the urine specific gravity prior to excretory urography is below 1.040, radiographic contrast agents may cause a significant increase which is not due to renal conservation of water in excess of solute. Care should be taken not to misinterpret such findings as evidence of adequate renal function. To avoid contrast medium–induced errors in urinalysis, at least 24 hours should be allowed to elapse before samples are collected for analysis.

[b]Albustix®, Ames Co., Elkhart, IN 46515.

REFERENCES

1. Bishop EJ: A method of visualizing the urinary tract and a basis for assessing renal function in small animal radiography. *JAVMA* 123:187-192, 1953.
2. Drury F, Dyce KM: The radiography of the normal urinary tract of the dog. *Vet Rec* 65:647-649, 1953.
3. Tennile NB, Thornton GW: Intravenous urography studies in the unanesthetized dog. *Vet Med* 53:29-40, 1958.
4. Ackerman N: Intravenous pyelography. *JAAHA* 10:277-284, 1974.
5. Bartels JE: Feline intravenous urography. *JAAHA* 9:349-353, 1973.
6. Borthwick R, Robbie B: Large volume urography in the cat. *J Small Anim Pract* 12:579-583, 1971.
7. Borthwick R, Robbie B: Urography in the dog by an intravenous transfusion technique. *J Small Anim Pract* 10:465-470, 1969.
8. Kneller SK: Role of the excretory urogram in the diagnosis of renal and ureteral disease. *Vet Clin North Am* 4:843-861, 1974.
9. Lord PE, Scott RC, Chan KF: Intravenous urography for the evaluation of renal diseases in small animals. *JAAHA* 10:139-152, 1974.

10. Root CR: Contrast radiography of the urinary system, in Ticer JW (ed): *Radiographic Technique in Small Animal Practice.* Philadelphia, WB Saunders Co, 1975, pp 396-414.

11. Walker RG, Douglas SW: The use of contrast media in the diagnosis of urinary tract abnormalities in the dog with particular reference to infusion urography: A report of two cases. *Vet Rec* 87:287-289, 1970.

12. Watters JW: Urinary tract radiography—Kidney and ureters. *Compend Contin Educ Pract Vet* 2:224-231, 1980.

13. Zontine WJ: Radiographic interpretation: Excretory urogram. *Mod Vet Pract* 56:106-111, 1975.

14. Biery DN: The upper urinary tract, in O'Brien TR (ed): *Radiographic Diagnosis of Abdominal Disorders in the Dog and Cat.* Philadelphia, WB Saunders Co, 1978, pp 481-542.

15. Feeney DA, Barber DL, Osborne CA: Advances in canine excretory urography, in *Proceedings 30th Gaines Veterinary Symposium.* White Plains, NY, Gaines Dog Research Center, 1981, pp 8-22.

16. Feeney DA, Thrall DE, Barber DL, et al, Normal canine excretory urogram: Effects of dose, time and individual dog variation. *Am J Vet Res* 40:1596-1604, 1979.

17. Saxton HM: Review article: Urography. *Br J Radiol* 42:321-346, 1969.

18. Barber DL, Finco DR: Radiographic findings in induced bacterial pyelonephritis in dogs. *JAVMA* 175:1183-1190, 1979.

19. Finco DR, Stiles NS, Kneller SK, et al: Radiologic estimation of kidney size of the dog. *JAVMA* 159:995-1002, 1971.

20. Barrett RB, Kneller SK: Feline kidney mensuration. *Acta Radiol Suppl* 319:279-280, 1972.

21. Johnston GR, Feeney DA, Osborne CA: Radiographic findings in urinary tract infection. *Vet Clin North Am* 9:749-774, 1979.

22. Feeney DA, Barber DL, Osborne CA: The functional aspects of excretory nephrography: A review, submitted to *Vet Radiol.*

23. Feeney DA, Osborne CA, Jessen CR: Effects of radiocontrast agents on the urinalysis with emphasis on specific gravity. *JAVMA* 176:1378-1381, 1980.

The Excretory Urogram: Part II
Interpretation of Abnormal Findings

D. A. Feeney, DVM, MS
Assistant Professor
Department of Small Animal
Clinical Sciences
College of Veterinary Medicine
University of Minnesota
St. Paul, Minnesota

D. L. Barber, DVM, MS
Assistant Professor
Department of Anatomy and
Radiology
College of Veterinary Medicine
University of Georgia
Athens, Georgia

G. R. Johnston, DVM, MS
Assistant Professor

C. A. Osborne, DVM, PhD
Professor and Chairman

Department of Small Animal
Clinical Sciences
College of Veterinary Medicine
University of Minnesota
St. Paul, Minnesota

The excretory urogram may be used to obtain qualitative information about the functional status of canine and feline kidneys by observation of the sequential trends in nephrographic opacity. Comparisons of the degree of initial nephrographic opacification and subsequent trends in nephrographic opacification during excretory urography may suggest the presence of conditions such as contrast medium–induced renal failure, contrast medium–induced systemic hypotension, acute renal obstruction, polyuric renal disease, and glomerular dysfunction. Observation of the size, shape, and distribution of parenchymal opacification of the kidneys during urography assists in diagnosis of renal neoplasms, renal cysts, renal infarcts, hematomas, hydronephrosis, and chronic generalized renal disease (end-stage kidneys). Comparison of structural alterations with the size and shape of the renal pelvis and its diverticula may permit diagnosis of pyelonephritis, hydronephrosis, renal neoplasia, and/or renal calculi.

Excretory urography is an integral part of the evaluation of most patients with suspected urinary tract disease. It is used to evaluate the size, shape, and position of various components of the urinary tract.[1-7] Specific situations in which excretory urography is indicated include following severe abdominal trauma and cases of hematuria, dysuria, incontinence, polyuria, oliguria, anuria, and palpable abnormalities.[1,3,7,8] Excretory urography may also be used for evaluation of the upper and lower urinary tract in the presence of abdominal masses of undetermined origin. Involvement (or noninvolvement) of urinary tract structures can be assessed, and the relationship of the masses to the urinary structures may assist in identifying the site or sites of their origin.

Excretory urography may be used in patients with or without azotemia to evaluate renal size or to determine if outflow obstruction has occurred. In humans, failure to correct dehydration prior to administration of radiopaque contrast agents has been associated with adverse reactions involving the kidneys.[9] Occurrence of adverse reactions is more frequent in dehydrated patients with diabetes mellitus, myeloma, and combined renal and hepatic failure than in other dehydrated patients.[9] Based on reports in humans, it has been recommended that excretory urography only be performed on adequately hydrated patients.[3,6]

In general, the radiographic quality (opacification and contrast

Originally published in Volume 4, Number 4, April 1982

enhancement) of the excretory urogram decreases as the degree of renal dysfunction becomes more severe.[10] For this reason, increased doses of radiographic contrast medium have been recommended to improve the quality of the urogram during moderate to severe renal dysfunction.[3,11] Some pathophysiologic alterations in renal function may be associated with specific variation in the sequence of opacification of the kidney during urography (Table I). The radiographic appearance and pathophysiology of these functional abnormalities have been described elsewhere in detail.[3,16] The opacity of the collecting system (pelvis, ureters, and bladder) generally decreases in patients with renal failure because of an obligatory increase in urine volume that reduces the concentration of contrast medium in urine. Reduced opacification of the excretory pathway is not pathognomonic for primary renal failure, however, since it may be associated with an inadequate dosage of contrast medium and nonrenal causes of polyuria.

Contrast medium–induced renal failure has been reported in humans,[17-19] dogs,[3] and cats.[20] The pathophysiology of this disease has not been precisely determined, but it appears to be complex. Possible mechanisms include renal vasoconstriction, direct toxicity to renal tubules, renal vascular occlusion secondary to contrast-induced red blood cell aggregation, and obstruction of renal tubules by Tamm-Horsfall mucoprotein.[17,18] In humans, diabetes mellitus, preexisting renal disease, multiple myeloma, dehydration, and advanced age have been associated with increased risk of contrast medium–induced renal failure.[17-19] The clinical course is usually transient (2 to 37 days) in human patients. It is initially characterized by oliguria and progressive azotemia, followed by increased urine flow rates and subsequent return of normal renal function.[17-19] Although this disorder has not been documented in large numbers of dogs and cats, it is presumed to be potentially reversible. Changes in creatinine clearance have been reported in dogs following contrast medium administration, but the wide degree of renal function impairment among dogs was interpreted to suggest variation in individual susceptibility.[21]

The Nephrogram

Opacification of the renal parenchyma following intravenous injection of contrast medium is termed the

TABLE I

NEPHROGRAPHIC OPACIFICATION PATTERNS ASSOCIATED WITH COMMON RENAL DISORDERS*

Pattern	Associated Disorders
Sequential decrease in nephrographic opacity	
A. Good initial opacification followed by progressive decrease in opacity	None[12]
B. Poor initial opacification followed by progressive decrease in opacity	Primary polyuric renal failure Inadequate contrast medium dose Others
Sequential persistence in nephrographic opacity	
A. Fair to good initial opacification followed by persistent opacity	Acute renal tubular necrosis[13] Contrast medium–induced renal failure[14] Systemic hypotension due to radiocontrast agents[13] Others
B. Poor initial opacification followed by persistent opacity	Primary glomerular dysfunction[13] Severe generalized renal disease Others
Sequential increase in nephrographic opacity	
A. Fair to good opacification followed by progressive increase in opacity	Systemic hypotension due to radiocontrast agents[13,20] Acute renal obstruction (probably due to precipitated Tamm-Horsfall mucoprotein in renal tubules)[13] Contrast medium–induced renal failure[14] Others
B. Poor initial opacification followed by progressive increase in opacity	Acute extrarenal obstruction[13] Systemic hypotension existing prior to contrast medium administration[15] Renal ischemia (arterial or venous)[13] Others

*Modified from Feeney DA, Barber DL, Osborne CA: The functional aspects of the nephrogram in excretory urography: A review. *Vet Radiol* 23:42–45, 1982.

nephrogram. The components (vascular and tubular) that contribute to the nephrogram have been described.[3,22]

An early vascular nephrogram is a reliable index of renal perfusion. A tubular nephrogram is indicative of the presence of functional renal parenchyma. The normal sequence of opacification and appearance of the normal nephrogram have been described.[3,22] The opacity of the nephrogram is proportional to the dose (in milligrams of iodine) of contrast medium administered.[12] However, the degree of opacity and trends of opacity (e.g., increase, decrease, or persistent) following intravenous administration of contrast medium may be influenced by renal perfusion, nephron function, and patency of the renal outflow tract.[3,4]

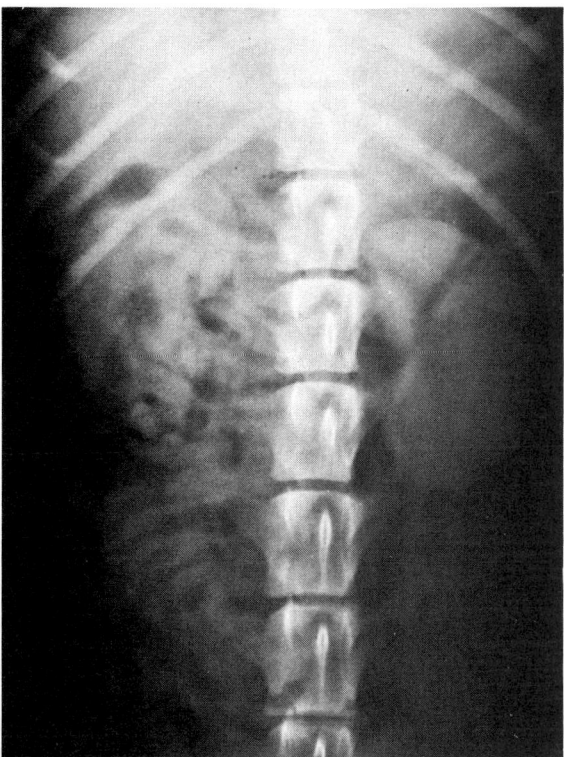

Figure 1A

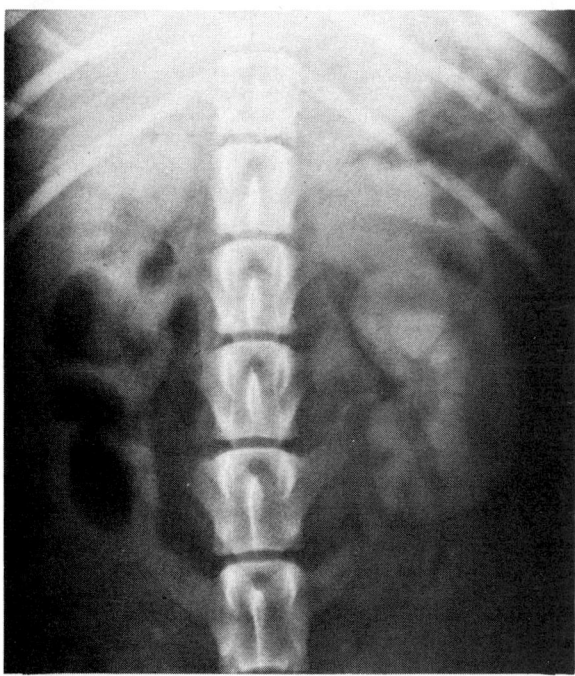

Figure 1B

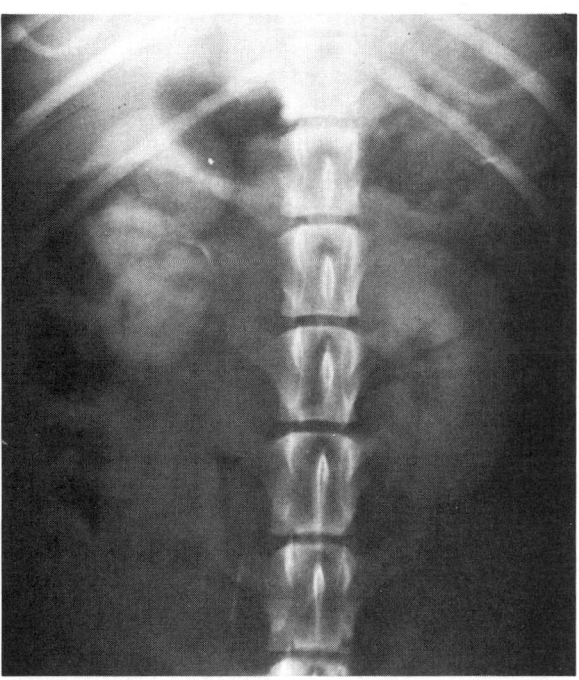

Figure 1C

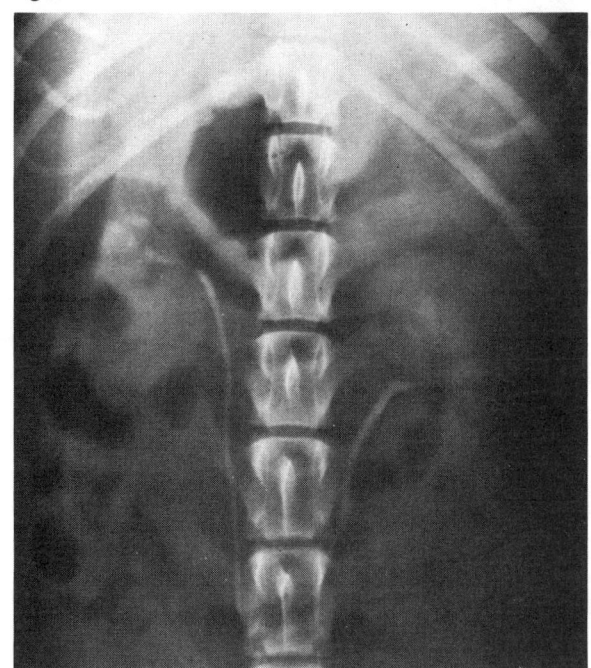

Figure 1D

Figure 1—Excretory urogram of a mature male beagle during systemic hypotension and collapse which occurred following bolus intravenous injection of sodium iothalamate. Ventrodorsal radiographs made at **(A)** 15 seconds, **(B)** 5 minutes, **(C)** 20 minutes, and **(D)** 40 minutes postinjection. Note persistent slightly increasing nephrographic opacity and lack of normal pelvic and ureteral opacification from **A** to **D**. (From Feeney DA, Barber DL, Osborne CA: Advances in canine excretory urography, in *30th Gaines Veterinary Symposium (1981)*. White Plains, NY, Gaines Dog Research Center, 1981, pp 8-22. Reprinted with permission.)

As a general rule, nephrographic appearance should be assessed on each radiograph for variations in opacification, shape, size, and the interface between areas of nonuniform opacification. In addition, after contrast medium injection, the opacity of the nephrograms should be compared in chronologic order to ascertain the sequence of nephrographic opacification. When present, opacification of the collecting system occurs as the nephrogram begins to fade. The maximum degree of opacity of the nephrogram in patients with renal dysfunction is usually observed during the initial vascular phase.[22]

Possible nephrographic patterns found during excretory urography in humans, dogs, and cats are summarized in Table I. In general, the initial opacification refers to findings on 10-second and 5-minute post-contrast medium injection radiographs. *Persistent opacity* and *progressive* changes in opacity (in the table) refer to radiographs obtained 20 minutes or more after injection (including circumstances when radiographs are made 12 to 24 hours after contrast medium injection). Subsequent opacification of the renal pelves, pelvic diverticula, and ureters (pyelogram) is dependent on a number of factors (see discussion in the section about the pyelogram).

An example of an abnormal trend in nephrographic opacity is contrast medium–induced hypotension (Table I). A mature beagle given the routine dose of contrast medium collapsed seconds later. Therapy for hypovolemic shock was immediately initiated and continued throughout the radiographic sequence. Radiographs were obtained during this contrast medium–induced reaction (Figure 1). Note the persistence of, and tendency toward, increased nephrographic opacity through the 20-minute postinjection radiograph. Almost no opacification of pyelographic structures occurred until the animal returned to a nearly normal physiological status 40 minutes following contrast medium injection.

Alterations in renal parenchyma may often be detected by studying nephrographic appearance. An algorithm has been developed in which renal size, renal capsular surface characteristics, and distribution of opacification were used to identify probable causes of specific nephrographio findings (Figure 2). Diseases (such as amyloidosis) that are highly variable in appearance have not been included because they have no predictable trend in architectural alterations.

Localized alterations in nephrographic appearance are usually associated with neoplasms, renal infarcts, solitary renal cysts, hematomas, and/or abscesses.[3] Differentiation of these disorders may be facilitated by examining the interface between normal and abnormal

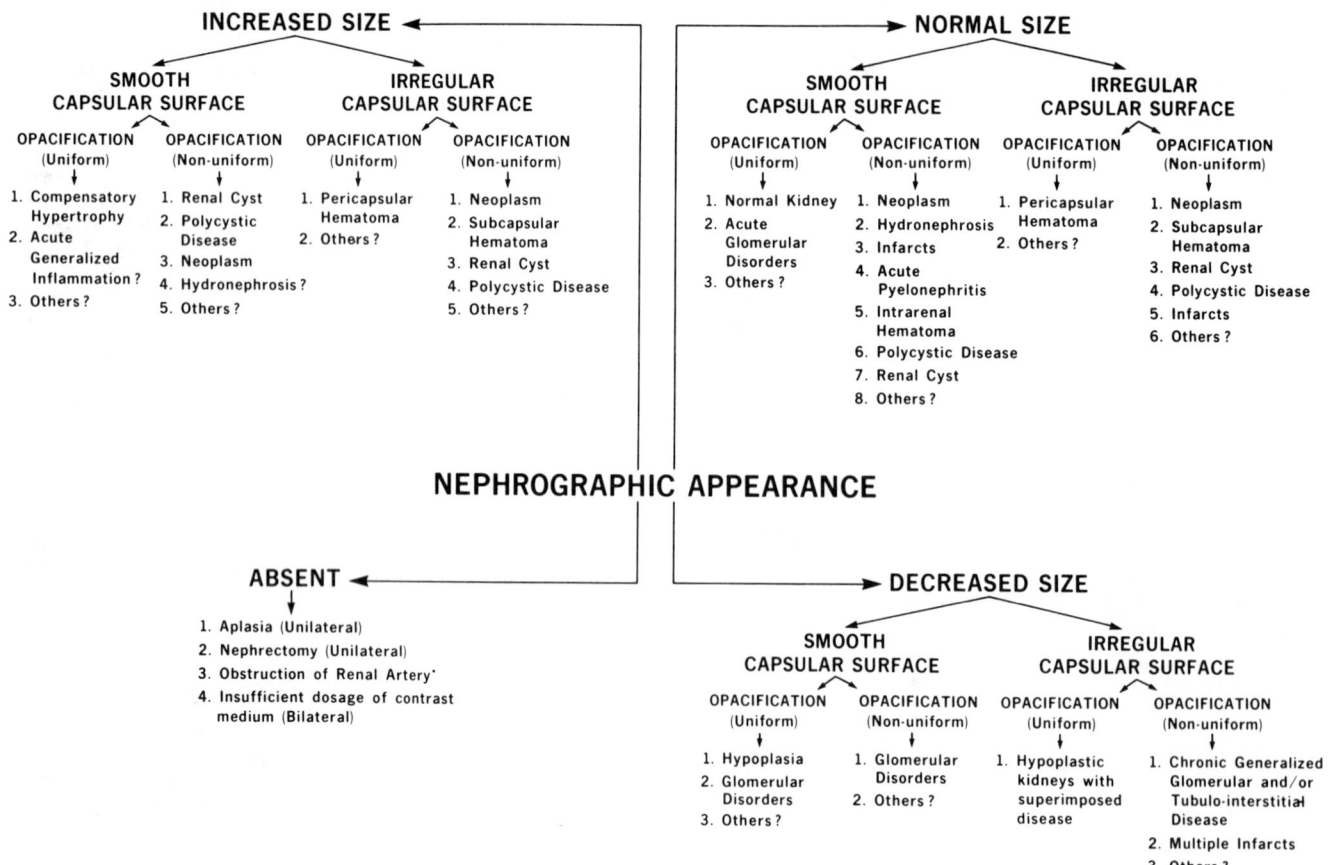

Figure 2—Algorithm for interpretation of nephrographic appearance following intravenous injection of radiographic contrast medium. *Bilateral obstruction of renal arteries would result in death within a few days. (From Feeney DA, Barber DL, Osborne CA: Advances in canine excretory urography, in *30th Gaines Veterinary Symposium (1981)*. White Plains, NY, Gaines Dog Research Center, 1981, pp 8-22. Reprinted with permission.)

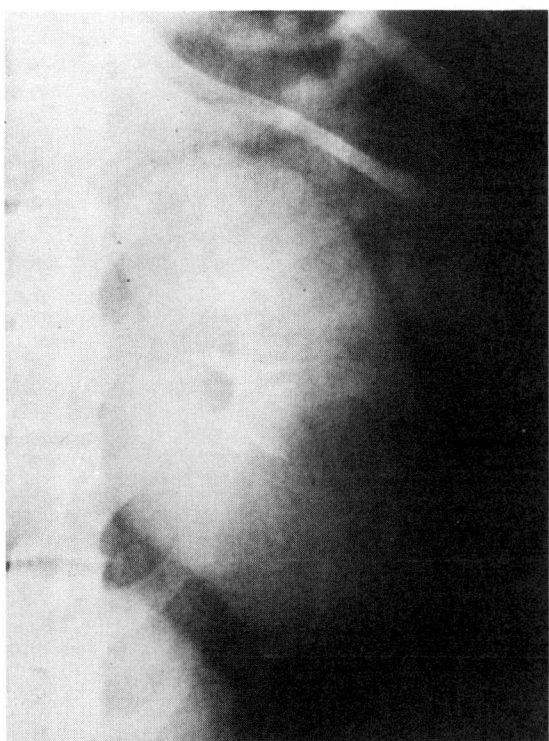

Figure 3—Excretory urogram of a dog with a solitary renal cyst of caudal pole of the kidney. Ventrodorsal view. Note spherical, smoothly marginated area of decreased opacity. (Courtesy of J. Lebel, Colorado State University)

regions. Smooth margins at the interface between lesions and normal kidney are usually associated with renal cysts (Figure 3), whereas an irregular interface is usually associated with neoplasms (Figure 4), infarcts, or hematomas.[3] Moderate hydronephrosis due to ureteral obstruction is an example of a localized parenchymal alteration caused by an abnormality in the collection system (Figure 5).

Generalized alterations in nephrographic appearance are usually associated with advanced hydronephrosis, diffuse infiltrative processes, e.g., lymphosarcoma and feline infectious peritonitis (Figure 6), polycystic disease (Figure 7), congenital renal diseases such as renal dysplasia associated with Lhaso apsos (Figure 8) and Norwegian elkhounds, and chronic generalized renal disorders (Figure 9). Ranking these possible diagnoses in order of probability may be facilitated by knowledge of renal size, capsular surface characteristics (Figure 2), and the history and breed.

The Pyelogram

Opacification of the renal pelves, pelvic diverticula, and ureters is termed the *pyelogram*. Opacification of these structures is due to excretion of contrast medium after it has been filtered and concentrated by nephrons. Detection of concentrated contrast medium in normal renal pelves and ureters three to five minutes after contrast medium administration indicates that renal function is present and that no complete obstruction of the outflow tract exists. Opacity of pyelographic components is related to the dose of contrast medium, state of hydration, degree of renal function, and volume of urine containing contrast medium in the excretory pathway.[9,10,12,23] There is little change in the normal pyelographic appearance following initial opacification except for minor variation in the size of the structures.[12]

Pyelographic alterations caused by common renal diseases are described in Table II. Pyelographic abnormalities in unanesthetized dogs are best assessed on radiographs made 5, 20, and 40 minutes post-contrast

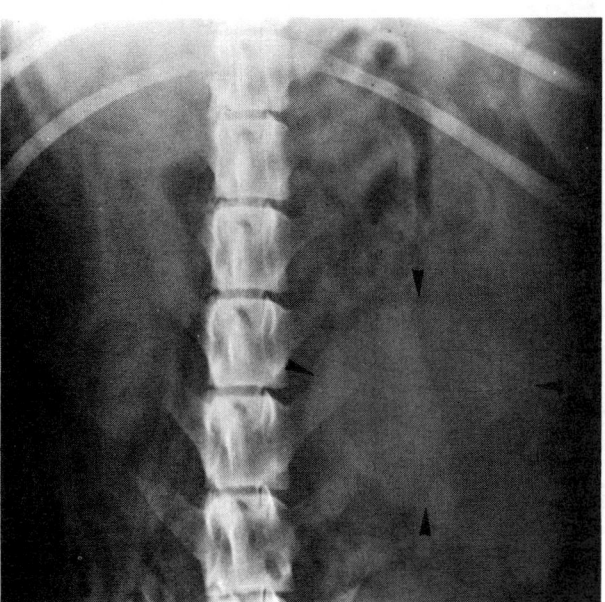

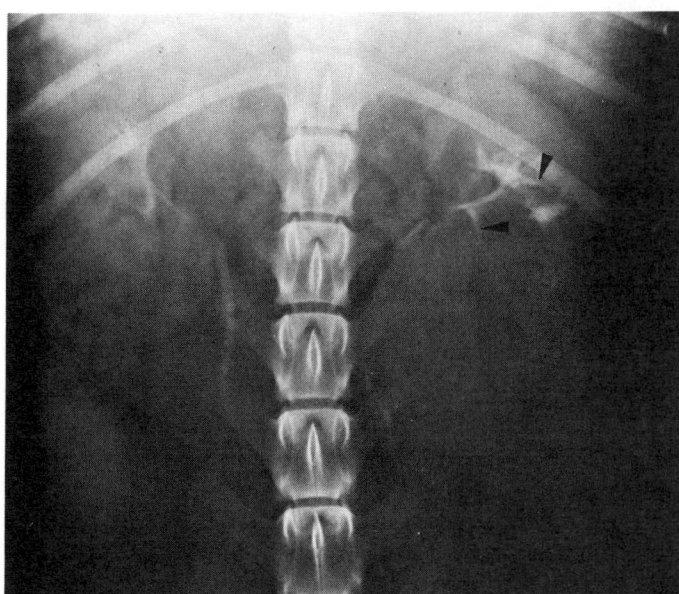

Figure 4—Excretory urogram of a dog with a solitary renal adenocarcinoma of the left kidney. **(A)** Note enlargement of the caudal pole (*arrows*) of the left kidney on survey ventrodorsal radiograph. **(B)** The left renal pelvis is distorted (*arrows*), and the size and shape of the caudal pole of the left kidney are abnormal on this 5-minute postinjection radiograph. Left ureter has been displaced medially by the neoplasm.

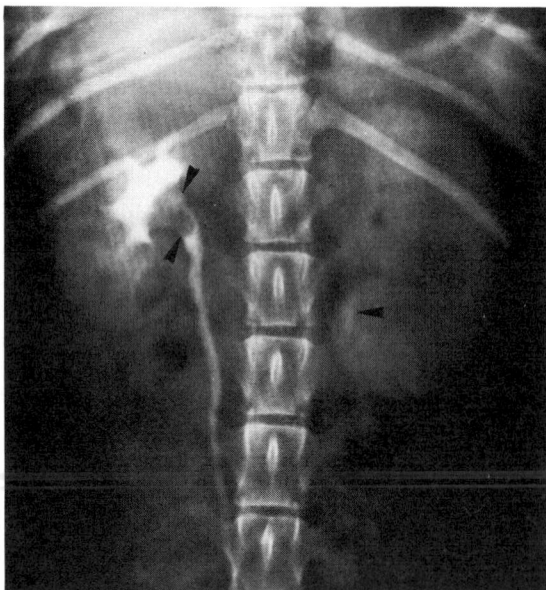

Figure 5—Excretory urogram of a dog with a right renal pelvic calculus and a left ureteral calculus radiographed 20 minute after intravenous injection of contrast medium. Ventrodorsal view. The calculus produces a triangular filling defect (*arrows*) in the dilated pelvis and proximal ureter of the right kidney. The left kidney is enlarged and/or has a perihilar void in nephrographic opacity due to a dilated, nonopacified renal pelvis. A ureteral calculus (*arrow*) located at the medial aspect of the caudal pole of the left kidney caused ureteral obstruction. (From Feeney DA, Barber DL, Osborne CA: Advances in canine excretory urography, in *30th Gaines Veterinary Symposium (1981)*. White Plains, NY, Gaines Dog Research Center, 1981, pp 8-22. Reprinted with permission.)

medium injection. Localized distortions of pyelographic structure are usually associated with renal cysts, neo-

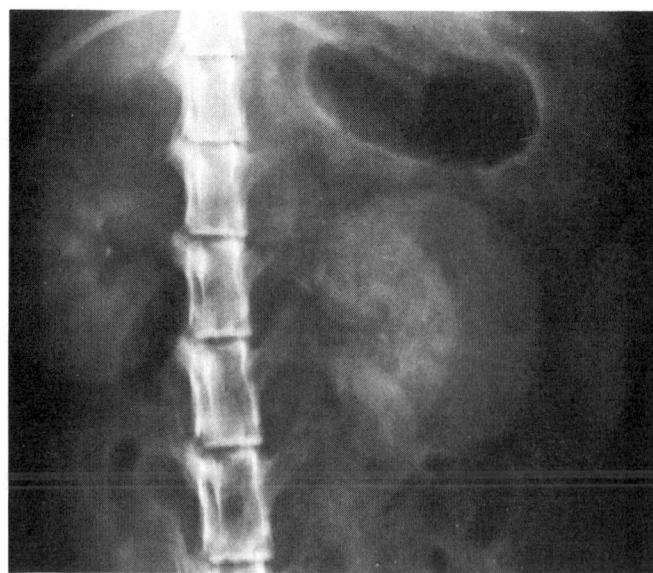

Figure 6—Excretory urogram of a two-year-old cat with mild bilateral renal enlargement due to feline infectious peritonitis. Ventrodorsal view five minutes after contrast medium administration. Uniform nephrographic opacity with poor pyelographic opacity is present. The loss of serosal-surface clarity is due to the presence of peritoneal fluid.

plasms (Figure 4), hematomas, and infarcts.[3] Generalized distortions of pyelographic structure are usually caused by inflammatory disease such as pyelonephritis (Figure 10) and outflow obstruction due to hydronephrosis, or pelvic and/or ureteral uroliths. Uroliths are often associated with obstruction and inflammation (Figure 5).[3] Congenital anomalies such as aperistaltic megaloureter

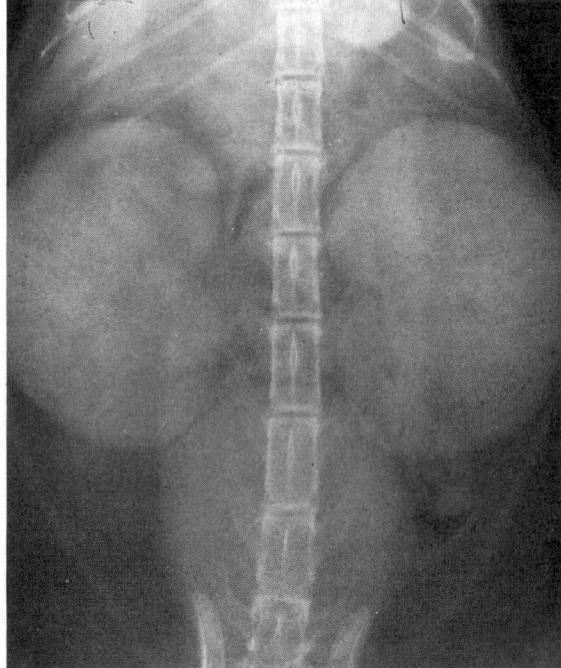

Figure 7A

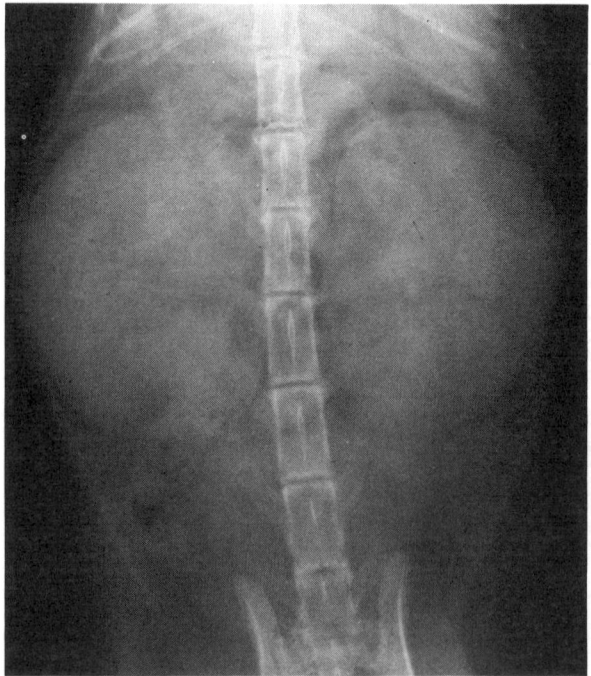

Figure 7B

Figure 7—Excretory urogram of an 11-month-old cat with polycystic kidneys. Ventrodorsal views. **(A)** Note the irregular (patchy) opacification of the enlarged kidneys with no definite renal pelvic opacification, five minutes after contrast medium administration. **(B)** Note the decreased nephrographic opacity and filling of the urinary bladder with poorly concentrated contrast medium 40 minutes after contrast medium administration. Pyelographic opacity is poor as a result of poor renal function, not obstruction.

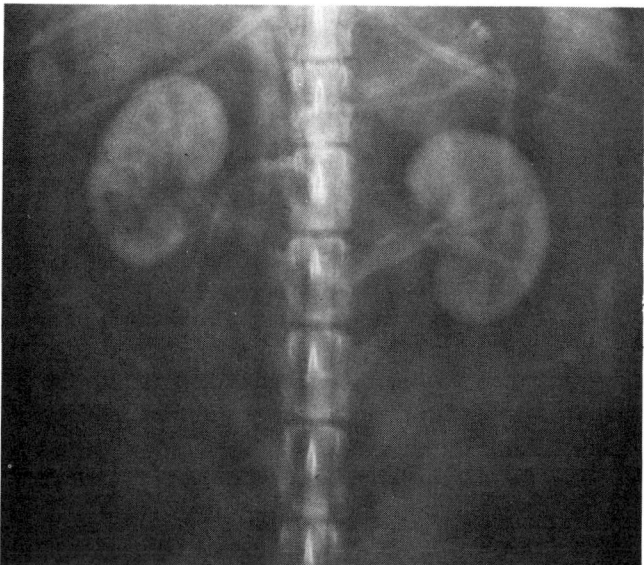

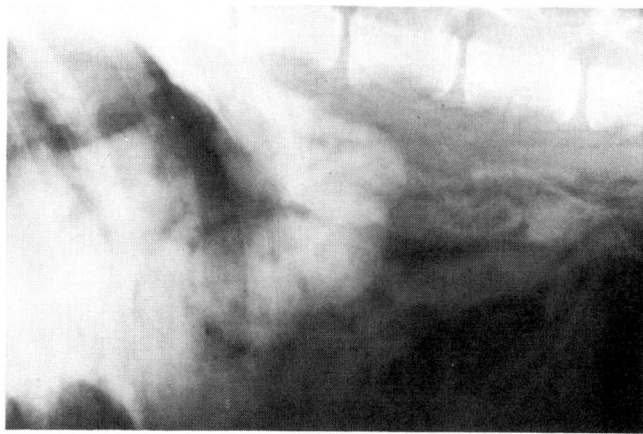

Figure 9—Close-up lateral view of an excretory urogram of end-stage canine kidneys obtained five minutes following contrast medium administration. Note poor opacification, decreased size, and irregular shape of kidneys.

Figure 8—Excretory urogram of a one-year-old male Lhasa apso with chronic progressive generalized renal disease of probable familial origin. Ventrodorsal views. **(A)** Note small kidneys with thin cortices, capsular irregularity, and poor opacification of the right caudal pole on 10-second post-contrast medium injection film.

TABLE II

PYELOGRAPHIC CHARACTERISTICS OF COMMON RENAL DISEASES*

I. Pyelonephritis
  A. Acute
    Pelvic dilatation
    Proximal ureteral dilatation
    Absent or incomplete filling of diverticula
  B. Chronic
    ± pelvic dilatation with irregular borders
    Proximal ureteral dilatation
    Short blunt diverticula

II. Hydronephrosis
  Pelvic dilatation
  Dilatation of pelvic diverticula (Note: Diverticula may not be distinguishable if pelvic dilatation is severe)
  Ureteral dilatation

III. Neoplasia
  A. Of renal parenchyma
    Distortion or deviation of renal pelvis, sometimes with dilatation
    Distortion or deviation of pelvic diverticula
  B. Of renal pelvis
    Distortion or dilatation of renal pelvis
    Filling defects in renal pelvis

IV. Uroliths
  Filling defects in renal pelvis
  Uroliths usually radiolucent compared to contrast medium
  May be changes associated with pyelonephritis
  ±pelvic dilatation

*From Feeney DA, Barber DL, Osborne CA: Advances in canine excretory urography, in *30th Gaines Veterinary Symposium (1981)*. White Plains, NY, Gaines Dog Research Center, 1981, pp 8-22. Reprinted with permission.

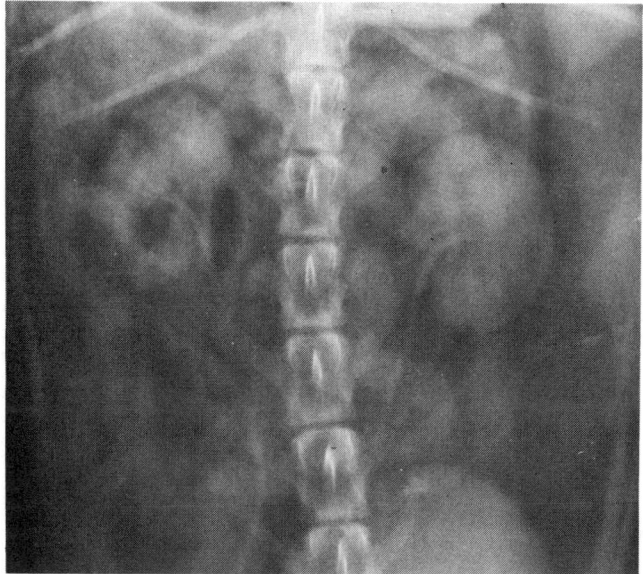

Figure 8—**(B)** Note small kidney with fading nephrogram and poor pyelographic opacification at five minutes after contrast medium administration.

and ectopic ureter may also cause pyelographic changes which resemble or are associated with pyelonephritis (Figure 11). Space-occupying infiltrative diseases such as lymphosarcoma and feline infectious peritonitis may compress the renal pelves and pelvic diverticula (Figure 6),[5] causing distortion and poor opacification. However, alteration of the renal pelves and/or pelvic diverticula with concomitant enlargement of the kidneys is indicative of primary diffuse renal involvement.

Failure of pyelographic opacification following a normal or abnormal nephrogram may be associated with decreased glomerular filtration rate, renal tubular dysfunction, intra- or extrarenal obstruction, premature

radiography after contrast medium administration, anuria, oliguria, hypotension, and/or hypovolemia. These factors may cause a delay of minutes to hours from the time of nephrographic opacification to the time of pyelographic opacification. Any delay in pyelographic opacification beyond three to five minutes after contrast medium injection is reason to suspect an abnormality. Such delay should be interpreted in light of laboratory evaluation of renal function and the status of the patient (e.g., collapsed, depressed, alert).

Evaluation of Excretory Urograms

For optimum consistent results the authors recommend the following sequence of evaluation of excretory urograms. Portions of this sequence may be deleted or modified, depending on the portion of the urinary tract to be specifically examined.

1. Determine that the patient is properly hydrated.
2. Following proper patient preparation confirmed by diagnostic quality survey radiographs, intravenously inject contrast medium at a dosage of 800 mg of iodine per kilogram of body weight.[22]
3. a. Make a ventrodorsal radiograph at 5 to 20 seconds, 5 minutes, 20 minutes, and 40 minutes following bolus intravenous injection of contrast medium.
   b. Make a lateral radiograph 5 minutes following injection.
   c. Make oblique ventrodorsal radiographs 3 to 5 minutes following injection to delineate ureteral termination (bladder, urethra, vagina, or other possible terminating sites).
4. Observe the chronologic sequence and distribution of nephrographic opacity.
   a. Maximum uniform renal opacification should occur immediately after injection, followed by progressive loss of opacity. If this trend is not observed, see Table I.
   b. The renal parenchymal opacity should be uniform with a smooth capsular surface and normal size.[22] If this is not observed see Table II.
5. Observe the chronologic sequence of opacification and size of the pyelographic structures (renal pelves, pelvic diverticula, ureters).[22]

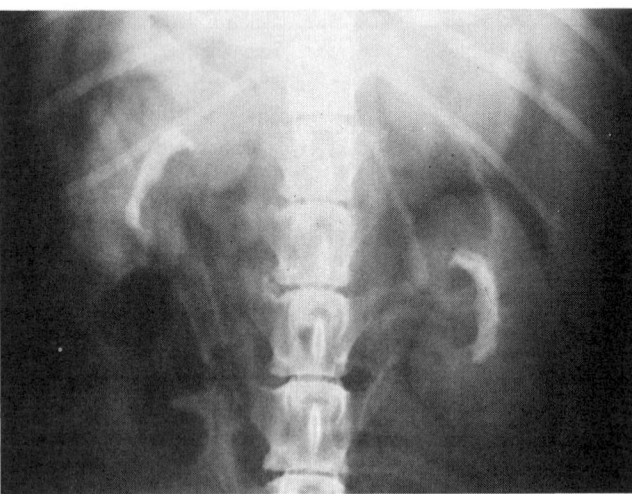

Figure 10—Close-up ventrodorsal view of an excretory urogram of canine kidneys with chronic pyelonephritis obtained 40 minutes after contrast medium administration. Note increased size of renal pelves with short blunted pelvic diverticula. Scalloped renal margins are due to renal scarring.

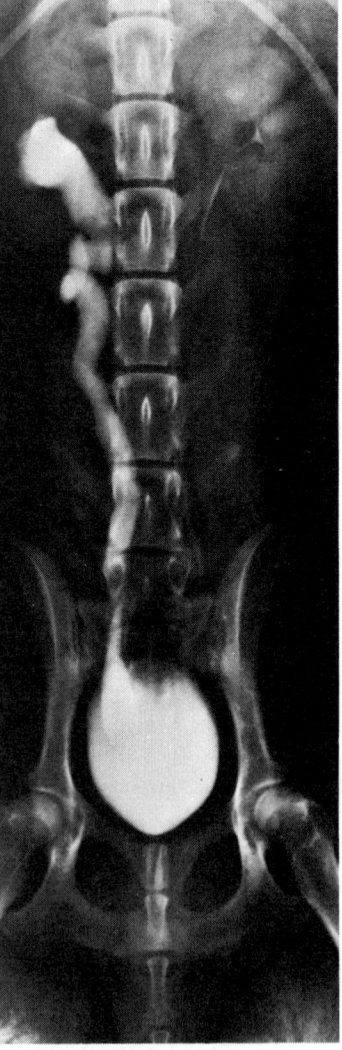

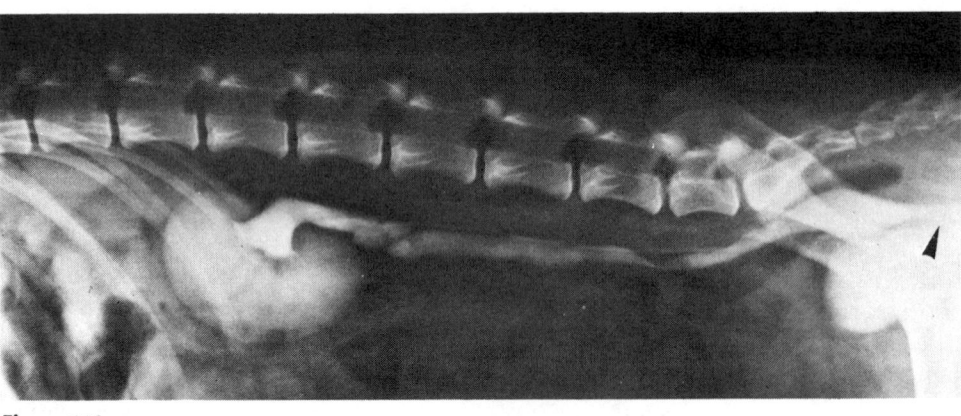

Figure 11A

Figure 11B

Figure 11—Excretory urogram of a 1½-year-old Siberian husky with a right ectopic ureter. **(A)** Lateral view obtained five minutes after contrast medium administration. Note dilated renal pelvis and ureter without dilated pelvic diverticula (often associated with pyelonephritis) on the right side. The dilated ureter continues caudally past the trigone (*arrow*). **(B)** Ventrodorsal view obtained 40 minutes after contrast injection. The termination of the abnormal right ureter is not visualized, but contrast medium deposition on the hair of the hindlegs is highly suggestive of incontinence.

a. The pyelogram should be observed 1 to 3 minutes following peak nephrographic opacity and should slowly fade during the following several hours. If not, reexamine the nephrogram (Table I).

b. Measure the width of the renal pelves, pelvic diverticula, and ureters as previously described.[12,22] If abnormal, see Table II.

6. If diseases of the urinary bladder are suspected but retrograde studies are impossible or contraindicated, examine the urinary bladder 30 to 40 minutes postinjection. Lateral, ventrodorsal and, if necessary, oblique views should be obtained at this time to facilitate evaluation of the urinary bladder.

REFERENCES

1. Ackerman N: Intravenous pyelography. *JAAHA* 10:277-284, 1974.
2. Bartels JE: Feline intravenous urography. *JAAHA* 9:349-353, 1973.
3. Feeney DA, Barber DL, Osborne CA: Advances in canine excretory urography, in *Proceedings 30th Gaines Veterinary Symposium.* White Plains, NY, Gaines Dog Research Center, 1981, pp 8-22.
4. Johnston GR, Feeney DA, Osborne CA: Radiographic findings in urinary tract infection. *Vet Clin North Am* 9:749-774, 1979.
5. Kneller SK: Role of the excretory urogram in the diagnosis of renal and ureteral disease. *Vet Clin North Am* 4:843-861, 1974.
6. Root CR: Contrast radiography of the urinary system, in Ticer JW (ed): *Radiographic Technique in Small Animal Practice.* Philadelphia, WB Saunders Co, 1975, pp 396-414.
7. Watters JW: Urinary tract radiography—Kidneys and ureters. *Compend Contin Educ Pract Vet* 2(3):224-231, 1980.
8. Barber DL, Finco DR: Radiographic findings in induced bacterial pyelonephritis in dogs. *JAVMA* 175:1183-1190, 1979.
9. Saxton HM: Review article: Urography. *Br J Radiol* 42:321-346, 1969.
10. Thrall DE, Finco DR: Canine excretory urography: Is quality a function of BUN? *JAAHA* 12:446-450, 1976.
11. Lord PF, Scott RC, Chan KF: Intravenous urography for the evaluation of renal diseases in small animals. *JAAHA* 10:139-152, 1974.
12. Feeney DA, Thrall DE, Barber DL, et al: Normal canine excretory urogram: Effects of dose, time and individual dog variation. *Am J Vet Res* 40:1596-1604, 1979.
13. Fry IK, Cattell WR: The nephrographic pattern during excretory urography. *Br Med Bull* 28:227-232, 1972.
14. Older RA, Kobobkin M, Cleeve DM, et al: Contrast-induced acute renal failure. *Am J Roentgenol* 134:339-342, 1980.
15. Newhouse JH, Pfister RC: The nephrogram. *Radiol Clin North Am* 17:213-226, 1979.
16. Feeney DA, Barber DL, Osborne CA: The functional aspects of the nephrogram in excretory urography: A review. *Vet Radiol*, in press.
17. Ansari Z, Baldwin DS: Acute renal failure due to radiocontrast agents. *Nephron* 17:28-40, 1976.
18. Byrd L, Sherman RL: Radiocontrast-induced acute renal failure. *Medicine* 58:270-278, 1979.
19. Van Zee BE, Hoy WE, Talley TE, Jaenike JR: Renal injury associated with intravenous pyelography in non-diabetic and diabetic patients. *Ann Intern Med* 89:51-54, 1978.
20. Biery DN: The upper urinary tract, in O'Brien TR (ed): *Radiographic Diagnosis of Abdominal Disorders in the Dog and Cat.* Philadelphia, WB Saunders Co, 1978, pp 481-542.
21. Feeney DA, Osborne CA, Jessen CR: Effect of multiple excretory urograms on glomerular filtration of normal dogs. A preliminary report. *Am J Vet Res* 41:960-963, 1980.
22. Feeney DA, Barber DL, Johnston GR, Osborne CA: The excretory urogram: Part I. Techniques, normal radiographic appearance, and misinterpretation. *Compend Contin Educ Pract Vet* 4(3):233-243, 1982.
23. Feeney DA, Barber DL, Culver DH, et al: Canine excretory urogram: Correlation with base-line measurements. *Am J Vet Res* 41:279-283, 1980.

Urethrography and Cystography in Cats Part I. Techniques, Normal Radiographic Anatomy, and Artifacts

Gary R. Johnston, DVM, MS
Daniel A. Feeney, DVM, MS
Carl A. Osborne, DVM, PhD

Department of Small Animal Clinical Sciences
University of Minnesota
College of Veterinary Medicine
St. Paul, Minnesota

The feline urologic syndrome (FUS) (cystitis, urethritis, and urethral obstruction syndrome) is the most common disorder of the urinary tract of cats. Investigations into possible causes have primarily been related to viral, bacterial, or dietery factors that may influence the disease. The radiographic findings in cats with FUS have not been adequately reported. This shortcoming is related to the absence of a standardized technique for cystography and urethrography in cats. The purpose of this article is to (1) describe simple inexpensive techniques of cystography and urethrography in cats, (2) illustrate the normal radiographic appearance of the feline cystogram and urethrogram, and (3) describe and illustrate the technical pitfalls of cystography and urethrography that may simulate the radiographic appearance of inflammatory or neoplastic disease.

The clinical manifestations, incidence, pathogenesis, and medical and/or surgical management of FUS have been described.[1-16] Although a great quantity of information about FUS has been published, the use of different criteria by different investigators in defining this syndrome has resulted in some confusion. The syndrome is primarily encountered in male cats, but females are also affected. The site of urethral obstruction in male cats has been reported to be near the bulbourethral gland,[2] in the membranous (postprostatic) urethra,[2] in the penile urethra,[2] and/or at the tip of the glans penis.[17] Urethral obstruction rarely occurs in female cats. The lumen of the male cat's urethra narrows at the ischiatic arch caudal to the bulbourethral gland and is reported to be a frequent site of obstruction.[2,16,17] However, this report has not been verified in a large series of patients by radiographic techniques. Case reports and textbook reviews of FUS suggest sporadic occurrence of lesions elsewhere, but their frequency of occurrence and significance remain unclear.

Techniques

The paucity of information related to the radiographic appearance of the lower urinary tract (especially the urethra) of cats with FUS is related, at least in part, to technical difficulty in obtaining diagnostic contrast urethrocystograms. To better define the radiographic appearance

Originally published in Volume 4, Number 10, October 1982

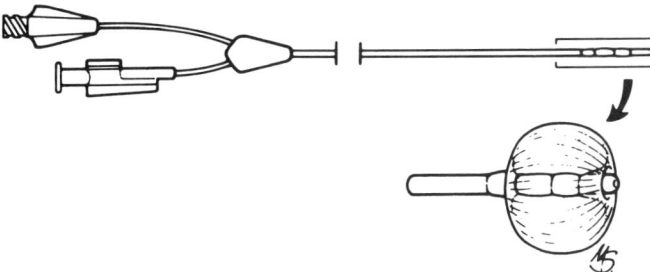

Figure 1—Swan-Ganz flow-directed balloon catheter used for retrograde urethrography in cats.

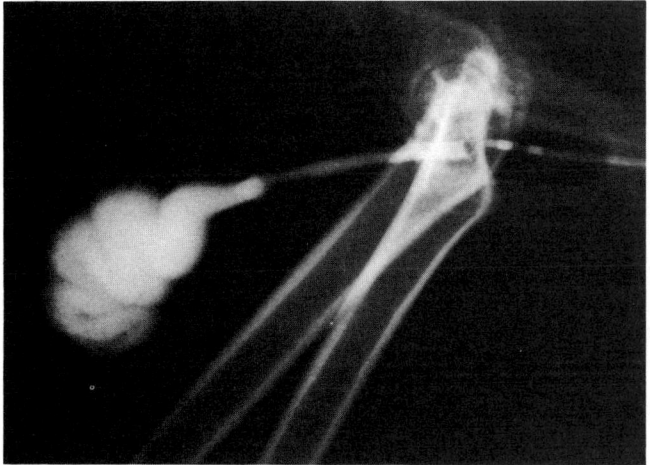

Figure 2—Lateral radiograph of a normal retrograde urethrogram on an adult female domestic shorthair cat. The use of a sterile aqueous lubricant as a diluent increases the viscosity of the contrast medium and facilitates distention of the urethral lumen. The incomplete mixing of the aqueous lubricant and diluted contrast medium with the urinary bladder contents frequently results in a wavy layered radiographic appearance of the positive contrast medium.

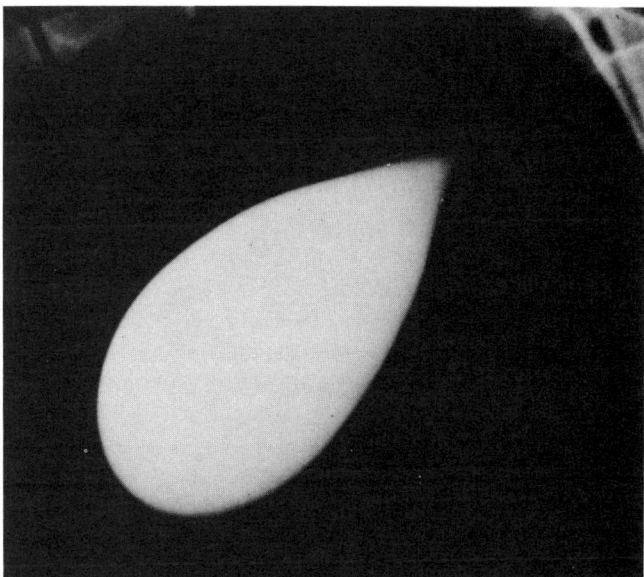

Figure 3—Normal positive contrast cystogram on a two-year-old castrated male domestic shorthair cat. The normal feline urinary bladder varies in configuration depending on the degree of urinary bladder distention. Note smooth mucosal contrast medium margin and tear-shaped configuration.

of the lower urinary tract of cats with FUS and to localize the site(s) of various abnormalities, a standard protocol for survey and contrast radiographic technique was devised to permit detailed evaluation of the urinary bladder and urethra and to permit comparison of the diagnostic usefulness of different techniques. To obtain radiographs of diagnostic quality within the same time frame, the following sequence was adopted: (1) survey radiography, (2) pneumocystography, (3) double contrast cystography, (4) positive contrast retrograde urethrocystography, and (5) positive contrast antegrade (voiding) urethrography.

Patient Preparation

Proper preparation of the patient is essential to optimal radiographic visualization of urinary tract lesions. Because some radiographic alterations are subtle, it is essential that intestines contain no ingesta and little or no gas. This is especially important if contrast procedures are to be performed. Overnight fasting and a cleansing enema are recommended prior to elective radiography. Water should be available throughout the fasting period.

Pharmacologic restraint is usually necessary to obtain satisfactory films and to minimize the possibility of iatrogenic trauma to the urethra and/or urinary bladder. The authors routinely use ketamine hydrochloride[a] or thiamylal sodium.[b]

Survey lateral and ventrodorsal radiographs should be obtained for evaluation of patient preparation, radiographic technique, and lesions that may be obscured or distorted by contrast radiography.

Prior to contrast radiography the bladder should be emptied by manual compression or with the aid of a 3.5 French catheter.[c] Failure to empty urine from the bladder may simulate bladder-wall thickening during pneumocystography. A "jet stream" encountered during positive contrast retrograde urethrography also may simulate mural thickening because of the incomplete mixing of the positive contrast medium and urine.

Pneumocystography

The authors recommend that the technique of pneumocystography incorporate both partial and complete distention of the urinary bladder with negative contrast media of air, CO_2, or nitrous oxide to aid in detection of small mural lesions. Although embolization may occur following injection of air into the lower urinary tract,[18] in the authors' experience with thousands of cases it has been rare. A lateral radiograph should be obtained after 5 to 8 ml of negative contrast medium have been infused into the urinary bladder via a catheter. Lateral views of a partially distended bladder have been

[a]Ketaset®, Bristol Laboratories, Syracuse, NY 13201.
[b]Bio-tal®, Bio-Ceutic Laboratories, Inc., St. Joseph, MO 64502.
[c]Sovereign Sterile Disposable Feeding Tube and Urethral Catheter, Sherwood Medical Industries Inc., St. Louis, MO 63103.

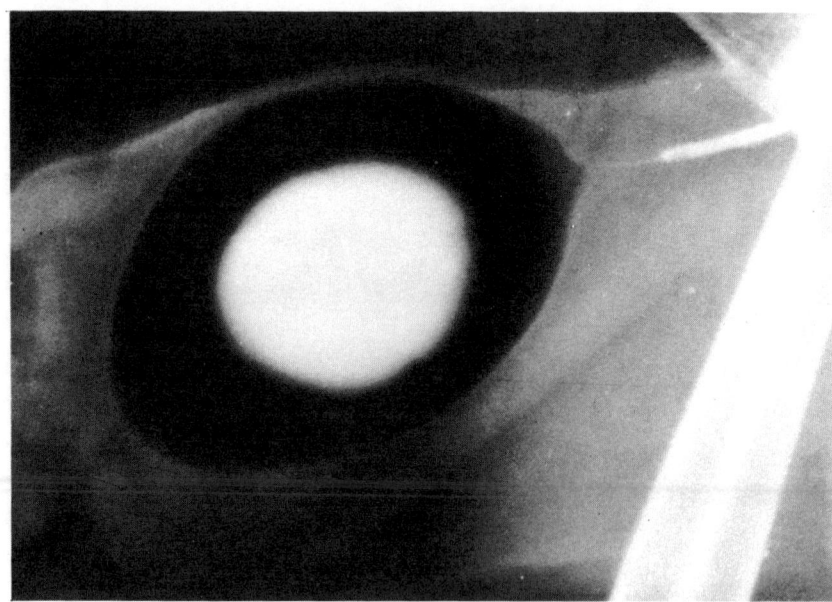

Figure 4—Normal double contrast cystogram of a 14-year-old spayed female domestic shorthair cat. With adequate urinary bladder distention, the urinary bladder wall should have a smooth uniform thickness. The positive contrast medium in the double contrast cystogram should have a smooth interface with the mucosa of the urinary bladder.

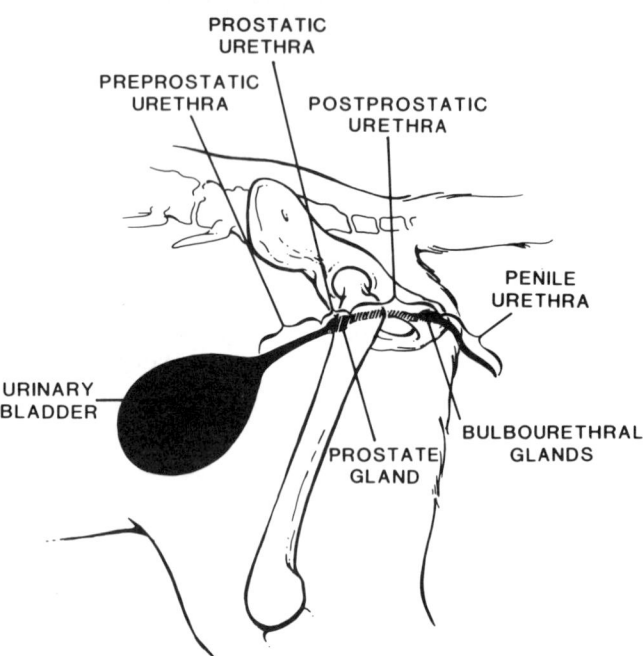

Figure 5—Drawing of the normal urethra and bladder of a male cat. Anatomical areas of the urethra illustrated in this drawing are not all identifiable on radiographs.

beneficial in demonstrating small urachal diverticula that were not obvious after complete distention of the bladder. Following complete distention of the bladder lumen, lateral and ventrodorsal radiographs should be obtained. Maximum distention of the urinary bladder varies in cats with FUS. Volumes of 15 to 45 ml may be obtained without spontaneous voiding in sedated or anesthetized cats. However, absolute values for volume distention should be used with caution because of possible iatrogenic bladder rupture and air embolism. Digital palpation of the bladder, and signs of patient discomfort including abdominal compression and flexion of the rear legs should be used to determine whether the degree of bladder distention is sufficient.

Some cats with inflammatory lower urinary tract disease may be unable to tolerate complete distention of the urinary bladder. If spontaneous voiding occurs following partial distention of the bladder lumen, further attempts to distend the bladder with negative contrast medium are likely to result in spontaneous micturition. Removal of the bladder contents and infusion of 1 to 2 ml of lidocaine hydrochloride[d] may provide sufficient topical anesthesia to permit the desired degree of distention.

Double Contrast Cystography

Following pneumocystography, a double contrast cystogram can be obtained by infusion of 0.25 to 0.75 ml of positive contrast medium into the bladder lumen via a catheter. The authors prefer undiluted meglumine diatrizoate[e] or meglumine iothalamate,[f] although other aqueous organic triiodinated compounds used for intravascular injections may be used. Lateral and ventrodorsal radiographs should be obtained, as described in the section on pneumocystography. This small quantity of contrast material accumulates in the dependent portion of the urinary bladder and facilitates detection of radiolucent free intraluminal filling defects. It also aids in detection of dependent mucosal irregularities that cannot be identified by survey radiography or pneumocystography. Because no effort is made to coat the entire mucosal surface with contrast medium, small mucosal abnormalities may not be observed. If subtle mucosal lesions are suspected, additional views which are intermediate in position to lateral and ventrodorsal views (so-called oblique views) should be obtained. Distention of the bladder lumen with positive contrast

[d]Xylocaine® 2%, Astra Pharmaceutical Products Inc., Worcester, MA 01606.
[e]Hypaque® Meglumine 60%, Winthrop Laboratories, New York, NY 10016.
[f]Conray®, Mallinckrodt Chemical Works, St. Louis, MO 66134.

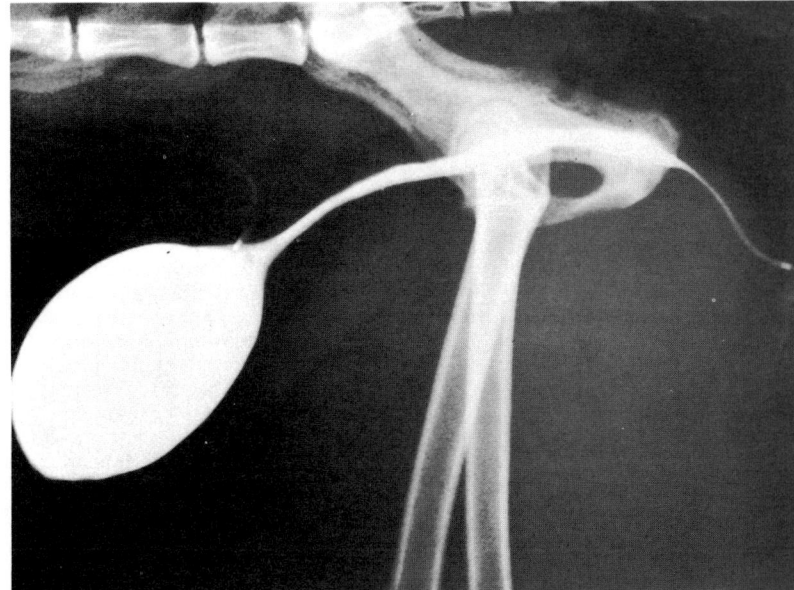

Figure 6A

Figure 6—Normal urethrogram of a four-year-old castrated male domestic shorthair cat. The normal radiographic appearance of the urethra varies depending on the technique of urethrography. Note bilateral vesicourethral reflux. (**A**) Normal retrograde urethrogram.

Figure 6—(**B**) Normal antegrade (voiding) urethrogram performed by external bladder compression using a wooden spoon.

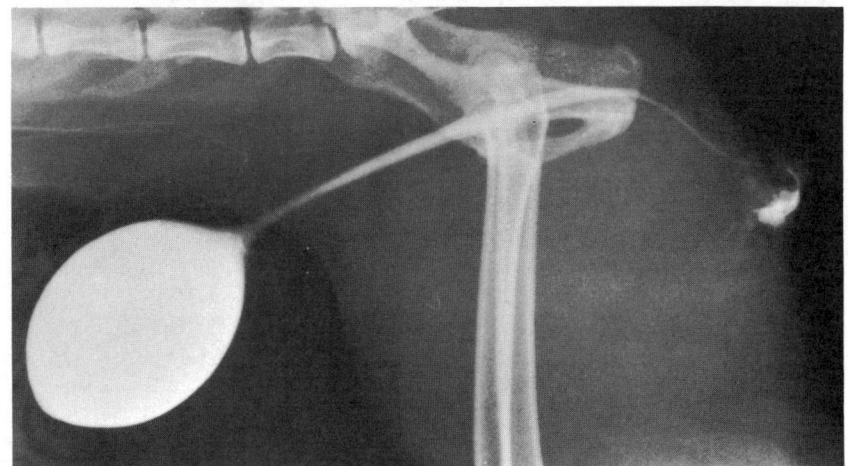

Figure 6B

medium (positive contrast cystography) may also be considered.

Positive Contrast Retrograde Urethrocystography

Positive contrast cystography and/or urethrocystography should follow pneumocystography and double contrast cystography for the evaluation of urethral and bladder lesions. Intraluminal, mural, and extraluminal urethral lesions are best defined by positive contrast urethrography. In addition, the positive contrast cystogram or urethrocystogram can detect small urachal diverticula that may not be detectable with negative contrast agents. Mucosal tears and lacerations are better demonstrated by the positive contrast media. Positive contrast media also eliminate the risk of fatal air embolization.

Following double contrast cystography, the bladder contents should be removed. A sufficient quantity of a 5% solution of aqueous positive contrast medium should be infused into the urinary bladder to induce moderate

distention of its lumen. The urinary catheter should then be removed. Lateral and ventrodorsal views of the lower urinary tract should be obtained. Alternatively, they may be obtained following distention of the urethra with contrast medium.

Moderate distention of the urinary bladder with positive contrast medium is required to provide sufficient intraluminal pressure to ensure maximum distention of the proximal portion of the urethra during retrograde urethrography. (Complications of this procedure will be discussed in Part II of this article.) The volume of contrast medium required to distend the bladder lumen should be similar to that required to distend it with gas during pneumocystography.

Several techniques for contrast urethrography may be considered. Retrograde or antegrade studies utilizing balloon or nonballoon catheters are recommended for male cats. A 4 French balloon catheter[g] (Figure 1) or a

[g]Swan-Ganz, Flow Directed Balloon Catheter, Edwards Laboratories, Santa Ana, CA 92711.

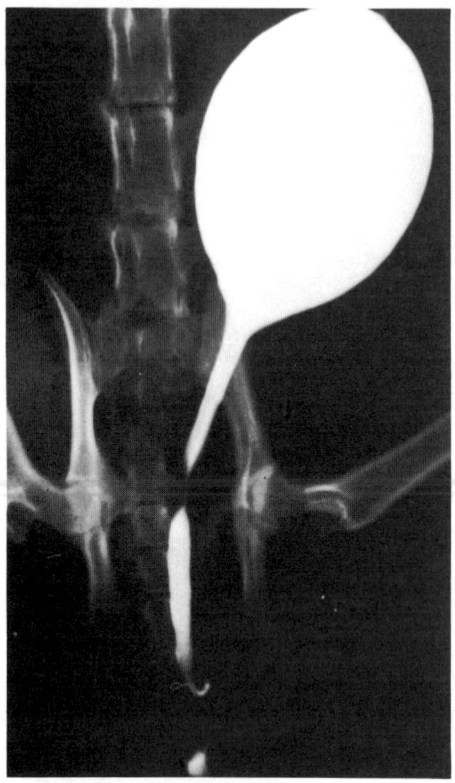

Figure 7A

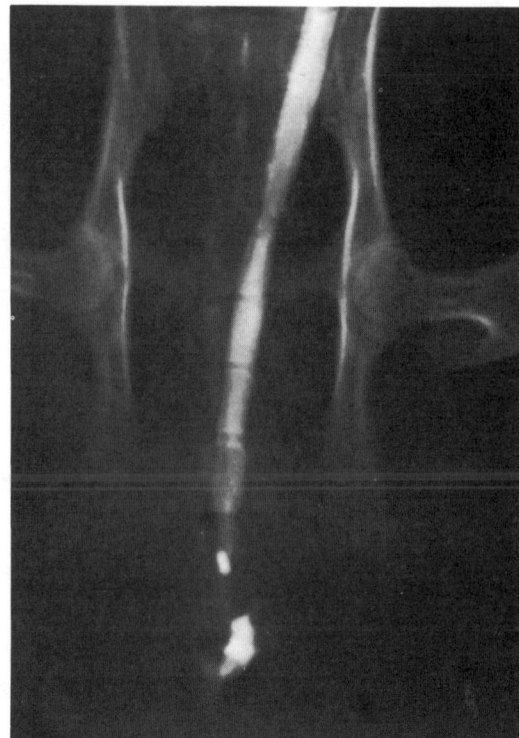

Figure 7B

Figure 7—Ventrodorsal radiographs of positive contrast retrograde urethrograms on a two-year-old male Siamese cat. (**A**) An abrupt narrowing of the prostatic urethra which simulates a partial urethral obstruction is frequently encountered with retrograde urethrography. (**B**) The prostatic urethral luminal narrowing encountered during retrograde urethrography subsequently distended during antegrade urethrography. Suspected urethral strictures should be confirmed and differentiated from spasm by using both retrograde and antegrade urethrography.

Figure 8—Lateral radiographs of a retrograde urethrogram on a nine-year-old spayed female domestic shorthair cat. (**A**) Two milliliters of positive contrast medium infused into the urinary bladder resulted in insufficient intravesical pressure to distend the urethral lumen.

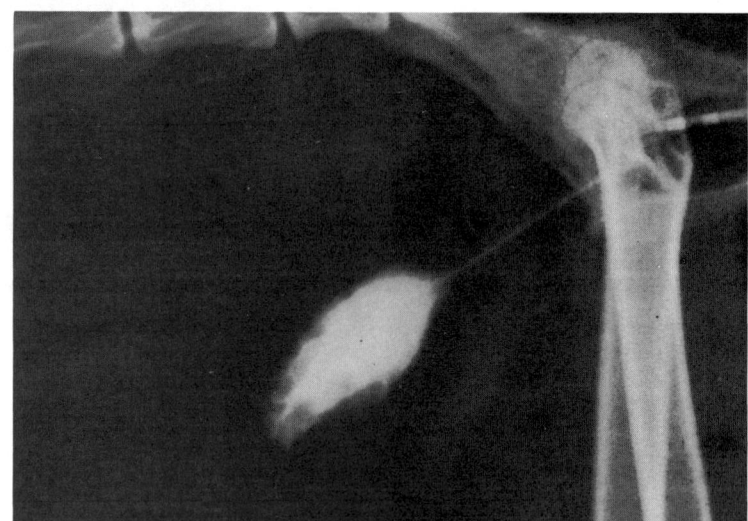

Figure 8A

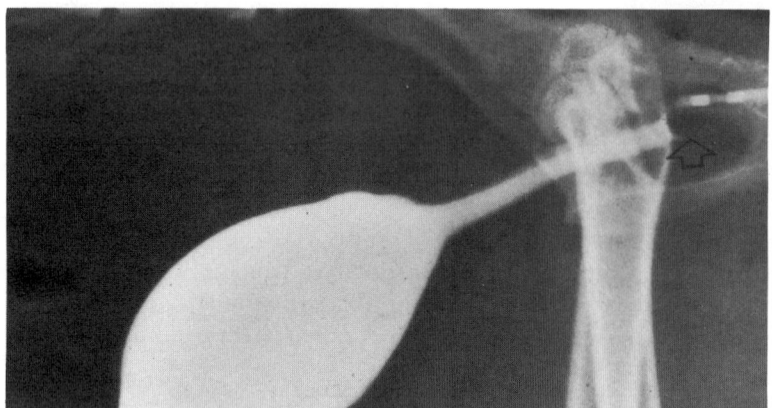

Figure 8B

Figure 8—(**B**) Greater distention of the urinary bladder with positive contrast medium via an inflated balloon catheter (*arrow*) resulted in sufficient intravesical hydrostatic pressure to ensure urethral distention.

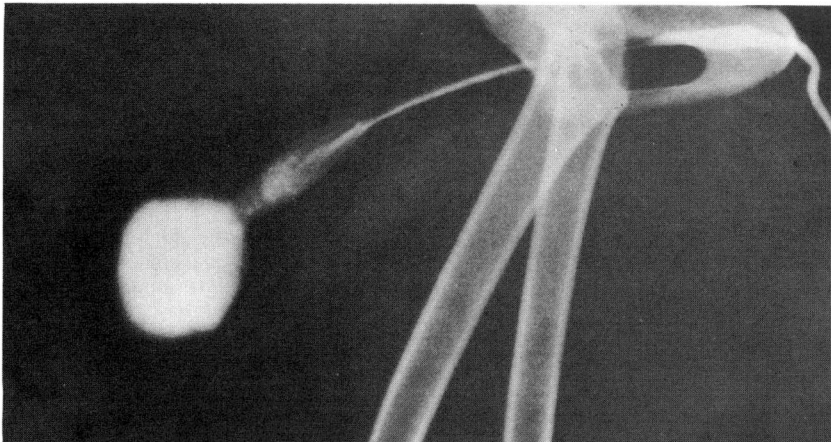

Figure 9A

Figure 9—This series of urethrograms was obtained on a four-year-old male domestic shorthair cat. (**A**) Inadequate urinary bladder distention prior to urethrography has resulted in incomplete luminal distention of the proximal urethra. Failure to remove the contents of the urinary bladder also resulted in a "jet stream" effect of the positive contrast medium, which mimics a mural lesion.

Figure 9—(**B**) Further infusion of positive contrast media into the urinary bladder provided sufficient intravesical hydrostatic pressure to ensure distention of the proximal urethral lumen. Mixing of the urine with the contrast medium has eliminated the previously encountered pseudomural filling defect.

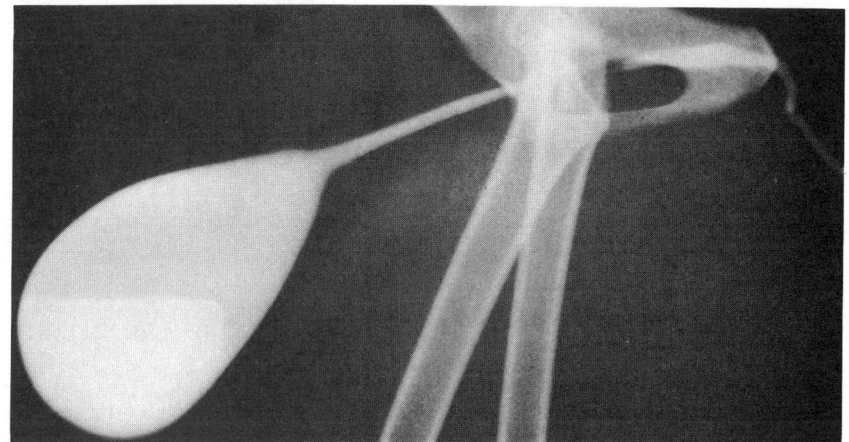

Figure 9B

3.5 French tomcat urethral catheter[h] has been satisfactory. Balloon-tipped catheters have a distinct advantage over other types of urethral catheters in that they prevent reflux of contrast medium through the urethral orifice, thus ensuring proper filling of the urethral lumen proximal to the inflated balloon. Retrograde urethrography in male cats in which a urethral catheter is secured in the penile urethra by external digital compression is not recommended because of potential exposure of personnel to ionizing radiation. Retrograde urethrography of female cats can be performed with the aid of a 4 or 5 French balloon catheter.[g] Satisfactory retrograde urethrograms of the female urethra cannot be obtained with other types of urethral catheters because of reflux of contrast medium around the catheter with subsequent loss through the urethral orifice.

The aqueous organic iodinated contrast media used for contrast cystography are also recommended for contrast urethrography. However, the contrast medium should be diluted 1:3 with sterile distilled water or saline. Reduction of the radiodensity of the contrast medium aids in detection of filling defects that otherwise may be obscured by using undiluted contrast media.

Sterile aqueous lubricants[i,j] may be mixed with contrast medium (one part contrast medium to one part sterile saline or distilled water to one part aqueous lubricant) to increase its viscosity and promote distention of the urethral lumen (Figure 2).

The lumen of the balloon catheter should be filled with contrast medium prior to its placement in the urethra to prevent artifacts caused by air bubbles. Care should also be used with balloon catheters to prevent iatrogenic trauma and infection of the urinary tract.

To perform retrograde positive contrast urethrocystography in male cats, the penile urethra is exteriorized and a 4 French balloon catheter is inserted approximately 1.5 cm into the urethral lumen. Lubrication of the catheter tip with an anesthetic lubricant[k] facilitates catheter placement. Inflation of the balloon with 0.5 ml of air helps stabilize the catheter's location. The balloon should not be placed just inside the urethral orifice because the small diameter of the penile urethra at this site will prevent sufficient inflation of the balloon to maintain the catheter's position.

---

[h]Sovereign Open End Tom Cat Catheter, Sherwood Medical Industries Inc., St. Louis, MO 63103.

[i]K-Y jelly®, Johnson & Johnson Products, New Brunswick, NJ 08903.
[j]Lubafax®, Burroughs Wellcome Co., Research Triangle Park, NC 27709.
[k]Xylocaine 2% Jelly, Astra Pharmaceutical Products Inc., Worcester, MA 01606.

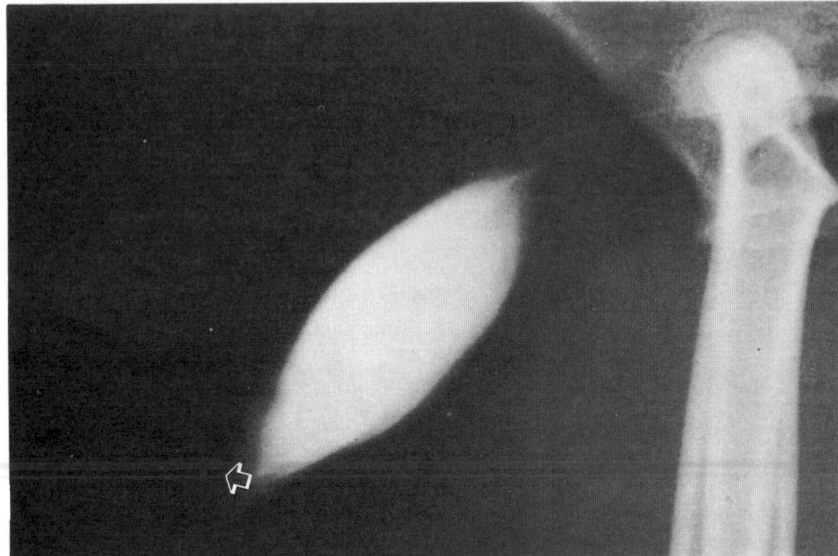

Figure 10—Lateral positive contrast cystogram on a four-year-old spayed female domestic shorthair cat. (**A**) Improper catheter placement and incomplete distention have resulted in abnormal bladder configuration due to either smooth muscle spasms or catheter pressure. The catheter extends to the cranial tip of the bladder (*arrow*).

Figure 10A

Figure 10—(**B**) Subsequent catheter withdrawal to the trigone area and further bladder distention resulted in a smooth contour of the urinary bladder wall except for a small remnant of the urachal diverticulum (*arrow*). Pooling of contrast medium in the vagina and vestibule distal to the external urethral orifice is a normal finding with voiding cystourethrography.

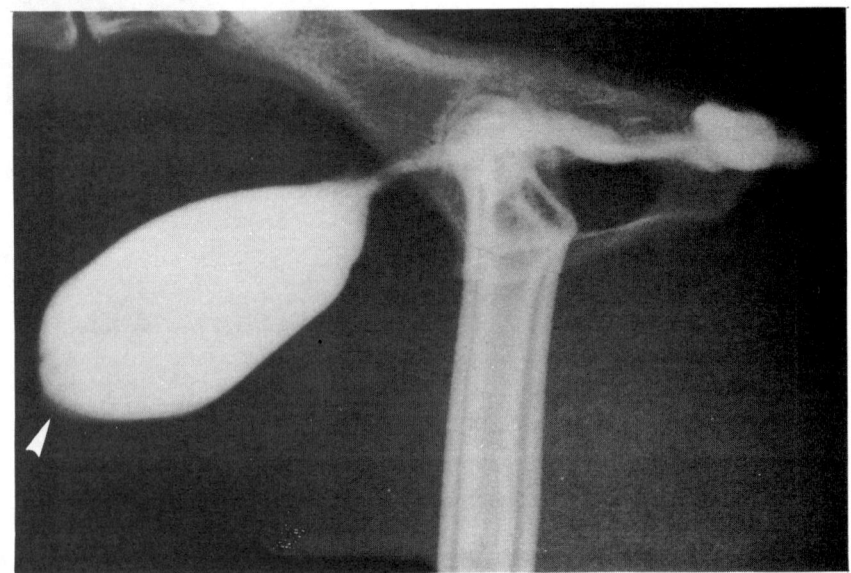

Figure 10B

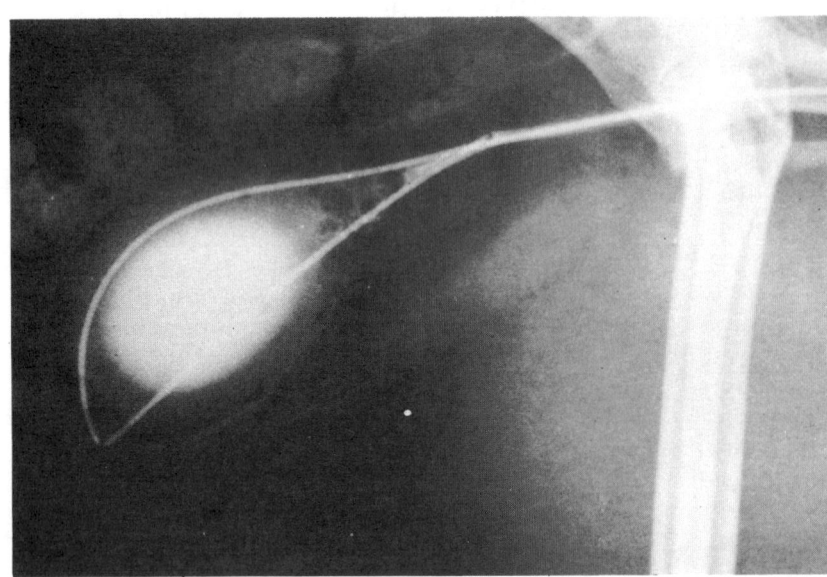

Figure 11—Lateral cystogram on an eight-year-old castrated male domestic longhair cat. Improper placement of nonflexible urethral catheter may cause catheter kinking and may result in bladder and/or urethral trauma. A cystotomy was necessary for removal of the catheter.

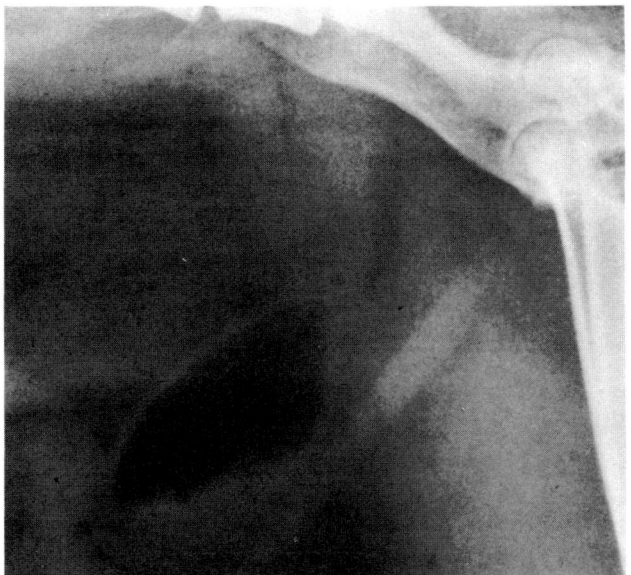

Figure 12A

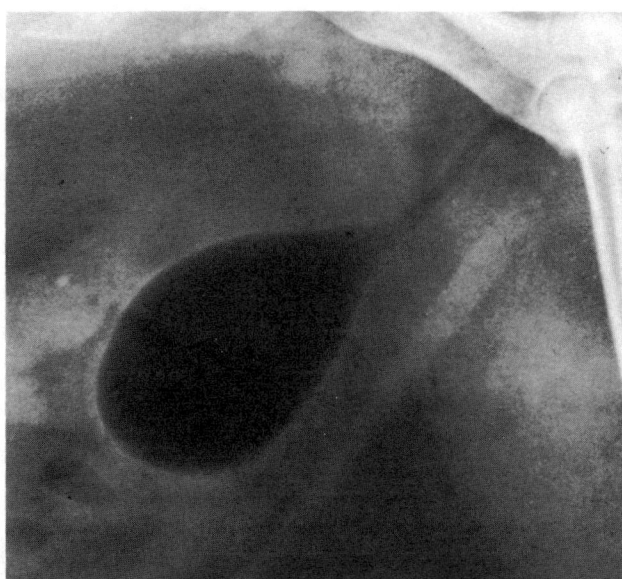

Figure 12B

Figure 12—Inadequate distention of the urinary bladder during cystography or urethrography can result in mural pseudolesions simulating inflammatory or neoplastic disease. This series of pneumocystograms was of an eight-year-old domestic shorthair cat. **(A)** Inadequate urinary bladder distention during pneumocystography resulted in an area of cranioventral thickening suggestive of neoplastic or inflammatory disease. **(B)** Subsequent gas distention of the urinary bladder during pneumocystography has eliminated the previously suspected mural lesion.

Injection of 2 to 3 ml of iodinated contrast medium ensures complete filling of the urethral lumen but may not cause maximal distention. To facilitate maximal distention of the urethral lumen, the radiographs should be obtained slightly before injection of contrast medium through the catheter has been completed.

The procedure for retrograde positive contrast urethrocystography in female cats is similar to that described for male cats. The tip of the balloon catheter should be placed just inside the external urethral orifice. Positioning of the catheter may be verified with the aid of a small otoscope speculum.

Positive Contrast Antegrade (Voiding) Urethrography

Use of balloon catheters for retrograde positive contrast urethrography in nonobstructed cats prevents radiographic evaluation of the portion of the urethra occupied by and distal to the balloon. This portion of the urethra may be visualized by antegrade positive contrast urethrography if necessary. If positive contrast cystography precedes this phase of the study, the bladder will have been filled with contrast medium. If not, the bladder lumen should be distended with an appropriate quantity of aqueous iodinated contrast medium injected via a urinary catheter. Contrast medium can be forced into the urethra with abdominal compression using a wooden spoon placed over the abdomen at a site adjacent to the bladder. Abdominal compression can be induced at the appropriate time by pressing the handle downward. Exposure of the lateral view of the entire lower urinary tract at the time of induced micturition enables evaluation of the distal urethra and the competence of vesicoureteral valves. External abdominal compression

with a wooden spoon may produce some distortion of the bladder and proximal urethra.

Antegrade positive contrast urethrocystography may also be considered for evaluation of the urethral lumen of cats that are difficult to catheterize or whose urethral lumina are obstructed. The technique does not require balloon catheters. The urinary bladder is distended with contrast medium either by excretory urography or percutaneous transabdominal bladder infusion via cystocentesis using a 22-gauge, 3-in. spinal needle.[1] Following distention of the bladder, antegrade urethrography can be performed in the manner described for cats without urethral obstruction. Contrast medium may be forced into the urethral lumen by external abdominal bladder compression or by spontaneous initiation of the micturition reflex which can be induced by gradual distention of the urinary bladder during light-plane anesthesia of the cat. Although external abdominal compression of the bladder with a wooden spoon is preferred, some degree of distortion of the bladder and proximal urethra commonly occurs. Appropriate caution should be used to prevent iatrogenic bladder rupture.

Selection of Technique

To compare the diagnostic usefulness of the various radiographic techniques for evaluating the urinary bladder and urethra, each of the described procedures was performed. Although the procedures complement each other and together permit extensive and complete evaluation of the lower urinary tract, it is impractical and usually unnecessary to perform all of the described studies. The authors' recommendations include a min-

---

[1]Spinal Needle, Becton-Dickinson, Rutherford, NJ 07070.

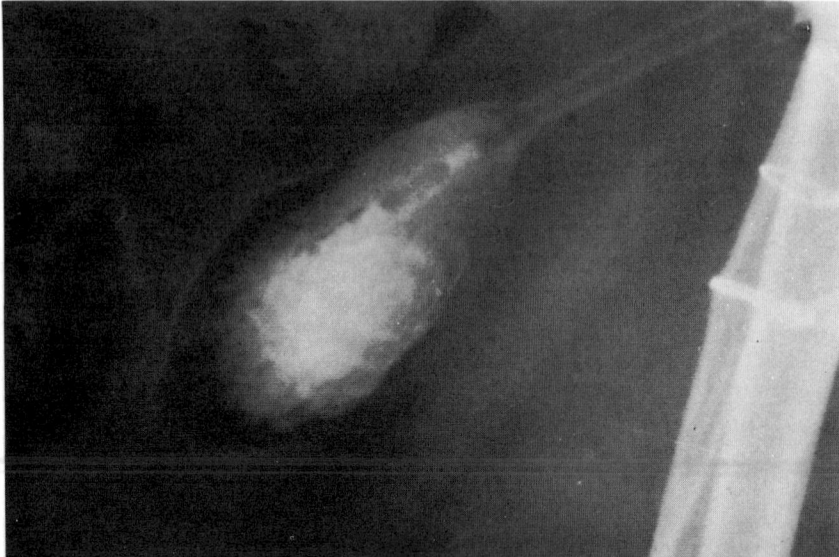

Figure 13A

Figure 13—Lateral radiograph of a double contrast cystogram of a six-year-old spayed female domestic shorthair cat. (**A**) Inadequate urinary bladder distention has resulted in an irregular mucosal contrast medium pattern in the dependent portion of the bladder. Diffuse bladder-wall thickening also appears to be present. These findings mimic inflammatory disease of the urinary bladder.

Figure 13—(**B**) Subsequent distention of the urinary bladder has resulted in a normal mucosal pattern and bladder wall thickness.

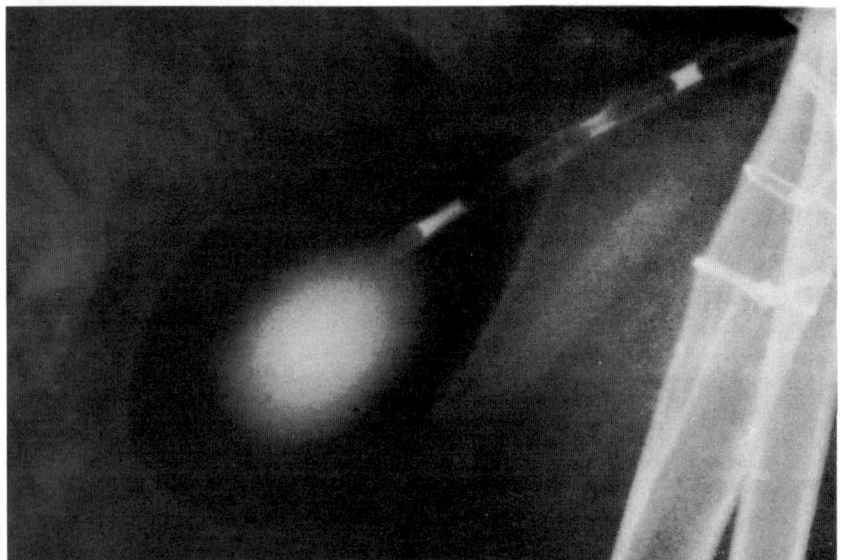

Figure 13B

imum of eight radiographs: a ventrodorsal and lateral view for two survey radiographs, two for double contrast cystography, two for retrograde urethrography, and two lateral radiographs for antegrade urethrography and partial-distention pneumocystography. They have not evaluated pneumourethrography or double contrast urethrography as diagnostic techniques for urethral disorders because all urethral lesions were considered adequately demonstrated by positive contrast antegrade or retrograde urethrography.

Normal Radiographic Anatomy
Urinary Bladder

The normal feline urinary bladder may be ovoid, ellipsoid, or teardrop-shaped depending on its degree of distention (Figures 3 and 4). The wall of the urinary bladder is normally smooth and has a uniform thickness when distended (Figures 3 and 4). In double contrast cystograms, positive contrast medium in the dependent portion of the bladder lumen has a smooth contour at its interface with the bladder wall (Figure 4).

Urethra

The urethra of male cats may be divided into several anatomical regions on the basis of location and microscopic appearance. They are the (1) preprostatic urethra, (2) prostatic urethra, (3) postprostatic urethra, and (4) penile urethra (Figure 5). Radiographically, the urethra may be divided into (1) the intrapelvic urethra (including preprostatic, prostatic, and postprostatic urethra) and (2) the penile urethra (Figure 6). The normal prostatic urethra is occasionally seen as a narrowed area in the mid-pelvic urethra (Figure 7). Provided adequate pressure is induced in the bladder lumen by distention with contrast medium, the normal urethra of male cats has a continuous and uniformly smooth luminal surface. However, the normal diameter of the urethral lumen is variable. The maximum diameter of the penile urethra

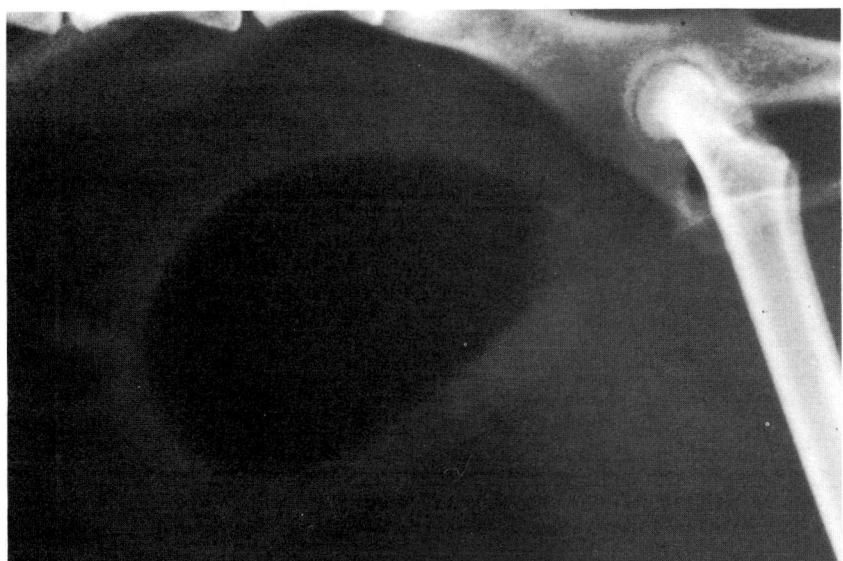

Figure 14A

Figure 14—Lateral radiographs of a four-year-old spayed female domestic shorthair cat. (**A**) Intraluminal filling defects with a fluid density may be obscured in the dependent portion of the urinary bladder with a pneumocystogram.

Figure 14—(**B**) Double contrast cystogram demonstrates two filling defects (blood clots) in the dependent portion of the urinary bladder which were not visible by pneumocystography or survey radiography.

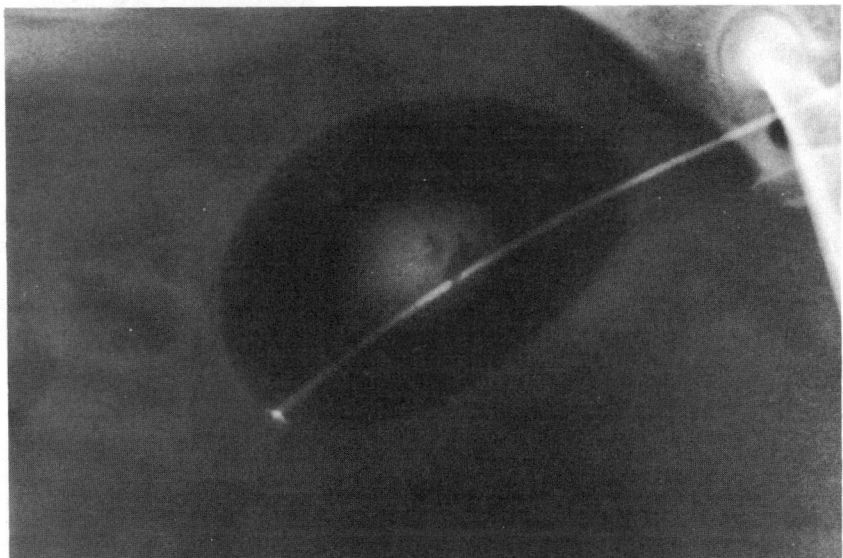

Figure 14B

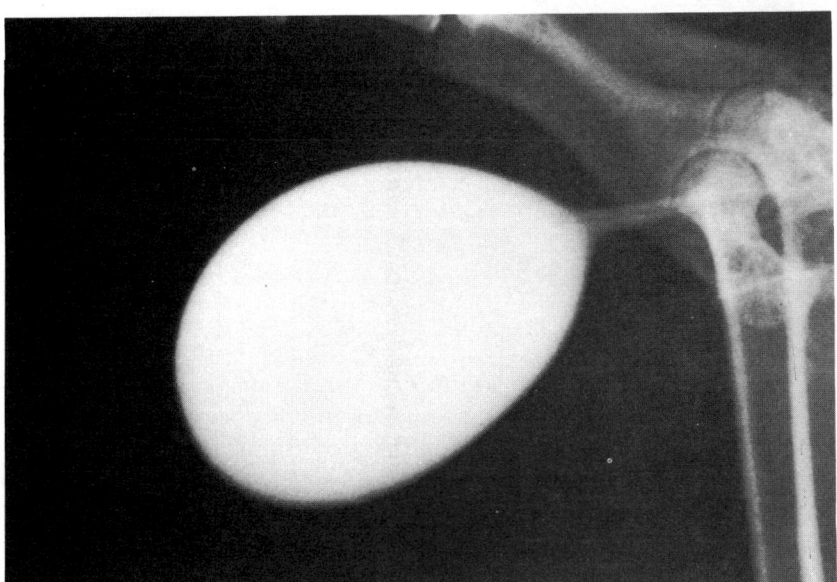

Figure 14C

Figure 14—(**C**) Use of undiluted positive contrast medium for urethrocystography also obscures the two filling defects in the dependent bladder previously seen with double contrast cystography.

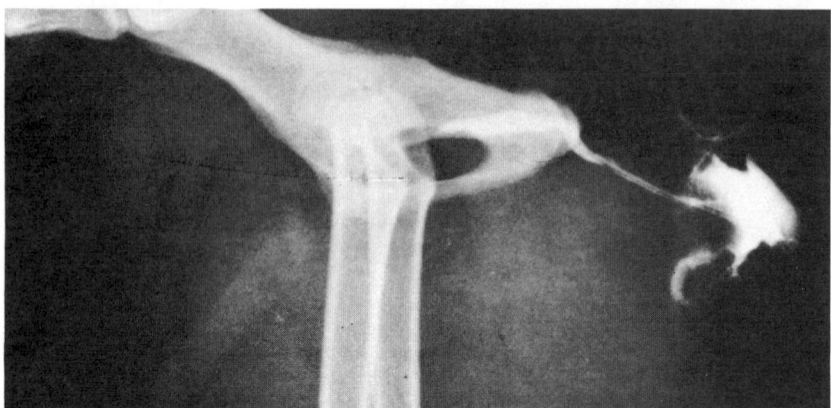

Figure 15A

Figure 15—Retrograde urethrograms on the cat in Figure 9. (**A**) The use of a nonballoon catheter for the retrograde injection of positive contrast medium resulted in pericatheter reflux of contrast medium and incomplete luminal distention of the proximal urethra. Incomplete filling of the proximal urethra could be misinterpreted as luminal obstruction.

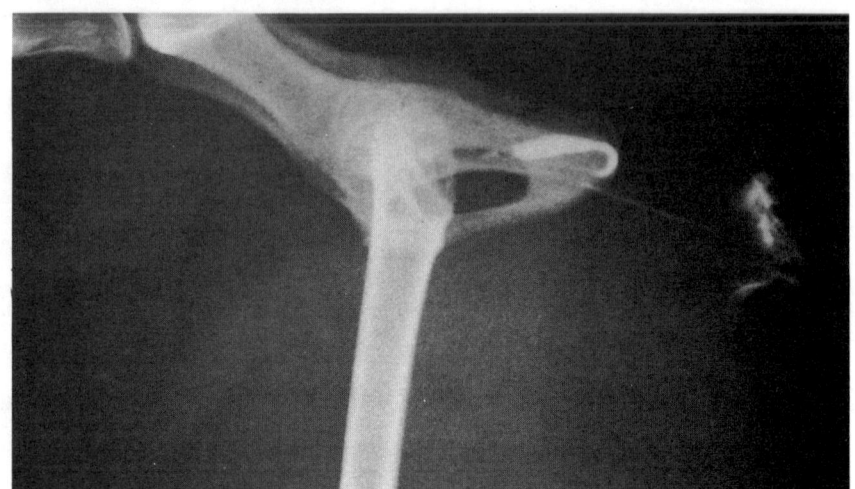

Figure 15—(**B**) Excessive external catheter pressure has caused a flexure in the penile urethra which has resulted in a partial obstruction of the urethral lumen and predisposes to incomplete luminal filling of the proximal urethra and pericatheter reflux.

Figure 15B

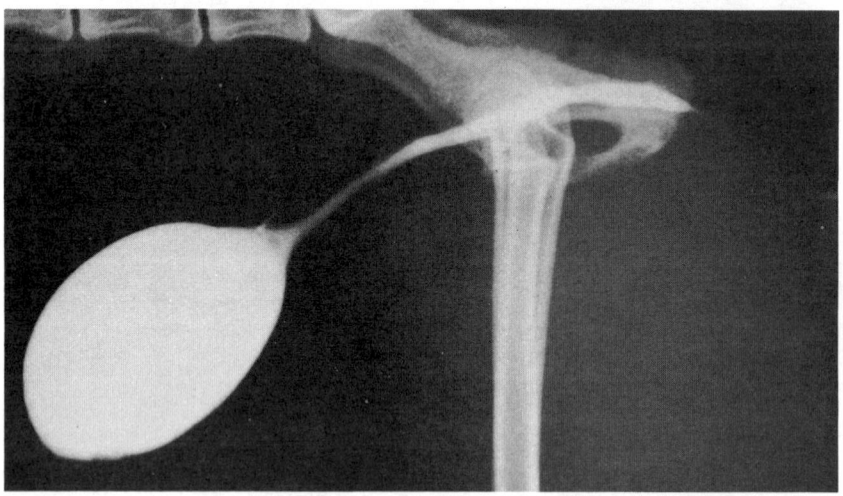

Figure 16—Retrograde urethrogram on the cat in Figure 6. Normal retrograde urethrogram with exposure occurring after the injection of contrast medium was completed. The incomplete filling of the penile urethra was a technical artifact resulting from failure to expose the x-ray film during the contrast medium injection. The filling defect at the bladder neck is an air bubble.

normally occurs at the level of the ischiatic arch. The diameter of the penile urethra becomes progressively smaller toward the external urethral orifice (Figure 6).

The urethra of normal female cats has a uniform diameter throughout its length (Figure 8). As in male cats, the mucosal surface is normally smooth.

Artifacts

Artifacts caused by improper technique during cys-

tography or urethrography may result in radiographic findings that mimic inflammatory or neoplastic conditions. Failure to remove the bladder contents prior to cystography or urethrography may result in pseudointraluminal or mural filling defects following infusion of the positive or negative contrast medium (Figure 9). For cystography, the catheter tip should be placed near the bladder neck, because improper catheter placement can result in an abnormally shaped urinary bladder

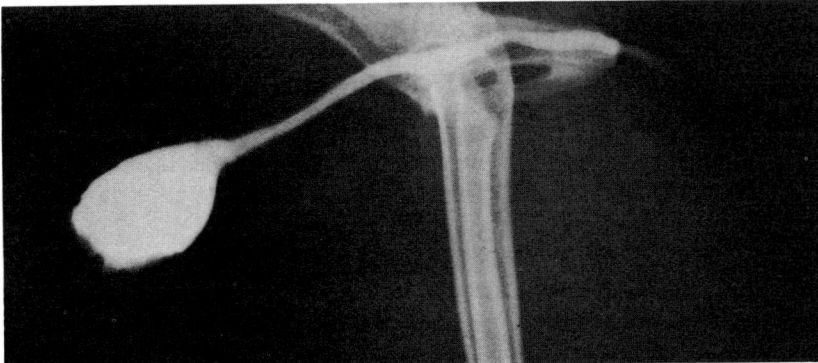

Figure 17A

Figure 17—Antegrade (voiding) contrast urethrocystograms on the cat in Figure 12. (**A**) Variations in urethral diameter are frequently encountered in voiding cystourethrography and may be caused by peristaltic contractions and/or urethral spasms. Note irregular thickening of the bladder wall caused by underdistention of the urinary bladder.

Figure 17—(**B**) Subsequent voiding cystourethrography performed by external abdominal bladder compression with a wooden spoon eliminated the variations in urethral diameter previously seen. The filling defect in the bladder is an air bubble. A slight amount of vesicoureteral reflux is present.

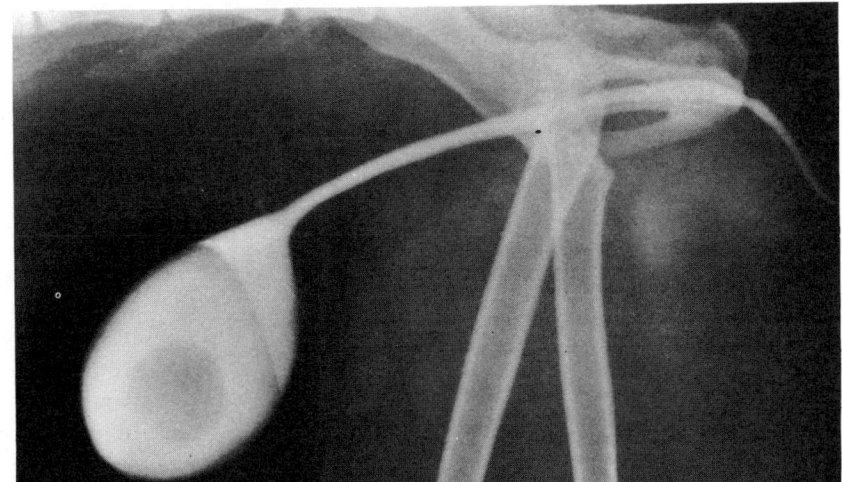

Figure 17B

(Figure 10) or catheter kinking (Figure 11). Inadequate urinary bladder distention, the most common technical pitfall, is associated with normal thickening of the bladder wall that often cannot be distinguished from abnormal bladder-wall thickening. Mural thickening associated with incomplete filling of the bladder may appear diffuse or localized and may simulate inflammation or neoplasia (Figures 12 and 13). Inadequate bladder distention may also result in an abnormally shaped urinary bladder because of extramural compression by contiguous structures. Normal mucosal irregularity suggesting inflammatory and/or neoplastic disease may also be encountered with inadequate bladder distention during double contrast or positive contrast cystography (Figures 8 and 13). A positive contrast cystogram obtained without a preceding pneumocystogram and double contrast cystogram may inhibit visualization of free intraluminal filling defects in the dependent portion of the urinary bladder (Figure 14). Excessive volumes of positive contrast media used in double contrast cystograms may similarly mask free intraluminal filling defects in the dependent portion of the urinary bladder.

Incomplete luminal distention of the urethra commonly occurs during retrograde urethrography of male and female cats. Incomplete urethral distention can be focal, segmental, or generalized and may be caused by technique or urethral disease. Voluntary contractions of the urethralis muscle at the ischiatic arch, smooth-muscle spasms, and peristaltic contractions are the most common causes of focal luminal narrowing and must be differentiated from a urethral stricture. The most common cause of segmental or generalized incomplete urethral distention is inadequate intravesical hydrostatic pressure prior to retrograde urethrography (Figures 8 and 9). Pericatheter reflux of contrast medium around nonballoon catheters is also a common cause of regional or segmental incomplete urethral distention (Figure 15A). Pericatheter reflux of contrast medium with nonballoon catheters used for retrograde urethrography may be influenced by excessive cranial catheter placement, which can result in an iatrogenic flexure of the penile urethra and subsequent partial or complete luminal obstruction (Figure 15B). A slight reduction in prostatic urethral luminal diameter may be encountered with retrograde injection and is considered normal (Figure 7A). Subsequent evaluation of the prostatic urethra with antegrade urethrography by external bladder compression further distends the prostatic urethral lumen (Figure 7B). Incomplete luminal filling in any part of the urethra may occur if the film is exposed after injection of the contrast medium (Figure 16).

Antegrade urethrography associated with spontaneous micturition around the urethral catheter or following gradual overdistention of the urinary bladder may

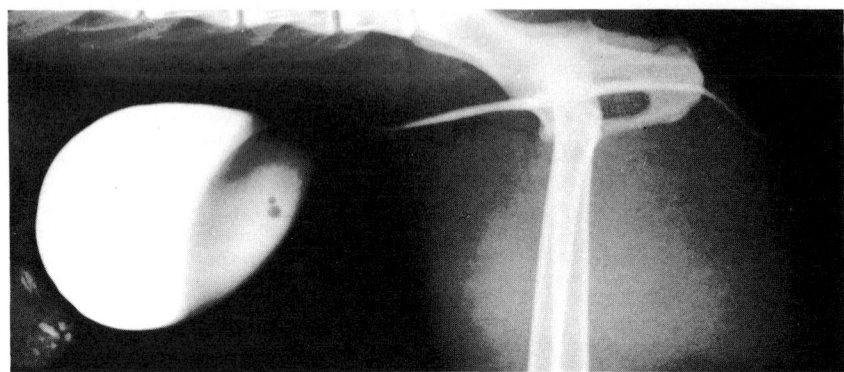

Figure 18—Lateral radiograph of an antegrade urethrogram on a six-year-old male domestic shorthair cat. Improper placement of the wooden spoon for abdominal compression has resulted in compression of the proximal urethra, which simulates urethral disease. Several air bubbles are present in the bladder.

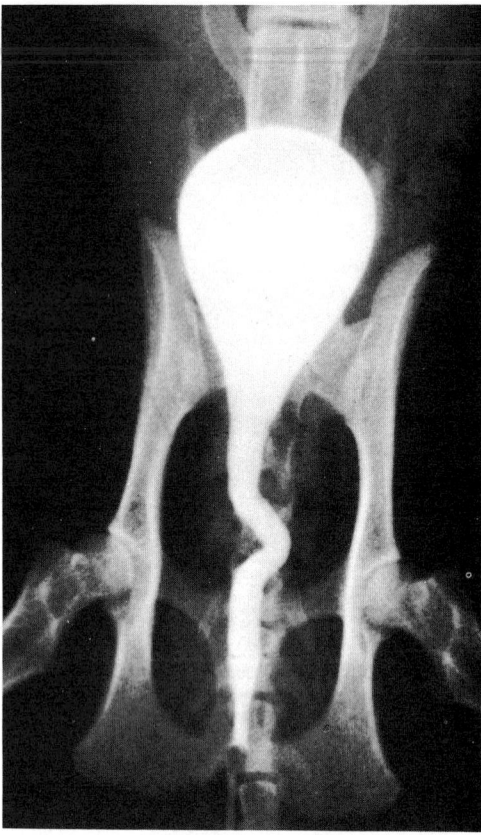

Figure 19—Ventrodorsal radiograph of a retrograde urethrogram on a three-year-old female domestic shorthair cat. The pressure of the abdominal contents on the distended urinary bladder has resulted in caudal displacement of the bladder and a secondary intrapelvic urethral flexure. Flexures, which may mimic extraurethral lesions, can be differentiated by subsequent urethrography with elevation of the caudal abdomen.

Although adequate distention of the urinary bladder is necessary to ensure urethral distention, iatrogenic urethral flexures may occur because of caudal bladder displacement by cranial abdominal contents. These urethral flexures may mimic urethral displacement by extraurethral lesions and may require further radiographic evaluation (Figure 19).

If a focal urethral stricture is suspected on the initial retrograde urethrogram, a second retrograde study preceded by intraluminal infusion of 0.25 to 0.75 ml of lidocaine hydrochloride may help differentiate a stricture from a urethral spasm. If the focal luminal narrowing persists, antegrade urethrography performed by external bladder compression will distend a nonstrictured urethra.

REFERENCES

1. Foster SJ: "Urolithiasis" syndrome in male cats. A statistical analysis of the problem with clinic observations. *J Small Anim Pract* 8:201-211, 1967.
2. Jackson OF: The treatment and subsequent prevention of struvite urolithiasis in cats. *J Small Anim Pract* 12:555-568, 1981.
3. Osborne CA, Lees G: Feline cystitis, urethritis, urethral obstruction syndrome. *Mod Vet Pract* 59:173-180; 349; 357; 513-520; 669-673, 1978.
4. Feline urolithiasis: Interim report. *Vet Rec* 96:298-299, 1975.
5. Jungreis T: Bladder stones in female cats. *Feline Pract* 5:7, 1975.
6. Pierce D: Feline urolithiasis: A case study. *Feline Pract* 4:30-31, 1974.
7. Lewis LD, Chow FHC, Taton GF, Hamer DW: Effect of various dietary mineral concentrations on the occurrence of feline urolithiasis. *JAVMA* 172:559-563, 1978.
8. Reif JS, Bovee K, Gaskell CJ, Batt RM, Maguire TG: Feline urethral obstruction: A case-control study. *JAVMA* 170:1320-1324, 1974.
9. Rich LJ: Current concepts of feline urethral obstruction. *Vet Clin North Am* 1:245-250, 1971.
10. Rich LJ, Dysart K, Chow FHC,, Hamer DW: Urethral obstruction in male cats: Experimental production by addition of magnesium and phosphate to the diet. *Feline Pract* 4(5):44-47, 1974.
11. Willeberg P: Interaction effects of epidemiologic factors in feline urologic syndrome. *Nord Vet Med* 28:193-200, 1976.
12. Gaskell PJ: Therapy for FUS. *J Small Anim Pract* 19:301, 1978.
13. Robinette JD: Silicone rubber prosthesis for replacement of the urethra of male cats. *JAVMA* 163:285-288, 1973.
14. Whitehead JE: Urolithiasis in the feline. *SAC* 1:307-319, 1961.
15. McCully RM, Lieberman LL: Histopathology in a case of feline urolithiasis. *Can Vet J* 2:52-61, 1961.
16. Richards DA, Hinci PJ, Morse EM: Feline perineal urethrostomy—A new technique for an old problem. *JAAHA* 8:66-73, 1972.
17. Meier FW: Urethral obstruction and stenosis in the male cat. *JAVMA* 137:67-70, 1960.
18. Zontine WJ, Andrews LK: Fatal air embolization as a complication of pneumocystography. *J Am Vet Radiol Soc* 19:8, 1978.

result in some areas of incomplete urethral distention because of peristaltic contractions or urethral spasms (Figure 17). Some distortion of the urinary bladder or urethra may occur with external bladder compression (Figure 18). Use of balloon catheters for retrograde injection of contrast media, use of sterile aqueous lubricants as diluents, or use of antegrade urethrography with external bladder compression will distend the urethra and facilitate differentiation of incomplete urethral distention (Figures 7, 9, and 17).

Order Information and Order Form

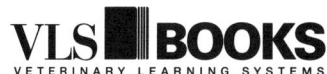

Copy this form and send to:

Veterinary Learning Systems
425 Phillips Boulevard Ste 100
Trenton, NJ 08618-1496

Orders by FAX: (609)882-6357
Orders by telephone: (609)882-5600

ITEM	PRICE	SHIPPING	SUBTOTAL
***COMPENDIUM* COLLECTIONS**			
Renal Disease in Small Animal Practice	$52.00	+$3*	
Abdominal Disease in Equine Practice	$43.00	+$3*	
Radiology in Practice	$44.00	+$3*	
Gastroenterology in Practice	$54.00	+$3*	
Lameness in Equine Practice	$49.00	+$3*	
Infectious Disease in Food Animal Practice	$48.00	+$3*	
Veterinary Laboratory Medicine in Practice	$48.00	+$3*	
Feline Medicine and Surgery in Practice	$56.00	+$3*	
Emergency Medicine and Critical Care in Practice	$48.00	+$3*	
Exotic Animal Medicine in Practice Volume 1	$36.00	+$3*	
Exotic Animal Medicine in Practice Volume 2	$28.00	+$3*	
Exotic Animal Medicine in Practice Volumes 1 and 2	$59.00	+$6*	
***VETERINARY TECHNICIAN* COLLECTION**			
Exotic Animals: A Veterinary Handbook	$32.00	+$3*	
Nursing Care in Veterinary Practice	$32.00	+$3*	
ORIGINAL TEXTS AND MANUALS			
Atlas of Feline Ophthalmology	$75.00	+$3*	
Pet Skin and Haircoat Problems:			
Tests and Treatment for Veterinary Technicians	$39.00	+$3*	
A Guide to Equine Joint Injection	$28.00	+$3*	
A Guide to Equine Hoof Wall Repair	$28.00	+$3*	
Dermatology for the Small Animal Practitioner: Exotics • Feline • Canine	$55.00	+$3*	
Food Animal Surgery	$44.00	+$3*	
VIDEOS			
Techniques in Avian Medicine: Part I	$49.95	+$3*	
Techniques in Avian Medicine: Part II	$49.95	+$3*	
Techniques in Avian Medicine: Parts I and II	$85.00	+$3*	
Exotics Video: Snakes, Birds, Ferrets, and Pocket Pets	$36.00	+$3*	

JOURNALS

Compendium on Continuing Education for the Practicing Veterinarian® $56.00

US - 1 Year/12 Issues

Veterinary Technician® $35.00

US - 1 Year/11 Issues

Perspectives—A Resource for Women in Veterinary Medicine™ $34.00

US - 1 Year/11 Issues

* US shipping price per book. Foreign orders add $5 per book for shipping.

TOTAL

Name:

Street:

City: /State /Zip:

Telephone: (   )

D94136

Urethrography and Cystography in Cats Part II. Abnormal Radiographic Anatomy and Complications

Gary R. Johnston, DVM, MS
Daniel A. Feeney, DVM, MS
Carl A. Osborne, DVM, PhD

Department of Small Animal Clinical Sciences
University of Minnesota
College of Veterinary Medicine
St. Paul, Minnesota

The feline urologic syndrome (FUS) is a common urinary tract disorder which affects male and female cats. Many of these cats have a variety of radiographic abnormalities in the urinary tract that may play a role in the cause or may contribute to the recurrent nature of the disease. These anatomical abnormalities can be visualized by uroradiographic contrast procedures. In Part I of this two-part article, the techniques of cystography and urethrography and the normal radiographic appearance of each technique were described. The technical and interpretative pitfalls of these procedures were also discussed. In Part II, the radiographic abnormalities encountered during survey and contrast uroradiography are discussed and illustrated. The complications associated with cystography and urethrography in cats are also described.

Radiographic Abnormalities

Detection of radiographic abnormalities necessitates careful systematic evaluation of both survey radiographs and special uroradiographic procedures. Failure to obtain survey radiographs or to adequately interpret these films prior to cystography or urethrography procedures may lead to an incorrect or incomplete diagnosis.

Survey Radiography

Radiographic evaluation of cats with FUS begins with the systematic evaluation of survey radiographs for abnormalities of size, shape, location, and radiographic density. Abnormalities encountered on survey radiographs do not negate the necessity for further evaluation with cystography and urethrography. Abnormal survey radiographic findings may be suggestive of a lesion that can only be adequately demonstrated with a contrast study.

A markedly distended urinary bladder on survey radiographs is compatible with lower urinary tract obstruction or may be normal. An abnormally enlarged proximal urethra may be suggested on a lateral survey radiograph by the presence of an increased fluid density ventral to the descending colon (Figure 1). An abnormally shaped urinary bladder may also be seen in cats with lower urinary tract disease. The presence of

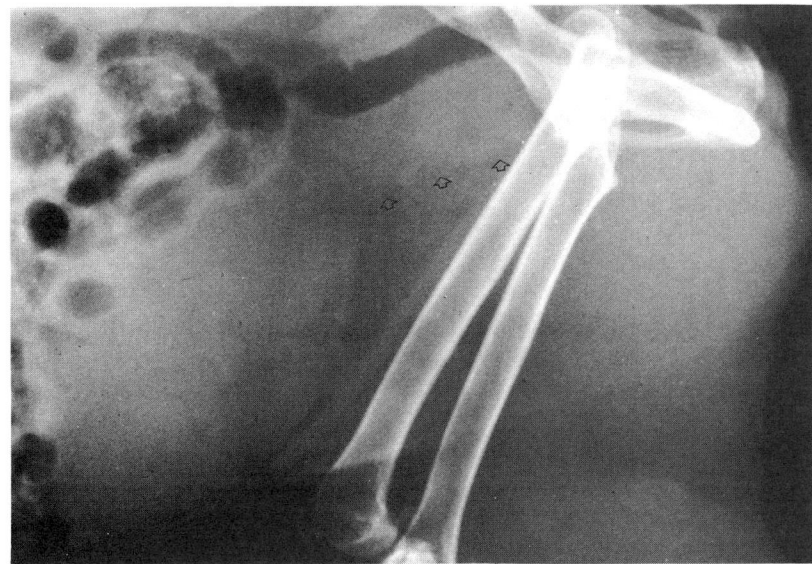

Figure 1—An area of increased fluid density *(arrows)* ventral to the descending colon represented an enlarged proximal urethra in an adult male domestic short-haired cat with urethral obstruction. Compare with Figure 20.

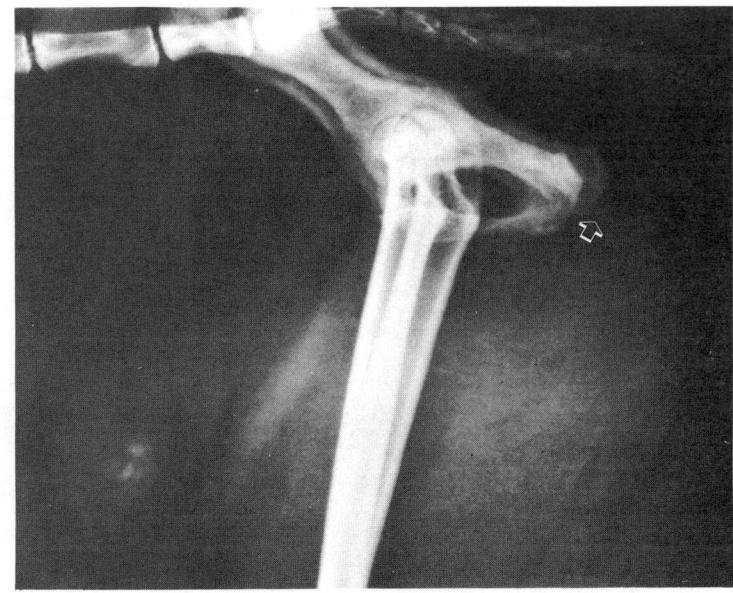

Figure 2—A wedge-shaped protruding fluid density from the cranioventral bladder margin suggestive of a diverticulum, multiple radiopaque cystic uroliths, and a solitary radiopaque urethral calculus *(arrow)* are visible in a five-year-old neutered male domestic short-haired cat with dysuria and stranguria. Compare with cystograms in Figures 10B and 12.

a urachal diverticulum or a persistent urachal ligament of the urinary bladder may be suggested by the radiographic presence of a wedge-shaped protruding fluid density from the cranioventral bladder margin on a lateral recumbent view (Figure 2). However, caution must be used when evaluating abnormalities of urinary bladder shape because superimposed fluid-filled bowel may simulate bladder diverticula. An abnormal location of the urinary bladder may be due to an inguinal or other type of abdominal hernia. Abnormalities such as radiopaque uroliths (Figures 2 and 3), intravesical foreign bodies, and mural calcification of the urinary bladder can have abnormal radiographic densities involving the urinary bladder and/or urethra identified on survey radiographs. Radiopaque uroliths may be single (Figures 3A and 3B) or multiple (Figures 2 and 3C) and may vary in size, shape, and location within the urinary bladder and urethra. Radiolucent densities within the bladder may be visible on survey radiographs.

Free intraluminal gas is the most common of these and appears as a smooth round radiolucent density in the bladder silhouette, its location being controlled by positioning (Figure 4). Free intraluminal gas is commonly the result of prior catheterization or transabdominal cystocentesis. Gas located within the bladder wall, emphysematous cystitis, may be more difficult to identify radiographically but usually appears within any or all layers of the bladder wall. Emphysematous cystitis may be secondary to diabetes mellitus or bacterial cystitis. Intraluminal and intramural gas must be differentiated from superimposed gas-filled bowel.

Contrast Uroradiography

Evaluation of cystograms and urethrograms should be systematic and should follow the careful evaluation of survey radiographs. Diagnostic impressions gained from the survey radiographs should be verified with cystography or urethrography. Abnormal radiographic

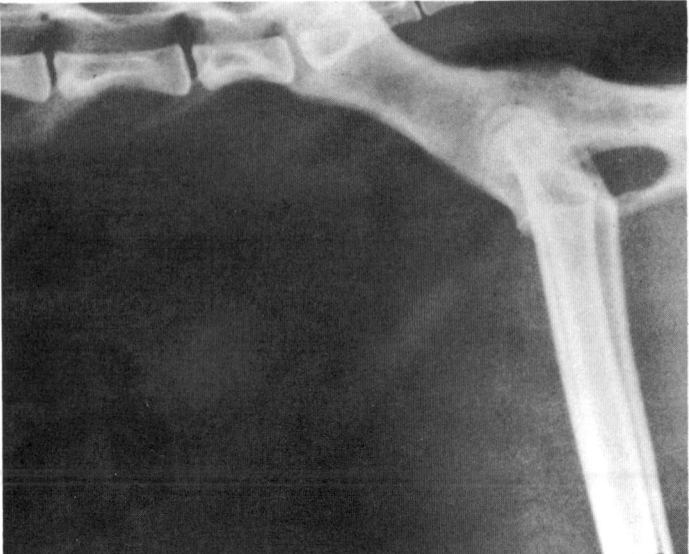

Figure 3A

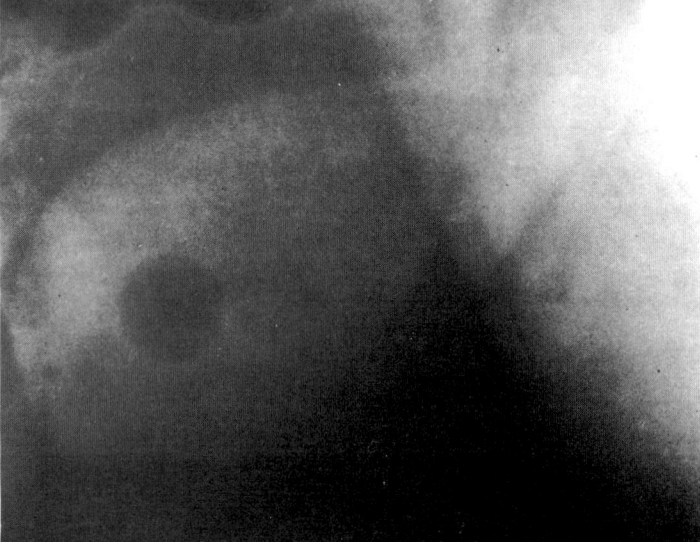

Figure 3C

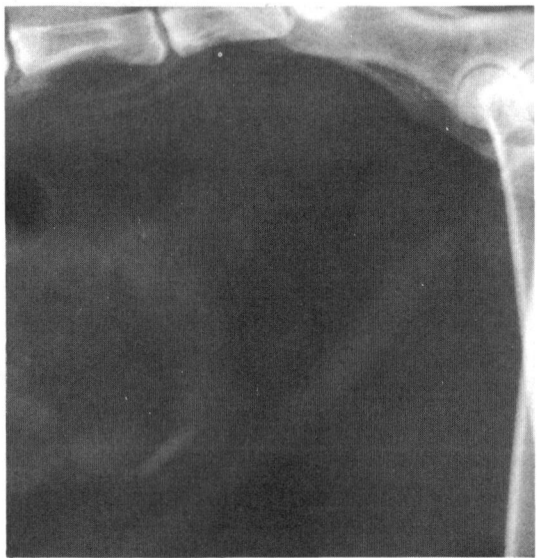

Figure 3B

Figure 3—Uroliths vary in size, number, shape, and location within the urinary bladder and urethra. **(A)** A large spheroidal solitary cystic urolith in a three-year-old male domestic short-haired cat with renal failure. **(B)** Solitary pumpkin-seed-shaped urolith in a 10-year-old spayed female domestic long-haired cat with lower urinary tract disease. Subsequent cystography localized the calculus within the urinary bladder. **(C)** Multiple sandlike cystic uroliths are visible in a one-year-old male Siamese cat with urethral obstruction of three days duration.

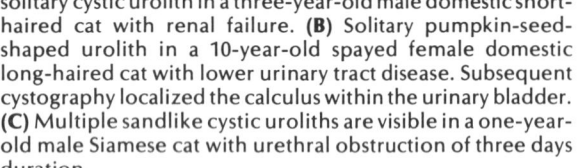

Figure 4—The gas density located in the center of the urinary bladder silhouette on the lateral recumbent survey radiograph represents free intraluminal gas. Prior bladder catheterization, transabdominal cystocentesis, and pneumocystography are common causes of free intraluminal urinary bladder gas.

findings will be described for the following structures: ureters, urinary bladder, and urethra.

Ureters

Vesicoureteral reflux (VUR), although incompletely described, has been reported during cystography and urethrography in cats.[1,2] Information is insufficient to derive meaningful conclusions about the incidence of VUR in normal cats. VUR was encountered in 20 of 53 (37.7%) male and female cats with FUS examined by the authors (Figure 5). Although VUR might theoretically predispose cats with FUS to ascending bacterial infection, this is considered unlikely because of the low incidence of bacterial urinary tract infection present in cats. Focal dilatation of the distal ureter in cats with VUR may be encountered in cats with FUS (Figure 6). Whether this represents a normal variation in anatomy related to overdistention of the urinary bladder or is related to inflammatory ureteral or bladder disease is not known. Other causes of focal or diffuse ureteral dilatation include ureteral ectopia, ureteral calculi, ureteral strictures, and ureteroceles.

Urinary Bladder

The radiographic findings encountered in cats with

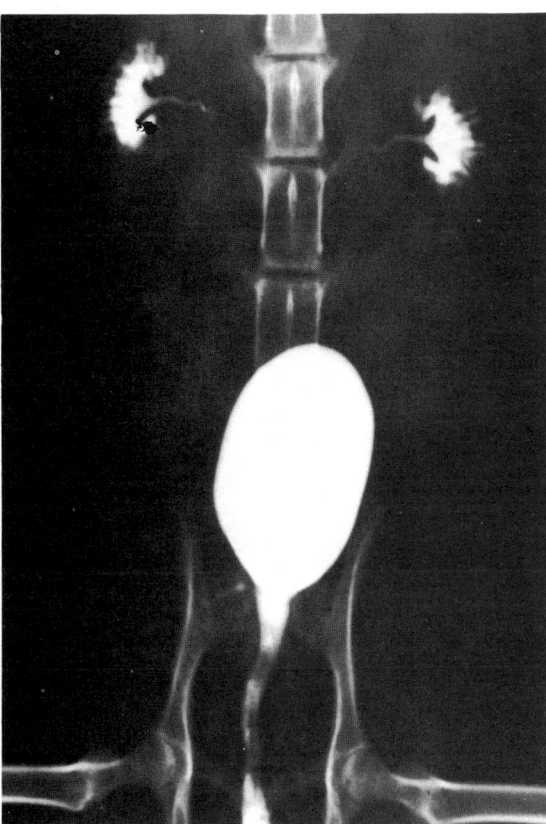

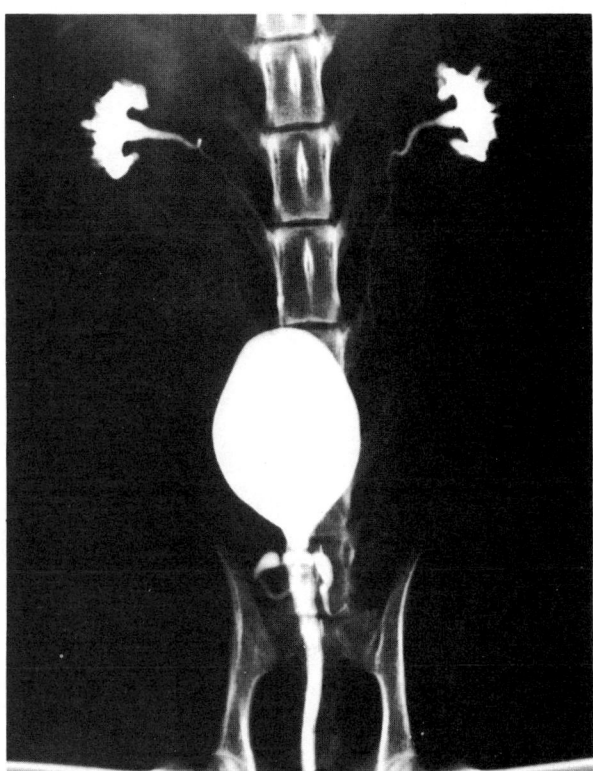

Figure 5—Bilateral vesicoureteral reflux of iodinated contrast medium was encountered during retrograde urethrocystography in a 14-month-old neutered male domestic short-haired cat. The cat had hematuria and dysuria of four months duration and two prior episodes of urethral obstruction. This radiographic finding may or may not be indicative of ascending urinary tract infection.

Figure 6—Bilateral focal dilatation of the distal ureters is present with bilateral vesicoureteral reflux during positive contrast cystourethrography in a six-year-old neutered male domestic short-haired cat with intermittent hematuria of several months duration. A perineal urethrostomy had been performed three months previously for episodes of hematuria, dysuria, and stranguria. The cause of localized ureteral dilatation is unknown but may be related to overdistention of a normal urinary bladder or ureteral disease.

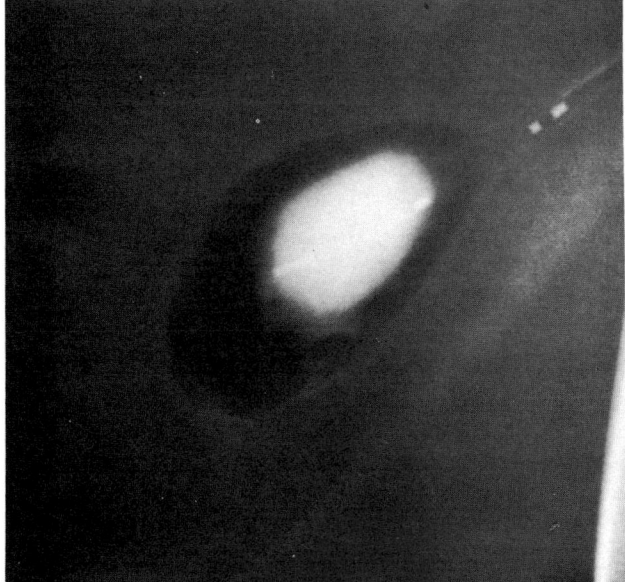

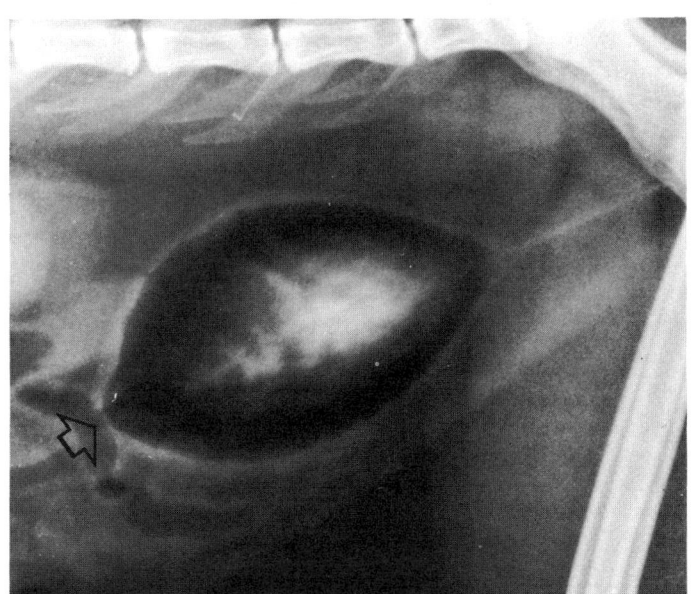

Figure 7A
Figure 7B

Figure 7—Mucosal irregularity is frequently present in cats with acute or chronic lower urinary tract disease secondary to neoplastic, infectious, or noninfectious disease. It is best visualized with double contrast cystography and is seen as either a focal or diffuse lesion. **(A)** Focal mucosal irregularity of the cranioventral bladder wall with ulceration was present in an eight-year-old spayed female Siamese cat with hematuria and dysuria of one week duration. **(B)** Diffuse mucosal irregularity and bladder wall thickening are visible in a five-year-old castrated male domestic short-haired cat with hematuria and dysuria of two weeks duration. One episode of urethral obstruction occurred two weeks prior to double contrast cystography. Note the presence of a urachal diverticulum on the cranioventral margin of the urinary bladder *(arrow)*.

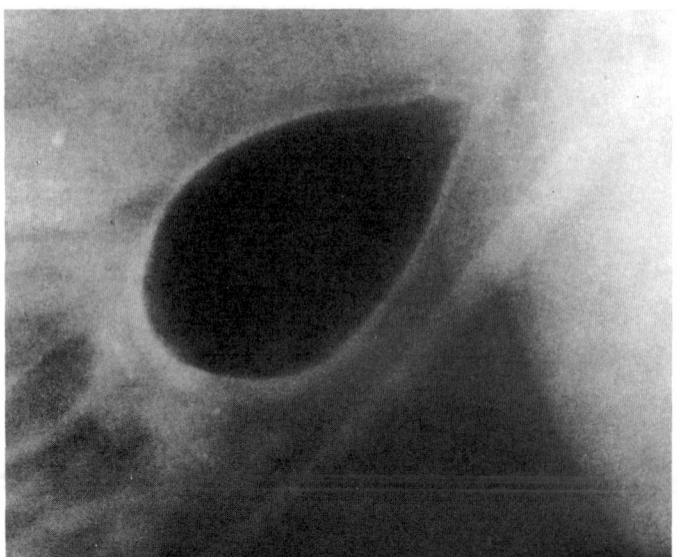

Figure 8A

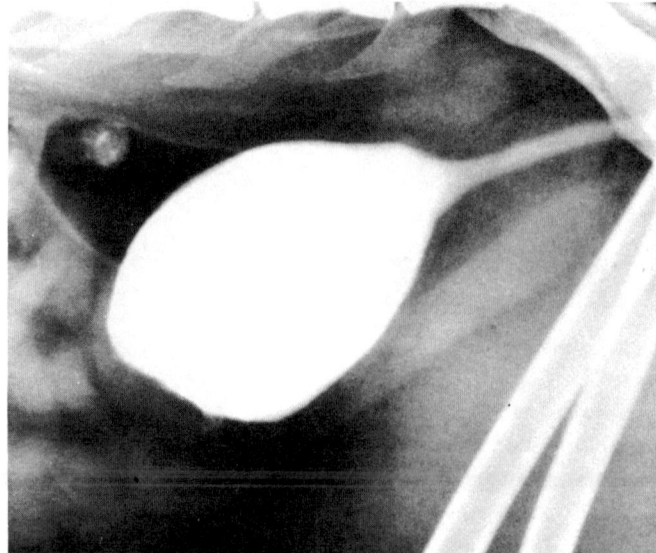

Figure 8B

Figure 8—Mural thickening of the bladder is frequently encountered in cats with lower urinary tract disease and can be due to infectious, noninfectious or neoplastic causes. **(A)** Cranioventral bladder wall thickening is present on pneumocystography in an eight-year-old neutered male cat with hematuria, dysuria, and sterile urine. The cat had a noninfectious, inflammatory cystitis. **(B)** Cranioventral thickening of the bladder wall is visible in an adult male domestic short-haired cat with dysuria and hematuria of two weeks duration. When the clinical signs persisted during medical management of lower urinary disease, the owner requested euthanasia. A transitional cell carcinoma was found.

FUS can vary from no visible radiographic abnormality to severe diffuse involvement of the urinary bladder. For convenience, the radiographic abnormalities encountered in the authors' series of cats with FUS will be described as mucosal or mural lesions or luminal defects.

Mucosal Lesions—Mucosal irregularity may be caused by inflammatory or neoplastic disease. Caution must be exercised in evaluating for mucosal irregularity, because inadequate distention of the urinary bladder can simulate mucosal disease. Although mucosal irregularity can be seen with pneumocystography or positive contrast cystography, subtle lesions are more visible with double contrast cystography. Mucosal lesions are characterized by an irregular interface between the contrast medium and the bladder in the dependent portion of the urinary bladder. Mucosal irregularity may be focal or diffuse (Figure 7). Mucosal ulcerations may be seen in conjunction with mucosal irregularity and are characterized by the ulcerated surface being coated with contrast medium (Figure 7A). Contrast media will also coat the surface of blood clots, and this can simulate ulcerations.

Mural Lesions—If inadequately distended, the normal urinary bladder wall may appear thickened. However, urinary bladder wall thickening may be abnormal and caused by infectious, noninfectious, or neoplastic disease. Therefore, its significance must be evaluated in light of the clinical signs, urine culture, urinalysis, cytology, clinical duration, degree of bladder distention, and prior urethral or bladder instrumentation. Cats with an acute lower urinary tract disease may not have mural or mucosal lesions. The most common location for thickening is the cranioventral bladder wall (Figure

8). Cranioventral bladder thickening is frequently encountered in cats with urachal diverticula. Diffuse mural thickening may be encountered in cats with either acute or chronic lower urinary tract disease. Prolonged bladder distention due to urethral obstruction may result in hemorrhage, edema, and inflammation which can cause diffuse mural thickening (Figure 9). Diffuse cystitis may also be encountered in cats with chronic lower urinary tract disease (Figures 9B and 9C). Diverticula of the urinary bladder may be encountered in male and female cats with lower urinary tract disease and may be congenital or acquired. However, congenital urachal diverticula are considered the most common and may be patent or nonpatent.[4-6] Urachal diverticula have been proposed as significant predisposing factors to lower urinary tract disease.[7] The incidence of urachal anomalies in cats without urinary tract disease is unknown. Pneumocystography or double contrast cystography can demonstrate most urachal diverticula (Figures 7B and 9C), although the smaller diverticula may not be identified unless a positive contrast study is performed (Figure 10). Some urachal diverticula can be difficult to demonstrate by contrast cystography even when a wedge-shaped cranioventral prominence is encountered on survey radiographs. These diverticula may represent stretching of the urachal ligament that attaches the urinary bladder cranioventrally. Urachal diverticula vary markedly in size and shape. They may be wedge-shaped (Figure 7B), pointed (Figure 10A), conical (Figure 10B), or round and cystlike (Figures 9C and 11) and may be associated with attached or free uroliths (Figures 9C and 11A).

Luminal Filling Defects—Luminal filling defects,

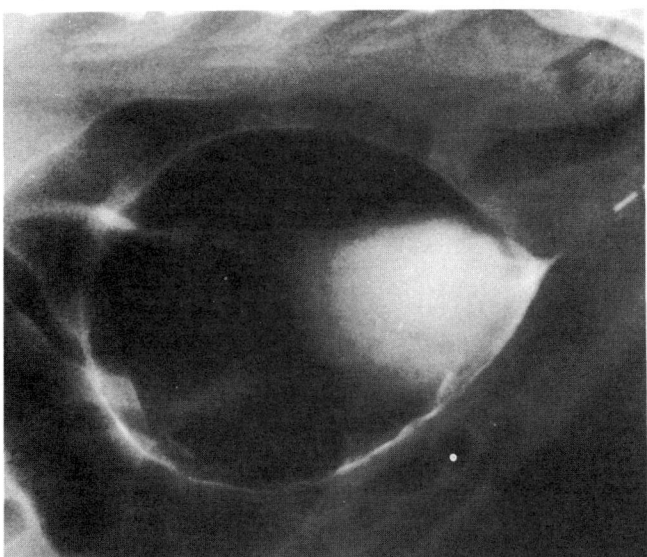

Figure 9A

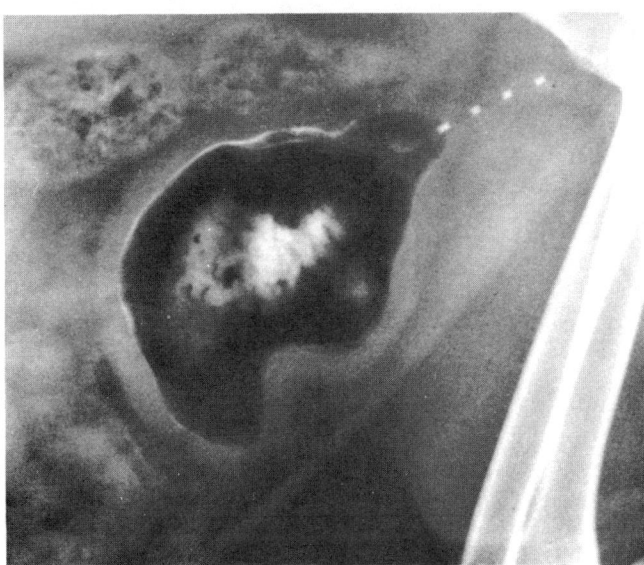

Figure 9B

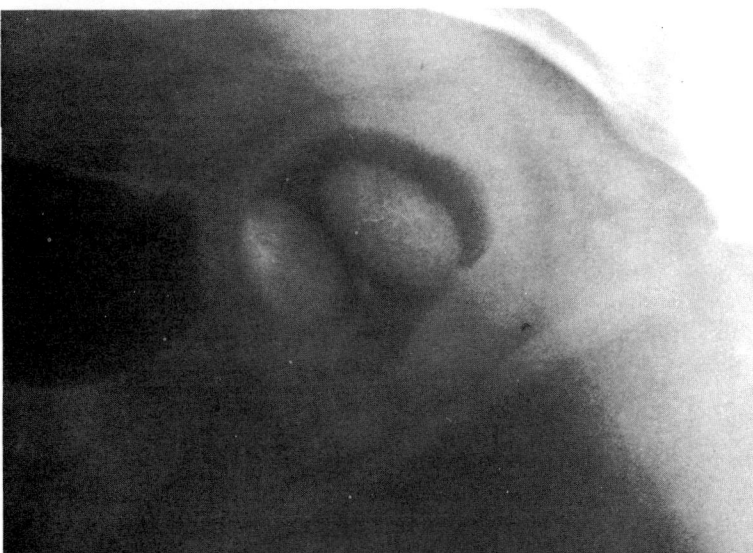

Figure 9C

either free or attached, may be encountered during cystography in cats with lower urinary tract disease. Filling defects are any materials within the bladder that alter normal filling. The differential features of the common filling defects encountered in cats with FUS are listed in Table I.

Free luminal filling defects encountered during cystography in cats with lower urinary tract disease include uroliths (Figures 9C, 11A, and 12), blood clots (Figures 9B and 13), air bubbles (Figure 14), and mucus or matrix plugs (Figures 9B and 15). Uroliths (Figures 11A and 12) and blood clots (Figure 16) may also be attached filling defects. Attached filling defects less frequently encountered during cystography in cats with lower urinary tract disease include neoplasms, submucosal hematomas (Figure 17), polypoid cystitis, ureteroceles and adherent fluid-dense calculi.

Urethra

Urethral abnormalities encountered in the authors' series of cats with FUS include urethral calculi (Figures 10B and 18), urethral strictures (Figure 19), and urethral dilatation (Figures 19 and 20). Female cats are infrequently obstructed by urethral calculi when compared with males. All urethral abnormalities in the authors' prospective evaluation of cats with FUS were confined to males.

Complications

Complications encountered during contrast procedures used for evaluating cats with FUS may be caused

Figure 9—Diffuse thickening of the urinary bladder wall may be encountered in acute or chronic infectious, noninfectious, or neoplastic disease. (**A**) Diffuse mural thickening is seen with double contrast cystography in a six-year-old male domestic short-haired cat five days following relief of urethral obstruction. Overdistention of the urinary bladder of cats may result in urothelial ulcerations, submucosal hemorrhage, edema of the bladder wall, and impaired bladder wall integrity.[3] Radiographically, these lesions are characterized by an increased thickness of the bladder wall. (**B**) Diffuse mural thickening, multiple blood clots, uroliths, and a bladder wall invagination are present in a three-year-old neutered male domestic short-haired cat with hematuria and dysuria of two weeks duration. A perineal urethrostomy for urethral obstruction had been performed five months previously. A second episode of urethral obstruction preceded the survey and uroradiographic contrast studies by four days. A catheterized urine sample was positive for *Proteus mirabilis*. A chronic, necrotic, transmural cystitis was diagnosed histologically. (**C**) Lateral pneumocystogram in a five-year-old male cat with lower urinary tract disease. A perineal urethrostomy had been performed three years previously because of urethral obstruction. Diffuse bladder wall thickening, reduced bladder wall distensibility, two radiopaque cystic uroliths, and a urachal diverticulum are evident. Removal of the penile urethra may alter the normal defense mechanism of the lower urinary tract and predispose the animal to ascending urinary tract infection. Diverticula and other defects may further predispose to urinary tract infection by causing stasis and retention of urine.

TABLE I
Differential Radiographic Characteristics of
Intraluminal Filling Defects of the Urinary Bladder

Radiographic Criteria	Air Bubbles	Calculi	Sebaceous or Mucous Plugs	Blood Clots
Size	Small to large	Small to large	Small	Small to large
Number	Single, multiple or coalescent	Single or multiple	Single or multiple	Single or multiple
Shape	Commonly round; if coalescing, ovoid or polyhedral	Spheroidal, ovoid, polygonal, pumpkin seed	Spheroidal, ovoid, polygonal, linear	Spheroidal, ovoid, polygonal, linear
Margination	Smooth and distinct	Smooth or irregular, distinct or indistinct	Smooth or irregular, distinct or indistinct	Indistinct and irregular
Location	Commonly at periphery of contrast puddle; if large and coalescing, anywhere	Center of contrast puddle or attached to bladder wall	Center of contrast puddle or attached to bladder wall	Center of contrast puddle or attached to bladder wall
Density				
Survey radiography	Radiolucent	Water-dense (radiolucent) calculi: nondetectable Radiopaque calculi: radiopaque or nondetectable (if small)	Nondetectable	Nondetectable
Pneumocystography	Radiolucent	Water-dense calculi: nondetectable or radiopaque (if attached) Radiopaque calculi: radiopaque	Nondetectable	Nondetectable or radiopaque (attached)
Double contrast cystography	Radiolucent	Water-dense calculi: radiolucent Radiopaque calculi: radiolucent	Radiolucent	Radiolucent
Positive contrast urethrocystography	Radiolucent	Water-dense calculi: radiolucent or nondetectable Radiopaque calculi: radiolucent or nondetectable	Nondetectable	Nondetectable

by the materials or the techniques of cystography and urethrography. These potential complications may compromise the normal defense mechanisms of the urinary system and predispose the patient to urinary tract infection. Fatal complications have not been encountered in the authors' series of cats with FUS.

Materials
Contrast Media
Positive Contrast Media—Meglumine diatrizoate and meglumine iothalamate are triiodinated contrast agents used for cystography and urethrography. Systemic reactions to these radiopaque contrast media are rarely encountered during cystography and urethrography. Local tissue reactions to positive contrast agents have been reported and are related to hyperosmolarity, total volume, method of injection, and duration of contact with the urothelium.[8-12] Concentrations of 5 to 10% of a positive contrast medium are recommended for cystography and are reported to produce minimal inflammatory reaction of the urinary bladder.[8]

Negative Contrast Media—Negative contrast media such as air, carbon dioxide, and nitrous oxide are used in contrast evaluation of lower urinary tract disease. Fatal vascular embolization, an uncommon complication, following pneumocystography with air in dogs and cats, has been reported.[13,14] Carbon dioxide and nitrous oxide are recommended in the presence of urothelial disruption because of their greater solubility in blood compared to that of air. Fatal vascular embolization was not encountered in the authors' series of cats evaluated by pneumocystography or double contrast cystography utilizing air. One case of fatal air embolization following pneumocystography with air was referred to the University of Minnesota Veterinary Hospital for necropsy (Figures 21 and 22).

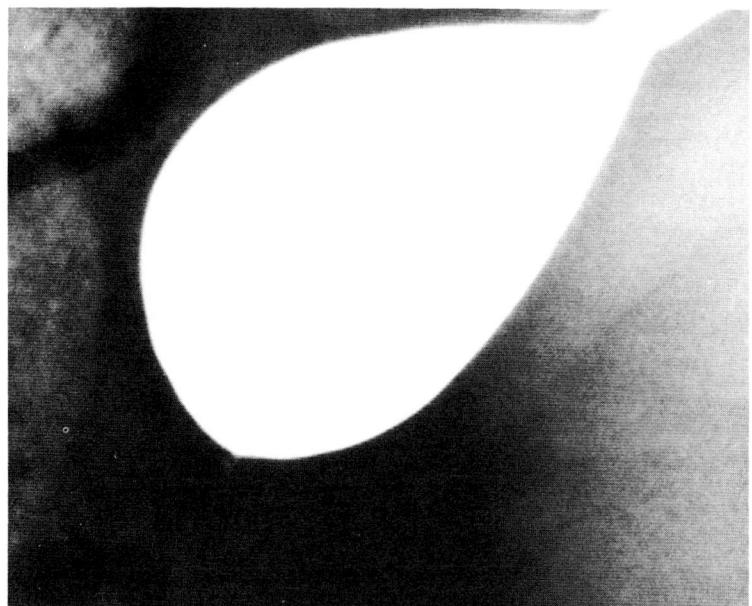

Figure 10A

Figure 10—Some diverticula may be difficult to demonstrate radiographically by pneumocystography or double contrast cystography. (**A**) A small diverticulum was encountered during positive contrast urethrocystography in this one-year-old female Manx cat with intermittent hematuria of one month duration. (**B**) Lateral positive contrast cystogram of the cat in Figure 2. Note cranioventral thickening of the bladder wall in association with a urachal diverticulum and the urethral calculus (*arrow*). Note also that the cystic uroliths visible on the survey radiograph (Figure 2) are obscured by the positive contrast medium.

Figure 11—Urinary bladder diverticula vary in shape, size, and location. (**A**) A cranioventral cystlike diverticulum with cystic uroliths is present in a nine-year-old neutered male domestic long-haired cat. The cat had intermittent lower urinary tract disease of five years duration and no prior history of urethral obstruction. (**B**) A craniolateral cystlike diverticulum is visible in a four-year-old spayed female domestic short-haired cat with hematuria and dysuria of six weeks duration. A surgical biopsy from the resected diverticulum indicated mucosal ulcerations with edema, hyperemia, and hemorrhage. A Gram's stain from the diverticulum revealed no bacteria.

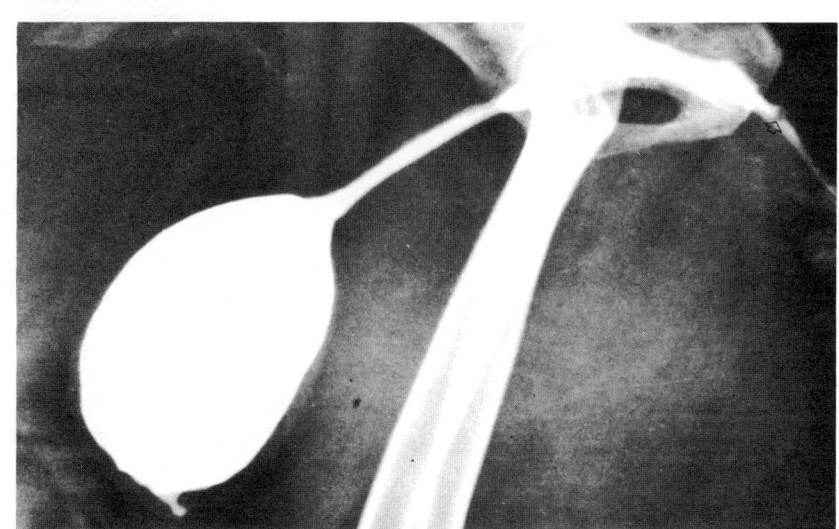

Figure 10B

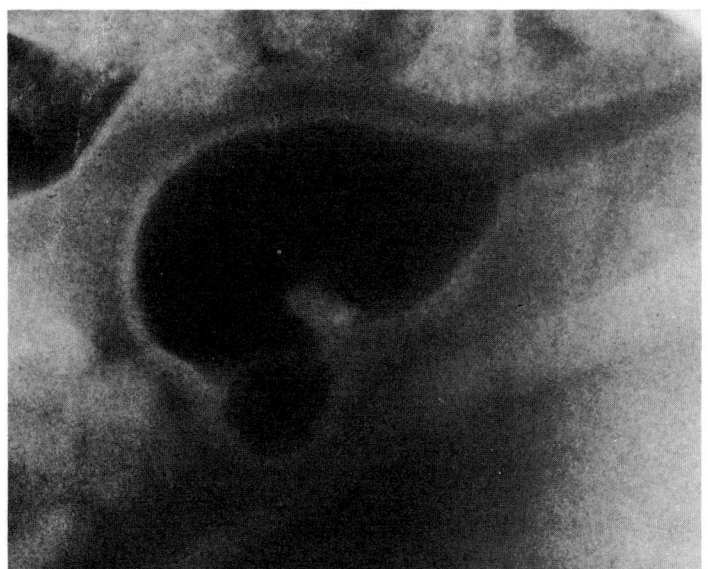

Figure 11A

Figure 11B➤

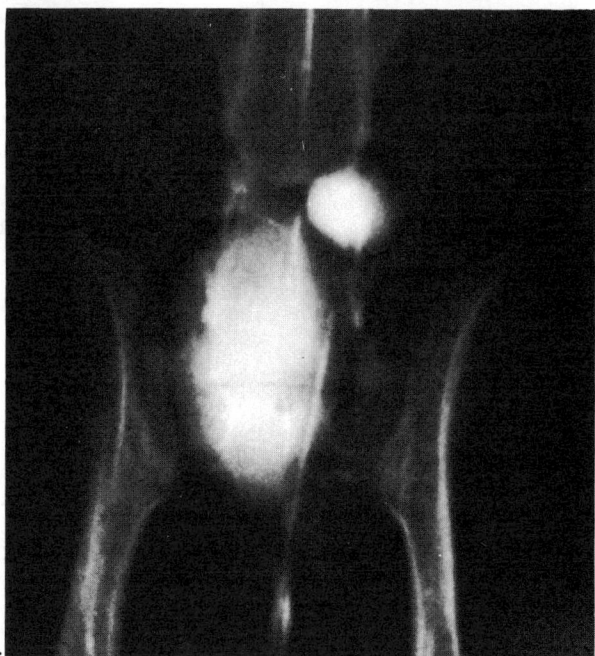

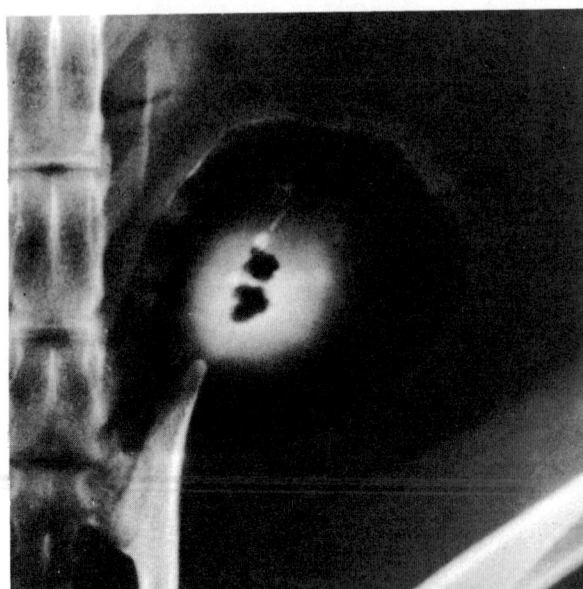

Figure 12—Multiple cystoliths are visible with double contrast cystography in the cat described in Figures 2 and 10B. Variations in radiographic density of calculi are related to their location in relationship to positive or negative contrast media. The urinary bladder wall is also thickened and irregular.

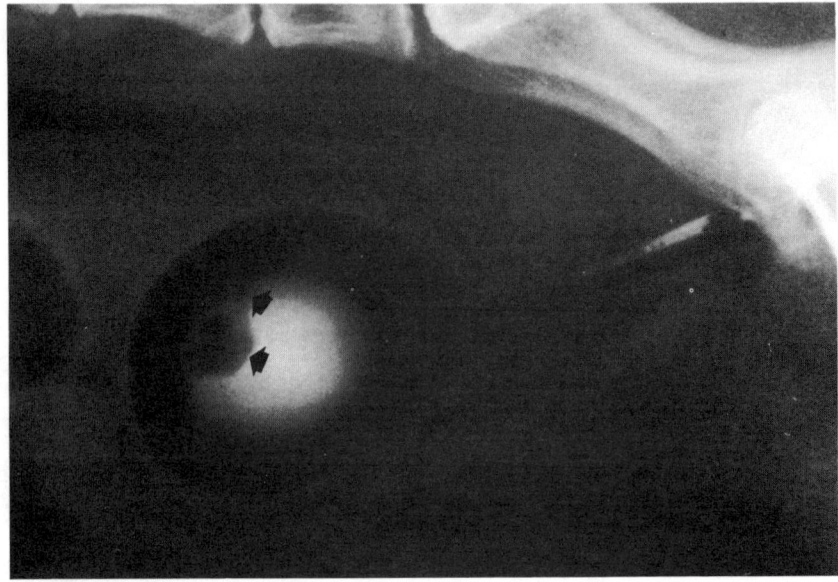

Figure 13—Two free intraluminal filling defects (*arrows*) were visible with double contrast cystography in a six-year-old neutered male Persian cat with intermittent hematuria and dysuria of three years duration. Physical palpation, survey radiography and pneumocystography failed to demonstrate the filling defect. The irregular shape, indistinct borders, and fluid-dense composition of the filling defect are most compatible with blood clots.

Figure 14—Air bubbles appear as free intraluminal filling defects with positive contrast cystography. Their appearance and location vary depending on the type of contrast medium used and their number and degree of coalescence. Solitary air bubbles are spheroidal and best identified during double contrast cystography at the periphery of the contrast puddle (see Figure 27A). Multiple air bubbles may appear anywhere in the bladder lumen and may be spheroidal, ovoid, or polygonal depending on the degree of coalescence.

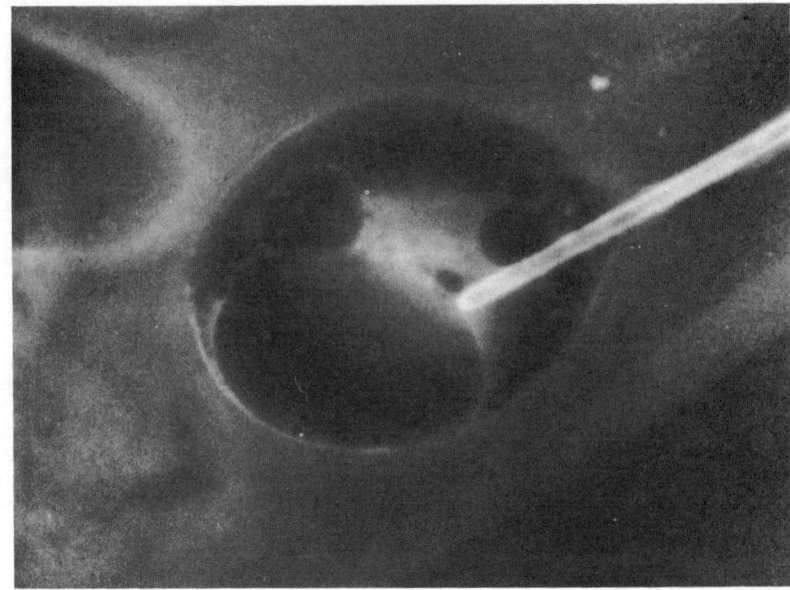

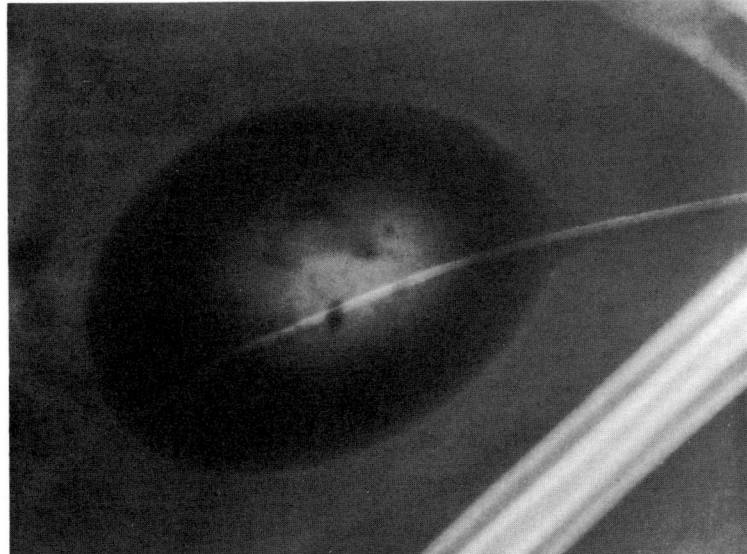

Figure 15—Filling defects are visualized with double contrast cystography in an adult male domestic long-haired cat with hematuria and pollakiuria of six weeks duration. Their variable shapes and irregular, indistinct borders suggest that they are blood clots or mucous plugs. Inability to detect these filling defects during survey radiography and pneumocystography attests to their water density. Mucous and sebaceous plugs, small calculi, and blood clots may be difficult to differentiate radiographically.

Figure 16—Blood clots visible with cystography may be free intraluminal filling defects (Figure 13) or attached to the bladder wall. Tangential radiographic projections are recommended to optimally demonstrate the site(s) of attachment. Attached filling defects are seen with double contrast cystography in a four-year-old neutered male cat with intermittent hematuria of approximately two years duration. Failure to identify the filling defect by survey radiography or pneumocystography indicates their water composition. Inflammatory polyps or fluid-dense attached calculi must also be considered as radiographic differential diagnoses for the three peripherally located filling defects. The centrally located linear filling defect is a blood clot.

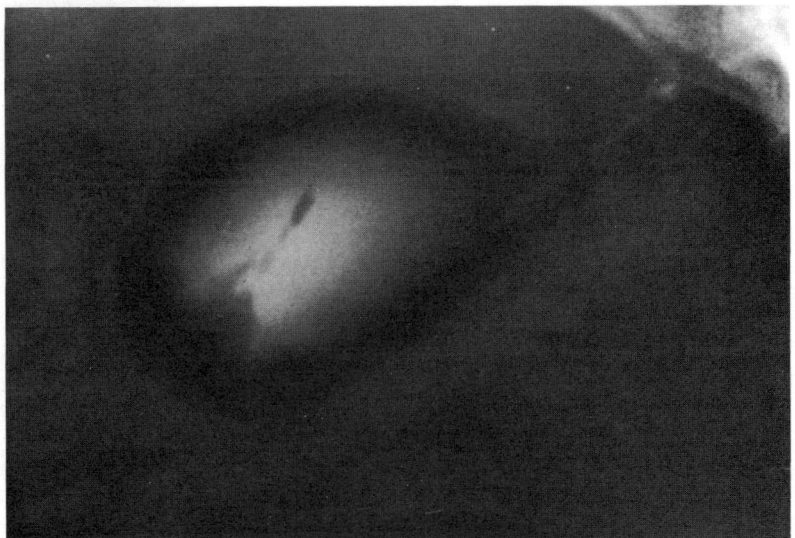

Figure 17—A large soft-tissue-density filling defect is visible with pneumocystography in an 18-month-old neutered male Persian cat with lower urinary tract disease. The histologic diagnosis following surgical resection was an organizing ulcerative submucosal hematoma.

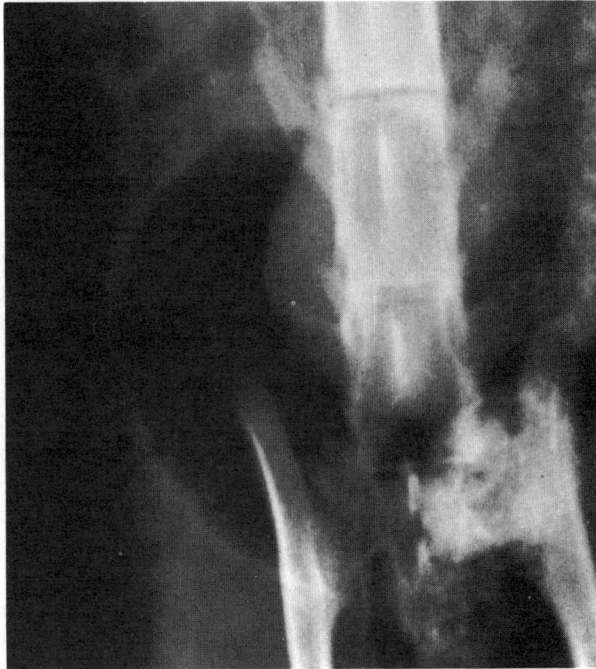

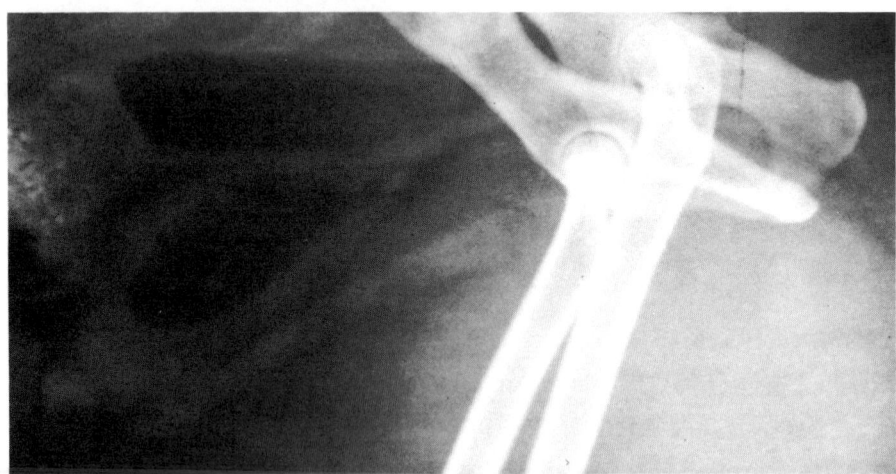

Figure 18—Mutliple cystic calculi and a solitary preprostatic urethral calculus are visible with pneumocystography in a two-year-old male Persian cat with recurrent hematuria following cystotomy for removal of the uroliths. Recurrent urolithiasis must be suspected in cats with clinical recurrence of disease. Although the penile urethra is reported as the most common site of obstruction by calculi, other areas of the urethra may be involved. A perineal urethrostomy may be ineffective if the urethra proximal to the urethrotomy is the site of obstruction.

Figure 19—Positive contrast retrograde urethrogram of an eight-month-old male domestic short-haired cat with urinary incontinence and one prior episode of urethral obstruction. Excretory urography excluded ureteral ectopia as the cause of incontinence. Marked urethral dilatation proximal and distal to a stricture in the mid-pelvic urethra is present. On postmortem examination, the stricture was considered congenital.

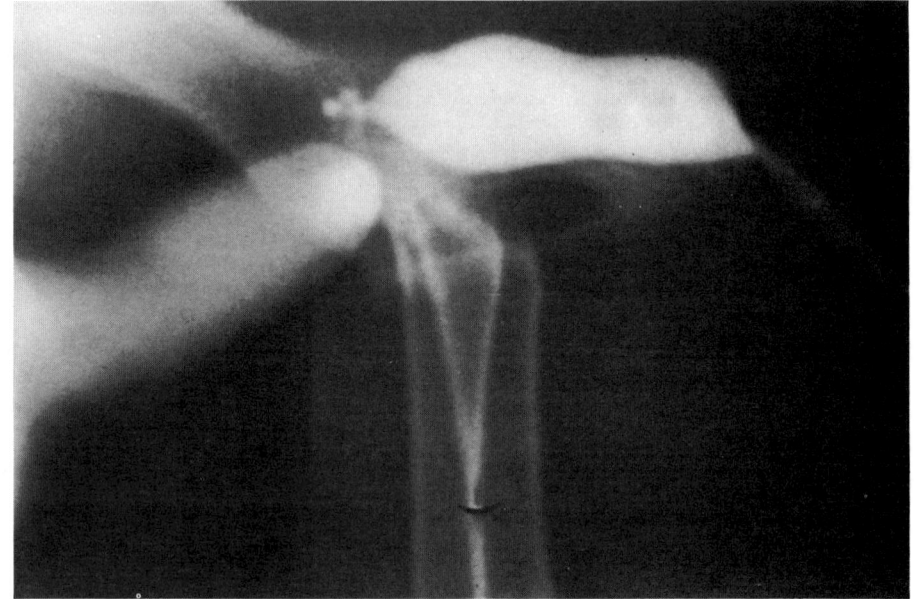

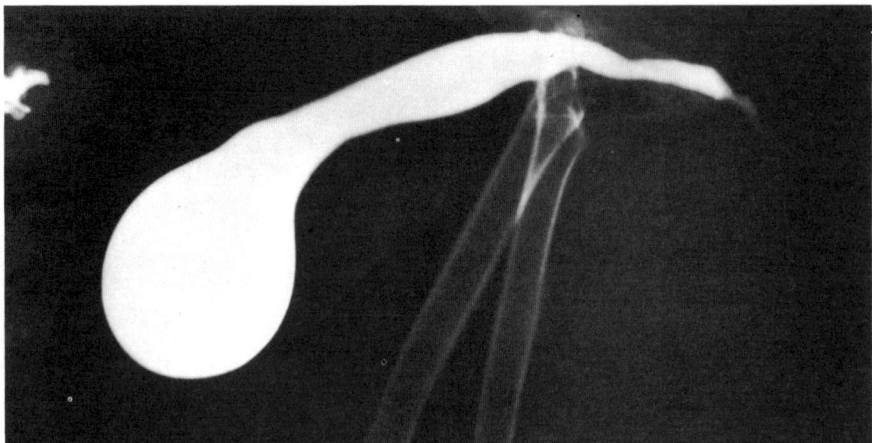

Figure 20—Generalized urethral dilatation is demonstrated with retrograde urethrocystography in the cat described in Figure 1. Histologic diagnosis was a mild inflammatory cystitis. No microscopic urethral lesions were visible. It is not known if the urethral dilatation represented a sequela to chronic partial urethral obstruction or if it was congenital.

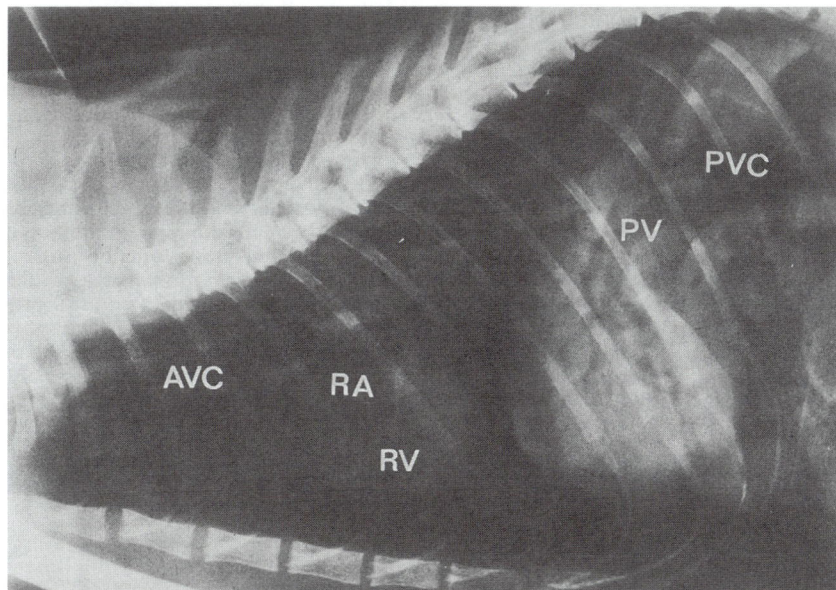

Figure 21—Postmortem radiograph of a four-year-old female domestic short-haired cat that died of vascular air embolism following pneumocystography. Gas is located in the following vascular structures: cranial vena cava (*AVC*), caudal vena cava (*PVC*), hepatic portal veins (*PV*), right atrium (*RA*), and right ventricle (*RV*).

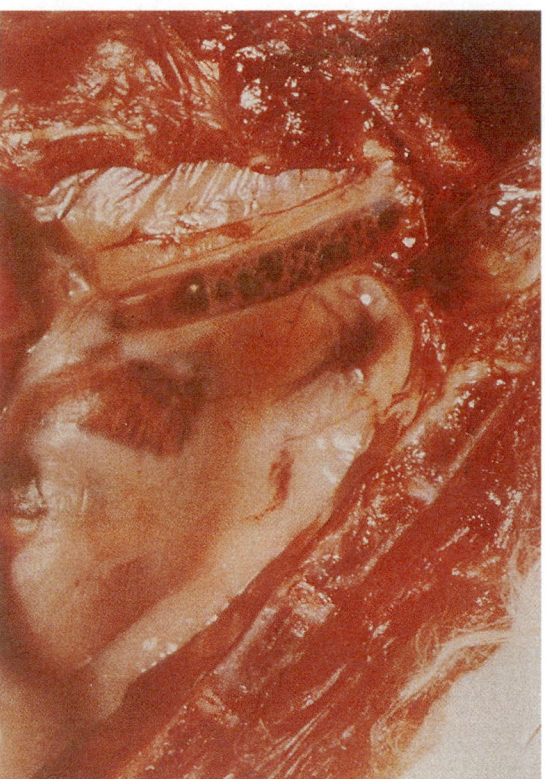

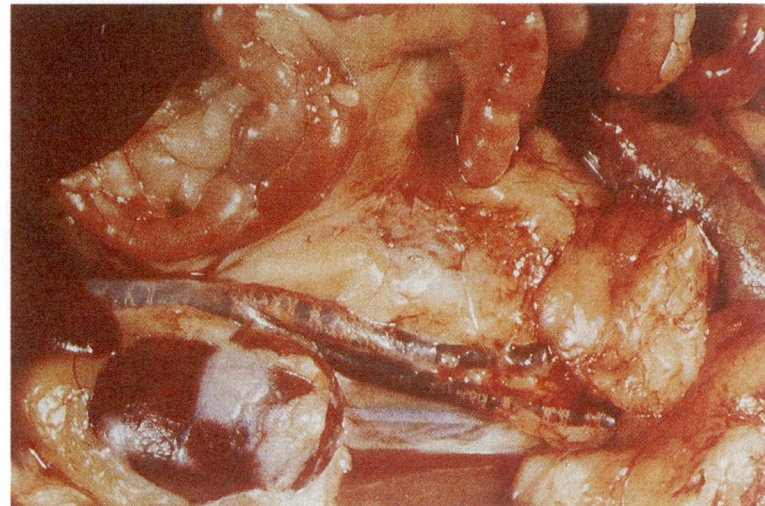

Figure 22B

Figure 22—Necropsy photographs from the cat described in Figure 21. (**A**) Lateral thorax. (**B**) Ventrodorsal abdomen. Note presence of air bubbles in the cranial vena cava (**A**) and portal vein (**B**). The reason for the air in the portal circulation is unknown.

Figure 22A

Figure 23—Submucosal urethral hemorrhages are visible in the distal urethra of a normal adult male cat. These lesions were encountered one day following inflation of a balloon catheter for 15 minutes duration in the distal urethra. This is usually considered a reversible complication of balloon catheter urethrography.

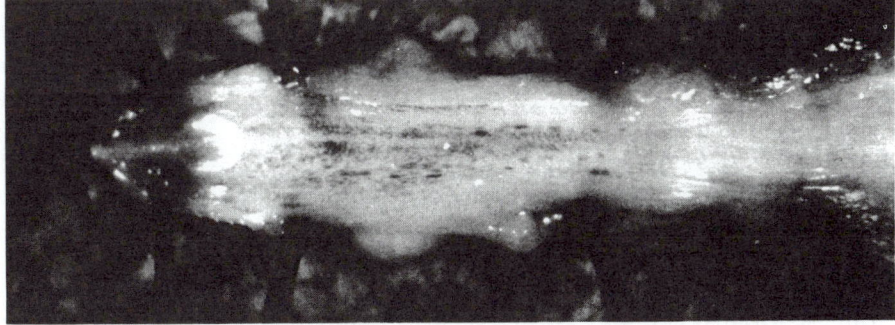

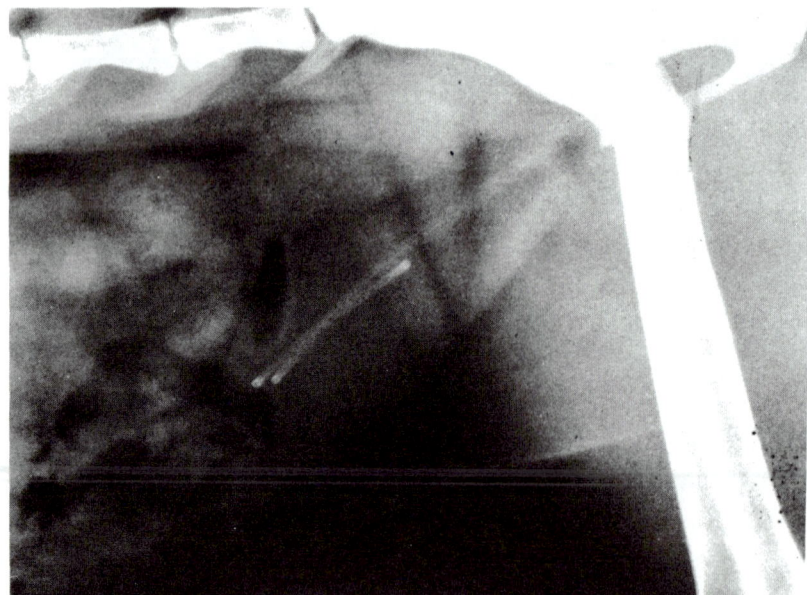

Figure 24—This one-year-old male domestic short-haired cat removed its own stay sutures, which allowed a retrograde migration of the catheter into the bladder. Failure to locate the indwelling catheter by visual examination should alert the clinician that further investigation should be made with survey radiography. Indwelling catheters, particularly in male cats, may allow for ascending bladder infection and a concurrent catheter-induced urethritis.

Figure 25—Granulomatous cystitis, character-ized histologically by multinucleated giant cells with cytoplasmic inclusions and associated mononuclear inflammatory cell reactions, was encountered in a normal adult female cat fol-lowing retrograde urethrography where an aqueous lubricant was used as a diluent for the positive contrast medium. Leakage of contrast material into the bladder wall was evident radi-ographically. (Periodic acid-Schiff stain, original magnification, × 160).

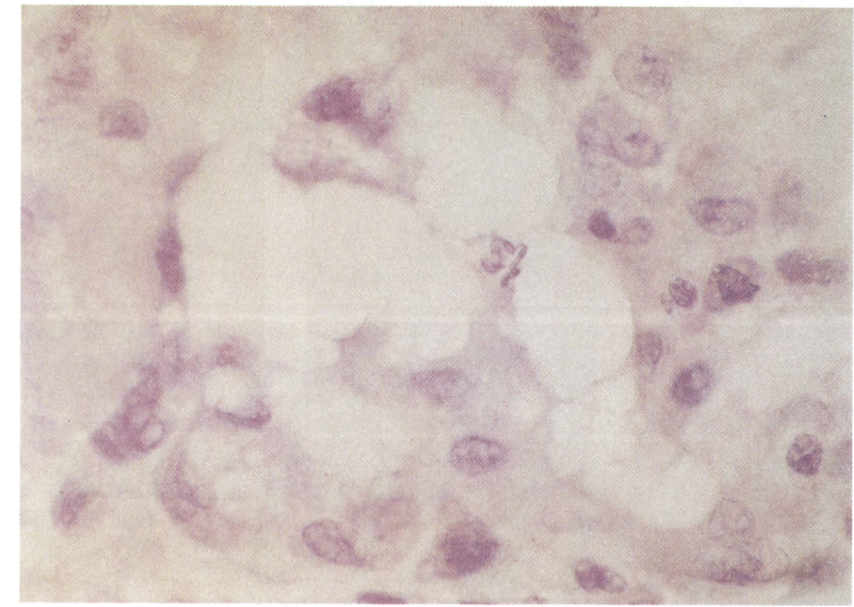

Catheters

Balloon Catheters—Despite the extensive use of bal-loon-tipped retention catheters for urethrography, there is a paucity of information concerning their potential complications. Submucosal urethral hemorrhages have been reported in the area occupied by an inflated balloon catheter in dogs and cats one day following balloon inflation for 15 minutes (Figure 23).[3] Similar lesions were not encountered in dogs or cats examined 14 days post-balloon inflation[3] for 15 minutes duration, which indicates the reversibility of the urethral lesions resulting from the inflated balloon catheter.

Nonballoon Catheters—Complications resulting from nonballoon catheters may be related to several variables including patient susceptibility, catheter material, catheter size, duration of catheterization, method of urine drainage, and concomitant use of antimicrobial agents.[15]

Catheter kinking or improper placement of a stiff, nonflexible urethral catheter may result in iatrogenic trauma to the urinary bladder or urethra. Mucosal ulcerations and submucosal hemorrhage may reduce the natural defense mechanisms of the lower urinary tract and predispose to infection. Urethral trauma has

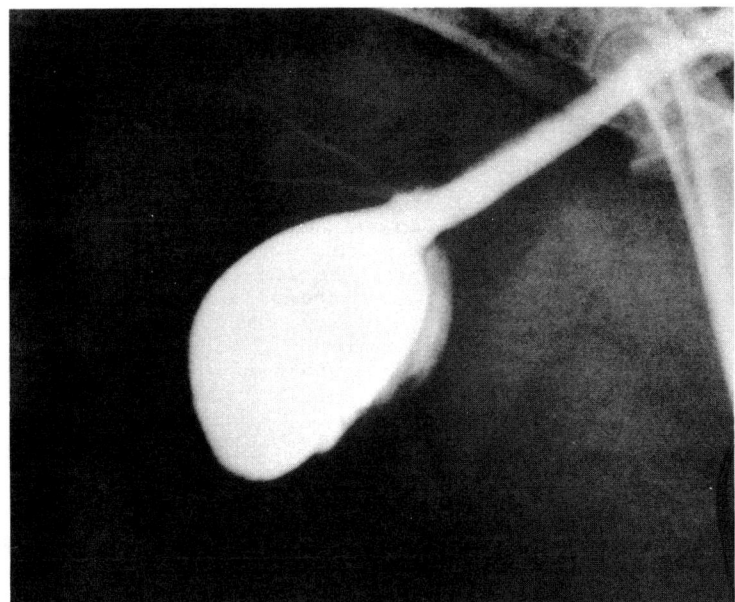

Figure 26A

Figure 26—Acute overdistention of a normal or abnormal urinary bladder during cystography or urethrography in cats can result in (**A**) mural leakage, with confinement of the contrast medium inside the serosal surface, or (**B**) complete disruption of the bladder wall, with escape of the bladder contents into the peritoneal cavity. Cats with lower urinary tract disease may be predisposed to urinary bladder discontinuity because of existing inflammatory disease. Infusion of the urinary bladder in cats with FUS should proceed slowly with external palpation, pericatheter reflux, and retrograde pressure on the syringe plunger as criteria for maximum bladder distention. Note bilateral ureterovesical reflux in **A**.

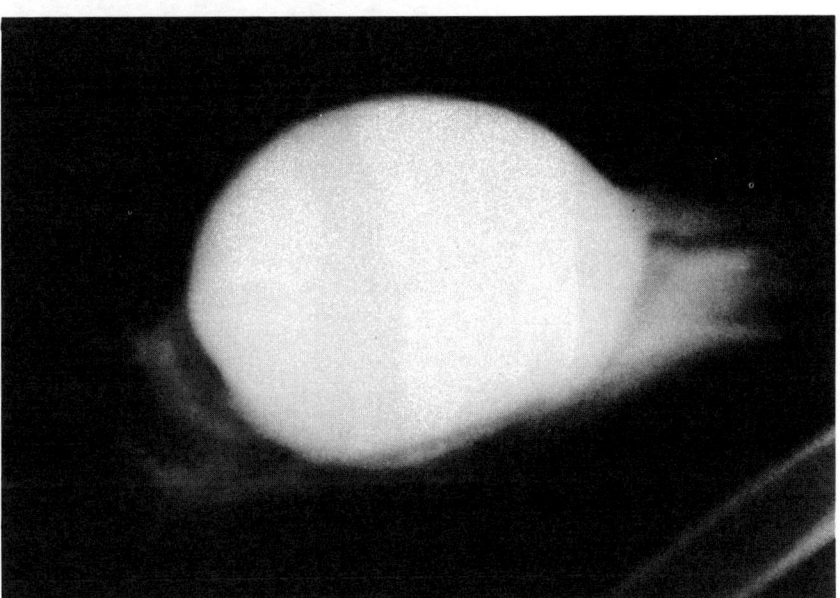

Figure 26B

been infrequently encountered in cats with FUS evaluated by the authors. Coating the catheter with an aqueous lubricant prior to insertion has reduced the occurrence of this complication. The use of soft rubber catheters also minimizes urethral or bladder trauma.

Suture material used to secure an indwelling catheter may be removed by the obstinate patient, and this may result in a retrograde migration of the urethral catheter into the urinary bladder (Figure 24).

Aqueous Lubricants

Surgical lubricating jellies are used to facilitate urethral instrumentation and add viscosity to radiopaque contrast media. Two reports have implicated surgical lubricants in the cause of urethral foreign body granu-lomas in humans following urethral instrumentation.[16,17] Experimental injection of an aqueous lubricant in laboratory animals has evoked a similar tissue response.[18,19] A similar tissue response in dogs and cats was encountered following retrograde urethrography where an aqueous lubricant was used as a diluent (Figure 25).[3] It is not known whether the granulomatous reaction encountered in these tissues was caused by the aqueous lubricant or other unknown factors. The information, although limited, suggests that these products are not as innocuous as they have been previously suspected to be.

Topical Anesthetics

Topical anesthetics are used to facilitate human and

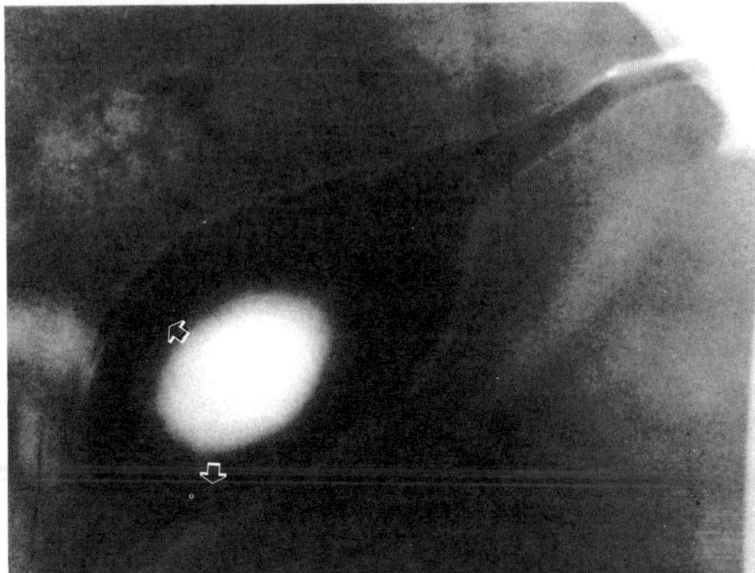

Figure 27A

Figure 27—Emphysematous cystitis may be encountered with bacterial cystitis and other bladder diseases or may be iatrogenic and related to improper use of urinary catheters. Emphysematous cystitis may vary from focal elevations of the urothelium (**A**), to diffuse transmural involvement of the entire wall of the urinary bladder (**B**). Note the presence of air bubbles (*arrows*) at the periphery of the contrast puddle in **A**.

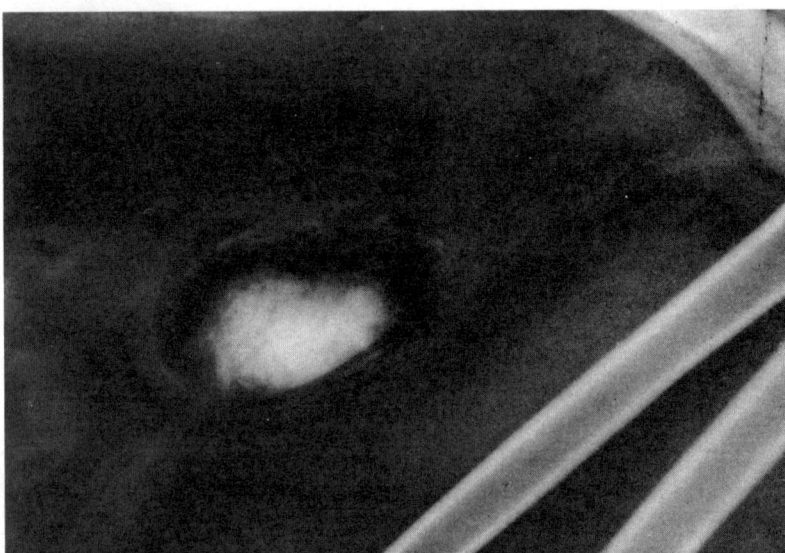

Figure 27B

veterinary urologic procedures. Lidocaine hydrochloride is available as a urologic jelly or as an aqueous preparation. Systemic reactions to lidocaine hydrochloride are characterized by central nervous system excitation and cardiovascular depression but are infrequently encountered in humans.[20] Systemic toxicity to lidocaine hydrochloride is variable, depending on the route and speed of administration. Blood levels have not been determined after application of lidocaine to urothelial membranes. To avert potential complication, doses less than 4.5 mg/kg (2 mg/lb) are recommended for cats. Adverse reaction to intravesical infusion of lidocaine hydrochloride has not been encountered by the authors.

Techniques of Urethrocystography
Overdistention
Acute distention of the urinary bladder during cystography or urethrocystography may result in lesions to the urinary bladder and/or urethra. High intravesical pressure and rapid distention of the urinary bladder may impair circulation and can lead to ischemia, venous stasis, and tissue necrosis.[21,22] Overdistention may result in tears in the urothelium, connective tissue, smooth muscle, and blood vessels, thereby predisposing to bladder wall discontinuity.[22] These lesions may compromise the defense mechanisms of the urinary tract and predispose to lower urinary tract infection. Intravesical volumes recommended for cystography and urethrography in dogs and cats vary from 6.6 to 11.1 ml/kg (3 to 5 ml/lb). These volumes may be excessive for cats with lower urinary tract disease and may result in bladder rupture. Radiographically, bladder rupture may vary from mural leakage, with confinement of the contrast medium inside the serosal surface, to complete mural tears, with escape of contrast medium into the peritoneal space (Figure 26).

Macroscopic hematuria is the most frequently encountered complication immediately following cystography and urethrography in male and female cats with FUS. However, the hematuria is temporary and usually subsides in three to five days. Similar findings have been reported in normal dogs and cats following acute bladder distention during retrograde urethrography.[3]

Emphysematous Cystitis

Iatrogenic emphysematous cystitis due to the radiographic procedures has been encountered in cats and may range from focal to diffuse elevation of the urothelium to a transmural involvement of all layers of the urinary bladder (Figure 27). Catheter trauma to the urinary bladder mucosa or concurrent inflammatory bladder disease may predispose to vascular embolization of a negative contrast medium. The patient should be closely monitored for cardiovascular collapse if emphysematous cystitis is identified.

Iatrogenic Urinary Tract Infection

Iatrogenic urinary tract infection (UTI) is a serious potential complication of cystography and urethrography in dogs and cats. Potential pathogenic microbes may enter the urinary bladder by several routes. Transport of microbes by the catheter into the bladder during catheterization is considered the common route of infection.[15] Presence of the normal bacterial flora in the distal urethral mucosa results in the transport of some organisms into the bladder whenever a urinary catheter is used but can be minimized by the use of sterilized catheters and aseptic catheterization techniques. Microbes may also ascend through the catheter lumen when a nonsterile catheter or syringe serves as a source of microbial contamination. Motile bacteria may enter the urinary bladder in the absence of retrograde flow if a continuous column of urine exists in the catheter between the source of contamination and the bladder.[15] Motile bacteria may also ascend the urethral lumen around the outside of the urethral catheter. Compromise of the normal bladder defense mechanisms by catheter trauma or overdistention may further predispose to infection.

Radiographic evaluation of male cats with indwelling urethral catheters for relief of urethral obstruction presents several potential problems to the clinician. Cathe-

ter-induced urethritis and bacterial cystitis have been reported in male cats after placement of indwelling urethral catheters.[15,23] These cats may represent a high-risk population predisposed to urinary tract infection because of the presence of the indwelling catheter.

REFERENCES

1. Kipnis RM: Vesicoureteral reflux in a cat. *JAVMA* 167(4):288-292, 1975.
2. Farrow CS: Retrograde urography in the cat. *VM SAC* 69:435-437, 1974.
3. Johnston GR: *Retrograde Contrast Urethrography in the Dog and Cat: Complications and Morphologic Evaluation.* Master thesis, University of Minnesota, 1979.
4. Green RW, Bohning RH, Jr: Patent persistent urachus associated with urolithiasis in a cat. *JAVMA* 158:489, 1971.
5. Hansen JS: Patent urachus in a cat. *VM SAC* 67:379, 1972.
6. Hansen JS: Persistent urachal ligament in a cat. *VM SAC* 67:1090, 1972.
7. Hansen JS: Urachal remnant in the cat: Occurrence and relationship to the feline urological syndrome. *VM SAC* 72:1735-1746, 1977.
8. Breton L, Pennock PW, Valli VE: The effects of Hypaque 25% and sodium iodide 10% in the canine urinary bladder. *J Am Vet Radiol Soc* 19:116, 1978.
9. McAlister WH, Palmer K: The histologic effects of four commonly used media for excretory urography and an attempt to modify the responses. *Radiology* 99:511, 1971.
10. McAlister WH, Shackelford GD, Kissone J: The histologic effects of 30% Cystokon, Hypaque 25%, and Renografin-30 in the bladder. *Radiology* 104:563, 1972.
11. Neustein DH, Herman JR: New urethral anesthetic, clinical evaluation employing new method. *NY State J Med* 67:1401, 1967.
12. Sie CM, Dunbar JS, Wright VJ, Hardwick DF: Contrast media used in cystourethrography. *Invest Urol* 12:434, 1975.
13. Ackerman N, Wingfield WE, Corley EA: Fatal air embolization associated with pneumourethrography. *JAVMA* 160:1616, 1972.
14. Zontine WJ, Andrews LK: Fatal air embolization as a complication of pneumocystography in two cats. *J Am Vet Radiol Soc* 19:8, 1978.
15. Lees GE, Osborne CA: Urinary tract infections associated with the use and misuse of urinary catheters. *Vet Clin North Am* 9(4):713-727, 1979.
16. Climie ARW: Periurethral granuloma due to lubricating jelly. *Harper Hosp Bull* 20:226, 1962.
17. Reed RJ, Smith JL, Sternberg WH: Granulomas induced by surgical lubricating jelly. *Am J Clin Pathol* 36:41, 1961.
18. Blaine G: Experimental observations on absorbable alginate products in surgery. *Ann Surg* 125:102, 1947.
19. Richards CE: Visco-Rayopake in cystourethrography. *J Urol* 58:185, 1947.
20. Covino BG: Systemic toxicity of local anesthetic agents. *Anesth Analg* 57:387, 1978.
21. Finkbeinder A, Lapides J: Effect of distention on blood flow in the dog's urinary bladder. *Invest Urol* 12:210, 1974.
22. Mehrotra RML: An experimental study of the vesical circulation during distention and in cystitis. *J Pathol Bacteriol* 66:79, 1953.
23. Lees GE, Osborne CA, Stevens JB, Ward GE: Adverse effects of open indwelling urethral catheterization in clinically normal male cats. *Am J Vet Res* 42:825, 1981.

Retrograde Vaginocystography: A Contrast Study for Evaluation of Bitches with Urinary Incontinence

KEY FACTS

- Retrograde vaginocystography is a relatively simple technique that requires minimal equipment.
- The technique is a valuable diagnostic aid, especially in cases of urinary incontinence, vaginal discharge, dysuria, or vaginal abnormalities that prevent digital or instrumental examination.
- Room air can be used for the double-contrast cystography but carries the risk of gas embolization; introduction of air should be avoided during vaginocystography because air bubbles inadvertently allowed to enter the vagina may be mistaken for a space-occupying lesion.
- Contraction of the constrictor vestibuli muscle under light anesthesia resembles a stricture and should not be interpreted as a pathologic lesion.

University of Guelph

Renee Leveille, DVM   Matthew A. O. Atilola, DVM, MS, PhD

URINARY problems in bitches are commonly encountered in small animal practice. Clinical examination of the vagina and urethra of bitches, however, is often unsatisfactory.[1] Digital vaginal examination may be restricted by differences in the length or diameter of the vagina and the examiner's digit. Although endoscopy is a valuable diagnostic aid in examining the caudal reproductive tract,[2] lesions of the vaginal and urethral lumina can prevent catheterization or adequate insertion of the endoscope.

Radiographic procedures are often used for localization or verification of diseases originating in or affecting the urogenital tract, investigation of underlying cause of a recurrent urinary tract problem, qualitative assessment of organ function to determine prognosis, and assessment of therapeutic response.[3] A single abnormal presentation on survey radiographs usually is not pathognomonic of a specific disorder but can suggest several different diseases. Radiographic signs on survey film often indicate a need for contrast studies to substantiate findings and to define the disease process more clearly.[4,5]

Retrograde vaginocystography has often been described in the British literature[6-9] but infrequently in North America.[4,7] This article describes the use of retrograde vaginocystography as a contrast study to define abnormalities of the lower urinary tract in bitches.

STUDY POPULATION

Between January 1983 and January 1989, 12,654 dogs were presented to the Small Animal Hospital of the Ontario Veterinary College in Guelph, Ontario, Canada. Of the dogs, 169 (1.3%) bitches were examined for urinary incontinence. The seven bitches in this report were selected on the basis of the diagnostic imaging procedures performed. Four dogs were examined by intravenous urography and retrograde vaginocystography (cases 3 through 6) and three dogs by retrograde vaginocystography only (cases 1, 2, and 7).

From the recorded histories, the age, breed, duration of clinical signs, and the nature of urinary incontinence were determined. Table I summarizes the clinical course of seven cases in which retrograde vaginocystography was performed.

TABLE I
Patients in Which Retrograde Vaginocystography was Performed

Case	Age (years)	Sex	Breed	Clinical Signs	Duration	Radiologic Diagnosis
1	1	Intact female	German shepherd	Urinary incontinence, vaginal discharge, pollakiuria	10 months	*Retrograde vaginocystography:* vaginal structure and possible short urethra, cystitis
2	1	Intact female	Tibetan terrier	Urinary incontinence, recurring urinary infection, pollakiuria, hematuria, dysuria	3 months	*Retrograde vaginocystography:* vaginitis
3	3	Intact female	Golden retriever	Urinary incontinence, perivulvar dermatitis	2 years	*Intravenous urography and retrograde vaginocystography:* left ectopic ureter
4	0.5	Intact female	Labrador retriever	Urinary incontinence	3 months	*Intravenous urography:* dilated left renal pelvis and ureter; *retrograde vaginocystography:* left ureter enters the vagina
5	5	Spayed female	English springer spaniel	Urinary incontinence	5 years (intermittent)	*Intravenous urography and retrograde vaginocystography:* no abnormal findings
6	7.5	Intact female	Husky	Urinary incontinence	5 months	*Intravenous urography:* dilation of right ureter; *retrograde vaginocystography:* right ectopic ureter
7	14	Spayed female	Irish terrier	Urinary incontinence, hematuria, pyuria, behavior change	1 week	*Retrograde vaginocystography:* no ectopic ureter seen

TECHNIQUE

As for any routine contrast radiographic examination of the abdomen, the bitches were prepared by cleansing the colon and rectum with an enema 24 hours and 3 hours before the procedure. The procedure was performed with standard general anesthetic protocol. Preliminary lateral and ventrodorsal abdominal radiographs preceded contrast cystography and provided evidence of gastrointestinal cleaning as well as satisfactory exposure technique. All catheters and equipment were sterilized and the genitalia cleaned before the lower urinary tract was catheterized.

The procedure was completed in two steps: first was double-contrast cystography; second was vaginourethrography. The bitch was positioned in dorsal recumbency (frog-leg position) for the double-contrast cystogram. A small Foley catheter (10 to 12 gauge) with an inflatable cuff was inserted within the bladder neck. The bladder was emptied, and about 10 ml of a 50% solution of an iodinated contrast medium was introduced. The dog was placed in lateral recumbency and then dorsal recumbency in order to spread the contrast material evenly over the mucosa. Nitrous oxide or carbon dioxide was then introduced. Lateral and ventrodorsal radiographic projections were obtained.

The Foley catheter was removed and the distal tip cut to preserve the cuff. The catheter was then filled with contrast medium before insertion into the vagina in order to avoid introducing air bubbles. The catheter was positioned in the vestibule and the cuff reinflated to prevent leakage of the contrast medium from the vulva. Sometimes it was necessary to close the vulvar lips with tissue forceps to prevent the catheter from slipping out. The dose of 1 ml/kg was injected slowly. Excessive pressure was avoided to prevent vaginal rupture.[9]

THE LATERAL radiographic view, which was exposed at the end of the injection, was the most informative. Ventrodorsal and oblique projections made variable contribution to the studies.

RESULTS

Retrograde bladder filling from ectopic ureters can occur.[7,8,10,11] In our series, the duration of the clinical signs ranged from one week to two years and had been reported as an intermittent problem by some owners.

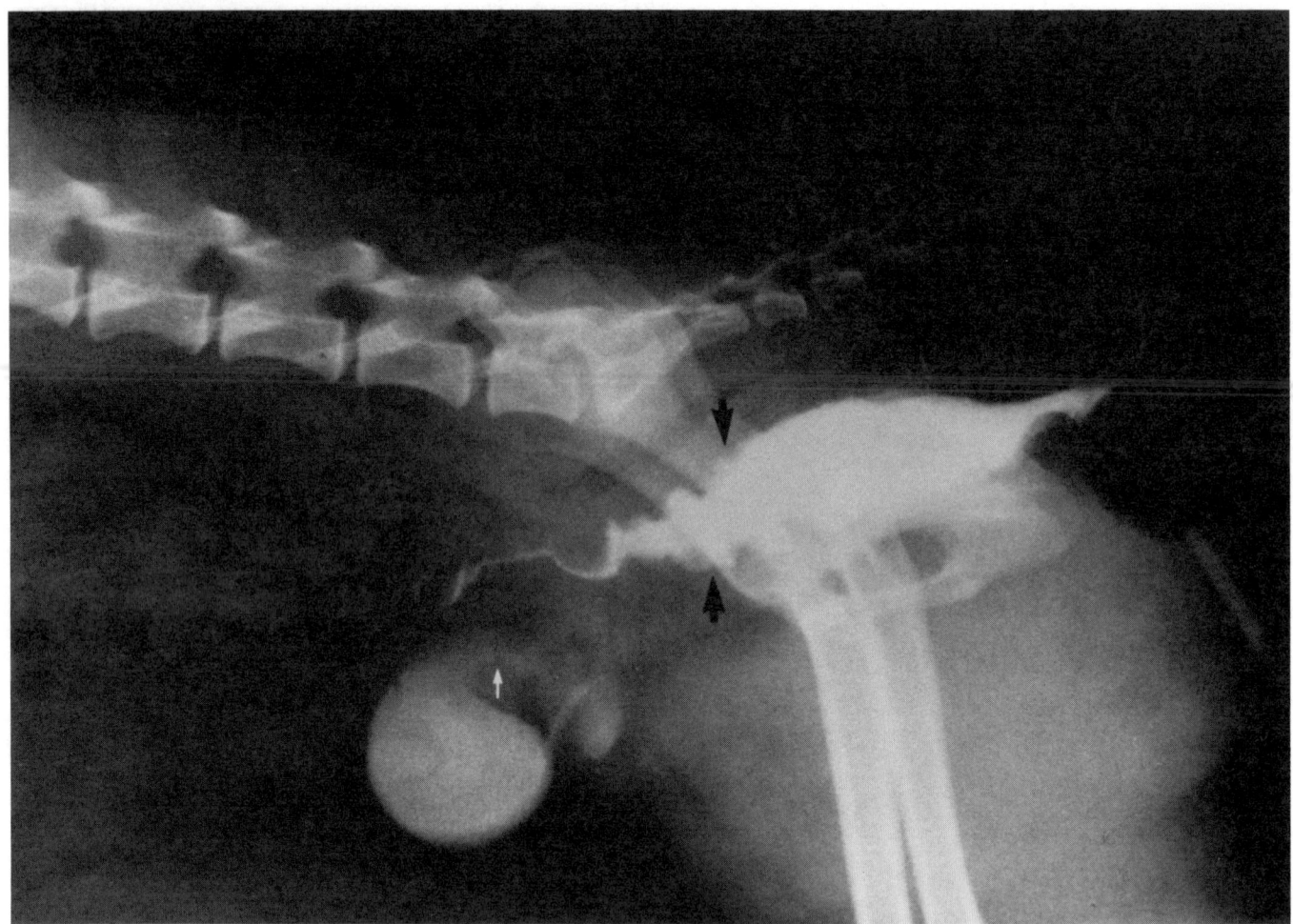

Figure 1—Abnormal retrograde vaginocystography of a one-year-old, intact female Tibetan terrier with vaginitis (case 2). Note the irregular appearance of the vaginal mucosa (*black arrows*). An artifactual luminal defect in the bladder resulting from lack of distention is shown (*small arrow*). A cystography performed afterward eliminated the possibility of mass lesion.

The exact location of the ectopic ureteral orifices was not clearly shown by intravenous urography in cases 3, 4, and 6. Intravenous urography did, however, reveal hydroureter and dilation of the ipsilateral renal pelvis in cases 4 and 6 (Figure 1).

Unlike intravenous urography, retrograde vaginocystography was successful in determining the opening of the ectopic ureter in cases 3, 4, and 6. Each ectopic ureter was confirmed at surgery. In case 7, at necropsy, there was no evidence of ectopic ureter; and the hematuria and pyuria were suspected to originate from an ascending infection.

DISCUSSION

Ectopic ureter is the most frequently diagnosed cause of congenital urinary incontinence.[8] The incidence of unilateral or bilateral ectopia of the ureters in dogs is unknown, and the condition apparently is most common in bitches.[10,12-15] Failure to recognize the condition in male dogs is likely because of lack of incontinence.[10] Confirmation of a tentative diagnosis of ectopic ureter is best made by using positive-contrast radiography of the urinary tract.[12]

Evaluation of the urinary tract by intravenous urography is indicated to confirm the presence of ectopic ureter and to determine whether other abnormalities of the kidneys and ureters are present. Although intravenous urography is an important diagnostic aid, visualization of the urethra and the exact site of termination of the ureters may be difficult.[5]

WHEN an abnormal orifice is detected in the vagina or suspected to be in the urethra, catheterization of the orifice followed by retrograde urethrography can be attempted; but its value is reduced because the catheter in the urethral lumen may obscure or distort a lesion. Voiding urethrography, a commonly used procedure in human patients, has been used in dogs for urethral examinations; but

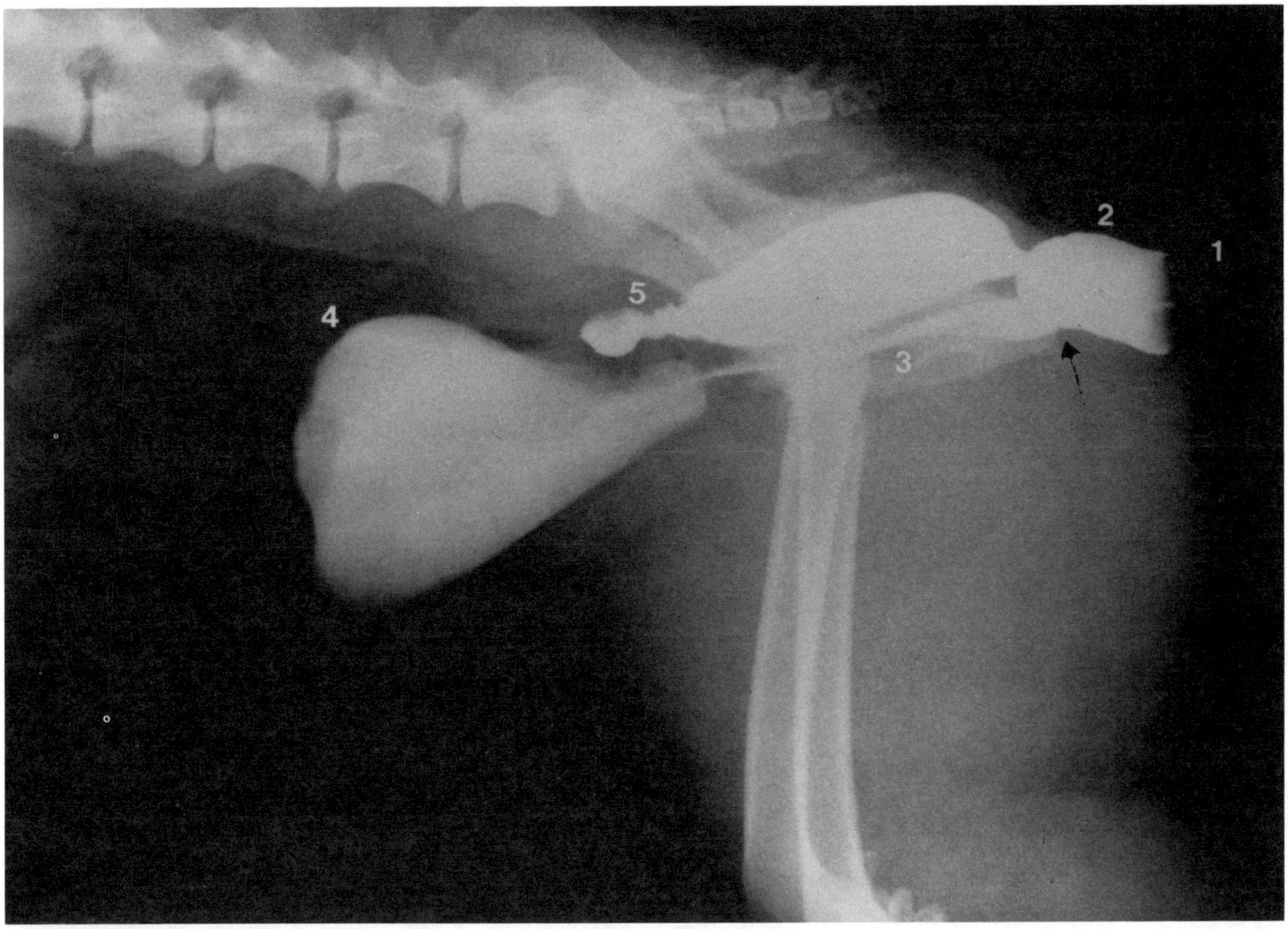

Figure 2—Normal retrograde vaginocystography of a five-year-old, spayed female English springer spaniel (case 5). The *arrow* points to the normal stricture attributable to the contraction of the constrictor vestibuli muscle. *1* = inflated cuff of the Foley catheter, *2* = vagina, *3* = urethra, *4* = bladder (not fully distended), and *5* = cervix.

the difficulty in performing the examination usually results from an inconsistent ability to stimulate urination.[16]

Retrograde vaginocystography has been very helpful in evaluating the terminal orifice of ectopic ureters, the entire length of the urethra, and the vaginal contour (Figure 2). Retrograde vaginocystography is a relatively simple technique that requires minimal equipment. The catheterization of small females may present some difficulties, as in case 7, in which only a vaginogram could be performed.

Room air can be used for the double-contrast cystography; however, it carries the risk of gas embolization.[4] Introduction of air and inadequate anesthesia should be avoided during vaginocystography because air bubbles inadvertently introduced into the vagina may be mistaken for a space-occupying lesion. Contraction of the constrictor vestibuli muscle under light anesthesia does resemble a stricture and should not be interpreted as a pathologic lesion (Figure 2). In estrous bitches, the required dose to fill the vagina is likely to be considerably higher than expected. The effects of endogenous hormones may also explain the larger volume needed in intact bitches.[9]

THE RISK of pyelitis or other urogenital infection is considered minimal with this technique. No side effects were observed in any of the patients. Even when retrograde vaginocystography is diagnostic, intravenous urography is indicated for evaluation of possible additional abnormalities, such as hydroureter and renal hypoplasia.[4]

Although there are many indications for retrograde vaginocystography, investigation of ectopic ureter is the most common[7,8] (Figures 3 and 4). It is also useful in cases of sphincter incompetence and other urethral anomalies because it allows the length and width of the urethra to be assessed, as seen in cases 1 and 5.[17,18] The procedure can be used in patients with other pathologic conditions or malformations, such as ureterovaginal fistula or bilateral dila-

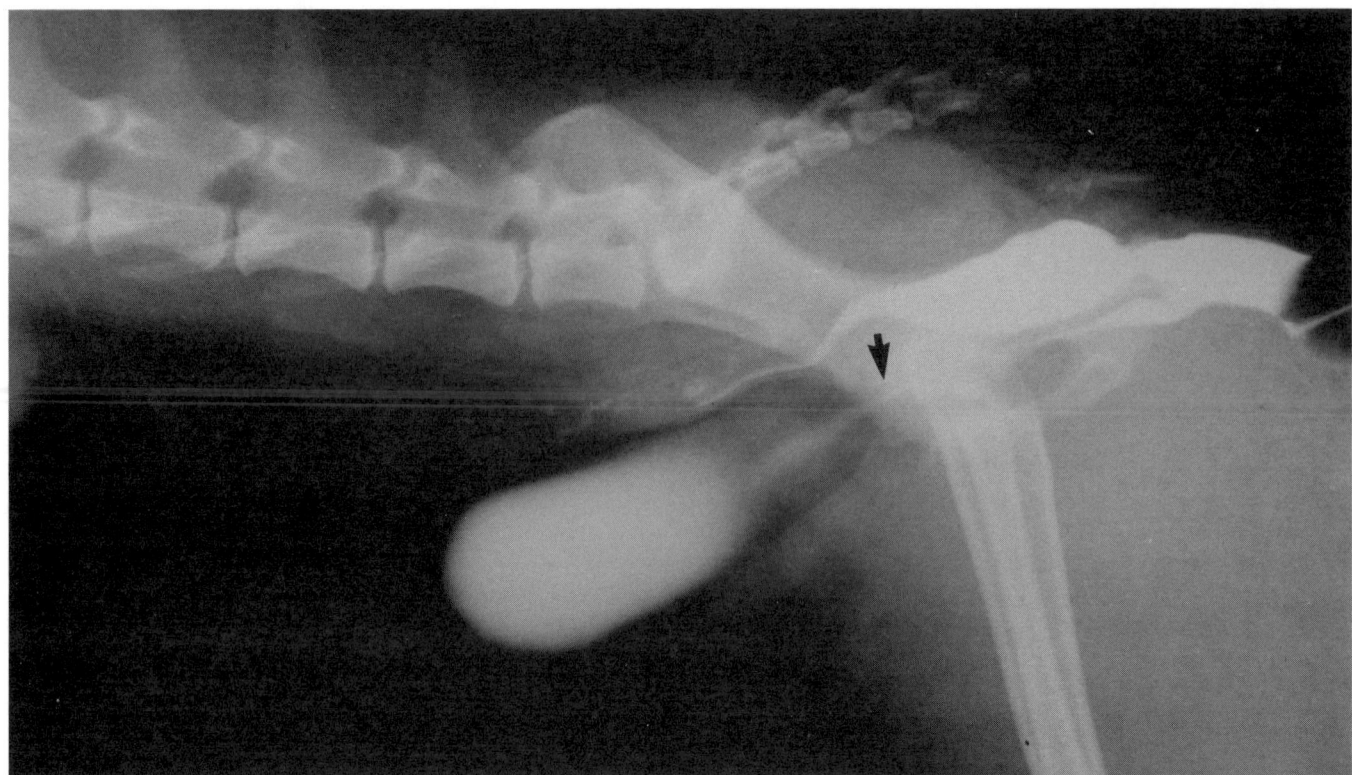

Figure 3—Abnormal retrograde vaginocystography of a two-year-old, intact female golden retriever (case 3). The *arrow* indicates the ectopic ureter.

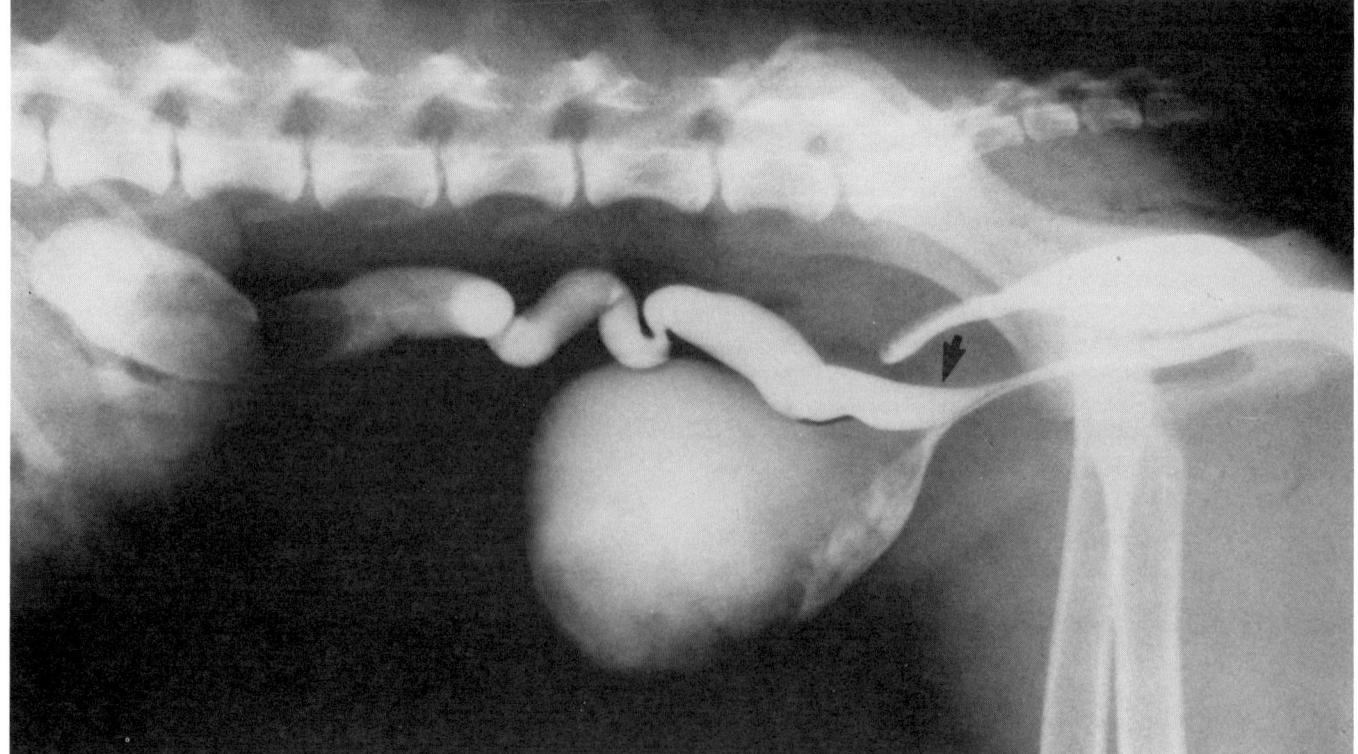

Figure 4—Abnormal retrograde vaginocystography of a six-month-old, intact female Labrador retriever (case 4). The *arrow* indicates the hydroureter and ectopic ureter.

tation of the vagina (intersexuality), and in bitches with vaginal discharge and in which a residual portion of uterus and patency of the cervix can be demonstrated. In addition, retrograde vaginocystography may demonstrate urethral filling defects, rectovaginal fistulae, and vaginal tumors[9] as well as other causes of incontinence (cases 1, 2, 5, and 7).

CONCLUSION

We have found that satisfactory results can be obtained with retrograde vaginocystography; this finding supports a previous report.[7] When adequately performed, vaginocystography can provide essential information about bitches with urinary incontinence. Its accuracy and simplicity make it useful in investigating cases of urinary incontinence, vaginal discharge, dysuria, and physical abnormalities of the canine female lower urinary tract.

About the Authors
When this article was being prepared, Dr. Leveille was affiliated with the Department of Clinical Sciences, Ontario Veterinary College, University of Guelph, Guelph, Ontario, Canada. She is currently affiliated with the Department of Veterinary Clinical Sciences, College of Veterinary Medicine, The Ohio State University, Columbus, Ohio. Dr. Atilola is affiliated with the Department of Clinical Sciences, Ontario Veterinary College, University of Guelph.

REFERENCES

1. Adams WM, Biery DN, Millar HC: Pneumovaginography in the dog: A case report. *J Am Vet Radiol Soc* 19:80, 1978.
2. Lindsay FEF: The normal endoscopic appearance of the caudal reproductive tract of the cyclic and noncyclic bitch: Postuterine endoscopy. *J Small Anim Pract* 24:1, 1983.
3. Feeney DA, Johnston GR: Urogenital imaging: A practical update. *Semin Vet Med Surg [Small Anim]* 1:144–164, 1984.
4. O'Brien TR: Upper urinary tract and radiology of the bladder and urethra, in *Radiographic Diagnosis of Abdominal Disorders in the Dog and Cat.* Philadelphia, WB Saunders Co, 1981, pp 481–694.
5. Adams WM, DiBartola SP: Radiographic and clinical features of pelvic bladder in the dog. *JAVMA* 182:1212–1217, 1983.
6. Douglas SW, Hertage ME, Williamson HD: Contrast media technique, in *Principles of Veterinary Radiography,* ed 4. London, Bailliere Tindall, 1987.
7. Holt PE, Gibbs C, Pearson H: Canine ectopic ureter—A review of twenty-nine cases. *J Small Anim Pract* 23:195–208, 1982.
8. Webbon PM: The radiological investigation of congenital urinary incontinence in the bitch. *Vet Annu* 22:199–206, 1982.
9. Holt PE, Gibbs C, Latham J: An evaluation of positive-contrast vaginourethrography as a diagnostic aid in the bitch. *J Small Anim Pract* 25:531–549, 1984.
10. Smith CW: Bilateral ectopic ureter in a male dog with urinary incontinence. *JAVMA* 177:1022–1024, 1980.
11. Osborne CA, Dieterich HF, Hanlon GF, et al: Urinary incontinence due to ectopic ureter in a male dog. *JAVMA* 166:911–914, 1975.
12. Owen R: Canine ureteral ectopia—A review. Incidence, diagnosis and treatment. *J Small Anim Pract* 14:419–427, 1973.
13. Osborne CA, Perman V: Ectopic ureter in a male dog. *JAVMA* 154:273–278, 1969.
14. Lennox JS, Eger CE, Owen RR: Clinical experiences with the combined technique of ureterovesicular anastomosis for treatment of ectopic ureters. *JAAHA* 12:406–410, 1976.
15. Haynes HM: Ectopic ureter in dogs: Epidemiologic features. *Teratology* 10:129–132, 1974.
16. Ticer JW, Crispin PS, Ackerman N: Positive-contrast retrograde urethrography: A useful procedure for evaluating urethral disorders in the dog. *Vet Radiol* 21:2–11, 1980.
17. Holt PE: Importance of urethral length, bladder neck position and vestibulovaginal stenosis in sphincter mechanism incompetence in the incontinent bitch. *Res Vet Sci* 39:364–372, 1985.
18. Mahaffey MB, Barsanti JA, Barber DI, Crowell WA: Pelvic bladder in dogs without urinary incontinence. *JAVMA* 184:1477–1479, 1984.

KEY FACTS

- Cystoscopy in female dogs can provide valuable information on the diagnosis of various urologic problems.
- Surgical procedures used to manage many urologic problems can be eliminated by the use of cystoscopy.
- Purchase of cystoscopic equipment may be economically impractical except at referral centers where many patients with urologic disease are seen.

Cystoscopy in Female Dogs

David F. Senior, BVSc
  Diplomate, ACVIM
Deborah A. Sundstrom, BS

Department of Medical Sciences
College of Veterinary Medicine
University of Florida
Gainesville, Florida

Endoscopic equipment is commonly used for diagnosis and treatment of various diseases in veterinary medicine. Cystoscopy, however, although performed on occasion, has not been widely used in veterinary practices[1-5]; the indications for its use have not been sufficiently frequent to warrant purchase of the necessary equipment. Furthermore, most urologic problems have been managed by open surgery, which has enjoyed good client acceptance. Recent advances in human endourology have eliminated the use of open surgery in the diagnosis and treatment of many conditions. Veterinary clients have begun to question the need for open surgery and to wonder why pets with urinary tract disease could not be managed with endoscopic techniques. Cystoscopy has many uses in human patients.[6] Many of these procedures are possible in dogs, although most have only been performed to a limited extent or on an experimental basis (Table I).

The primary instrument of human endourology is the rigid cystoscope. Improved optics have made the quality of the image seen remarkably good. This instrument is well suited for use in female dogs. Cystoscopy with a rigid cystoscope has been performed experimentally in male dogs by passing the instrument through a urethrostomy incision; however, this procedure has not been widely adopted in veterinary practice.[1,3,4] A fiberoptic bronchoscope passed into the bladder via the urethra also has been used experimentally in male dogs.[4] Although the quality of the image is not as good with bronchoscopes as it is with rigid cystoscopes, diagnosis, biopsy, and photography can still be performed. The following discussion provides guidelines for the use of rigid cystoscopes in female dogs.

Technique

Cystoscopy in female dogs is performed with the dog under general anesthesia and positioned in dorsal recumbency. Introduction of the cystoscope and the examination are much easier when the dog's hindquarters are placed slightly beyond the end of the examination table. A V-shaped support can be used to prevent rolling, and the patient can be elevated caudally to make the examination angle more comfortable for the clinician, provided the position does not interfere with adequate respiration. The hindlimbs and tail can be tied out of the way, but this is not usually necessary. Excessive or dirty hair around the vulva should be clipped; the patient's perineum should then be

Originally published in Volume 10, Number 8, August 1988

TABLE I
Potential Uses for Cystoscopy

Bladder disease
    Examination for lower urinary tract disease[4]
    Biopsy and resection (of polyps and neoplasms)
    Transurethral prostatectomy[3]
    Correction of urethral stricture
    Removal of bladder stones[a]
        Lithotripsy[5]
        Stone basketry[5]

Ureteral disease
    Correction of stricture[a]
    Stone basketry[a]

Renal disease
    Cannulation of ureters[1,2,9,11]
        Culture of ureteral urine[a]
        Retrograde pyelography[12]
        Renal cytology; brush biopsy[a]
        Retrograde nephrostomy[11]
        Differential glomerular filtration rate estimation[a]

[a]To date, used only in humans.

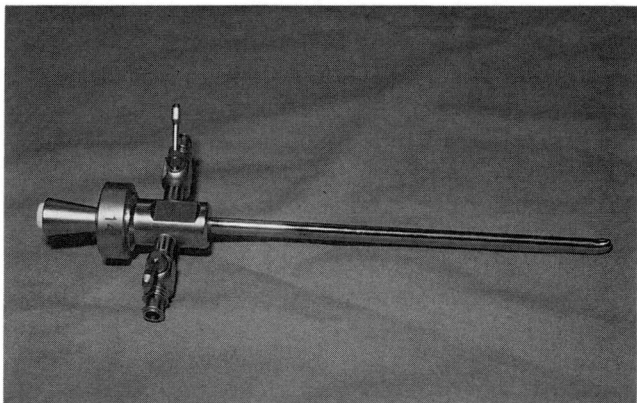

Figure 1A

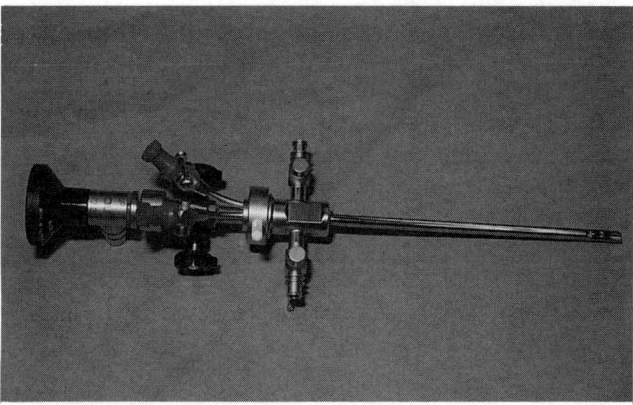

Figure 1B

Figure 1—(**A**) Cystoscope sheath with obturator in place. (**B**) Cystoscope sheath with Albarran operating bridge and telescope in place.

prepared according to a standard surgical scrub routine. The vulva can be rinsed with an antiseptic douche before the caudal body, legs, and tail are draped, leaving the vulva exposed.

All equipment for dilation and cystoscopy should be sterilized, organized, and placed on a sterile drape. Cystoscopic equipment (Figure 1) is made in two lengths, adult and pediatric. In dogs weighing more than 10 to 15 kg, a 17 to 21 French, adult-length cystoscope is suitable. In smaller dogs, a 14 to 15 French, pediatric-length cystoscope can be used. The instrument has an obturator that makes passage of the sheath through the urethra atraumatic. The Albarran operating bridge is designed to deflect instruments (e.g., catheters, biopsy forceps, or electrocautery electrodes) as they are passed through the sheath. Telescopes with several different viewing angles are available; the 30° and 70° viewing angles enable visualization of the entire bladder and urethra and are suitable for most operative procedures.

After preparation of the patient and organization of the necessary instruments, introduction of the cystoscope into the bladder can begin. Instruments that will be passed through the urethra should be coated liberally with a suitable sterile lubricant. The urethral os can be visualized adequately using a 3-inch Killian nasal speculum and head lamp. Urethral dilation, with a balloon dilator (Diaflex™ Urethral Dilator Catheter, Model 7500-01, female—American Edwards Laboratories) that is left in place for 30 to 60 seconds, may be necessary before passing the cystoscope sheath. The dilator should be deflated and withdrawn, and then the cystoscope sheath with an obturator in place should be gently advanced into the bladder. Once the sheath is in place, the obturator can be withdrawn and the Albarran bridge and telescope can be locked in place inside it. Irriga-

tion and drainage lines and the light cable can be connected, and the bladder examination can begin (Figure 2).

Initially, the bladder is best observed while it is being filled with irrigation fluid, because small lesions may become flattened and less obvious once the bladder wall is stretched.[7] Any physiologic salt solution is a satisfactory irrigation fluid for routine examination. For electrohydraulic shock-wave lithotripsy, however, 0.01% saline is preferable because it allows better transmission of shock waves.[5] For tissue preservation during biopsy and for optimum electrocautery, a 1.5% glycine solution is the irrigant of choice.[4] Overdistention of the bladder produces submucosal petechial hemorrhages that may confuse interpretation of the findings and may cause bladder rupture, particularly if the bladder wall is weakened by an infiltrative neoplasm. Several rinses with irrigation fluid may be necessary before the fluid medium is sufficiently clear for good visualization and photography, particularly when there is inflammation with lots of cellular debris or hemorrhage.

During placement of the cystoscope, a small quantity of air is always introduced into the bladder. When the dog is in dorsal recumbency, the air bubble remains at the uppermost ventral region of the bladder.

The entire bladder wall should be examined systematically by successive advances and retractions of the cystoscope followed by partial rotation of the instrument. In this way, even small lesions will not be missed. Useful landmarks include the cranial pole, trigone and neck of the bladder, the air bubble, and ureteral orifices. The ureteral orifices should be located and their positions should be noted. Urine can be observed intermittently flowing out of the ureteral orifices. The bladder neck and urethra are best examined by slowly withdrawing the cystoscope while the irrigation fluid is running.

Results and Discussion

Cystoscopy was performed 39 times in 35 female dogs for experimental purposes and for investigation of urologic disease in some of the patients. Experimental procedures that required cystoscopy included development of a retrograde nephrostomy technique (12 dogs), investigation of

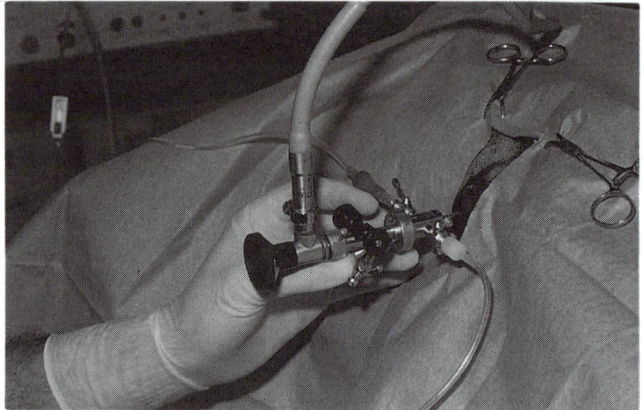

Figure 2—Cystoscope with an irrigation line, a drainage line, and light supply placed in an adult mixed-breed female dog weighing 20 kg.

the detrimental effects of extracorporeal shock-wave lithotripsy (8 dogs), electrohydraulic shock-wave lithotripsy (2 dogs, 4 procedures), and a study of the effects of extreme urethral dilation (8 dogs). Clinical patients (5 dogs) were examined cystoscopically for visualization and biopsy of intravesicular masses (2 dogs, 3 procedures), transurethral polyp resection (1 dog), location of ureteral openings (1 dog), and investigation of hematuria (2 dogs). No problems related to the cystoscopy were seen following the procedures.

We have used several methods of urethral dilation, including the use of filiforms with followers in two dogs, Van Buren urethral sounds in 12 dogs, and a urethral balloon dilator in 23 dogs. The most satisfactory instrument for us has been the urethral balloon dilator, because with it, the dilation is a one-step procedure that can be completed with relatively little trauma. In another study, satisfactory dilation was achieved using an Otis urethrotome (without the urethrotome blade).[4] The necessity for dilation and the extent to which the canine female urethra can be safely dilated without permanent trauma and residual effects on urethral function are not yet known.

In previous studies in which urethral size was calibrated, four beagles weighing 10 to 15 kg had urethral sizes of 15 to 17 French, and 12 mongrel dogs weighing 16 to 23 kg (mean of 18.5 kg) had urethral sizes of 18 to 22 French.[4,8] Two dogs in the latter study underwent urethral dilation to 45 French with a Killian dilator and showed no histologic abnormalities 2½ to 3 months later, although clinical signs during the postdilation period were not reported.[8] In another study, 16 and 21 French cystoscopes were passed into the bladder of 15- to 25-kg dogs without previous urethral dilation.[2] No adverse postoperative signs were reported. Most procedures can be performed through a 19.5 French cystoscope, and dilation beyond 30 French would be unnecessary for even the largest instruments.

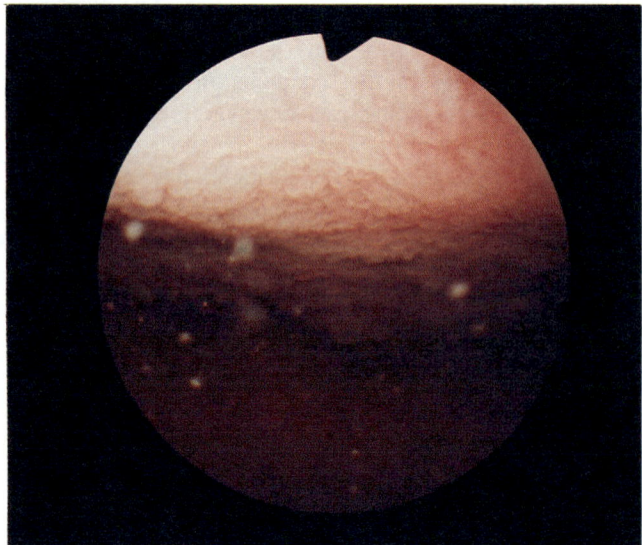

Figure 3A

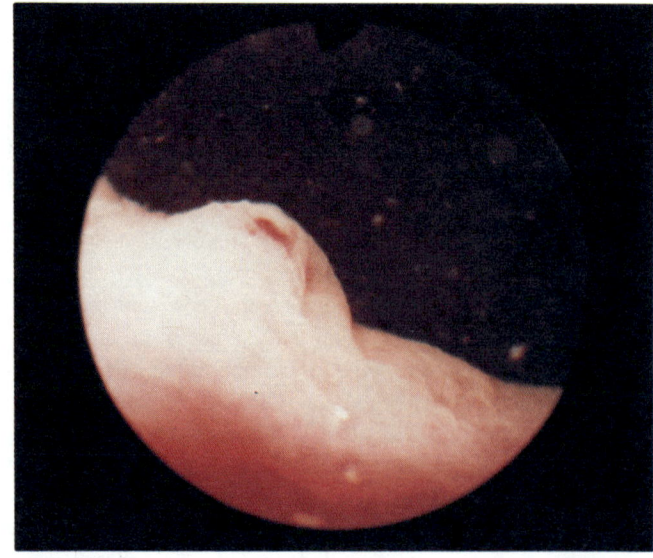

Figure 3B

Figure 3—(**A**) Normal appearance of the partially distended ventral bladder wall. (The small white spots in the lower half of the field are mucosal particles suspended in the irrigation fluid.) (**B**) Normal appearance of a ureteral orifice.

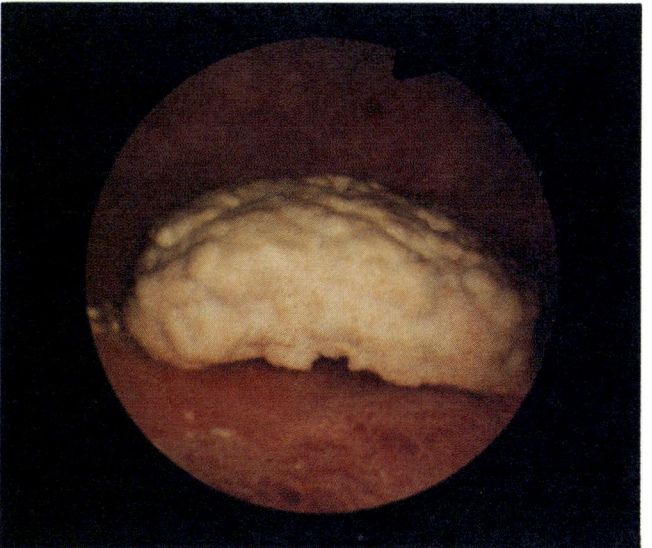

Figure 4A

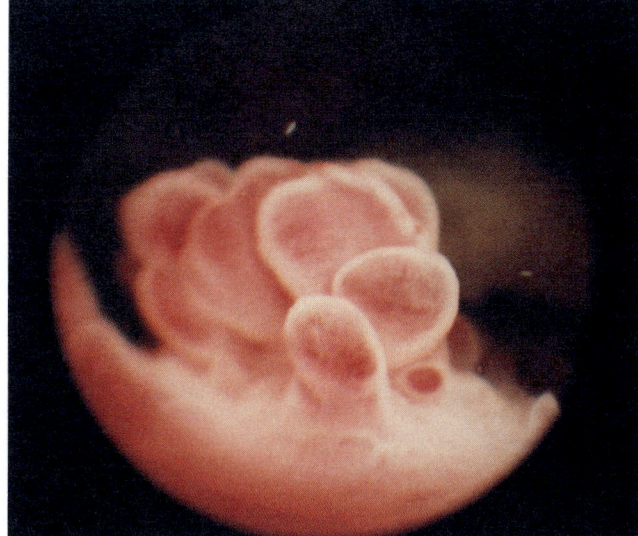

Figure 4B

Figure 4—(**A**) Cystic calculus composed of struvite in the bladder of a two-year-old mixed-breed female dog. (**B**) An inflammatory polyp in the bladder of a two-year-old mixed-breed female dog.

When distended, the normal bladder viewed through a cystoscope has a flat, pale, blanched appearance with a fine vascular pattern (Figure 3). When contracted, the mucosa shows irregular folds and develops a more reddish hue. Such abnormalities as stones, inflammatory polyps, and neoplasms are easily seen (Figure 4). The location of the ureters can be evident cystoscopically to confirm a suspected diagnosis of ureteral ectopia. In one dog suspected of having ureteral ectopia, contrast radiographic results were equivocal; cystoscopically, however, we were able to locate precisely the ureteral openings.

Various instruments are available for passage through the cystoscopes, including forceps for grasping, biopsy, and cutting; stone baskets; and electrodes for electrocautery. Electrohydraulic shock-wave lithotripsy, ureteral cannulation for urine collection, and diagnostic retrograde pyelography also can be performed with a cystoscope.[1,2,5,9]

Any new procedure should have significant advantages in safety, efficacy, and benefits to the patient before it replaces existing methods as the procedure of choice. Other important considerations in selecting a diagnostic or treatment method include the time required to complete the procedure and the cost of equipment. Routine bladder examination and biopsy can be performed safely with a cystoscope. Until the clinician becomes skilled in transurethral resection, resection of superficial polyps and tumors may be more time-consuming with a cystoscope than it would be by open surgery. More invasive tumors are not resectable with a cystoscope. The value of ureteral catheterization in canine clinical patients is not yet established; but its use in humans indicate that the procedure might be useful in dogs. Uses for retrograde ureteral catheterization in humans include localization of the site of infection, retrograde pyelography, placement of a ureteral stent for

---

Equipment Used in Canine Female Cystoscopy[a]

Cystoscope sheath with obturator
Albarran operating bridge
Telescope: 5° and 70°[b]
Light source
Light cable
Forceps: Grasping
        Cutting
        Biopsy
Stone baskets[b]
Electrocautery lead[b]
Ellick evacuator and adapter[b]

---

[a]The price range for the basic necessary equipment, in 1988 U.S. dollars, is between $6000 and $7000. The price range for the optional equipment listed is between $2000 and $3000.
[b]Optional equipment.

---

drainage of an obstructed kidney, removal of ureteral stones with a stone basket, brush biopsy of the renal pelvis, renal clearance studies of individual kidneys, and identification of ureters during surgery.[6,10]

The purchase of new cystoscopic equipment, which is expensive, may be economically impractical except at referral centers where many patients with urologic disease are seen. The basic equipment necessary as well as optional extras used in comprehensive cystoscopic examination, diagnosis, and treatment are listed in the box on this page. Used cystoscopes may be less expensive; light sources and light-carrying cables could be adapted for cystoscopy from other endoscopic equipment.

Contraindications for cystoscopy in humans are few, although it is recommended that such acute inflammatory processes as cystitis, prostatitis, or urethritis be resolved before cystoscopy is attempted.[6]

REFERENCES

1. Vermooten V: Cystoscopy in male and female dogs. *J Lab Clin Med* 15:650–657, 1930.
2. Ensor RD, Boyarsky S, Glenn JF: Cystoscopy and ureteral catheterization in the dog. *JAVMA* 149:1067–1072, 1966.
3. Trindade JCS, Lautenschlager MFM, de Araujo CG: Endoscopic surgery: A new teaching method. *J Urol* 126:192, 1981.
4. Cooper JE, Milroy EJG, Turton JA, et al: Cystoscopic examination of male and female dogs. *Vet Rec* 115:571–574, 1984.
5. Senior DF: Electrohydraulic shock-wave lithotripsy in experimental canine struvite bladder stone disease. *Vet Surg* 13:143–145, 1984.
6. Leadbetter GW: Diagnostic urologic instrumentation, in Harrison JH, Gittes RF, Perlmutter AD, et al (eds): *Campbells Urology*, ed 4. Philadelphia, WB Saunders Co, 1978, pp 358–374.
7. Gill WB, Huffman JL, Lyon FS, Bagley DH: In vivo urothelial surface histology by microscopic chromocystoscopy. *J Urol* 130:669–671, 1983.
8. Tanagho EA, Lyon RP: Urethral dilatation versus internal urethrotomy. *J Urol* 105:242–244, 1971.
9. Senior DF, Newman RC: Retrograde ureteral catheterization in female dogs. *JAAHA* 22:833–837, 1986.
10. Chaussy C, Schmiedt E, Jocham D, et al: First clinical experience with extracorporeally induced destruction of kidney stones by shock waves. *J Urol* 127:417–420, 1982.
11. Hunter PT, Hawkins IF, Finlayson B, et al: Hawkins-Hunter retrograde transcutaneous nephrostomy: A new technique. *Urology* 22:583–587, 1983.
12. Newman RC, Finlayson B, Hackett RL, et al: ESWL—Effect on canine renal and neurological tissue, in Gravenstein JS, Peter K (eds): *Extracorporeal Shock Wave Lithotripsy for Renal Stone Disease: Technical and Clinical Aspects*. Stoneham, MA, Butterworths, in press.